Chronic Fatigue Syndrome: Causes, Diagnosis and Treatment

Chronic Fatigue Syndrome: Causes, Diagnosis and Treatment

Editor: Augustin Hughes

AMERICAN
MEDICAL PUBLISHERS
www.americanmedicalpublishers.com

AMERICAN
MEDICAL PUBLISHERS
www.americanmedicalpublishers.com

Cataloging-in-Publication Data

Chronic fatigue syndrome : causes, diagnosis and treatment / edited by Augustin Hughes.
p. cm.
Includes bibliographical references and index.
ISBN 978-1-63927-978-4
1. Chronic fatigue syndrome. 2. Chronic fatigue syndrome--Etiology. 3. Chronic fatigue syndrome--Diagnosis.
4. Chronic fatigue syndrome--Treatment. 5. Epstein-Barr virus diseases. I. Hughes, Augustin.
RB150.F37 C47 2023
616.047 8--dc23

American Medical Publishers,
41 Flatbush Avenue,
1st Floor, New York,
NY 11217, USA

ISBN 978-1-63927-978-4 (Hardback)

Contents

Preface

Over the recent decade, advancements and applications have progressed exponentially. This has led to the increased interest in this field and projects are being conducted to enhance knowledge. The main objective of this book is to present some of the critical challenges and provide insights into possible solutions. This book will answer the varied questions that arise in the field and also provide an increased scope for furthering studies.

Chronic Fatigue Syndrome (CFS) or myalgic encephalomyelitis (ME) is a complicated disorder characterized by unexplained extreme fatigue that stays for at least six months. The cause for such condition cannot be correlated with any underlying medical condition. The fatigue increases with physical or mental activity and it does not improve with rest. The common symptoms include fatigue, problems with memory or concentration, sore throat, and headaches. Several factors may cause CFS. Potential reasons involve viral infections, immune system problems, hormonal imbalances, and physical or emotional trauma. CFS cannot be diagnosed as there is no single test for this purpose. In some medical conditions such as anemia, diabetes, and hypothyroidism, fatigue is the common symptom. The exact condition causing fatigue can be diagnosed by lab tests. Counselling therapy, exercise, and proper resolution of sleep problems can help in relieving the CFS. Exercise that starts at a very low intensity and increases very gradually over time may be helpful in improving long-term function. This book contains some path-breaking studies related to CFS. It provides significant information of the clinical aspects of chronic fatigue syndrome to help develop a good understanding for its diagnosis and treatment. Those with an interest in this field would find this book helpful.

I hope that this book, with its visionary approach, will be a valuable addition and will promote interest among readers. Each of the authors has provided their extraordinary competence in their specific fields by providing different perspectives as they come from diverse nations and regions. I thank them for their contributions.

Editor

1

Long Term Follow up of Young People with Chronic Fatigue Syndrome Attending a Pediatric Outpatient Service

*Katherine S. Rowe**

Department of General Medicine, Royal Children's Hospital, Melbourne, VIC, Australia

Correspondence:
Katherine S. Rowe
kathy@roweresearch.com

Aim: To determine the reported duration of illness, the functional and educational long-term outcomes, predictive factors for recovery and seek feedback regarding management in pediatric/adolescent myalgic encepahalomyelitis/chronic fatigue syndrome (ME/CFS).

Methods: A cohort observational study of 784 young people, mean age 14.6 (6–18) years, with ME/CFS diagnosed at a specialist pediatric hospital and receiving regular care, was conducted with follow-up for a mean 8 (range 1–21) years after onset. Baseline symptoms, history, depression and anxiety questionnaires were available from 418. The remaining 366, did not have similar standardized baseline information. Questionnaires requested functional rating, persistent symptoms, duration of illness if "recovered," social engagement and school/work attendance. Feedback was sought regarding management, support services, useful information, helpful interventions or personnel and use of alternative therapies. Reported recovery and function were compared with baseline information and between the two groups.

Results: Follow-up data were returned from 81.8%. There was no significant difference in functional score (if reported recovery) or illness duration related to provision of baseline data. The mean duration of illness was 5 (range 1–15) years in the 50% who reported recovery. By 5 years 38% and by 10 years 68% reported recovery. At 10 years the mean functional score was 8/10 (range 2–10) with 5% scoring <6. Depression, anxiety or severity of illness at diagnosis was not predictive of non-recovery. Designing and monitoring their own management plan that included educational, social, physical and enjoyable activities, as well as having symptom management and understanding professionals were highly valued. However, remaining engaged in an education system that flexibly accommodated their illness and aspirations was consistently reported as crucial for long term functioning.

Conclusions: ME/CFS in young people has a mean duration of 5 years (1–15) with 68% reporting recovery by 10 years. All improved functionally with 5% remaining very unwell and a further 20% significantly unwell. There were no obvious baseline predictors for recovery. However, depression, anxiety, orthostatic intolerance and to a lesser extent pain at follow up were identified as hampering recovery or function. Supportive professionals, remaining engaged in education and management strategies were identified as helpful.

Keywords: chronic fatigue syndrome, ME/CFS, adolescent, follow up study, child, functional outcome, duration of illness

INTRODUCTION

Questions that either parents or young people ask soon after receiving a diagnosis of Myalgic Encephalomyelitis/Chronic Fatigue Syndrome (ME/CFS) are: "how long will the illness last"; "is there way of telling whether they will recover," and "what can be done to manage the illness in the best way possible?"

ME/CFS is a condition of unknown etiology that commonly follows an infection in young people. There is a new onset of fatigue that has been present for at least 3–6 months and is not relieved by rest and not explained by other medical conditions. Post-exertional malaise, cognitive difficulties, unrefreshing sleep are present, in addition to a variety of somatic symptoms such as pain, (headache, abdominal or muscle pain), as well as flu-like symptoms without high fever and often symptoms associated with orthostatic intolerance.

Challenges to providing answers to these questions include: confirming that those followed up have a diagnosis of ME/CFS not just fatigue; ensuring that the maximum proportion of those who are diagnosed are included in the follow up; having a range of severity at diagnosis; and having an adequate cohort size with regular follow up, for sufficient length of time, in order to be confident that a realistic estimate has been obtained. Retention rates in follow up studies may also be affected by those who recover or those who remain very unwell, who may not wish to remain in contact with the medical profession. Hence perceptions of outcomes remain distorted. In addition, young people in early adult life are mobile, move away from home and frequently change their name, or transition to adult services, so following up a pediatric cohort has added challenges.

Carter et al. (1), describe outcomes for "chronic fatigue" in adolescents. However, this was at a time when ME/CFS was not well recognized in young people. Norris et al. (2) use the term "chronic disabling fatigue" identified from a survey and without clinical assessment, for their outcome study. Similarly Rimes et al. (3) used repeated community surveys to both diagnose fatigue and chronic fatigue syndrome for their estimates of outcomes but the small yields mean the findings are difficult to interpret. Krilov et al. (4) indicated that half the cohort had fatigue for only 1–6 months when first seen and 70% were followed up for 1–4 years afterwards to provide their estimate of duration of illness. Gill et al. (5) followed 34 (69% of cohort) who were retrospectively diagnosed with CFS or idiopathic fatigue for up to 4.5 (1–8) years. Van der Werf et al. (6) followed a cohort of young people with short duration of illness for 12 months. However, Bell et al. (7) followed 35 (76%) of a well-defined group for 13 years. Hence information regarding outcomes in ME/CFS in young people is scarce due to differentiating chronic fatigue from ME/CFS and ensuring that sufficient numbers are followed for an adequate period of time.

Differences in how recovery is reported and what that means to the young person add other variables. Measures of fatigue (8), symptom presence and functional outcomes, (9, 10), self-report (6), or a combination of global functioning and self-report have been used (7) thus making comparisons difficult. In describing a 2 year follow up of 54 young people, van Geelen et al. (9) reported that 50% improved in symptoms but the majority were reportedly missing more than one third of school. Hence it is important to document function and symptoms as well as perceptions of recovery. Parslow et al. (11) have been investigating what aspects of defining recovery are important to young people with ME/CFS. Understanding what a young person considers as "recovery" in a chronic illness can be problematic, but even more so in a condition that impacts every aspect of their development (social, educational, physical, and emotional) during adolescence. Without careful consideration of these aspects of development, it can be very difficult to interpret outcomes meaningfully.

Although most studies have attempted to assess the natural history of the condition, other studies have reported long term outcomes following interventions. Five year follow-up post-trial of intravenous immunoglobulin in young people (12), indicated that the mean functional outcome of the placebo group at 5 years matched that of the intervention group 6 months after the final infusion suggesting a significant number had recovered by that time (13). Other interventions that have been helpful (14) and have assisted with improving function, have not necessarily reported "recovery" (15). There have not been other convincing treatments that have altered the course of the illness (10). Although a variety of management strategies such as adaptive pacing, graded exercise, cognitive behavior therapy (14) can be helpful, the evidence for significant improvement is scarce and hampered by difficulties in comparing outcome measures according to clinical presentation, patient characteristics, case criteria and degree of disability (16). Managing some of the co-morbid or contributing conditions such as orthostatic intolerance (17) has also modified function. However, follow up after these interventions has often been for a short period of time, so realistic estimates of the duration of chronic illness is problematic.

This study sought to provide answers to the three common questions. How long does it last? Is there any way of predicting how long it will last, and what is helpful from the young person's viewpoint in managing the illness?

This study is an observational cohort study of 784 consecutive patients, diagnosed with ME/CFS after referral to an outpatient service at a specialized pediatric tertiary referral hospital, who received supportive medical care and were followed for a mean 8 (range 1–21) years.

The aims of this study were: (1) to document the long term functional and educational outcomes of a cohort of 784 young people with ME/CFS, 418 of whom provided standardized baseline medical and psychological information and additional follow up data on up to 6 occasions, 2–16 years after diagnosis; (2) to determine the duration based on self-reported recovery including the proportion reporting recovery at 5 and 10 years; (3) to identify any predictors of recovery based on baseline information obtained, and (4) to obtain feedback regarding useful management.

The objectives of the study were: (1) to describe the demographic, medical and psychological characteristics of the cohort, including the medical management; (2) to follow up the entire cohort for reported recovery, functional and educational outcomes and feedback regarding management; (3) to compare the functional and reported recovery between the group providing baseline data and the group that did not, to determine if there was a systematic bias; (4) to investigate whether there is an association between questionnaire identified depression and anxiety, or antinuclear antibody presence and reported recovery; and (5) to obtain feedback regarding management.

METHODS

Characteristics of the Cohort and Description of Routine Medical Care

Setting

The Royal Children's Hospital is a specialized secondary and tertiary referral pediatric and adolescent hospital that services metropolitan Melbourne and all rural areas for the state of Victoria including bordering areas in neighboring states. Furthest distances require 4–5 h of car travel. Referrals are received from family doctors or from specialist pediatricians. Victoria has a population of 5.8 million and is multicultural with successive waves of immigrants or refugees from different parts of the world contributing to the mix. There is a universal health system that ensures citizens can access health care free of charge to the family. Twenty-six per cent of its citizens are born overseas from 200 countries, speaking 260 different languages, with an additional 30% having at least 1 parent born overseas (18). The hospital clinics reflect this demographic. More than 70 languages are spoken in the hospital.

Chronic Fatigue Syndrome Clinic

The clinic has been functioning since 1989. In the early years of the clinic, the Holmes definition and Fukuda criteria for CFS were available (19–21). However, acceptance of the diagnosis in young people was uncommon in the medical fraternity, and it was uncertain if the illness was similar to that in adults. Nonetheless, it was well recognized that Epstein Barr Virus (EBV) infection (or glandular fever) could run a prolonged course during adolescence with comparable symptoms. Irrespective of whether EBV was confirmed, it was assumed in some cases, that this was the cause. Alternative explanations that were often entertained were depression, "stress," school refusal or somatization disorder or the possibility of undisclosed family difficulties. Parents who were anxious due to concern about the unexplained change in the young person were often considered to be contributing to their illness. Hence many who attended the clinic had experienced unsatisfying encounters with the medical profession.

Accurate documentation of the presentation was therefore important as described below. Ninety two patients diagnosed in the first 5 years using Holmes et al. (19) definition participated in an intravenous immunoglobulin trial (12) and were followed up separately every second year for a 5-year follow up post-trial (13) who were not included, but used for comparison in this study. Symptom patterns and characteristics of the patient group for the first 189 have also been reported elsewhere (22). Those analyses indicated that reported symptomatology was very consistent among the young people in this population, and the presence of post-exertional malaise (PEM), unrefreshing sleep, cognitive difficulties, persistent fatigue and pain (headache, muscle, abdominal) were all almost universally reported. Sore throats and glands, feeling hot and cold, and symptoms later recognized as associated with orthostatic intolerance were very common.

As immunoglobulin was a scarce resource requiring approval by a government agency, a decision was made to not allow intravenous immunoglobulin to be available for ME/CFS for young people due to some adverse effects (12), as well as inconclusive trials in adults (23–25). Thus, options for treatment reverted to general management strategies for chronic illness. We relied on feedback from young people to inform us regarding what was helpful in their management. The service has since expanded to several pediatricians and access to a 4-week self-management program run by the Victorian Pediatric Rehabilitation Service at the hospital.

Participants

A diagnosis of Chronic Fatigue Syndrome was made in 784 young people following an extensive history, examination, and routine investigations to exclude alternative diagnoses and confirm the presence of key symptoms identified from the earlier study (22). PEM, unrefreshing sleep and cognitive symptoms were required in addition to the Fukuda criteria (20). Other conditions including school refusal, somatization disorder, eating disorders, isolated significant depression or anxiety, connective tissue disorders, celiac disease or endocrine disorders were specifically checked. An adolescent psychosocial (HEADSS) screen was also conducted where appropriate (26). Passive standing test was not routinely performed initially. However, upon recognition of the association of orthostatic intolerance with ME/CFS this assessment was included.

Routine screening investigations included celiac screen, thyroid function and antinuclear antibody. The laboratory reported antinuclear antibody titers of 1:40 and above until 2008, when titers of 1:160 or above were considered significant. Serology for EBV or Cytomegalovirus (CMV) was routinely assessed or if there was any likelihood of overseas or tropical infections, or being in areas where Ross River Virus, Q fever (coxiella burnetti), Barmah forest virus were endemic, serology for exposure was also checked.

Ethics and Informed Consent

Institutional ethics approval was obtained for the baseline questionnaires and informed consent was obtained from the young person. For the follow up study, ethics approval was obtained to contact the last known address to obtain consent to forward a questionnaire for feedback on management strategies, progress of the illness and rates of reported recovery. If the young person was still at home their verbal consent was obtained or if their parents were still at the address they either provided a forwarding address or offered to forward the questionnaire which included documentation for informed consent. Occasionally the family was contacted from information in the national or state telephone directory.

Baseline Information

The baseline demographic and symptom questionnaire used by Lloyd et al. (25) and Rowe (12) (**Appendix 1**) in their immunoglobulin trials, was given to 489 of the 784 young people (mean 14.8 age 7–18) (with 55 concurrently receiving the De Paul Pediatric questionnaire). This included type of onset, family history and presence of co-morbid conditions. In addition, scales for depression (27, 28), anxiety (29), General Health Questionnaire (30) and Parental Bonding Questionnaire (31) were completed. Initially the Child Behavior Checklist (Achenbach) and Family environment scale (Moos) were included, but discarded as noncontributory after assessing 150 young people. The Parental Bonding Questionnaire was also not included after the CFS group showed no difference in scores with a matched community sample. Any abnormal laboratory findings were documented. The symptom pattern, severity and frequency were compared with questionnaire responses from an earlier separate sample (22) from the same clinic to confirm consistency in reported symptoms across time. The baseline information was collated using descriptive statistics (Statistica 13 -Statsoft –TIBCO).

Routine Care Offered at the Clinic

Initial appointment

Following diagnosis, the young person was asked: to rate the most troublesome symptom/s that he/she would like help with; to outline his/her aspirations prior to illness; to describe current school attendance, interests, and previous participation in sport, the family situation and supports including parental work schedule, and means of transport to school or activities. The young person was provided with a brief explanation of our current knowledge, a plan for managing the most severe symptoms, and an outline of a management plan that the young person would devise.

Management plan designed by the young person

The rationale for the management plan was to minimize the impact of chronic illness while accommodating the specific issues associated with ME/CFS. As ME/CFS affects the educational, physical, social and emotional aspects of their life, it was considered important to not neglect any of these areas. This should include some proactive social contact, academic input, physical activity and a commitment to attend something enjoyable outside of home on a regular basis. None of these activities was to be neglected but the proportion did not have to be equal. The plan needed to be sustainable for at least a month before it was reviewed. For example, some physical activity is required to prevent becoming so de-conditioned that they were not sure whether they were weak and fatigued because they were unwell or because muscles weren't being used. Social contact is important to ensure that the social learning that occurs during adolescence (how to respond in different situations, what behavior is acceptable and how to interpret different social situations and how to understand one's peers) is not neglected. It can be very daunting later when it is expected that these skills have been acquired. Academic engagement is important so that they feel that their life chances have not been destroyed. The regular enjoyable activity outside of home is something that they have chosen to go to because it is "worth it" and will not result in a prolonged recovery. It removes any prevarication regarding whether they feel well enough, whether they would cope or whether it would be easier not to go. Only if they are unable to move out of bed do they not attend. This hopefully prevents the reluctance to make decisions, to be adventurous or to be reliable.

In addition, young people generally have not had to learn to prioritize their activities during their teenage years but this skill is needed as developing adults. It is explained that they need to acquire this useful skill much earlier than most. Some activities, for example, attending school for an enjoyable subject could fulfill social, academic, and enjoyable activities and also require some physical activity. If their important social network was outside of school then there needed to be an effort to engage with that group for a period of time that was manageable. If some young people felt that "life was not worth living" if they couldn't play sport, as this was their main social connection, then adjustments could be made so that they could be part of the team by "coming off the bench" for a few minutes or not having a requirement to actively train, or else they could be moved to a team position that did not require a lot of stamina. On the other hand, for some, physical activity may be a few activities of daily living spaced over the day, or once they are able to do some activity and have increased their strength they often chose a variety of activities that they enjoy.

Their aspirations (prior to becoming unwell) played a key role in the decisions regarding their education. Attending school for set hours, rather than for specific subjects was difficult to sustain. Reduction in the school subject load to include subjects and teachers they liked, as well as subjects that were pre-requisites for what they wanted to do as a career was crucial. Trying to keep up with all subjects when only minimal information was given was a source of unnecessary stress, and this rarely succeeded. A planned timetable ensured that the arrangements could provide some consistency and predictability for the family and be manageable for the young person. If the symptoms were severe, the extent of "academic input" may be reduced to reading about a hobby or reading a story that they were already familiar with.

It was explained to the young person that these consequences of illness can be more damaging than the illness itself and can occur with any chronic illness. Neglecting these areas creates significant hurdles to recovery such as: navigating social anxiety and social learning; entering the workforce without a potentially enjoyable, satisfying or more lucrative, less physically demanding job; needing to increase strength, or not having the confidence or resilience to know how they are able to manage their life. The young person was asked to estimate how this could be achieved within the bounds of the amount of energy available over the period of a week. The young person was to make the decisions over the next few weeks and to discuss their plan with their parents.

Symptom management

Due to concerns with medication in young people and the risks of multiple medications, only the most severe one or two symptoms were treated. Often treating one symptom such as sleep disturbance, and allowing them to take control of their life with the management plan reduced the severity of some of the other troublesome symptoms. Despite the prominent fatigue, malaise and concentration difficulties, the complaints of headache and sleep disturbance or dizziness and nausea due to orthostatic intolerance, could often be managed effectively.

Difficulties with sleep initiation, sleep phase shift, frequent waking and disturbing nightmares were actively managed with sleep hygiene techniques and melatonin or low dose tricyclic medications such as dothiepin or amitryptiline. Simple migraine prophylactic medications such as pizotifen or periactin were anecdotally effective in reducing the severity of headache and simple measures with increasing salt and fluid including electrolyte drinks and encouraging lower limb exercises and gentle exercise could assist with orthostatic intolerance. Similarly, muscle pain and fibromyalgia could be helped by reducing sleep disturbance and encouraging gentle exercise or physical therapy.

Residual difficulties with concentration, recognition of depression, persistent severe dysmenorrhea associated with exacerbation of CFS symptoms, ongoing nausea, abdominal discomfort, persistent orthostatic symptoms were addressed after review and the implementation of the management plan.

Review appointments

A 6-week follow up appointment was scheduled for review of their plan, including whether the logistics were sustainable, to check on residual symptoms, and whether the symptom management was appropriate. Any further queries from the young person were addressed. Once a decision had been made regarding the schedule for education, appropriate explanation, documentation, advocacy, extra support, special provision or special consideration and tailoring a specific education program to ensure maximum possible opportunity to participate, was provided or requested from the education authorities. Sometimes there was a combination of Distance Education and school attendance for 1–2 subjects, or attendance for a few classes with Visiting Teacher assistance. If necessary, the minimum requirements were negotiated to ensure the year level was passed and that they could progress with their peers. Additional details regarding educational strategies used by the Visiting Teacher Service have been documented (32). If adjustments to sport schedules were required, these were provided and coaches and staff were usually very accommodating once they understood the reasons for the requests.

Generally 3-monthly reviews were arranged to assess progress, educational issues, symptom management and review of goals. They were seen more frequently if necessary. Occasionally young people were followed up by a local pediatrician.

In addition, parents often needed help navigating the difficult adolescent period and uncertainties regarding assisting with the tasks of adolescent development in the context a chronic illness that is generally not well understood. Parents are not sure if they should be defending, protecting and trusting the young person's judgment, or cajoling, setting limits and allowing the young person to make mistakes. Many parents had put their life "on hold" to care for the young person with the attendant complications for the whole family, and this often added significant stressors. For many young people doing some small chores that did not require much effort was important to be part of the family and reduce tensions with siblings.

Follow Up Study

Participants

The cohort of 784 (mean age 14.8, range 6–18 years) diagnosed with ME/CFS over a 20 year period from 1991 was followed up between January 2008 and June 2011 to document reported outcomes. Initial contact via last known address, parental contact or national telephone directory provided verbal information and consent for forwarding questionnaires.

Content of Questionnaire

The follow up questionnaire (**Appendix 2**) asked about proportion of work or school attended, use of educational support, Visiting Teacher service, disability support, educational level achieved, illnesses experienced, exacerbations of ME/CFS, reported recovery and duration of illness if recovered. Feedback was sought regarding useful or helpful information, useful or helpful personnel (medical or otherwise), use of alternative therapies and their perceived effectiveness, and whether anything could have been handled better during their illness. Any family history of ME/CFS was also asked. Both the Bell CFIDS Disability Scale (33) and a global rating 1–10/10 (with 10 being "back to normal") were used in the first 4 feedback questionnaires and in the final follow-up a global rating was also requested. During review appointments they had been frequently asked for a global rating following their description of function considering social connection, physical activity, education/work participation, symptom presence and recovery after any activity. The young person's rating was compared with concurrent physician and parental ratings based on their descriptions. A scale was developed based on their descriptions and rating (**Appendix 3**). A comparison between the distribution of ratings on the Bell and Global scale was conducted.

Comparison of Functional Rating and Reported Recovery

As additional data had been obtained from follow up questionnaires documenting the progress of the illness and providing feedback from those who had completed baseline information ($n = 418$), consistency in reporting outcomes could be checked.

The functional rating for both those who reported recovery and those who did not, was plotted to identify any overlap.

Comparison of Reported Recovery and Functional Outcomes Between Two Groups

The demographics, proportion followed up, functional outcomes and reported duration of illness for both groups were compared to identify whether a systematic bias was introduced when young people return or fail to return baseline information. Returning information may reflect level of engagement, severity of illness or exercising choice.

Association Between Questionnaire-Identified Baseline Depression, Anxiety, and Clinical Features With Outcomes

Mean baseline depression and anxiety scores were compared between those who reported recovery and those who did not using student's t-test. Presence of questionnaire-identified depression and anxiety were also compared with reported recovery outcomes. The presence of antinuclear antibody titers and outcomes were investigated using Chi square test. Statistica 13 (Statsoft –TIBCO) was used for all analyses.

Feedback Regarding Management

Descriptive data regarding useful management, helpful information, helpful professionals, use of alternative therapies, and ways to improve management were collated and categorized.

RESULTS

Baseline Demographics, Medical and Psychological Characteristics of Cohort

Demographics

A total of 784 young people with mean age of onset of ME/CFS 14.8 (range 6–18) years and M:F ratio of 1:3, were diagnosed with ME/CFS. The mean duration of illness prior to being diagnosed was 13.6 months (range 4 months—7 years). Socioeconomic status reflected the population based on Socioeconomic Index for Areas (SEIFA) data compared with census data across two census periods (18, 34). The rural/urban mix was proportionate to the population of Victoria however the ethnic mix was neither representative of the population of the state nor of the clientele of the hospital. Despite Victoria having successive immigration waves from over 200 countries, 80% of CFS patients had an Anglo-Celtic background (currently approximately 25% of the population), but predominantly Scottish/Irish descent, and another 11% were of northern European descent (Dutch and Scandinavian which is <0.5% of the population). Middle Eastern, African and young people of Asian descent were significantly underrepresented.

History Information

From 489 baseline history and psychological questionnaires distributed, 418 (85.5%) provided baseline history information. Fifty five were also given concurrent DePaul Pediatric questionnaires (35), of which 35 were returned (63.6%).

Onset

Eighty percent reported a defined onset following an infection, (most commonly EBV in 40% of cases), but a variety of other infections were documented such as CMV (10%), Mycoplasma, Toxoplasmosis, Varicella, Rubella, Parvo virus, Salmonella, Ross River virus, with 25% having documented serological change at the onset. Gastroenteritis and respiratory infections were commonly reported. Surgery for tonsillectomy or appendectomy in 2% and vaccination in 0.9% was identified as associated at the onset. Occasionally ME/CFS was diagnosed after a neurological insult or following a trivial infection in athletes who were overtraining (1–2%). Gradual onset was more commonly associated with orthostatic intolerance in young people with hyperflexible joints.

The peak onset was during winter with lower frequency at the beginning and end of the school year during summer and spring. Only 59% of the cohort ($n = 683$) had evidence of previous exposure to EBV and 35% of those tested ($n = 600$) had positive IgG for CMV. There was no difference in the prevalence of positive serology for either CMV (33% cf 36%) or EBV (58% cf 59%) between the groups with and without documented baseline information.

Symptom pattern

Symptoms of prolonged fatigue, persistent headache, needing excessive amounts of sleep, poor concentration, disturbed sleep, excessive muscle pain and fatigue after activity were reported in 90–100% of cases. Other pain, cognitive, "immunological symptoms" like sore throats, sore glands and felling hot and cold were reported by 60–80% of young people. Likely orthostatic symptoms, such as nausea, disturbed balance, difficulty focusing, tingling, anxiety and chest pain were reported frequently (more than 50%) also. The remaining 12 symptoms were reported in low frequency and also are not generally associated with ME/CFS (**Figure 1**). The most common 8 symptoms were reported with the same frequency and almost identical severity compared with the earlier separate sample (22). The remaining symptoms were comparable and again significantly different from the community sample of age and gender matched adolescents. Fatigue, concentration difficulties, motivation and pain were identified as limiting activity (**Figure 2**) whereas depression was less so.

Fifty eight per cent reported a continuous pattern of illness with fluctuating severity, 14% continuous at same level of severity, 12% relapsing and remitting pattern, 9.5% relapsing in past now continuous and 6.5% continuous in past and now relapsing.

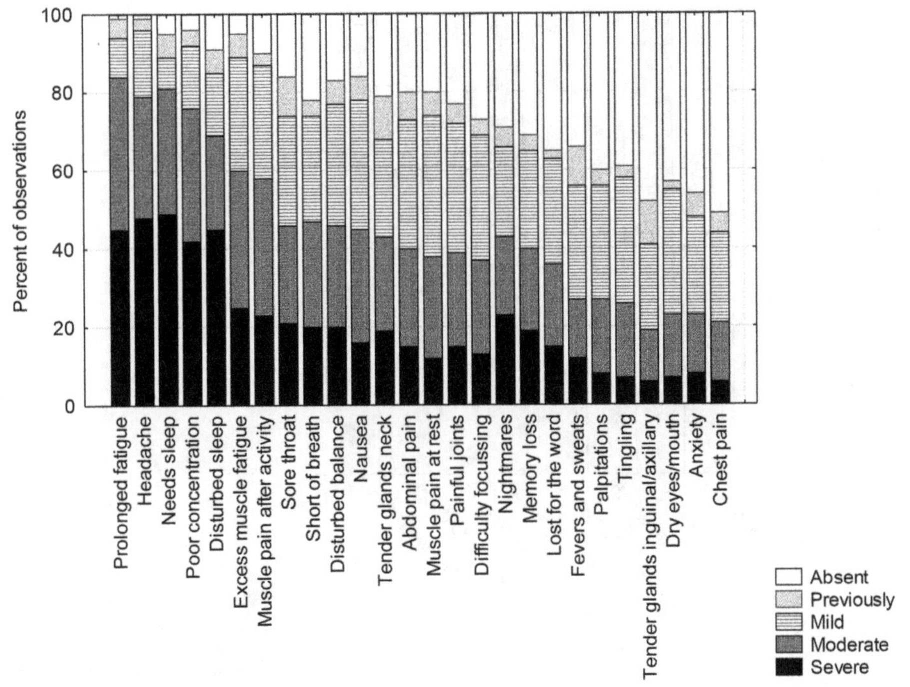

FIGURE 1 | Frequency and severity of symptoms in young people with ME/CFS ($n = 418$).

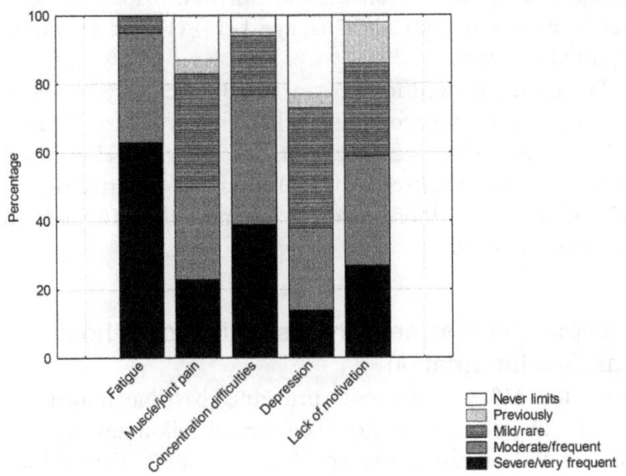

FIGURE 2 | Rating of symptoms limiting functioning.

Baseline depression (Beck), anxiety (Spielberger) and General Health Questionnaires

The mean total score on the Beck was 13.8 sd 8.9 (range 1-51) ($n = 370$). On this scale, scores between 0 and 10 indicate "normal ups and downs" experienced by 45%, 10–20, "mild mood changes" (35%), 20–30, moderate depression (15%), 30–40, significant depression (4%) and >40 severe (1%). Items related to "ability to work," "tiredness," "sleep disturbance," "ability to make decisions," and "feeling dissatisfied" scored highly (mean for each item 1.3–1.7, range 0–3), and as they are associated with CFS, the scores may as a consequence be inflated. Twenty per cent of the cohort scored more than 20 while 5% were in the moderately severe range. Less than 1% reported anhedonia symptoms (feeling "hopeless," "bad or worthless," "disgusted with themselves," or "feeling as if they deserved to be punished"). Direct questions regarding aspects of depression, motivation, concentration and effects on functioning revealed a consistency in responses within the baseline questionnaire (**Figure 2**), It was noted that 25%, at least "some of the time" (**Figure 3**) thought that their family "would be better off if they were dead" however less than half these were moderately depressed based on the Beck where 1% reported suicidal thoughts. Community surveys of adolescents in Victoria have noted 18% (CI 17–20) of young people report significant depressive symptoms (36). Thus, the rates of depression in this clinical sample were reported at only marginally higher rate than the adolescent population. Higher scores were associated with severity of symptoms, not feeling supported by family, the medical profession or school. The mean score, however, was significantly different from a small community sample of age and gender matched young people (**Table 1**).

The mean "state" scores for the Spielberger was 43.9 sd 12.6 (range 21–79) ($n = 273$) and the mean score for the "trait" was 45.1 sd 12.8 (range 21–80) ($n = 259$). The mean total score was 88.9 sd 24.9 (range 40–157) which was higher than the previous clinical sample and significantly different from the community sample. Approximately 30% of the young people with ME/CFS experienced moderate levels of anxiety when diagnosed.

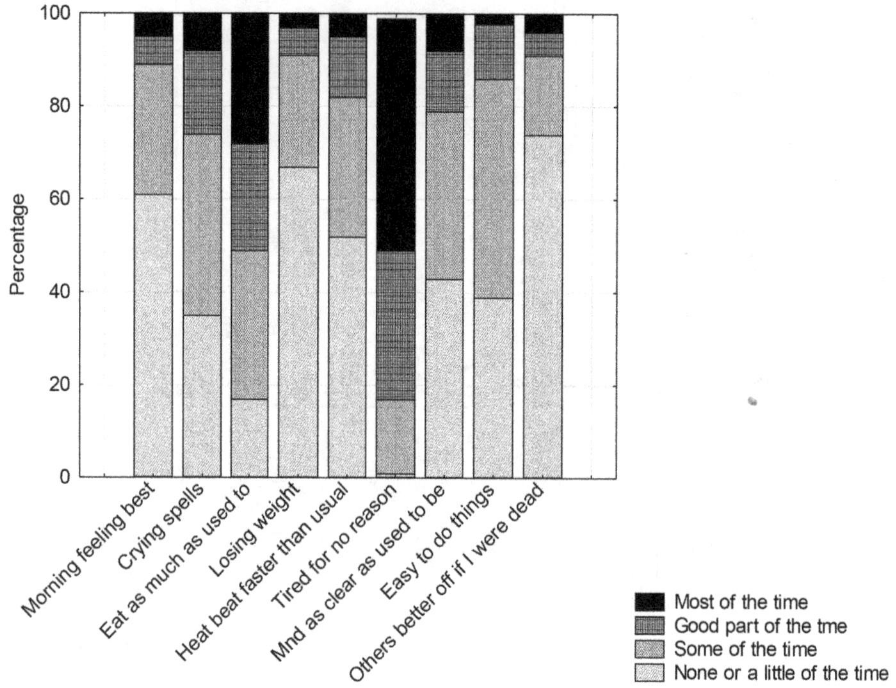

FIGURE 3 | Rating of frequency of specific symptoms in ME/CFS.

The mean General Health Questionnaire score of 16.0, sd 3.01 (range 9–27) was similar to the previous clinical group but significantly different from the community sample (**Table 1**).

Anti-nuclear antibody titers

Thirteen percent of the sample ($n = 442$) had a titer between 1:40 and 1:80, however the reporting level changed in 2008 from 1:40 to 1:160. Twenty one per cent of the sample ($n = 499$) had a significantly positive titer comprising 10% with 1:160 (mildly positive), 9% between 1:320 and 1:640 (moderately positive), and 2% between 1:1,280 and 1:2,560 (strongly positive). The described patterns were speckled (65.5%), homogeneous (3.2%), nucleolar (15%) and mixed speckled/homogeneous (15.9%). The high titers were not associated with clinical signs or any other markers of connective tissue disorders such as high sedimentation rate, positive antibodies to double stranded DNA, or extractable nuclear antibodies, and this was confirmed by a rheumatologist. The proportion of positive titers is at least double the expected rate in this age group, and although it not unknown to have moderately strong positive titers without evidence of connective tissues disorders in pediatric rheumatology clinics, the proportion of moderate to strongly positive titers is much greater than expected (personal communication-J Akikusa, Royal Children's Hospital, Aug 2018).

Follow Up Study

Duration of Illness

From the total group of 784 (M:F ratio of 1:3) and mean age 22.5 years sd 4.6 (range 7–35.7) data were obtained from 81.8%. The mean duration of follow up was 8 years sd 4.3 (range 1–21 years). Mean duration of illness for total group was 5 years ($n = 298$) sd 2.7 (range 1–15) (**Figure 4**) and 47% reported recovery.

For those followed for <5 years 29.8% (55 of 185) reported recovery and for those followed for longer than 5 years, 127 of 456 (27.9%) reported recovery occurring before 5 years. However, for those followed for between 5 and 10 years, 54% reported recovery (233/431), and for those followed for more than 10 years 68% reported recovery.

Comparison Between Groups With and Without Baseline Information

From the 418 young people providing baseline information, 364 (87.1% return rate) provided formal follow up data on a total of 971, mean 2.5 (range 1–7) occasions. One third ($n = 122$) provided one response and the remainder ($n = 242$) provided a mean 3.5 (range 2–7) responses a minimum of 2 years apart. This enabled regular feedback concerning management and documentation of any relapses and confirmation of duration of illness close to the occasion rather than relying on memory.

From the remaining 366, 277 (75.6%) responses were obtained, and 30 provided formal follow up information on more than 1 occasion. The group without baseline information contained more young people who were still at secondary school, thus reflecting the difference in age distribution and use of services (t-test for independent samples $t = -3.33$ df 508 $p < 0.001$ F-ratio variances 1.68 $p < 0.00005$). There was also a significant difference in mean duration of follow up 7.6 years sd 4.5 (range 1–21.6) years compared with 8.3 (1–19) years (p

TABLE 1 | Comparison scores for Depression (Beck), Anxiety (Speilberger), and General Health Questionnaire (GHQ) for study group compared with previous clinical and community age and gender matched samples.

	Current clinical			Previous clinical[a]			Community sample[a]				
	n	mean	sd	n	mean	sd	n	mean	sd	*t*-value	*P*-value
Beck	370	13.8	8.9	159	12.5	7.0	65	5.3	5.7	7.97	<0.0005
Spielberger	259	88.9	24.9	118	85.4	22.4	65	69.6	17.7	5.28	<0.0005
GHQ	277	16.0	3.01	171	16.6	7.0	66	10.1	5.3	7.8	<0.0005

[a] *Rowe and Rowe (22).*

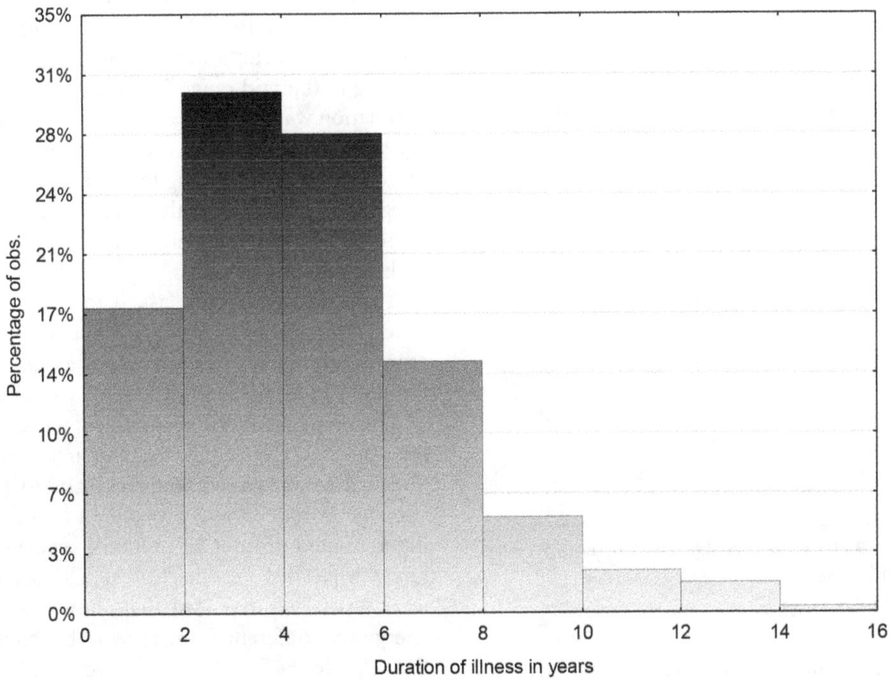

FIGURE 4 | Mean duration of illness for total group 5 years ($n = 298$) sd 2.7 (1–15).

< 0.05) and the proportion reporting recovery was significantly different 40% compared with 52% (Chi-square 6.8, $p < 0.01$).

As the majority of comparisons including: duration of illness (4.9 cf 5.1 years), functional score if reporting recovery (9.0 cf 8.8), duration of illness until help received (13.4 cf 13.8 months), proportion working or studying full time (61% cf 63%), proportion caring for children (5%) or not working or studying (5%) were not significantly different, the general comments and observations have been combined from the two groups (see **Table 2**).

Educational Outcomes

Only 5% of those followed up reported not working or studying, with 8% working or studying less than half time, 24% more than half time and 63% reported working or studying full time. Some of those reportedly not working or studying were traveling overseas prior to university whereas others remained very unwell or had other illnesses. Similarly, 62% reported that they were currently studying at either a secondary or tertiary level. Of the 66% who had undertaken a post-secondary course (tertiary education) half were still studying. Twenty per cent were also working part time while they were studying. Twenty per cent reported using the Visiting Teacher Service during their secondary education and 16.5% used Distance Education service either solely or supplementing their school attendance. Five per cent reported having children, some of whom were working outside of home as well.

For comparison, the 2011 census (18), indicated that 75% of 15–25 year olds complete secondary education and 60% undertake post-secondary education, with 6% unemployed, 9% not in the workforce and 26% in employment. The population census reported 85% of 15–25 year olds are fully engaged in either work or study or both.

A wide range of courses were undertaken by the cohort ranging from traditional University courses to ones with high entry criteria such as medicine, law and health sciences. Technical

TABLE 2 | Comparison data between study and comparison groups.

Total **cohort** n = **784** (M:F 1:3)
Mean **age 22.5** years (range 7–35.7 years)
Follow up (**FU**) data from **641** (**81.8%**)
Mean **length FU 8** (1–21) years
Proportion reporting **recovery 46.5%**
Mean **duration illness 5 years (1–15)** (n = 298)

	Study group who provided baseline data n = 418	Comparison group n = 366
N providing FU data (%)	**364** (87.1%)	**277** (75.6%)
M:F	23%:77%	27%:73%
Age at FU (range) years	23.2 (14.6–33)	21.9 (7–35.7)**
Mean length FU years	8.3 (1–19)	7.6 (1–21.6)*
Mean duration illness (months) until help/diagnosis	13.4 (3–72)	13.8 (3–84) (ns)
Proportion reporting recovery	52% (n = 188)	40% (n =110)#
Mean duration illness (years)	4.9 (1–14)	5.1 (1–15) (ns)
Mean functional score (if recovered)	9.0 (5–10)	8.8 (5–10) (ns)
Working/ studying full time	61%	63% (ns)
Using/used Visiting Teacher Service	20%	20%
Used Distance Education	11%	24%
Completed or undertaking post-secondary education	69%	62%
Not working/studying	5%	5%
Caring for children	5%	5%
Receiving Government Disability Support	26%	33%

*t-test $p < 0.05$ **t-test $p < 0.001$. #chi square 6.8 $p < 0.01$. Bolding indicates composition and outcomes for total cohort.

courses, diploma courses and some apprenticeships were also reported. Several had also completed Masters degrees and Ph.Ds. A very wide variety of occupations were reported from aeronautical engineering, health sciences, law, trades and with some working in the service industries. The majority of service industry jobs were part time for support while undertaking study. A very small percentage did not complete secondary education and this was reported associated with other illness, social circumstances or an unsupportive school.

Disability support from the government was received by 29% of the group. The majority was studying while receiving this or working part time. At the time, government policy allowed this support to enable part-time completion of a degree for those who were chronically unwell, without having to work as well. Of the 5% not studying or working outside of home, several were mothers, one was a carer for a parent, and others had an additional illness or were doing voluntary work.

ME/CFS Functional Score and Reported Recovery

As some young people found the concept of recovery difficult, they were asked to describe how they thought they were functioning with a rating of 10 being "very well" or "back to normal" and 1 being "bedridden." They were also asked what they meant by their score and it usually included a sense of the amount of activity, work or study that they were able to manage, what their stamina was like, how well they recovered from any activity, as well as social engagement and presence of symptoms. The young people were remarkably consistent in what they included in the scoring and how they described it. The clinician also rated the young person based on their reports and found high inter rater reliability for the scores (90%). Parents were generally also asked and they agreed in 80% cases. They often rated one point below the young person as they tended to compare them with how they "used to be." The descriptors of the global rating are in **Appendix 3**. Young people reported that the central part of the Bell CFIDS Scale was difficult to score and they preferred to use the global rating (ME/CFS Functional rating). Concurrent data were collected to allow comparison and this difference in scoring in the mid range (between 4 and 8) was confirmed. The correlation was 0.833 ($n = 252$), however the correlation between the two scales was less in the mid-range (0.65) with the ME/CFS Functional Rating tending to score higher. The Bell scale had an irregular distribution with scores 9 and 10 scoring with higher frequency but low frequencies in the mid-range and an increase at the lower end.

The study group was asked to assess their poorest level of functioning using the Bell scale and 98.7% scored <5 while 68% scored 2 or less. They were also asked their current level of functioning using the same scale as well as the functional rating.

The range of ME/CFS Functional score for those who reported that they had recovered was compared with those who reported they had not recovered. (**Figures 5** and **6**) There was a significant overlap. Some scored low due to other illnesses that they differentiated from CFS. Others reported that they did not know what was "normal" as it had been so long since they were well. They reported that "how a 22 year old spent their energy was different from 15 year, but they were not sure what that should be." Others, who reported themselves as "well," felt that they were managing well, but their parents made the comment that they "did not think that they had the stamina that they had demonstrated as an adolescent." Some needed to be "perfect" to describe themselves as "well" whereas others compared themselves with how they were when they were first unwell and were very grateful to be able to do what they were currently able to do. Some who felt they had recovered also scored lower, as they were caring for small children, were working part time and felt sleep deprived. Others admitted that they were dealing with depression as an additional issue. Hence many factors influenced whether recovery was reported, as well as whether the level of functioning was solely related to ME/CFS.

Reports of Recurrent Infections and Prolonged Recovery Afterwards

The majority reported a reduction in the number of infections and the fact that they rarely had upper respiratory infections when the rest of the family was unwell. They did notice that when they were starting to feel better they commonly had an increased number of upper respiratory infections over a year or two which then settled to a normal rate. This did trigger significant panic and low mood as the symptoms they experienced with these common illnesses reminded them of the early days of ME/CFS

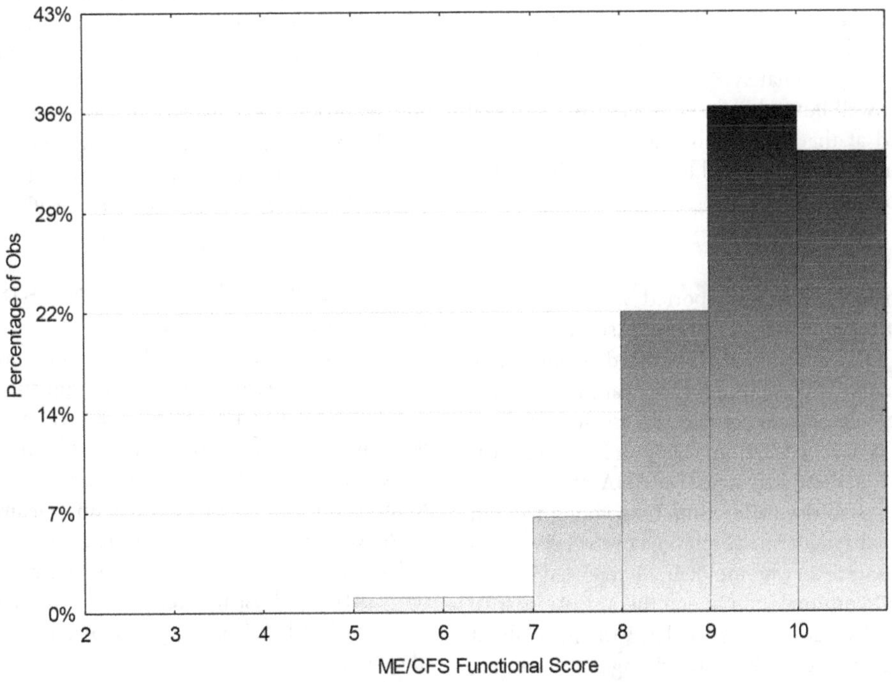

FIGURE 5 | Follow up global functioning score for those who indicated that they had recovered from ME/CFS for cohort (n = 298). Mean score 8.9 (range 5–10).

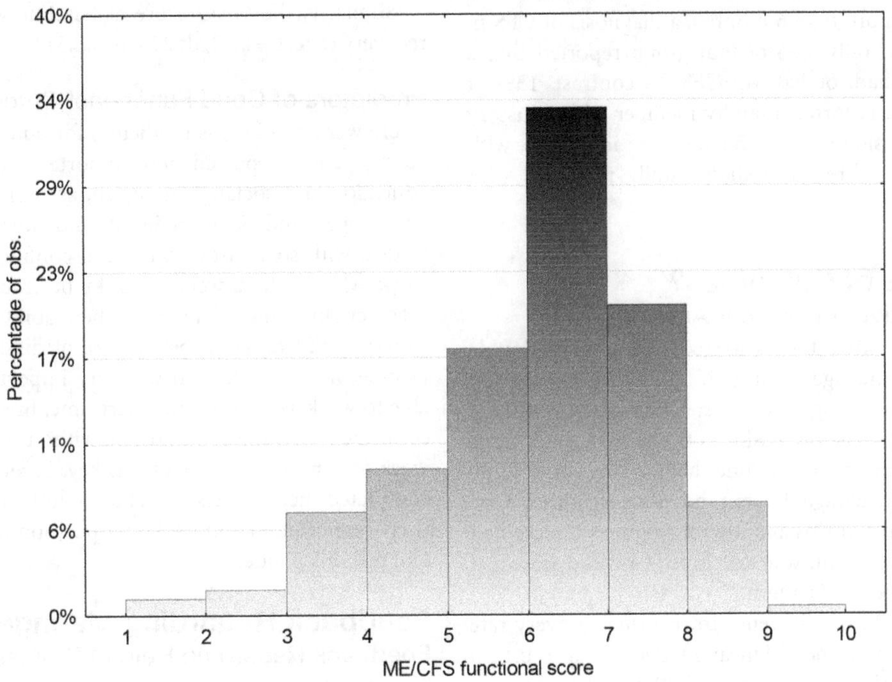

FIGURE 6 | ME/CFS Global functional score for those who reported that they had not recovered.

and they felt that they could not deal with prolonged illness again. As these illnesses commonly recurred on return to school they acknowledged that it made them more cautious about engaging again. They also clearly did not believe reassurance that feedback from others who had experienced similar events, indicated that recovery is generally short lived. Comments on feedback forms indicated the fear and anxiety was excessive but not warranted. Those who had had regular asthma prior to becoming ill, observed that they rarely had asthma when they were very unwell with ME/CFS. Approximately 5% had documented EBV infection when still unwell but only one young person who had significantly improved at that stage, had a prolonged recovery of several years. The remainder reverted to their usually level of functioning in <3 months.

Other Illnesses

The majority of associated illnesses reported were depression (rarely associated with depression at baseline), severe anxiety, panic disorder, and POTS and neurally mediated hypotension. There were individuals with agoraphobia, eating disorder, irritable bowel disease, celiac disease, Graves disease, Rheumatoid arthritis, and several developed Systemic Lupus Erythematosis (SLE) but all but one of these had negative ANA at the onset of CFS. Two struggled with drug addiction. One young woman had died at 22 from neuroendocrine carcinoma of the cervix and another had breast cancer at 23 who incidentally reported having a reduction in her CFS symptoms after chemotherapy. At least 10 young women disclosed sexual abuse years later, the majority of which occurred after they were unwell, thus adding to the trauma.

Members of Family With History of ME/ CFS

Although data from the baseline questionnaires indicated 17% had a close family member who had a prolonged recovery from an infection lasting more than 6 months, a diagnosis of CFS in the past or currently, only 12% of that group reported that a family member has had, or has ME/CFS. In contrast, 15% of the remaining cohort reported a family member with a history of ME/CFS. Parents, siblings and cousins were identified, with some families having three immediate family members with the diagnosis.

Any Predictors of Outcomes?

Presence of Positive Antinuclear Antibody Titers

The proportion of positive titers (>1:160) was at least double the expected rate in this age group (37, 38), and it is expected that titers increase with age. However, subsequently only 4 (0.5%) patients had diagnosed SLE. Of these, 2 had titers of 1:160 (speckled pattern) and one had a titer of 1:1,280 homogeneous pattern at age 15, but no other features. One with later rheumatoid arthritis and 2 with Sjogren's disease had negative ANA titers, while one who developed Grave's disease had a titer of 1:320 with speckled pattern.

There was no significant difference in reported recovery rate and level of ANA titer [General Linear model $F_{(1, 76)} = 0.12$ $p = 0.73$]. Those with high titers (1,280–2,560) reported recovery from CFS. Of those with a titer of 1:640 or higher, there were no follow up data available for 25% of them. Of the remainder, in ¼ the titer remained stable, ½ the titer reduced to normal or near normal, and ¼ the titer increased without any other clinical features of disease. Therefore, high titers were not associated with "non-recovery" and there was a suggestion that titers reduced with recovery.

Outcomes for Severe Symptoms at Outset

The rating for level of ill health early in the illness was a mean score of 1.9, sd 1.3 (range 0–5) with 98.7% scoring <5 and 68% 2 or less, using the Bell CFIDS score. At worst, the majority were bed ridden and unable to attend school at all, or at the most, attended for short periods during the week. Therefore, in this study the majority of young people had severe illness. Severity of illness was not predictive of "non-recovery."

Relationship of Identified Depression, Anxiety, or GHQ Scores to Outcomes

There was no difference in depression score at baseline between those that reported improvement (mean 14.46) and those that had not (mean 13.17) df 315. $t = -1.3$ $p = 0.18$. Although data were available on follow up from 86% of those with Beck data there was no significant difference in baseline score between the total group and those followed up ($\text{mean}_1 = 13.85$, $\text{mean}_2 = 13.78$; df 688 $p = 0.91$). If selected for higher depression scores at baseline (20% of sample) there was no difference in baseline score between those that reported recovery and those that did not (means 28 and 27.5) i.e., depression at baseline was not predictive of outcome.

There is also no difference in anxiety score at baseline between those who reported recovery and those who did not, so anxiety at baseline was not predictive of outcome using student t-test ($\text{mean}_1 = 28.1$, $\text{mean}_2 = 27.5$; $t = 0.4$ $p = 0.7$).

Similarly, the GHQ score at baseline was not predictive of recovery (t-test -0.62, df 233, $p = 0.5$).

Predictors of Good Functional Outcome

There were no obvious predictors for outcome. However, as the young people reported how important remaining engaged in education and socially connected, as well as feeling supported, encouraged and being believed, and how difficult it could be to deal with social isolation, social confidence and unsatisfying work when still unwell, it could be inferred that improving these circumstances improves their ability to cope with their situation and function better. Use of disability support during post-secondary education was very important, if they were not able to work as well as study part time. Ensuring that they could continue study at a reduced rate without having to try and find work to support themselves was key. Frequently when they had completed their studies and able to find a job, even if part time, they were often in a much better position to support themselves and feel independent.

Feedback Regarding Management

Feedback Regarding Helpful Professionals

Twenty three per cent of the group providing baseline information "did not find any professionals helpful," however only 17% of the remainder did not find professionals helpful despite our concerns that this group may contain a higher proportion of young people who did not engage with health services. Pediatrician, Visiting Teachers, cardiologists who were consulted because of orthostatic intolerance were most frequently cited, and less frequently physiotherapist, family doctors, some school staff, counselors, psychologist, massage therapist, sleep physician and gastroenterologist. The reasons they were found helpful related to "being taken seriously," "being believed," "providing support," "providing practical strategies," "alleviating symptoms," "providing educational liaison and advocacy," "dietary advice," and "managing other illnesses" that may also be present. The most common responses were appreciating "being understood," "feeling respected," "supported," "reassured," and "not feeling alone."

Feedback Regarding Helpful Information

The young people consistently indicated that the most helpful information was providing some management strategies to help them "feel in control of their life again." Managing symptoms and providing information regarding the importance of good routines particularly around sleeping and eating and activity was also appreciated, as well as understanding how to monitor their activities. Strategies for re-engaging with peers, assistance with liaising with schools as well as providing information regarding options to remain engaged in education were rated highly. General information about the illness prognosis and what had helped others, as well as up to date research information was useful. In addition to the hospital clinic, information was sourced from the internet, ME/CFS Society newsletters, and the support groups.

Could the Illness Have Been Handled Better?

There were some differences in feedback from the early questionnaires compared with the later ones mostly related to lack of awareness of the illness. They indicated the need for an earlier diagnosis, and more understanding by the community, the medical profession and by schools. They reported how important it is "to be believed" and to find "someone who understands." There were regular comments about the perceived arrogance of the medical profession and lack of understanding, and how distressing it was to be accused of "being lazy" or implying that it was "all in the mind." Lack of understanding and flexibility by educational institutions was reported as a major source of distress.

In later follow up returns, the comments regarding the need for general understanding of the illness and their plight, the need for earlier diagnosis and access to management strategies were similar. There were comments regarding self-management that they thought they could have managed better, such as managing stress, routines, pacing, depression, exercise and being more open to acknowledging the presence of depression especially as they were improving and re-engaging in society. There were comments regarding the need for resources to be available for the family, as well as regular but not necessarily frequent follow up appointments, and that contact with other young people in a similar situation would be helpful. Many commented that they also needed to be willing to ask for help.

Many indicated the need to be sensitive about when psychological assistance is offered. They were often not ready for that intervention as they felt they had enough to cope with. They were sensitive as to whether this was implying that psychological issues were the "cause." Many indicated that they were "miserable" and "fed-up with being unwell" but not depressed which on reflection was a healthy response to their situation. If they were happy and content with not being able to attend school, see friends, or do any physical activity it would be a cause for concern. Others reported that they struggled with motivation and seeing any end to the illness. Some had a family history of depression and were open to receiving assistance. It was noted that when many young people started to feel a little better they were willing to have strategies for managing stress and anxiety and also reassurance that they had developed resilience while learning to manage the illness, and if faced with challenges in the future would have the skills to cope. Some young people needed help with family issues. Others needed help with integrating back into school and dealing with the challenges of social interactions and social learning tasks of adolescence, particularly as they felt vulnerable and had lost some confidence.

Use of Alternative Therapies

Seventy per cent of the young people used alternative therapies and these included 40 different types, some trying up to 10 different ones. The therapies ranged from naturopathy, chiropractics, homeopathy, Chinese herbs, intravenous vitamins, Reiki, Qi Gong, Tai Chi, Yoga, Myotherapy, Bowen therapy, massage, hypnosis, cupping, aromatherapy, color therapy, meditation etc. There were very few therapies that were considered of any value by the young people. The only ones that approached a 30% positive response involved massage (under a variety of different guises) for those with muscle pain and "good dietary advice" often in young people with associated abdominal discomfort. The most common comment was that they "wished their parents had not wasted their money or their energy by taking them to people who had promised to cure them but didn't."

DISCUSSION

Demographics and Baseline Symptoms

The finding of M:F ratio of 1:3 is consistent with other studies showing a consistently higher proportion of females to males with CFS, for example, Reyes et al. (39), Rowe et al. (40), and Bell et al. (7). The observation in this study that the ethnic background characteristics are not consistent with the demographics of the state, nor the clientele of other general medical or adolescent health clinics in the hospital, is interesting in the light of reports of CFS occurring in community surveys in Japan (41), Korea (42), and the United Kingdom (43). However, each of these studies was in adults and associated with high rates of psychological distress and based on survey information rather than a clinical assessment of CFS. There may be ethnic and cultural differences in how CFS is reported, for example in Japan it is rare for infection to be recognized as the trigger, and chronic sleep deprivation and stress are noted to be associated with the condition, where it is commonly described as school phobia (personal communication, Prof. Miike, 2008). Shi et al. (44) reported likely CFS from surveys of Chinese students associated with despondency and anxiety regarding school. There was a predominance of males. There are few documented pediatric studies in other ethnic populations. Due to the universal health care system and the demographic of other medical clinics in the hospital, access to health care is unlikely to be the main explanation. This cohort reported a high rate of post infective onset, as well as higher than expected rates of positive antinuclear antibody serology without evidence of clinical connective tissue diseases. It is recognized that people of northern European descent have a higher proportion of autoimmune diseases both in ethnic variation in expression of autoimmune diseases such as SLE (45) and the prevalence of multiple sclerosis (46).

Of note, was the consistency with which this cohort of young people responded regarding the severity and frequency of symptoms that was comparable to the earlier cohort that was obtained when there was very little awareness of the condition in young people (47). The high rate of reported infections at the onset and the consistency in responses suggests a relatively homogeneous group. The rates of anxiety and depression were also comparable with the previous sample and higher than the community sample. It is noted that the baseline rate of reported depression was only marginally higher than a large concurrent adolescent survey in the state (36). Crawley et al. (48) and a review by Lievesley et al. (49) have reported increased prevalence of anxiety and depression in young people with CFS implying that this association may be contributing to the morbidity.

Follow Up Study

Outcomes

Follow up of this large well defined cohort with 87% of the study group providing data, has indicated that more than half the young people report recovery and many who do not report recovery, are also functioning well. The mean duration of illness was 5 years (range 1–15 years). By 10 years 68% reported recovery. The young people who reported recovery at 14 and 15 years could not identify any contributing factor. "It just happened." The duration of illness was comparable to the placebo arm in the 5-year follow up following the immunoglobulin trial and a mean of 8 years from onset (13). Sixteen percent were moderately unwell with 20% reporting "not quite back to normal" and the remaining 64% reporting recovery. Bell et al. (7) had a well characterized group also with a defined onset and likely post-infective, that was followed for approximately 13 years. Their findings were similar in that all had improved function and most considered that they had recovered except 20% remained unwell. Other follow up studies have been for short periods (1, 4, 6, 50); have not been diagnosed clinically (2); had half the cohort with fatigue of 1–6 months duration (4); the cohort was small in numbers (3); or the follow up did not have a high proportion participating (4, 5). Due to these differences, findings are difficult to compare. In this study, it is clear that there was variation in how young people defined recovery. There was a significant overlap in functional scores between those who had reported recovery and those that had not. In this study, as well as requesting an assessment as to whether they have recovered, an indication of their level of functioning that took into account stamina, recovery after activity, proportion of participation in work or school, whether the workload has been reduced, level of social contact and severity of symptoms. Early follow up questionnaires requested this in detail as well as using the Bell scale. Young people could consistently estimate their level of functioning. A global functional rating scale (**Appendix 3**) compiled from the surprisingly consistent descriptors of hundreds of young people with ME/CFS in the clinic has good inter-rater reliability. This however did not necessarily reflect their concept of whether they had recovered or not. They reported struggling with understanding what to expect as "normal functioning" as they had no frame of reference.

Other follow up studies have varied in how they have reported recovery making comparisons difficult. Differing measures such as measures of fatigue (8), symptom presence and functional outcomes, (9, 10), self-report (6) or a combination of global functioning and self-report have been used (7). Parslow et al. (11) have been investigating what aspects for defining recovery are important to young people with ME/CFS. Fatigue scales, Karnovsky scores, school attendance or physician's perspective (51) are useful markers of improvement but do not appear to capture the complexity of what is important to young people as well their tolerance level to the normal "ups and downs" of life and their satisfaction with what they are able to do.

In this follow up study there is a higher than expected rate of engagement in post-secondary education compared with the community rates, and a high proportion (95%) who are either working or studying part or full time. It was also noted that those who attended tertiary education, there was a much higher than community rate of completion of courses and lower than community rate of changing courses. In Victoria, there is a scheme available to apply for Special Entry Access to university if preparation for university entrance had been impacted by chronic illness, and usually very supportive Disability Liaison Units exist in universities to assist once enrolled. Universities recognize that young people who have faced adversity do not tend to waste their opportunities and their applications are usually given consideration.

It is noted that the proportion of young people with positive ANA is higher than expected without progressing to clinical autoimmune disease. There was a range of other illnesses reported which influenced the functional rating but were usually reported as separate from ME/CFS. Severe anxiety, depression, agoraphobia, eating disorder, although uncommon was linked with ongoing CFS. Presence of reported depression at follow up was linked with family discord or lack of support, difficulty with completing an education to equip for satisfying work, ongoing severe symptoms or disclosed history of sexual abuse that had often occurred after the onset of the illness.

Feedback

Regular feedback has helped inform our management and advice that we can offer young people. There has been a clear message about how important it is to the young person to be believed, to feel supported and to be provided with a management plan that enables them to have some control of their lives. Maintaining social connectedness and support for continuing education is crucial to ensure their aspirations remain. Similar to the reported feedback from young people in the UK, advocacy for school and ability to continue with education was valued (11). The education system in the state allowed for flexibility in workload, school attendance, mix of Distance Education and school based learning as well as access to a Visiting Teacher service whose brief is to help liaise and coordinate the learning program at school and at home until the young person is well enough to return to school full time. Appropriate documentation to access these services is required but experienced Visiting Teachers explaining to other teachers significantly improved cooperation and satisfaction on the part of student and staff.

Anecdotal information about the perceived value of various alternative therapies has been appreciated by young people. As few therapies have even reached expected level for placebo intervention, the time and money saved has been often been used to support an interest area that has contributed to enriching their life.

Feedback indicated the importance of being sensitive about when psychological assistance is offered as there were many situations where they were not receptive until later in the illness. Sometimes this was related to an implied attitude that ME/CFS is a "psychological illness" rather than a chronic illness with its attendant challenges.

If graded exercise was implied as a means to recovery and symptoms were made worse, the young person often withdrew from any medical assistance and frequently from school. Some interpreted the message as indicating that the problem was with their cooperation or motivation, not with what was being advocated. Several were very angry and suspicious of medical profession. At other times, intervention programs were very helpful when self-management strategies such as organizational skills, sleep hygiene, advocacy for appropriate school program and appropriate strengthening exercises and advice regarding how to monitor increases in activity including "boom/bust planning."

Many reported that they appreciated the plan that recognized the impact of illness on every aspect of their life and the fact that they could reduce this effect by not neglecting these areas. This approach was not disregarding the fact that they were ill or implying that their belief that they were unwell was hampering their recovery. If they felt they were believed, they did not have to prove it, and they just needed to find a way to survive it in good shape and feel that they were supported in doing so. Families certainly indicated that they were grateful and much less anxious when there was a negotiated plan and they were supported in dealing with the education authorities. Similarly, the education authorities reported being grateful for information and support.

Although a variety of management strategies such as adaptive pacing, graded exercise, cognitive behavior therapy can be helpful (14), the specifics of what this entails and whether it is implemented as an individualized program is often not clear. However, Burgess et al. (52) found a family focused individualized home based rehabilitation program was well received for those with severe CFS. Evidence for significant improvement is hampered by difficulties in comparing outcome measures according to clinical presentation, patient characteristics, case criteria and degree of disability (16). The routine care that occurred in this cohort does include aspects of these strategies but as no two management plans were the same, the details of how they were implemented were not standardized. What did seem important was that the young person was devising the plan with the support of the family and cooperation of the school.

Outcomes and Baseline Characteristics

Although many reports (3, 43, 49, 53, 54) imply that the presence of depression or anxiety at the onset could potentially influence the recovery or function, there was no convincing evidence in this study that the presence or absence of depression, anxiety or illness severity was associated with outcomes in this cohort. Neither the presence of positive ANA titer nor documented EBV infection was associated with outcomes. Nonetheless, depression, anxiety or other illness documented at follow up was reported as affecting function and occasionally was linked with ongoing CFS or else reported as a separate issue following recovery. Therefore, this study was not able to identify any predictor for recovery.

Strengths of This Study

The desire by young people to have answers to common questions ensured a high participation rate and frank responses from the large cohort over a long period of time. There was a very high proportion of the original cohort who willingly provided information despite the challenges in tracking such a mobile population. Despite little information in the public domain about the illness when some of the initial symptom inventory and background information data were collected, the consistency of responses indicates that the group is relatively homogeneous and consistent with earlier and later case definitions (19, 20, 35, 55) as well as being comparable to an earlier study group (12, 22). Although the comparison group in this cohort did not have comparable detailed baseline data nor the prospective repeated follow up questionnaires the 2 groups were only significantly different on age range and current education status but all other comparisons were comparable. Similarly, the concern that young people with severe CFS may not be represented in this study and therefore skew the findings, was not realized as some attended in wheel chairs and were clearly very limited, and the average functional score based on the Bell scale did indicate that at the beginning of the illness, they were severe.

The duration of illness and functional outcomes were also comparable between both groups, the placebo arm of the immunoglobulin trial as well as the Bell follow up study, which was a defined group for a prolonged period of time.

There was marked consistency in feedback comments. Regaining some control of their life by designing their own management plan was cited by the majority as the most helpful intervention.

Weaknesses

This study has provided information from only one center and may not be representative of outcomes in another area of the country or internationally. The high rate of post-infective/defined onset CFS has indicated a relatively homogeneous group so that the outcomes may not be applicable to other groups. In addition although the management principles were similar, the actual plan was very individualized and the effective component would not be easy to measure. The timing of the various activity increases and the nature of these activities as well as the timing of psychological assistance was also very varied and individual, based on the young person's situation and readiness both from an illness point of view as well as developmental stage. Similarly, standardized outcome measures that have been used in other studies were not used consistently as the young people did not feel that they were asking questions that were important to them. Similarly school attendance, as such, was not a satisfactory measure of their educational progress but the number of subjects, workload and quality and quantity of task completion was often more satisfactory.

Early in this study it is likely that the presence and significance of orthostatic intolerance may have been missed, although it was noted that those with a slower onset of symptoms (over several months) frequently had associated hyperflexible joints.

Although the regular attempts at formal follow up ensured that the time of recovery was reported close to the event, the proportion of the current sample returned at each time period was not high. As these data were initially collected as part of routine clinical care rather than a formal investigation of duration and predictive factors, the baseline data was not complete. It does however appear that there was little difference in outcomes and other characteristics when both study group and comparison group were part of the final follow up study. So the concerns that lack of completion of baseline data may affect outcomes by potentially reflecting lack of engagement, severity of illness, or not disclosing mental health issues were unfounded.

Further Study

In order to confirm if these estimates are able to be generalized, this study highlights the need for baseline questionnaire data that is not too onerous to be routinely collected in clinic cohorts. The data needs a severity or frequency scale, and an opportunity to indicate if the symptoms are currently not present, but were previously in the illness, as well as routine documentation of functional improvement and perception of recovery. Confirmation of the impact of depression and anxiety and illness severity at the outset and the perception that some of the contributing factors may be iatrogenic, and focusing on interventions that are important to young people would also be a fruitful area for further investigation. These factors may well vary depending on the sociocultural environment. The overlap between education and health and the importance of remaining engaged in education that was identified by young people as crucial for improved functional outcomes, as well as support and acceptance by family, medical personnel and schools and the importance of regular but not necessarily frequent follow up has been identified as areas that need further study. The impact of management of orthostatic intolerance on improving function warrants further study (17, 40). The suggestions that nonspecific autoimmune responses may be associated and that interventions such as intravenous immunoglobulin may be possible as a treatment option, warrants further investigation in a different cohort.

CONCLUSIONS

Follow up of this cohort indicated that a significant proportion reported recovery and this was confirmed with reported participation in school, work or social activities as well as the global score. The mean duration of illness was 5 years with a range of 1–15 years. Other features of this cohort indicated that there was a high proportion of reported and documented infectious trigger, the most common being EBV. The reported symptoms were very consistent across the group. The ethnic background of the cohort was not representative of the population nor the hospital clientele, and as 17% reported a close family member who had had a prolonged recovery following an infectious illness, had diagnosed ME/CFS in the past or currently, a possible genetic predisposition is likely. Moderate to strongly positive ANA titers were more common than expected and not associated with any other clinical indication of connective tissue disorders. Depression rates were marginally above adolescent baseline rates in Victoria. Higher scores were commonly associated with severity of symptoms, "not being believed" or difficulty negotiating an appropriate program at school. Anhedonia symptoms were rarely reported and these were often when there was a recognized strong family history of depression. There was no difference in outcome rates with those with moderately severe depression at first visit and those with none, however depression was more commonly reported in those with reduced global scores at follow up and those who reported they had not recovered. Additional illnesses were relatively common at follow up and either distinct or comorbid with ME/CFS (Fibromyalgia, anxiety, depression, severe orthostatic intolerance, IBS, fructose/lactose intolerance). There were no suicides reported.

Young people reported that management strategies that allowed them some control back over their lives, that reduced the uncertainty for families and ensured that they received the appropriate understanding and support were the most valuable intervention. Symptom management, especially sleep and headache were very helpful. There were many comments about needing to be believed and understood by the medical profession, teaching profession and family. Comments about alternative therapies usually reflected their parent's anxiety and desire to find something that might help rather than being helpful to the young person.

Many young people reported that they could have improved their self-management as well as acknowledging that they could have been more prepared to accept some help regarding some of the social and psychological issues that they had to face as they were returning back into active life, including dealing with their lack of confidence regarding their ability to cope with adversity or acquisition of social skills due to their absences from school. They acknowledged that this was offered but they were not necessarily ready to access the help.

Remaining engaged in education and therefore their ability to pursue their aspirations was identified as crucially important but involved significant advocacy support and creativity to ensure this occurred. There was a high proportion who reported engaged in or completing post-secondary education (higher than national rate) and more than 95% were working or studying part or full time.

The answers to the common questions are that the majority recover (68% by 10 years). The mean duration was 5 years with range 1–15 years. The functional outcome is generally good, however the duration of illness over such a crucial period of development means that attention to the impact it has on education, social, emotional and physical development was identified by the young people as key to how they coped with, and survived the experience. There was no obvious predictor for recovery at the onset, but there are many helpful interventions including management plan, symptom management and remaining engaged in education. The level of maturity and resilience demonstrated in the young people in the feedback during the follow up was inspiring.

AUTHOR CONTRIBUTIONS

The author confirms being the sole contributor of this work and has approved it for publication.

ACKNOWLEDGMENTS

The willingness and frank responses by the young people and their families in participating in these studies is gratefully acknowledged. The detective skills of Judy Moon in contacting so many in the follow up study, the assistance of Tessa Brewin in coordinating the clinic in the early years and the input of Fran Bailey as Physiotherapist, helping with realistic exercises has been invaluable. The assistance with analyses in the earlier studies by my late husband Ken is gratefully acknowledged. The data collection, writing, analyses, and patient care was the responsibility of the author.

REFERENCES

1. Carter BD, Edwards JF, Kronenberger WG, Michalczyk L, Marshall GS. Case control study of chronic fatigue in pediatric patients. *Pediatrics* (1995) 95:179–86.
2. Norris T, Collin SM, Tilling K, Nuevo R, Stansfeld SA, Sterne JA, et al. Natural course of chronic fatigue syndrome/myalgic encephalomyelitis in adolescents. *Arch Dis Child.* (2017) 102:522–8. doi: 10.1136/archdischild-2016-311198
3. Rimes KA, Goodman R, Hotopf M, Wessely S, Meltzer H, Chalder T. Incidence, prognosis, and risk factors for fatigue and chronic fatigue syndrome in adolescents: a prospective community study. *Pediatrics* (2007) 119:e603–9. doi: 10.1542/peds.2006-2231
4. Krilov LR, Fisher M, Friedman SB, Reitman D, Mandel FS. Course and outcome of chronic fatigue in children and adolescents. *Pediatrics* (1998) 102(2 Pt 1):360–6. doi: 10.1542/peds.102.2.360
5. Gill AC, Dosen A, Ziegler JB. Chronic fatigue syndrome in adolescents: a follow-up study. *Arch Pediatr Adolesc Med.* (2004) 158:225–9. doi: 10.1001/archpedi.158.3.225
6. van der Werf SP, de Vree B, Alberts M, van der Meer JW, Bleijenberg G, Netherlands Fatigue Research Group Nijmegen. Natural course and predicting self-reported improvement in patients with chronic fatigue syndrome with a relatively short illness duration. *J Psychosom Res.* (2002) 53:749–53. doi: 10.1016/S0022-3999(02)00324-0
7. Bell DS, Jordan K, Robinson M. Thirteen-year follow-up of children and adolescents with chronic fatigue syndrome. *Pediatrics* (2001) 107:994–8. doi: 10.1542/peds.107.5.994
8. Kawatani J, Mizuno K, Shiraishi S, Takao M, Joudoi T, Fukuda S, et al. Cognitive dysfunction and mental fatigue in childhood chronic fatigue syndrome–a 6-month follow-up study. *Brain Dev.* (2011) 33:832–41. doi: 10.1016/j.braindev.2010.12.009
9. van Geelen SM, Bakker RJ, Kuis W, van de Putte EM. Adolescent chronic fatigue syndrome: a follow-up study. *Arch Pediatr Adolesc Med.* (2010) 164:810–4. doi: 10.1001/archpediatrics.2010.145
10. Knoop H, Stulemeijer M, de Jong LW, Fiselier TJ, Bleijenberg G. Efficacy of cognitive behavioral therapy for adolescents with chronic fatigue syndrome: long-term follow-up of a randomized, controlled trial. *Pediatrics* (2008) 121:619–25. doi: 10.1542/peds.2007-1488
11. Parslow R, Patel A, Beasant L, Haywood K, Johnson D, Crawley E. What matters to children with CFS/ME? A conceptual model as the first stage in developing a PROM. *Arch Dis Child.* (2015) 100:1141–7. doi: 10.1136/archdischild-2015-308831
12. Rowe KS. Double blind placebo controlled trial to assess the efficacy of intravenous gammaglobulin for the management of Chronic Fatigue Syndrome in Adolescents. *J Psychiatr Res.* (1997) 31:133–47. doi: 10.1016/S0022-3956(96)00047-7
13. Rowe KS. 5-year follow-up of young people with Chronic Fatigue Syndrome following the double-blind randomised controlled intravenous gammaglobulin trial. *J Chronic Fatigue Syndr.* (1999) 5:97–107. doi: 10.1300/J092v05n03_08
14. Nijhof SL, Bleijenberg G, Uiterwaal CS, Kimpen JL, van de Putte EM. Effectiveness of internet-based cognitive behavioural treatment for adolescents with chronic fatigue syndrome (FITNET): a randomised controlled trial. *Lancet* (2012) 379:1412–8. doi: 10.1016/S0140-6736(12)60025-7
15. Nijhof SL, Priesterbach LP, Uiterwaal CS, Bleijenberg G, Kimpen JL, van de Putte EM. Internet-based therapy for adolescents with chronic fatigue syndrome: long-term follow-up. *Pediatrics* (2013) 131:e1788–95. doi: 10.1542/peds.2012-2007
16. Castro-Marrero J, Saez-Francas N, Santillo D, Alegre J. Treatment and management of chronic fatigue syndrome/myalgic encephalomyelitis: all roads lead to Rome. *Br J Pharmacol.* (2017) 174:345–69. doi: 10.1111/bph.13702
17. Rowe PC. Orthostatic intolerance and chronic fatigue syndrome: new light on an old problem. *J Pediatr.* (2002) 140:387–9. doi: 10.1067/mpd.2002.124318
18. Australian Bureau of Statistics. *Education and Work, Australia, Community Profiles* (2011). Available online at: www.abs.gov.au
19. Holmes GP, Kaplan JE, Gantz NM, Komaroff AL, Schonberger LB, Straus SE, et al. Chronic fatigue syndrome: a working case definition. *Ann Intern Med.* (1988) 108:387–9. doi: 10.7326/0003-4819-108-3-387
20. Fukuda K, Strauss S, Hickie I, Sharpe MC, Dobbins JG, Komaroff A. The chronic fatigue syndrome: a comprehensive approach to its definition and study. *Ann Intern Med.* (1994) 121:953–9. doi: 10.7326/0003-4819-121-12-199412150-00009

21. Lloyd A, Wakefield D, Boughton C, Dwyer J. What is myalgic encephalomyelitis? *Lancet* (1988) I:1286–7. doi: 10.1016/S0140-6736(88)92107-1
22. Rowe KS, Rowe KJ. Symptom patterns of children and adolescents with Chronic Fatigue Syndrome. In: Singh NN, Ollendick TH, Singh AN editors. Vol. 2, *International Perspectives on Child and Adolescent Mental Health*. New York, NY: Elsevier Science (2002). p. 395–415.
23. Peterson PK, Shepard J, Macres M, Schenck C, Crosson J, Rechtman D, et al. A controlled trial of intravenous immunoglobulin G in chronic fatigue syndrome. *Am J Med.* (1990) 89:554–60. doi: 10.1016/0002-9343(90)90172-A
24. Vollmer-Conna U, HIckie I, Hadzi-Pavlovic D, Tymms K, Wakefield D, Dwyer J, et al. Intravenous immunoglobulin is ineffective in the treatment of patients with Chronic fatigue Syndrome. *Am J Med.* (1997) 103:38–43. doi: 10.1016/S0002-9343(97)90045-0
25. Lloyd A, Hickie I, Wakefield D, Boughton C, Dwyer J. A double-blind placebo-controlled trial of intravenous immunoglobulin therapy in patients with the Chronic Fatigue Syndrome. *Am J Med.* (1990) 89:561–568. doi: 10.1016/0002-9343(90)90173-B
26. Goldenring JM, Cohen E.. H.E.A.D.S.S.-getting into adolescent heads. *Contemp Pediatr.* (1998) 5:75–90.
27. Beck AT, Ward CH, Mendelson M, Mock J, Erbaugh J. An inventory for measuring depression. *Arch Gen Psychiatry* (1961) 4:561–71. doi: 10.1001/archpsyc.1961.01710120031004
28. Beck AT, Steer RA, Garbin MG. Psychometric properties of the Beck Depression Inventory: Twenty-five years of evaluation. *Clin Psychol Rev.* (1988) 8:77–100. doi: 10.1016/0272-7358(88)90050-5
29. Speilberger CD, Gorsuch RL, Lushene PR, Vagg PR, Jacobs GA. *Self Evaluation Questionnaire State Trait. Manual for the State-Trait Anxiety Inventory* (1983). Palo Alto, CA: Consulting Psychologist Press.
30. Goldberg DP, Hilier VF. A scaled version of the general health questionnaire. *Psychol Med.* (1979) 9:139–45.
31. Parker G, Tupling H, Brown LB. A parental bonding instrument. *Br J Med Psychol.* (1979) 52:1–10. doi: 10.1111/j.2044-8341.1979.tb02487.x
32. Rowe KS, Fitzgerald P, Higgins R, Anderson G, Brewin T. Educational strategies for chronically ill students with a special section on Chronic Fatigue Syndrome. In: *Reprint in The Best of Set for the International Year of the Family-Families and School, No 10* (1994). Hawthorn, VIC: Australian Council for Educational Research.
33. Bell DS. *The Disease of a Thousand Names* (1991). New York, NY: Pollard Publications.
34. Australian Bureau of Statistics. *Education and Work, Australia* (2006). Available online at: www.abs.com.au
35. Jason LA, Jordan K, Miike T, Bell DS, Lapp C, Torres-Harding S, et al. A pediatric case definition for ME/CFS. *J Chronic Fatigue Syndr.* (2006) 13:1–44. doi: 10.1300/J092v13n02_01
36. State Government of Victoria. *Improving the Lives of Young Victorians in Our Community – A Summary Report.* Youth and Family Services Division (2000). Melbourne, VIC: Victorian Government Department of Human Services.
37. Malleson PN, Sailer M, Mackinnon MJ. Usefulness of antinuclear antibody testing to screen for rheumatic diseases. *Arch Dis Children* (1999) 77:299–304. doi: 10.1136/adc.77.4.299
38. Malleson PN, Mackinnon MJ, Sailer-Hoeck M, Spencer CH. Review for the generalist: the antinuclear antibody test in children-When to use it and what to do with a positive titer. *Pediatr Rheumatol Online J.* (2010) 8:27. doi: 10.1186/1546-0096-8-27
39. Reyes M, Nisenbaum R, Hoaglin DC, Unger ER, Emmons C, Randall B, et al. Prevalence and incidence of chronic fatigue syndrome in Wichita, Kansas. *Arch Int Med.* (2003) 163:1530–6. doi: 10.1001/archinte.163.13.1530
40. Rowe PC, Marden CL, Jasion SE, Cranston EM, Flaherty MA, Kelly KJ. Cow's milk protein intolerance in adolescents and young adults with chronic fatigue syndrome. *Acta Paediatr.* (2016) 105:e412–8. doi: 10.1111/apa.13476
41. Kawakami N, Iwata N, Fujihara S, Kitamura T. Prevalence of chronic fatigue syndrome in a community population in Japan. *Tohoku J Exp Med.* (1998) 186:33–41. doi: 10.1620/tjem.186.33
42. Kim CH, Shin HC, Won CW. Prevalence of chronic fatigue and chronic fatigue syndrome in Korea: community-based primary care study. *J Korean Med Sci.* (2005) 20:529–34. doi: 10.3346/jkms.2005.20.4.529
43. Bhui KS, Dinos S, Ashby D, Nazroo J, Wessely S, White PD. Chronic fatigue syndrome in an ethnically diverse population: the influence of psychosocial adversity and physical inactivity. *BMC Med.* (2011) 9:26. doi: 10.1186/1741-7015-9-26
44. Shi J, Shen J, Xie J, Zhi J, Xu Y. Chronic fatigue syndrome in Chinese middle-school students. *Medicine* (2018) 97:e9716. doi: 10.1097/MD.0000000000009716
45. Borchers AT, Naguwa SM, Shoenfeld Y, Gershwin ME. The geoepidemiology of systemic lupus erythematosus. *Autoimmun Rev.* (2010) 9:A277–87. doi: 10.1016/j.autrev.2009.12.008
46. Kingwell E, Marriott JM, Jetté N, Pringsheim T, Makhani N, Morrow SA, et al. Incidence and prevalence of multiple sclerosis in Europe: a systematic review. *BMC Neurol.* (2013) 13:128. doi: 10.1186/1471-2377-13-128
47. Rowe KS, Rowe KJ. Symptom patterns and psychological features of adolescents with chronic fatigue syndreome. *J Paediatr Child Health* (2005). 41:S9. doi: 10.1016/S1874-5911(02)80018-5
48. Crawley E, Hunt L, Stallard P. Anxiety in children with CFS/ME. *Eur Child Adolesc Psychiatry* (2009) 18:683–9. doi: 10.1007/s00787-009-0029-4
49. Lievesley K, Rimes KA, Chalder T. A review of the predisposing, precipitating and perpetuating factors in Chronic Fatigue Syndrome in children and adolescents. *Clin Psychol Rev.* (2014) 34:233–48. doi: 10.1016/j.cpr.2014.02.002
50. Rangel L, Garralda ME, Levin MR, Roberts H. The course of severe chronic fatigue syndrome in childhood. *J R Soc Med.* (2000) 93:129–34. doi: 10.1177/014107680009300306
51. Devendorf AR, Jackson CT, Sunnquist MA, Jason L. Defining and measuring recovery from myalgic encephalomyelitis and chronic fatigue syndrome: the physician perspective. *Dis Rehabil.* (2017). 1–8. doi: 10.1080/09638288.2017.1383518. [Epub ahead of print].
52. Burgess M, Lievesley K, Ali S, Chalder T. Home-based family focused rehabilitation for adolescents with severe Chronic Fatigue Syndrome. *Clin Child Psychol Psychiatry* (2018) 24:19–28. doi: 10.1177/1359104518794764
53. Fuller-Thomson E, Nimigon J. Factors associated with depression among individuals with chronic fatigue syndrome: findings from a nationally representative survey. *Fam Pract.* (2008) 25:414–22. doi: 10.1093/fampra/cmn064
54. ter Wolbeek M, van Doornen LJ, Kavelaars A, Heijnen CJ. Predictors of persistent and new-onset fatigue in adolescent girls. *Pediatrics* (2008) 121:e449–57. doi: 10.1542/peds.2007-1093
55. Jason LA, Barker A, Brown A. Pediatric myalgic encephalomyelitis/chronic fatigue syndrome. *Rev Health Care* (2013) 3:257–70. doi: 10.7175/rhc.v3i4.280

2

Chronotropic Intolerance: An Overlooked Determinant of Symptoms and Activity Limitation in Myalgic Encephalomyelitis/Chronic Fatigue Syndrome?

Todd E. Davenport[1,2], Mary Lehnen[1], Staci R. Stevens[2], J. Mark VanNess[2,3], Jared Stevens[2] and Christopher R. Snell[2]*

[1] Department of Physical Therapy, Thomas J. Long School of Pharmacy and Health Sciences, University of the Pacific, Stockton, CA, United States, [2] Workwell Foundation, Ripon, CA, United States, [3] Department of Health, Exercise, and Sport Sciences, College of the Pacific, University of the Pacific, Stockton, CA, United States

***Correspondence:**
Todd E. Davenport
tdavenport@pacific.edu

Post-exertional malaise (PEM) is the hallmark clinical feature of myalgic encephalomyelitis/chronic fatigue syndrome (ME/CFS). PEM involves a constellation of substantially disabling signs and symptoms that occur in response to physical, mental, emotional, and spiritual over-exertion. Because PEM occurs in response to over-exertion, physiological measurements obtained during standardized exertional paradigms hold promise to contribute greatly to our understanding of the cardiovascular, pulmonary, and metabolic states underlying PEM. In turn, information from standardized exertional paradigms can inform patho-etiologic studies and analeptic management strategies in people with ME/CFS. Several studies have been published that describe physiologic responses to exercise in people with ME/CFS, using maximal cardiopulmonary testing (CPET) as a standardized physiologic stressor. In both non-disabled people and people with a wide range of health conditions, the relationship between exercise heart rate (HR) and exercise workload during maximal CPET are repeatable and demonstrate a positive linear relationship. However, smaller or reduced increases in heart rate during CPET are consistently observed in ME/CFS. This blunted rise in heart rate is called chronotropic intolerance (CI). CI reflects an inability to appropriately increase cardiac output because of smaller than expected increases in heart rate. The purposes of this review are to (1) define CI and discuss its applications to clinical populations; (2) summarize existing data regarding heart rate responses to exercise obtained during maximal CPET in people with ME/CFS that have been published in the peer-reviewed literature through systematic review and meta-analysis; and (3) discuss how trends related to CI in ME/CFS observed in the literature should influence future patho-etiological research designs and clinical practice.

Keywords: myalgic encephalomyelitis (ME), exercise, exercise test, heart rate, chronotropic incompetence (CI), chronic fatigue syndrome

INTRODUCTION

Myalgic encephalomyelitis/chronic fatigue syndrome (ME/CFS) is estimated to affect 0.8 to 2.5 million people in the United States (1). Ninety percent of cases are thought to go undiagnosed (1), suggesting that people with ME/CFS are substantially under-counted, under-diagnosed, and under-treated. The hallmark clinical feature of ME/CFS is post-exertional malaise (PEM), which involves a constellation of substantially disabling signs and symptoms that occur in response to physical, mental, emotional, and spiritual over-exertion. A number of criteria for ME/CFS exist for clinical and research purposes (1–5). Criteria including PEM appear to have the best face validity to differentiate ME/CFS from other fatiguing health conditions (1, 6, 7). The pervasive nature of PEM in ME/CFS has led some working groups to revise diagnostic criteria for ME/CFS to highlight the multi-system deficits associated with exertion intolerance (1–3).

The importance of PEM in ME/CFS emphasizes the value of studies that document abnormalities in exercise response to advance understanding of the patho-etiology, potential biomarkers, and functional disability associated with ME/CFS. Heart rate is one objective measurement, which can be reliably obtained from wearable biometric technology. A large body of literature already exists that documents heart rate responses to exercise in ME/CFS and other fatiguing health conditions. The increasing availability and affordability of wearable biometric technology has led to the observation that wearables could be used for activity tracking and prediction of PEM, using cardiac function as an early proxy for future symptoms. Therefore, the purposes of this perspective are to (1) review the mechanisms for cardiac control during exercise; (2) review the literature related to heart rate responses and exercise in ME/CFS; and (3) discuss the potential implications for aberrant heart rate responses in ME/CFS and its relationship to interpreting the results of exercise testing paradigms and analeptic activity management.

THE RELATIONSHIP BETWEEN HEART RATE AND WORKLOAD IS REPEATABLE AND PREDICTABLE

Under normal conditions, the relationship between heart rate and workload increases linearly. Reliability of a measure is a precursor to validity. Exercise heart rates at maximal exertion and ventilatory anaerobic threshold (VAT) are highly reproducible in both non-disabled individuals and individuals with various health conditions (8–19). In addition, the relationship between workload and heart rate is normally very reproducible (20). That is to say, the correlation is subject to very low error variance. These observations suggest that deviations in the incremental increase in heart rate in response to each unit increase in workload might suggest pathology. In other words, variation in measurements during cardiopulmonary exercise testing (CPET) in people with ME/CFS may reflect true biological variance that can be functionally relevant and provide important patho-etiological clues about the nature of ME/CFS. In healthy people, peak VO_2 reflects a 4-fold increase over resting VO_2 (21), which is accomplished by a 2.2-time increase in heart rate, a 0.3-fold increase in stroke volume, and a 1.5-fold increase in arteriovenous oxygen difference (21). The elevation of one's heart rate is the largest contributor to both VO_2 and the ability to maintain exercise at maximal level workloads (21). Further, an increase in heart rate is a variable of great interest to clinicians and researchers when observing abnormal responses to exertion and predicting possible consequences due to those abnormal responses. A normal and intact heart rate response pattern to exertion is necessary because cardiac output (heart rate × stroke volume) must be matched to metabolic demands throughout the duration of exercise.

IMPAIRMENT IN CHRONOTROPIC RESPONSE IS MEASURABLE

Chronotropic intolerance (CI) is defined by a range of different criteria, including; failure to achieve age-predicted maximal heart rate, delays in achieving age-predicted maximal heart rate, inadequate heart rates at submaximal workloads, slowed post-exertion recovery heart rate, or heart rate fluctuations (21, 22). The prevalence of CI is poorly understood because it is non-uniformly defined. Gentlesk et al. (22) reported the prevalence of CI ranges from 3.1 to 11% in patients referred for exercise testing, >40% in a population of patients with pacemakers, and up to 60% in patients with atrial fibrillation (22). This variation in prevalence provides further evidence in support of the need for a clear definition and a standardized set of criteria so that diagnosis of CI may be made appropriately and populations can be compared (21).

CI is most often diagnosed using a percentage as the cutoff for distinguishing between normal and abnormal heart rate responses to incremental increases in workload during an exercise test (23). The most common percentages of age-predicted maximal heart rate that have been used range between 70 and 85% (23). CI also can be represented as a measure of heart rate reserve, which is the change in heart rate from rest to peak exercise measured during an exercise test (23). However, since the heart rate reserve equation is dependent upon the resting heart rate, it can be taken one step further to better represent an individual's heart rate response to exercise (23). In other words, chronotropic response can be calculated as a fraction of heart rate reserve achieved at maximal effort, given by $\frac{|\Delta HR_{rest\rightarrow peak}|}{(220-age)-HR_{peak}}$ (23). Failure to obtain ≥80% of the adjusted heart rate reserve during an incremental exercise test is the most common criterion used to distinguish CI (23). Some researchers prefer to take a more definitive route when measuring exertion. The ratio of the volume of carbon dioxide produced to the volume of oxygen consumed, or the respiratory exchange ratio, represents an objective measure of physiologic effort during exertion (23). It is generally accepted that a respiratory exchange ratio of >1.15 is indicative of intense, maximal exercise, while a ratio of <0.82 is indicative of a resting state. If an individual's respiratory exchange ratio is <1.05 at peak exercise, research suggests that this indicates either a submaximal level of effort or a premature termination of the exercise test and should be analyzed with caution (23). Similarly, in 1992, Wilkoff et al. (24) attempted to diagnose CI in a more objective manner through the use of the metabolic-chronotropic relationship, or the chronotropic index, which is the ratio between heart rate reserve and metabolic reserve during submaximal workloads. Wilkoff et al. (24) chose this method because it adjusts for age, physical fitness level, functional capacity, and it is unaffected by a researcher's choice of exercise test or protocol. Under normal conditions in healthy individuals, the percentage of heart rate reserve should match the percentage of metabolic reserve achieved during exertion to equal a chronotropic index of 1.0 with 95% confidence intervals of 0.8 and 1.3 (24). Therefore, if the metabolic-chronotropic relationship, or chronotropic index, is ≤0.8 from a given slope or single value throughout one stage of an incremental exercise test, then that is considered CI (24). The Wilkoff model for CI is given as $HR_{stage} = \frac{[(220-age)-HR_{rest}] * (METs_{stage}-1)}{(METs_{peak}-1) + HR_{rest}}$, and depends on age, resting heart rate, age-predicted maximal heart rate, age-predicted heart rate reserve, maximal heart rate observed during exercise testing, volume of oxygen consumed (VO_2–expressed as MET values; 3.5 ml/kg/min) at each stage and at peak exertion, and respiratory exchange ratio (24). Further, this equation can be combined with the previously discussed methods of age-predicted maximal heart rate, adjusted heart rate reserve, and respiratory exchange ratio to determine whether or not CI is present. For example, chronotropic index can be used as a deciding factor if a subject achieves an adequate peak respiratory exchange ratio of >1.09, but fails to achieve ≥80 or 85% of adjusted heart rate reserve or age-predicted maximal heart rate, or if a subject achieves a peak respiratory exchange ratio of <1.09 (21). One can see that there are a number of methods for distinguishing between a normal chronotropic response and CI, which is dependent upon a handful of variables. It is imperative that researchers work together to create a definition and criteria that are clearly defined to consistently identify CI.

FATIGUING HEALTH CONDITIONS INVOLVE IMPAIRED CHRONOTROPIC RESPONSES

Lauer et al. (25) examined prognostic implications of CI in 1,575 asymptomatic male participants from the Framingham Offspring Study. In order to be designated asymptomatic, participants were required to take part in an exercise treadmill test (25). Researchers followed the participants for an average of 7.7 years to investigate all-cause mortality and coronary heart disease events, including angina pectoris, coronary insufficiency, myocardial infarction, any type of coronary heart disease deaths, and coronary revascularization (25). The treadmill exercise test was terminated when participants achieved 85% of age- and sex-predicted maximal heart rate (25). Lauer et al. (25) also mentioned that treadmill tests were terminated upon "participant request, limiting chest discomfort, dyspnea, fatigue, leg discomfort, hypotension, an excessive increase in systolic blood pressure (i.e., peak systolic pressure ≥250 mmHg), ≥2 mm ST-segment depression, or significant ventricular ectopy. Researchers distinguished between normal and abnormal chronotropic responses using three different variables—the ability or inability to achieve 85% of his age- and sex-predicted maximal heart rate, an increase in heart rate from rest to peak, and the chronotropic index at stage 2 of the Bruce protocol (25). One thousand two hundred and forty-eight participants (79%) achieved 85% of their age-predicted maximal heart rates, while the remaining 327 participants (21%) failed to achieve 85% of the target heart rate (25). The participants that failed to reach the target heart rate were also at an increased risk for an ischemic ST-segment response to appear on an ECG, had a lower exercise capacity, and were related to higher occurrences of all-cause mortality and coronary heart disease events (25). The researchers found that increases in heart rate with exertion were inversely related to mortality risk and that an impaired chronotropic response index was also predictive of mortality (25).

EMPIRICAL DATA SUGGEST CHRONOTROPIC IMPAIRMENT IS PRESENT IN PEOPLE WITH ME/CFS

Our group (26, 27) and others (28–30) have measured heart rate responses to exercise in ME/CFS using CPET methodology that allows for careful characterization at peak exertion and VAT. The specific protocol our group has used for over 20 years was developed to capture the difference in underlying physiology between the average symptomatic state and potential cardiovascular, pulmonary, and metabolic decrements characteristic of PEM (26, 28, 31–33). To begin, patients are instructed to rest as much as possible before performing the first CPET, which measures a baseline of the individual and provides a physical stressor to induce PEM. A second CPET performed 24 h after the first is then conducted to measure the individual's response to exercise while in a post exertional state. Sedentary but otherwise non-disabled individuals exhibit high levels of reproducibility between tests (19, 34). Even individuals with various health conditions that present with fatigue demonstrate reproducible CPET measurements (9, 10, 13–17). However, the physiological correlates of PEM, which are typically exacerbated by exertion, are often indicated by variation outside expected intervals in successive exercise tests. Therefore, changes on the test are not related to poor reliability (i.e., "error variance"), but rather the biological variance associated with ME/CFS.

We conducted a systematic review to locate primary research articles published in the peer reviewed and so-called unpublished "gray literature" that described chronotropic responses to exercise during maximal cardiopulmonary exercise testing in people with ME/CFS, with or without comparison to matched control subjects. Maximal cardiopulmonary exercise testing was chosen because there are uniform criteria described for test cessation, and documented criteria exist to identify physiological performance at the ventilatory anaerobic threshold (VAT), which is the point at which non-oxidative or anaerobic metabolism begins to significantly contribute to energy metabolism with increasing exercise workloads (35, 36). Articles that reported

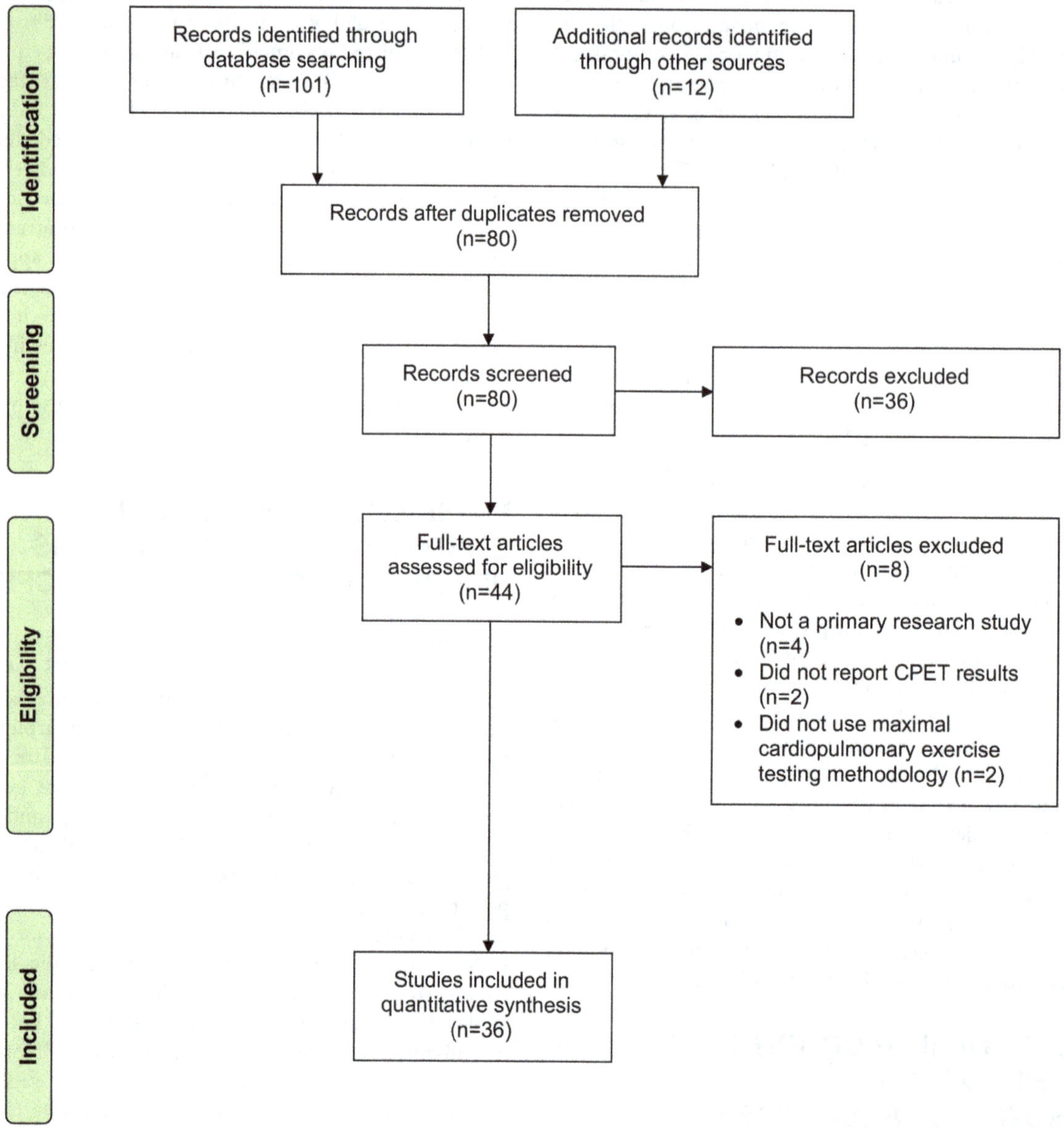

FIGURE 1 | Flow diagram describing the systematic review.

mean age of participants and heart rate at either peak exertion or VAT were included in the quantitative analysis. We searched Medline Complete, CINAHL, Academic Search Complete, SPORTDISCUS, and PsycINFO on 5 December 2018 using keywords [*(SU exercise tests) OR (exercise physiology) OR (cardiopulmonary system)*] *AND* [*(SU myalgic encephalomyelitis) OR (SU chronic fatigue syndrome)*]. We also conducted hand searches of reference sections and included other known papers that were not included in the search results. The systematic review revealed 36 articles that were included in the quantitative analysis (**Figure 1**).

CPET responses on a single test were assessed in the context of a single maximal CPET in patients with ME/CFS only (14 studies, including 1,169 patients with ME/CFS) compared with otherwise non-disabled individuals who were matched for gender and age (17 studies, including 961 patients with ME/CFS and 529 control subjects; **Tables 1–3**). Among these studies, 25 studies (28–30, 37–42, 47, 48, 52–60, 62, 63, 65–69) used the Fukuda et al. criteria (4), four studies (43–45, 51) used the Oxford criteria (5), five studies used the Holmes criteria (49, 50, 61, 64, 70), and one study (46) used the Fukuda et al. criteria, Canadian Consensus Criteria (2), and International Consensus Criteria (3). An additional four studies (30, 66) compared measurements obtained during a single CPET between men and women with ME/CFS (**Table 3**); three studies used the Fukuda criteria to identify ME/CFS (4). Three other studies (28, 46, 65) compared the responses of individuals

TABLE 1 | Heart rate measurements obtained at peak exertion during a single maximal cardiopulmonary exercise test in studies comparing subjects with myalgic encephalomyelitis/chronic fatigue syndrome ($n = 2,270$) to matched control subjects ($n = 594$).

Study	Case definition criteria	Control subjects				Patients with ME/CFS			
		n	Observed	Predicted	% Predicted	*n*	Observed	Predicted	% Predicted
HEART RATE AT PEAK EXERTION									
Bazelmans et al. (37)	Fukuda	20	173	186	93.0	20	165	187	88.2
Blazquez et al. (38)	Fukuda	–	–	–	–	32	129	180	71.7
Castro-Marrero et al. (39)	Fukuda	–	–	–	–	73	140	171	81.9
Cook et al. (40)	Fukuda	20	183	187	97.9	19	174	186	93.6
Cook et al. (41)	Fukuda	19	163	177	92.1	15	156	178	87.6
Cook et al. (42)	Fukuda	32	173	183	94.5	29	169	180	94.0
De Becker et al. (29)	Fukuda	204	171	184	92.9	427	151	183	82.5
Fulcher and White (43)	Oxford	30	182	183	99.5	66	171	183	93.4
Gallagher et al. (44)	Oxford	42	183	185	98.9	41	178	182	97.8
Gibson et al. (45)	Oxford	12	190	188	101.1	12	163	187	87.2
Hodges et al. (46)	Fukuda, CCC, ICC	10	161	181	89.0	10	154	183	84.2
Ickmans et al. (47)	Fukuda	13	165	191	86.4	30	145	184	78.8
Inbar et al. (48)	Fukuda	15	172	177	97.2	15	150	177	84.8
Keller et al. (28)	Fukuda	–	–	–	–	22	159	176	90.3
Kent-Braun et al. (49)	Holmes	–	–	–	–	6	–	–	93.0
Montague et al., (50)	Holmes	41	152	184	82.6	41	124	184	67.4
Mullis et al. (51)	Oxford	–	–	–	–	130	140	181	77.4
Nagelkirk et al. (52)	Fukuda	19	163	177	92.1	15	156	178	87.6
Nijs et al. (53)	Fukuda	–	–	–	–	64	140	180	77.8
Nijs et al. (54)	Fukuda	–	–	–	–	240	144	186	77.4
Nijs et al. (55)	Fukuda	–	–	–	–	77	140	179	78.2
Nijs et al. (56)	Fukuda	–	–	–	–	28	146	178	82.0
Nijs et al. (57)	Fukuda	–	–	–	–	16	159	182	87.4
Nijs et al. (58)	Fukuda	–	–	–	–	156	152	181	84.0
Nijs et al. (59)	Fukuda	–	–	–	–	36	146	181	80.7
Pardaens et al. (60)	Fukuda	–	–	–	–	116	142	181	78.5
Riley et al. (61)	Holmes	13	182	186	97.9	13	177	186	95.2
Robinson et al. (62)	Fukuda	6	173	176	98.3	6	177	175	101.1
Sargent et al. (30)	Fukuda	33	186	185	100.5	33	184	186	98.9
Shukla et al. (63)	Fukuda	10	179	173	103.5	10	159	171	93.0
Sisto et al. (64)	Holmes	22	178	187	95.2	21	161	186	86.6
Van Ness et al. (27)	Holmes	–	–	–	–	179	140	177	79.1
Vermeulen et al. (65)	Fukuda	15	167	184	90.7	15	158	184	86.4
Vermeulen and Vermeulen van Eck (66)	Fukuda	18	159	175	90.8	223	158	182	85.9
	Sample weighted mean	–	172.3	183.4	94.0	–	149.8	181.4	82.2
	95% confidence interval	–	171.3–173.3	182.9–183.8	93.6-94.4	–	149.2–150.4	181.3–181.6	81.9–82.5

n, sample size; ME/CFS, myalgic encephalomyelitis/chronic fatigue syndrome; CCC, Canadian Consensus Criteria; ICC, International Consensus Criteria.

with ME/CFS on two CPETs spaced 24 h apart. Two of the studies (28, 65) used the Fukuda et al. criteria (4) and one study (46) used a combination of the Fukuda et al. criteria (4), Canadian Consensus Criteria (2), and International Consensus Criteria (3). Raw HR data were extracted from each study at maximal exertion and VAT, as available. Age-predicted maximum HR values were calculated as $220 - mean\ age_{sample}$. Predicted VAT HR values were taken as 70% of predicted maximum HR (71, 72). Percentage of age-predicted maximum heart rate was computed by dividing the observed exercise heart rate by its respective age-predicted value.

Data from each study were pooled by calculating sample-weighted mean values for HR and 95% confidence interval (ConI) from the relevant studies, in order to conduct the

TABLE 2 | Heart rate measurements obtained at ventilatory anaerobic threshold during a single maximal cardiopulmonary exercise test in studies comparing subjects with myalgic encephalomyelitis/chronic fatigue syndrome ($n = 795$) to matched control subjects ($n = 353$).

Study	Case definition criteria	Control subjects				Patients with ME/CFS			
		n	Observed	Predicted	% Predicted	*n*	Observed	Predicted	% Predicted
HEART RATE AT VENTILATORY ANAEROBIC THRESHOLD									
Cook et al. (42)	Fukuda	32	112	128	87.4	29	109	126	86.5
De Becker et al. (29)	Fukuda	204	150	129	116.5	427	135	128	105.4
Hodges et al. (46)	Fukuda, CCC, ICC	10	137	127	108.1	10	134	128	104.6
Keller et al. (28)	Fukuda	–	–	–	–	22	114	123	92.5
Nagelkirk et al. (52)	Fukuda	19	110	124	88.7	15	111	125	88.8
Sargent et al. (30)	Fukuda	33	126	130	97.2	33	127	130	97.5
Sisto et al. (64)	Holmes	22	130	131	99.3	21	119	130	91.4
Vermeulen et al. (65)	Fukuda	15	111	129	97.7	15	110	129	85.6
Vermeulen and Vermeulen van Eck (66)	Fukuda	18	109	111	84.0	223	112	128	82.9
	Sample weighted mean	–	136.8	116.1	107.0	–	125.2	127.9	97.9
	95% confidence interval	–	135.1–138.4	115.4–116.8	105.9–108.1	–	124.5-125.9	127.7-128.0	97.4-98.4

n, sample size; ME/CFS, myalgic encephalomyelitis/chronic fatigue syndrome; CCC, Canadian Consensus Criteria; ICC, International Consensus Criteria.

TABLE 3 | Heart rate measurements obtained at peak exertion and ventilatory anaerobic threshold during a single maximal cardiopulmonary exercise test in studies comparing females ($n = 1,104$) and males ($n = 58$) with myalgic encephalomyelitis/chronic fatigue syndrome.

Study	Case definition criteria	Females with ME/CFS				Males with ME/CFS			
		n	Observed	Predicted	% Predicted	*n*	Observed	Predicted	% Predicted
HEART RATE AT PEAK EXERTION									
Blazquez et al. (38)	Fukuda	32	126	187	71.7	–	–	–	–
Castro-Marrero et al. (39)	Fukuda	73	140	171	81.8	–	–	–	–
Cook et al. (40)	Fukuda	19	174	186	93.6	–	–	–	–
De Becker et al. (29)	Fukuda	427	151	183	82.5	–	–	–	–
Ickmans et al. (47)	Fukuda	30	145	184	78.8	–	–	–	–
Montague et al. (50)	Unknown	20	126	187	67.4	11	119	180	66.1
Nijs et al. (58)	Fukuda	156	152	181	84.0	–	–	–	–
Nijs et al. (59)	Fukuda	36	146	181	80.7	–	–	–	–
Pardaens et al. (60)	Fukuda	116	142	181	78.5	–	–	–	–
Robinson et al. (62)	Fukuda	–	–	–	–	6	173	176	98.3
Sargent et al. (30)	Fukuda	17	183	186	98.4	16	184	186	98.9
Vermeulen and Vermeulen van Eck (66) (CFS Only)	Fukuda	178	158	177	89.3	25	155	178	87.0
	Sample weighted mean	–	150.1	180.8	83.0	–	158.0	180.4	87.5
	95% confidence interval	–	149.0–151.1	180.4–181.2	82.6–83.4	–	152.8–163.3	178.9–181.8	85.4–89.7
HEART RATE AT VENTILATORY ANAEROBIC THRESHOLD									
Sargent et al. (30)	Fukuda	17	131	130	100.6	16	122	130	93.7
Vermeulen and Vermeulen van Eck (66) (CFS Only)	Fukuda	178	112	128	87.4	25	104	125	83.5
	Sample weighted mean	–	113.7	128.3	88.6	–	110.0	126.8	87.5
	95% confidence interval	–	111.8–115.5	128.1–128.5	87.3–89.9	–	107.1–114.9	125.6–128.0	85.2–89.7

N, sample size; ME/CFS, myalgic encephalomyelitis/chronic fatigue syndrome.

following assessments: (1) to compare chronotropic responses to exercise in individuals with ME/CFS compared to matched control subjects, (2) to evaluate the effect of gender on HR responses to activity in individuals with ME/CFS, (3) to determine the effect of serial CPET on chronotropic response in individuals with ME/CFS, and (4) to estimate the effect of cardiovascular impairment on chronotropic response in individuals with ME/CFS. In addition, standardized mean difference and 95% ConI were calculated from studies that compared ME/CFS to matched control subjects, in order to estimate the magnitude of effect (73). A variance weighted summary also was calculated to pool the results across all studies. These results were used to generate forest plots for the data at peak exertion (**Figure 2**) and ventilatory anaerobic threshold (**Figure 3**). Q and I^2 statistics were assessed to determine the amount of statistical heterogeneity across studies (74). Pooled standard deviations were computed using a random effects model. Point estimates for pooled data were compared using independent samples *t*-tests. All analyses were considered statistically significant at $p < 0.05$.

Comparisons Between Patients With ME/CFS and Matched Control Subjects

There were 36 studies that reported heart rate responses at peak exertion in individuals with ME/CFS ($n =$ 2,270) and 21 studies involving matched control subjects ($n =$ 594; **Table 1**). Control subjects performed at 94.0% of age-predicted maximum HR (95%ConI: 93.6–94.4%), while individuals with ME/CFS performed at 82.2% (81.9–82.5%) of age-predicted maximum HR ($p < 0.0001$). Almost all the studies measured a decreased peak HR in individuals with ME/CFS. The standardized mean difference (*d*) for these data was −1.37 (95%ConI: −1.46 to −1.26), which indicates a very large effect, and 92% of the ME/CFS group had a peak exercise heart rate that was below the matched control group. This corresponded to an unstandardized mean difference of 11.2 fewer beats per minutes in patients with ME/CFS compared to matched control subjects (95%ConI: 6.9–15.4 bpm decrease). Significant heterogeneity was present in available studies ($Q = 113.8$, $p < 0.0001$; I^2: 82%), so these pooled difference estimates should be viewed with caution. Despite the heterogeneity present in this literature for each pooled effect size estimate, the high number of included studies and pooled sample size provides for substantial statistical power. Potential sources of variability in the published literature include the differences in case definitions used for ME/CFS, fitness levels of matched control subjects relative to patients with ME/CFS, testing modality (i.e., treadmill vs. bicycle), and statistical noise introduced by reliability of criteria to select peak performance between studies. Despite these methodological differences, published data indicate the presence of statistically significant and clinically relevant impairment in chronotropic response to exercise at peak exertion in individuals with ME/CFS compared to matched control subjects.

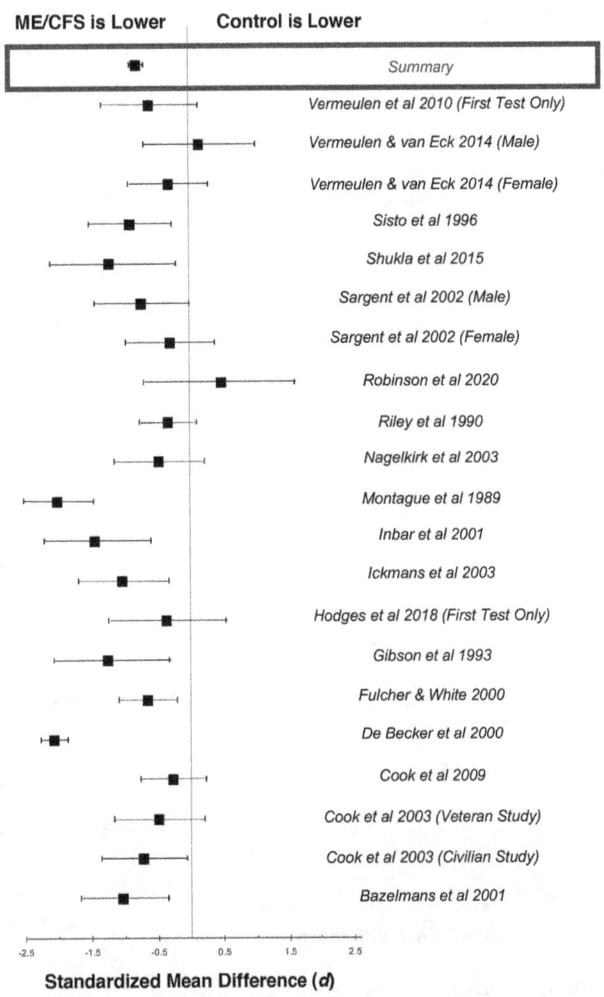

FIGURE 2 | Standardized mean differences (*d*) for heart rate at peak exertion during maximal cardiopulmonary exercise testing, comparing patients with ME/CFS ($n = 1{,}053$) and matched control subjects ($n = 569$). Boxes represent point estimates, and whiskers are 95% confidence intervals. Patients with ME/CFS had lower peak heart rates than matched control subjects (large effect size).

Twelve datasets from nine studies documented chronotropic responses at VAT in individuals with ME/CFS ($n =$ 795) compared to control subjects ($n = 353$; **Table 2**). Overall, control subjects performed at 107.0% (95%ConI: 105.9–108.1%) and individuals with ME/CFS performed at 97.9% (95%ConI: 97.4–98.4%) of their age-predicted heart rates ($p < 0.0001$). This finding indicates patients with ME/CFS, on average, remained relatively impaired when compared to age- and sex-matched control subjects. Seven of nine studies documenting chronotropic responses at VAT showed a decrease in patients with ME/CFS compared to matched control subjects, while the remaining two studies found slight increases. Overall, the standardized mean difference (*d*) for these data was −0.53 (95%ConI: −0.65 to −0.40), which indicates a moderate effect. Sixty-three percent of patients with ME/CFS had lower heart rates at VAT than matched controls in the context of a single test. These findings correspond to an unstandardized mean difference of 5.4 fewer

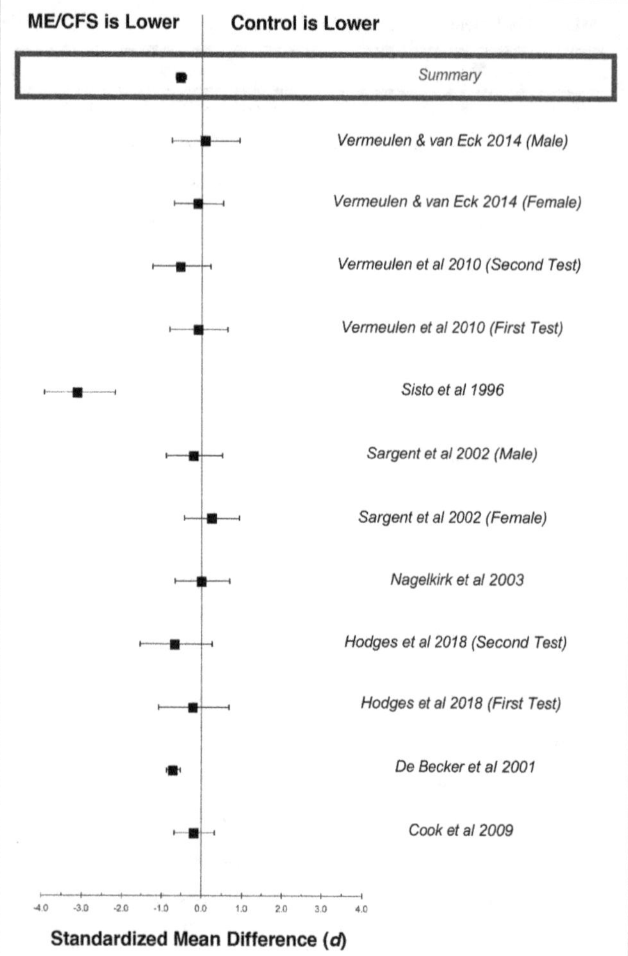

FIGURE 3 | Standardized mean differences (*d*) for exercise heart rate at ventilatory anaerobic threshold (VAT), comparing patients with ME/CFS ($n = 778$) and matched control subjects ($n = 378$). Boxes represent point estimates, and whiskers are 95% confidence intervals. Patients with ME/CFS had lower heart rates at VAT than matched control subjects (moderate effect size).

beats per minutes in patients with ME/CFS compared to matched control subjects (95%ConI: 1.5–9.2 bpm decrease). Moderate heterogeneity was present in available studies ($Q = 30.01$, $p < 0.01$; $I^2 = 60\%$). Like the peak exercise analysis, the relatively high pooled sample size provides substantial statistical power. However, it is notable that data evaluating heart rate at VAT from De Becker et al. (29) and Vermeulen and Vermeulen van Eck (66) differ by over 20 percentage points in people with ME/CFS (105.1 and 85.6%, respectively), and exert a large influence on sample-weighted means for observed heart rate and percent of predicted heart rate due to large sample sizes ($n = 427$ and $n = 204$, respectively). This observation highlights the need to consider the unique physiological characteristics of individual patients with ME/CFS. Some of the observed variation also may be attributed to heterogeneous methods used to select VAT used in the literature, indicating the need to identify and observe uniform methods of CPET analysis (75).

Comparisons Between Females and Males With ME/CFS

Articles describing two studies of CPET measurements in individuals with ME/CFS permitted abstraction of data by subject sex (30, 66), involving 1,104 females and 58 males with measurements at peak exertion and 41 males and 195 females with measurements at VAT (**Table 3**). Males demonstrated a significantly higher achievement of age-predicted maximum heart rate at peak exertion (females: 83.0%, 95%ConI: 82.6–83.4%; males: 87.5%, 95%ConI: 85.4–89.7%; $p < 0.0001$) but not VAT (females: 88.6%, 95%ConI: 87.3–89.9%; males: 87.5%, 95%ConI: 85.2–89.7%; $p = 0.476$). These data suggest that, although there may be important sex-related features in ME/CFS incidence, the expression of CI in ME/CFS appears homogeneous between sexes at submaximal workloads (75). Additional studies of sex-related difference in CI at peak levels of exertion are warranted, because male patients with ME/CFS appear under-represented in the literature to date.

Comparisons Between Measurements Obtained During Serial CPETs

There were three studies involving two CPETs conducted 24 h apart (28, 46, 65), comprising 47 patients with ME/CFS and 35 matched control subjects (**Table 4**). On the first CPET at maximal exertion, individuals with ME/CFS demonstrated a significantly lower heart rate response that was 87.9% of predicted by age (95%CI: 86.9–88.9%) compared to control subjects with a heart rate response of 90.0% of predicted by age (95%ConI: 89.5–90.5%; $p < 0.01$). On the second CPET at peak exertion, control subjects maintain the heart rate response to exercise compared to age-predicted norms (90.6%; 95%ConI: 90.1–91.1%) but individuals with ME/CFS demonstrated a significant decline compared to control subjects (84.3%; 95%ConI: 83.9–84.7%; $p < 0.05$). Although peak exertion is not common in daily life, sympathetic autonomic drive is maximal during peak exertion, so this observed difference may magnify subtle decrements in sympathetic autonomic drive that may only inconsistently be observed during lower levels of physical exertion.

During the first CPET at VAT, individuals with ME/CFS achieved 92.4% of predicted heart rate (95%ConI: 89.6–95.2) and control subjects achieved 95.0% of predicted heart rate (95%ConI: 88.9–101.0), which was not significantly different ($p = 0.387$). However, during the second CPET at VAT, individuals with ME/CFS decreased slightly (90.6%, 95%ConI: 88.1–93.6%) while matched control subjects increased (101.1%, 95%ConI: 94.5–107.6%), resulting in a significant difference in percentage of predicted HR achieved between groups on the second CPET ($p < 0.01$). The observed reduction of 10 beats per minute in patients with ME/CFS compared to matched control subjects in the post-exertional state also appears to be clinically important, because it represents a decrement in repeated submaximal functioning that is consistent with the relatively narrow physiological range for many usual

TABLE 4 | Heart rate measurements obtained at peak exertion and ventilatory anaerobic threshold during studies involving two cardiopulmonary exercise tests in individuals with myalgic encephalomyelitis/chronic fatigue syndrome ($n = 47$) and matched control subjects ($n = 35$).

Study	Case definition criteria	Test 1				Test 2			
		n	Observed	Predicted	% Predicted	*n*	Observed	Predicted	% Predicted
HEART RATE AT PEAK EXERTION IN PATIENTS WITH ME/CFS									
Hodges et al. (46)	Fukuda, CCC, ICC	10	154	183	84.2	10	151	183	82.5
Keller et al. (28)	Fukuda	22	160	176	90.9	22	150	176	85.2
Vermeulen et al. (65)	Fukuda	15	158	184	85.7	15	155	184	84.2
	Sample weighted mean	–	158.1	180.0	87.9	–	151.8	180.0	84.3
	95% confidence interval	–	157.2–159.0	178.8–181.3	86.9–88.9	–	151.1–152.6	178.8–181.3	83.9–84.7
MEASUREMENTS AT PEAK EXERTION IN CONTROL SUBJECTS									
Hodges et al. (46)	Fukuda, CCC, ICC	10	161	181	89.0	10	162	181	89.5
Vermeulen et al. (65)	Fukuda	15	167	184	90.8	15	168	184	91.3
	Sample weighted mean	–	164.6	182.8	90.0	–	165.6	182.8	90.6
	95% confidence interval	–	162.9–166.3	182.0–183.6	89.5–90.5	–	163.9–167.6	182.0–183.6	88.1–93.6
HEART RATE AT VENTILATORY ANAEROBIC THRESHOLD IN PATIENTS WITH ME/CFS									
Hodges et al. (46)	Fukuda, CCC, ICC	10	134	128	104.6	10	133	128	103.8
Keller et al. (28)	Fukuda	22	113	123	91.7	22	108	123	87.7
Vermeulen et al. (65)	Fukuda	15	110	129	85.4	15	112	129	87.0
	Sample weighted mean	–	116.5	126.0	92.4	–	114.5	126.0	90.9
	95% confidence interval	–	112.8–120.2	125.2–126.9	89.6–95.2	–	110.8–118.4	125.2–126.9	88.1–93.6
MEASUREMENTS AT VENTILATORY ANAEROBIC THRESHOLD IN CONTROL SUBJECTS									
Hodges et al. (46)	Fukuda, CCC, ICC	10	137	127	108.1	10	146	127	108.3
Vermeulen et al. (65)	Fukuda	15	111	129	86.2	15	118	129	91.6
	Sample weighted mean	–	121.4	128.0	95.0	–	129.2	128.0	101.0
	95% confidence interval	–	95.9–146.9	127.4–128.5	88.9–101.0	–	121.4–137.0	127.4–128.5	95.4–107.6

n, sample size; ME/CFS, myalgic encephalomyelitis/chronic fatigue syndrome; CCC, Canadian Consensus Criteria; ICC, International Consensus Criteria.

daily activities. The relatively small pooled sample sizes for this analysis suggest the need for future studies to examine test-retest effects in chronotropic and other responses to exercise, in the context of measurements obtained during standardized maximal CPET methodologies. The heterogeneity of findings at VAT on serial CPET also highlights the need to adhere to strict patient selection standards and a uniform methodology for conducting CPET and selecting VAT across future studies (75).

Comparisons Between Levels of Severity in ME/CFS

One article contained data 179 individuals with ME/CFS that allowed for analysis of chronotropic response based on cardiovascular impairment (**Table 6**) (27). In this study, subjects were classified according to the American Medical Association Guidelines for the Evaluation of Permanent Impairment (AMA) impairment level based on peak volume of oxygen consumed (VO_2). Classifications included no impairment ($n = 20$), mild impairment ($n = 67$), moderate impairment ($n = 72$), and severe impairment ($n = 20$). At maximal exertion, individuals with no impairment achieved 91.1% of age-predicted maximum HR. There was a general trend toward a declining percentage of age-predicted maximum HR with increasing AMA impairment level. Individuals with ME/CFS and mild AMA impairment reached 83.1% of age-predicted maximum HR, whereas those with moderate AMA impairment demonstrated 75.1% of age-predicted maximum HR, and individuals with severe AMA impairment only achieved 67.6% of age-predicted maximum HR. These data suggest the potential presence of a clinically important interaction between cardiovascular impairment and CI, in which functional impairment categories could be related to increasing levels of autonomic impairment.

RELEVANCE OF CI TO PATHO-ETIOLOGICAL STUDIES IN ME/CFS

Chronotropic responses during exercise result from a balance of neural and humoral influences on the intrinsic firing rate of sinoatrial (SA) and atrioventricular (AV) node cells (**Figure 4**). The normal discharge rate of sinoatrial node cells provides 100 beats per minute (76). In the resting state influence from parasympathetic fibers from the vagus nerve depresses heart rate to the normal range of 60–100 beats per minute. Parasympathetic effects on the SA and AV nodes are mediated through cholinergic inputs (76). Acetylcholine binds to muscarinic receptors on the cardiac muscle, SA node, and AV node (76). Sympatho-adrenal-medullary responses mediate the increase in heart rate commensurate with exercise workload. Sympathetic fibers innervate the myocardium, conduction system, SA node, and AV node, which act on cardiac structures

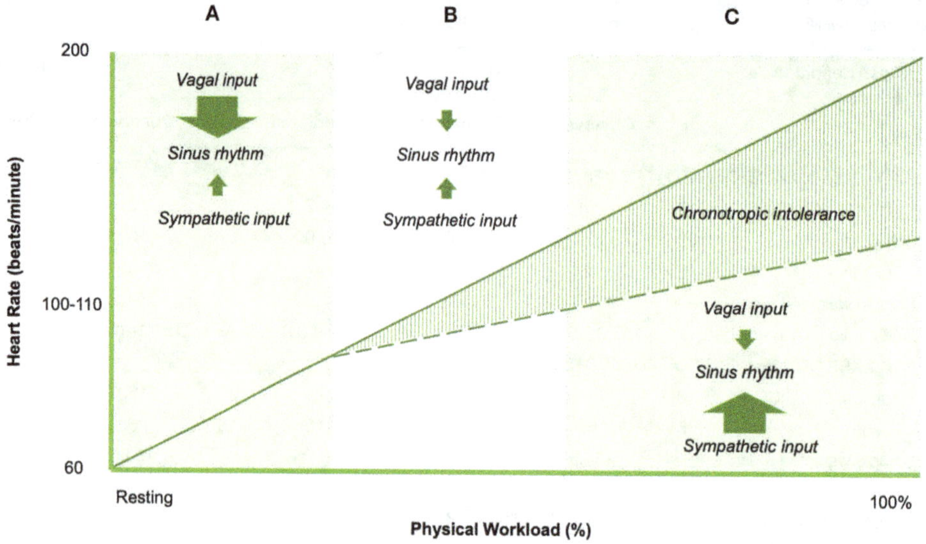

FIGURE 4 | Heart rate responses to exercise in non-ME/CFS (solid line) and ME/CFS (dashed line). Arrow sizes represent the direction and magnitude of the influence of the dominant controllers of heart rate in shaded region.

through the release of epinephrine at the neuromuscular junction (76) In addition, cardiac structures are responsive to circulating catecholamines from blood (epinephrine) (76). β_1-adrenoreceptors and β_2-adrenoreceptors are located on the myocardium, conduction system, SA node, and AV node, which bind epinephrine and norepinephrine (76). The net effect of adrenergic inputs is to increase heart rate above 100 beats per minute, such as during periods of distress or exercise. Following adrenergic/cholinergic binding on cardiac structures, local signal transduction is responsible for observed changes in heart rate (76).

The balance of cardiac neural control necessary for normal exercise-related changes in heart rate implicates the potential importance of impaired cardiac neural control to explain impairments in exercise-related heart rate change (77). Specifically, blunted changes in exercise-related heart rate could be linked to four major abnormalities of cardiac neural regulation. Down-regulation of β_1 and/or β_2 adrenoreceptors might result in adrenergic insensitivity, and limited rise in heart rate during exercise. Second, sympathetic fiber dysfunction could result in decreased norepinephrine output, which would reduce the adrenergic effects on cardiac structures and reduce exercise-related changes in heart rate. Third, diminished sympatho-adrenal-medullary activation may result in smaller rises in epinephrine. Finally, a relative dominance of vagus (cholinergic) inputs inhibit the influence of epinephrine and norepinephrine on local cardiac structures, and therefore blunt heart rate increases with increasing exercise workloads. This "cholinergic dominance" hypothesis would appear to be in line with existing conceptual work by Van Elzakkar (78). However, the specific mechanisms that cause or predispose to CI largely remain unclear. Intolerance of sympathetic autonomic endocrine signaling, myocardium, SA node, AV node, and

TABLE 5 | Raw and percent differences in metabolic equivalents between individuals with myalgic encephalomyelitis/chronic fatigue syndrome (ME/CFS) and matched sedentary individuals during serial cardiopulmonary exercise testing (CPET), based on re-analysis of data from Snell et al. (26).

	ME/CFS ($n = 51$)		Control ($n = 10$)
CPET1			
VO_2, Peak	21.51 (4.09) 20.34–22.71		25.04 (4.41) 22.35–27.73
METs, Peak (Calculated)	6.15 (1.17) 5.81–6.49		7.15 (1.26) 6.39–7.92
% Difference, Peak		−16.3%	
VO_2, VAT	12.74 (2.85) 11.92–13.55		13.83 (2.79) 12.00–15.67
METs, VAT (Calculated)	3.64 (0.81) 3.41–3.87		3.95 (0.78) 3.43–4.48
% Difference, Peak		−8.2%	
CPET2			
VO_2, Peak	20.44 (4.47) 19.25–21.63		23.96 (4.30) 21.27–26.65
METs, Peak (Calculated)	5.84 (1.28) 5.50–6.18		6.85 (1.23) 6.08–7.61
% Difference, Peak		−14.7%	
VO_2, VAT	11.36 (2.91) 10.39–12.01		14.12 (3.26) 12.29–15.96
METs, VAT (Calculated)	3.25 (0.83) 2.97–3.43		4.03 (.93) 3.51–4.56
% Difference, VAT		−19.4%	

Decremented performance was noted in individuals with ME/CFS on the second CPET at peak exertion and ventilatory anaerobic threshold, indicating the physiological correlates of post-exertional malaise. Measurements are expressed as mean (standard deviation) and 95% confidence interval. CPET, cardiopulmonary exercise test; HR, heart rate; ME/CFS, myalgic encephalomyelitis/chronic fatigue syndrome; METs, metabolic equivalents; VAT, ventilatory anaerobic threshold.

TABLE 6 | Chronotropic response to exercise measured during a single maximal cardiopulmonary exercise test in individuals with myalgic encephalomyelitis/chronic fatigue syndrome (ME/CFS), based on re-analysis of data from VanNess et al. (27).

	None ($n = 20$)	Mild ($n = 67$)	Moderate ($n = 72$)	Severe ($n = 20$)
PEAK EXERTION (MEASURED HEART RATE)				
Predicted HR	179	177	177	173
Actual HR	163	147	133	117
% Predicted	91.1	83.1	75.1	67.6
70% EXERTION (CALCULATED HEART RATE)				
Predicted HR	126	124	124	121
Actual HR	114	102	93	82
% Predicted	90.4	82.3	75.0	67.8

(The authors used the Holmes criteria to identify ME/CFS). At both peak exertion and ventilatory anaerobic threshold, the difference between age-predicted heart rate and observed heart rate increased as American Medical Association metabolic impairment category worsened. HR, heart rate.

conduction system all have been implicated in CI in various pathophysiological conditions (22, 79), and also have been suggested as a cause of PEM in ME/CFS (80, 81).

RELEVANCE OF CI TO EXERCISE TESTING AND ANALEPTIC MANAGEMENT FOR ME/CFS

One approach to circumvent potential challenges associated with maximal exercise testing is the use of submaximal exercise testing. Submaximal exercise paradigms have been proposed as a safer alternative to maximal cardiopulmonary exercise testing (82), because it is thought to be less likely to create severe, long-lasting symptoms in people with ME/CFS. One example of a submaximal test paradigm involves a sustained 25-min bout of work at 70% of age-predicted maximum heart rate (83). This type of "submaximal" physiological stressor has been used in a number of studies involving patients with ME/CFS. However, the presence of abnormal heart rate responses to exercise in people with ME/CFS suggests a potential to over-estimate workload based on predicted heart rate, which in turn, risks having subjects exert harder than intended during tests that are putatively "submaximal."

Although participants with ME/CFS in studies that use submaximal exercise test paradigms generally demonstrate averaged exercise heart rates that are statistically similar to control subjects, it seems notable that participants achieve statistical similarity at significantly lower averaged workloads and averaged VO_2 (83). Because cardiac, pulmonary, and metabolic measurements using submaximal protocols are not performed to peak exertion, it is impossible to determine the AMA impairment category or evaluate VAT for each subject, which prevents the estimation of potential effects of CI on actual exertion levels for patients with ME/CFS. In addition, it is possible that at least some patients with ME/CFS in studies using submaximal exercise paradigms could have been performing

TABLE 7 | Oxygen needs (expressed in METs) required to complete common activities of daily living (85), and assessment whether they occur under ventilatory anaerobic threshold (VAT) in individuals with myalgic encephalomyelitis/chronic fatigue syndrome (ME/CFS) and sedentary individuals.

Activity	MET requirement (ml/kg/hr)	Under VAT?		
		ME/CFS		Sedentary
		Pre PEM	Post PEM	
Circuit training	4.3	No	No	No
Driving automobiles	2.5	Yes	Yes	Yes
Folding laundry	2.3	Yes	Yes	Yes
Food preparation	**3.5**	**No**	**No**	**Yes**
Food shopping	2.5	Yes	Yes	Yes
Light bicycling	**3.5**	**No**	**No**	**Yes**
Light calisthenics	**3.5**	**No**	**No**	**Yes**
Lying quietly	1.0	Yes	Yes	Yes
Making the bed	**3.5**	**No**	**No**	**Yes**
Mild stretching	2.3	Yes	Yes	Yes
Moderate bicycling	**6.8**	**No**	**No**	**Yes**
Moderate cleaning	**3.5**	**No**	**No**	**Yes**
Playing with children	**3.5**	**No**	**No**	**Yes**
Scrubbing floors	**3.5**	**No**	**No**	**Yes**
Showering	2.0	Yes	Yes	Yes
Sitting quietly	1.3	Yes	Yes	Yes
Sleeping	0.95	Yes	Yes	Yes
Standing quietly	1.3	Yes	Yes	Yes
Sweeping	**3.3**	**Yes**	**No**	**Yes**
Vacuuming	**3.3**	**Yes**	**No**	**Yes**
Vigorous bicycling	8.8	No	No	No
Walking <2.0 mph	2.0	Yes	Yes	Yes
Walking 3.0 mph	**3.5**	**No**	**No**	**Yes**
Walking 3.5 mph	4.3	No	No	No
Washing dishes	2.5	Yes	Yes	Yes
Washing windows	**3.5**	**No**	**No**	**Yes**
Watering plants	2.5	Yes	Yes	Yes

Activities falling under the 95% confidence interval for VAT from data reported by Snell et al. (26) were considered under VAT. Likely differences in activity tolerance between individuals with ME/CFS and sedentary individuals appear in bold. ME/CFS, myalgic encephalomyelitis/chronic fatigue syndrome; METs, metabolic equivalents; PEM, post-exertional malaise; VAT, ventilatory anaerobic threshold.

maximal tests. For example, Cook et al. (83) published data on RER values for patients with ME/CFS and controls. The reported 99% confidence interval for averaged respiratory exchange ratio was 1.1 for people with ME/CFS but not control subjects. This observation suggests the potential for maximal exertion in some participants with ME/CFS but not control subjects (83), because RER values >1.15 are one criterion to determine a maximal CPET (84). These data point to important cautions about extrapolating the idea of submaximal tests to people with ME/CFS without individualized measurement and analysis.

Consideration of CI during submaximal exercise is critical to understanding the results of exercise studies using these putatively submaximal methodologies. The presence of CI suggests that it is difficult to determine whether each participant with ME/CFS receives a standardized dose of the physiologic stressor; indeed, the previously observed trend of CI makes it possible that the participants with ME/CFS who have more impairment may have received a proportionally greater stressor than participants with less impairment. For example, individuals classified as having no AMA impairment might be exerting submaximally at approximately 70% of age-predicted heart rate but individuals with moderate to severe AMA impairment actually might perform supra-maximally (33). Given the relatively low number of participants with ME/CFS in studies using submaximal exercise methodologies, careful standardization of the exercise stressor appears important to ensure that measures of blood chemistry, imaging and cognitive-perceptual data do not have outliers. Uniformity in sample characteristics and exercise stressor is made more important by the fact that neither sample size calculations nor tests of data normality are commonly reported in studies using submaximal methodologies.

Volume of oxygen consumed (VO_2) depends on a robust chronotropic response because heart rate rise during exercise increases cardiac output, and therefore the amount of oxygen available to tissues. Thus, CI may explain low achieved VO_2 at peak and VAT, especially when observed on a second CPET (26). These data suggest an interaction effect between group and test at VAT, in which there is a greater reduction in VO_2 at VAT in people with ME/CFS than matched, sedentary control subjects (26). We measured a 19.4% difference in VO_2 at VAT on a second CPET, which we believe reflects a clinically significant reduction in capacity for normal daily activities or ADLs (**Table 5**).

Many ADLs are conducted above VAT in people with ME/CFS (**Table 7**), which may predispose them to the development of PEM. A single bout of exercise may lower the VO_2 observed on a second test, which causes even more ADLs to exceed VO_2 at VAT in the post-exertional state. This observation is relevant because energy expenditures at, or close to VAT, represent vigorous activity and can be sustained for only short periods of time (**Table 7**). The International Labor Organization regard 30% or less of maximal VO_2 as the threshold for acceptable physiological demands over an 8-h work day. For a 12-h work day this is reduced to 23% or less and limited to physically light work. Extended working hours are not advisable when job-related mental or emotional stresses are high. Estimated energy expenditures for most occupations and life activities can be found in the online Compendium of Physical Activities (85).

CONCLUSION

This literature synthesis supports the presence of abnormally blunted HR responses to activity in people with ME/CFS, at both maximal exertion and submaximal VAT. Pathophysiological processes consistent with autonomic dysregulation should be prioritized for etiologic studies in ME/CFS, independent of distal pathogenic causes and proximal multi-system effects. The abnormal heart rate response to exercise in people with ME/CFS indicates that exercise testing based on a percentage of maximal heart rate cannot be considered "submaximal" in people with ME/CFS and presents a clear risk for supramaximal exertion during "submaximal" exercise tasks in the most severely involved individuals. Pacing self-management plans based on age-predicted heart rate thresholds should be viewed with caution, because the chronotropic response is impaired in people with ME/CFS. Threshold heart rates for effective analeptic management and the etiology of observed CI in people with ME/CFS should be formally established through adequately powered studies that involve serial maximal CPET methodologies.

AUTHOR CONTRIBUTIONS

All authors listed have made a substantial, direct and intellectual contribution to the work, and approved it for publication.

ACKNOWLEDGMENTS

The authors thank Mary Dimmock for her support of this work and acknowledge her contribution to accelerating ME/CFS education.

REFERENCES

1. Institute of Medicine. *Beyond Myalgic Encephalomyelitis/Chronic Fatigue Syndrome: Redefining an Illness.* Washington, DC: The National Academies Press (2015).
2. Carruthers BM, Jain AK, De Meirleir KL, Peterson DL, Klimas NG, Lerner AM, et al. Myalgic encephalomyelitis/chronic fatigue syndrome: clinical working case definition, diagnostic and treatment protocols. *J Chronic Fatigue Syndr.* (2003) 11:7–115. doi: 10.1300/J092v11n01_02
3. Carruthers BM, van de Sande MI, De Meirleir KL, Klimas NG, Broderick G, Mitchell T, et al. Myalgic encephalomyelitis: international consensus criteria. *J Intern Med.* (2011) 270:327–38. doi: 10.1111/j.1365-2796.2011.02428.x
4. Fukuda K, Straus SE, Hickie I, Sharpe MC, Dobbins JG, Komaroff A. The chronic fatigue syndrome: a comprehensive approach to its definition and study. International chronic fatigue syndrome study group. *Ann Intern Med.* (1994) 121:953–9. doi: 10.7326/0003-4819-121-12-199412150-00009
5. Sharpe MC, Archard LC, Banatvala JE, Borysiewicz LK, Clare AW, David A, et al. A report–chronic fatigue syndrome: guidelines for research. *J R Soc Med.* (1991) 84:118–21. doi: 10.1177/014107689108400224
6. Hawk C, Jason LA, Torres-Harding S. Differential diagnosis of chronic fatigue syndrome and major depressive disorder. *Int J Behav Med.* (2006) 13:244–51. doi: 10.1207/s15327558ijbm1303_8
7. King C, Jason LA. Improving the diagnostic criteria and procedures for chronic fatigue syndrome. *Biol Psychol.* (2005) 68:87–106. doi: 10.1016/j.biopsycho.2004.03.015
8. Balady GJ, Arena R, Sietsema K, Myers J, Coke L, Fletcher GF, et al. Clinician's Guide to cardiopulmonary exercise testing in adults: a scientific statement from the American Heart Association. *Circulation.* (2010) 122:191–225. doi: 10.1161/CIR.0b013e3181e52e69
9. Brown SE, Fischer CE, Stansbury DW, Light RW. Reproducibility of VO2max in patients with chronic air-flow obstruction. *Am Rev Respir Dis.* (1985) 131:435–8.
10. Covey MK, Larson JL, Alex CG, Wirtz S, Langbein WE. Test-retest reliability of symptom-limited cycle ergometer tests in patients with

chronic obstructive pulmonary disease. *Nurs Res.* (1999) 48:9–19. doi: 10.1097/00006199-199901000-00003

11. Cox NJ, Hendriks JC, Binkhorst RA, Folgering HT, van Herwaarden CL. Reproducibility of incremental maximal cycle ergometer tests in patients with mild to moderate obstructive lung diseases. *Lung.* (1989) 167:129–33. doi: 10.1007/BF02714939
12. Dideriksen K, Mikkelsen UR. Reproducibility of incremental maximal cycle ergometer tests in healthy recreationally active subjects. *Clin Physiol Funct Imaging.* (2017) 37:173–82. doi: 10.1111/cpf.12283
13. Hansen JE, Sun XG, Yasunobu Y, Garafano RP, Gates G, Barst RJ, et al. Reproducibility of cardiopulmonary exercise measurements in patients with pulmonary arterial hypertension. *Chest.* (2004) 126:816–24. doi: 10.1378/chest.126.3.816
14. Koufaki P, Naish PF, Mercer TH. Reproducibility of exercise tolerance in patients with end-stage renal disease. *Arch Phys Med Rehabil.* (2001) 82:1421–24. doi: 10.1053/apmr.2001.26076
15. Lehmann G, Kolling K. Reproducibility of cardiopulmonary exercise parameters in patients with valvular heart disease. *Chest.* (1996) 110:685–92. doi: 10.1378/chest.110.3.685
16. Marciniuk DD, Watts RE, Gallagher CG. Reproducibility of incremental maximal cycle ergometer testing in patients with restrictive lung disease. *Thorax.* (1993) 48:894–8. doi: 10.1136/thx.48.9.894
17. McKone EF, Barry SC, FitzGerald MX, Gallagher CG. Reproducibility of maximal exercise ergometer testing in patients with cystic fibrosis. *Chest.* (1999) 116:363–8.
18. Puente-Maestu L, Sanz ML, Sanz P, Nunez A, Gonzalez F, Whipp BJ. Reproducibility of the parameters of the on-transient cardiopulmonary responses during moderate exercise in patients with chronic obstructive pulmonary disease. *Eur J Appl Physiol.* (2001) 85:434–41. doi: 10.1007/s004210100486
19. Skinner JS, Wilmore KM, Jaskolska A, Jaskolski A, Daw EW, Rice T, et al. Reproducibility of maximal exercise test data in the HERITAGE family study. *Med Sci Sports Exerc.* (1999) 31:1623–28. doi: 10.1097/00005768-199911000-00020
20. Wasserman K, Hansen JE, Sue DY, Stringer W, Sietsema KE, Sun X-G, et al. *Principles of Exercise Testing and Interpretation: Including Pathophysiology and Clinical Applications.* 5th ed. Philadelphia, PA: Lippincott Williams & Wilkins (2011).
21. Brubaker PH, Kitzman DW. Chronotropic intolerance: causes, consequences, and management. *Circulation.* (2011) 123:1010–20. doi: 10.1161/CIRCULATIONAHA.110.940577
22. Gentlesk PJ, Markwood TT, Atwood JE. Chronotropic intolerance in a young adult: case report and literature review. *Chest.* (2004) 125:297–301. doi: 10.1378/chest.125.1.297
23. Kitzman DW. Chronotropic intolerance and functional capacity in cardiovascular disease. *Medgraphia.* (2012) 34:400–6.
24. Wilkoff BL, Miller RE. Exercise testing for chronotropic assessment. *Cardiol Clin.* (1992) 10:705–17.
25. Lauer MS, Okin PM, Larson MG, Evans JC, Levy D. Impaired heart rate response to graded exercise. Prognostic implications of chronotropic intolerance in the Framingham Heart Study. *Circulation.* (1996) 93:1520–6. doi: 10.1161/01.CIR.93.8.1520
26. Snell CR, Stevens SR, Davenport TE, Van Ness JM. Discriminative validity of metabolic and workload measurements for identifying people with chronic fatigue syndrome. *Phys Ther.* (2013) 93:1484–92. doi: 10.2522/ptj.20110368
27. Vanness JM, Snell CR, Strayer DR, Dempsey Lt, Stevens SR. Subclassifying chronic fatigue syndrome through exercise testing. *Med Sci Sports Exerc.* (2003) 35:908–13. doi: 10.1249/01.MSS.0000069510.58763.E8
28. Keller BA, Pryor JL, Giloteaux L. Inability of myalgic encephalomyelitis/chronic fatigue syndrome patients to reproduce VO(2)peak indicates functional impairment. *J Transl Med.* (2014) 12:104. doi: 10.1186/1479-5876-12-104
29. De Becker P, Roeykens J, Reynders M, McGregor N, De Meirleir K. Exercise capacity in chronic fatigue syndrome. *Arch Intern Med.* (2000) 160:3270–77. doi: 10.1001/archinte.160.21.3270
30. Sargent C, Scroop GC, Nemeth PM, Burnet RB, Buckley JD. Maximal oxygen uptake and lactate metabolism are normal in chronic fatigue syndrome. *Med Sci Sports Exerc.* (2002) 34:51–6. doi: 10.1097/00005768-200201000-00009
31. Davenport TE, Stevens SR, Baroni K, Van Ness M, Snell CR. Diagnostic accuracy of symptoms characterising chronic fatigue syndrome. *Disabil Rehabil.* (2011) 33:1768–75. doi: 10.3109/09638288.2010.546936
32. Davenport TE, Stevens SR, VanNess MJ, Snell CR, Little T. Conceptual model for physical therapist management of chronic fatigue syndrome/myalgic encephalomyelitis. *Phys Ther.* (2010) 90:602–14. doi: 10.2522/ptj.20090047
33. VanNess JM, Stevens SR, Bateman L, Stiles TL, Snell CR. Postexertional malaise in women with chronic fatigue syndrome. *J Womens Health (Larchmt).* (2010) 19:239–44. doi: 10.1089/jwh.2009.1507
34. Weston SB, Gabbett TJ. Reproducibility of ventilation of thresholds in trained cyclists during ramp cycle exercise. *J Sci Med Sport.* (2001) 4:357–66. doi: 10.1016/S1440-2440(01)80044-X
35. Reybrouck T, Ghesquiere J, Cattaert A, Fagard R, Amery A. Ventilatory thresholds during short- and long-term exercise. *J Appl Physiol Respir Environ Exerc Physiol.* (1983) 55:1694–700. doi: 10.1152/jappl.1983.55.6.1694
36. Reybrouck T, Ghesquiere J, Weymans M, Amery A. Ventilatory threshold measurement to evaluate maximal endurance performance. *Int J Sports Med.* (1986) 7:26–9. doi: 10.1055/s-2008-1025730
37. Bazelmans E, Bleijenberg G, Van Der Meer JW, Folgering H. Is physical deconditioning a perpetuating factor in chronic fatigue syndrome? A controlled study on maximal exercise performance and relations with fatigue, impairment and physical activity. *Psychol Med.* (2001) 31:107–14. doi: 10.1017/S0033291799003189
38. Blazquez A, Guillamó E, Alegre J, Ruiz E, Javierre C. Psycho-physiological impact on women with chronic fatigue syndrome in the context of their couple relationship. *Psychol Health Med.* (2012) 17:150–63. doi: 10.1080/13548506.2011.582124
39. Castro-Marrero J, Sáez-Francàs N, Segundo MJ, Calvo N, Faro M, Aliste L, et al. Effect of coenzyme Q10 plus nicotinamide adenine dinucleotide supplementation on maximum heart rate after exercise testing in chronic fatigue syndrome - a randomized, controlled, double-blind trial. *Clin Nutr.* (2016) 35:826–34. doi: 10.1016/j.clnu.2015.07.010
40. Cook DB, Nagelkirk PR, Peckerman A, Poluri A, Lamanca JJ, Natelson BH. Perceived exertion in fatiguing illness: civilians with chronic fatigue syndrome. *Med Sci Sports Exerc.* (2003) 35:563–8. doi: 10.1249/01.MSS.0000058360.61448.6C
41. Cook DB, Nagelkirk PR, Peckerman A, Poluri A, Lamanca JJ, Natelson BH. Perceived exertion in fatiguing illness: Gulf War veterans with chronic fatigue syndrome. *Med Sci Sports Exerc.* (2003) 35:569–74. doi: 10.1249/01.MSS.0000058438.25278.33
42. Cook DB, Nagelkirk PR, Poluri A, Mores J, Natelson BH. The influence of aerobic fitness and fibromyalgia on cardiorespiratory and perceptual responses to exercise in patients with chronic fatigue syndrome. *Arthritis Rheum.* (2006) 54:3351–62. doi: 10.1002/art.22124
43. Fulcher KY, White PD. Strength and physiological response to exercise in patients with chronic fatigue syndrome. *J Neurol Neurosurg Psychiatry.* (2000) 69:302–7. doi: 10.1136/jnnp.69.3.302
44. Gallagher AM, Coldrick AR, Hedge B, Weir WR, White PD. Is the chronic fatigue syndrome an exercise phobia? A case control study. *J Psychosom Res.* (2005) 58:367–73. doi: 10.1016/j.jpsychores.2005.02.002
45. Gibson H, Carroll N, Clague JE, Edwards RH. Exercise performance and fatiguability in patients with chronic fatigue syndrome. *J Neurol Neurosurg Psychiatry.* (1993) 56:993–8. doi: 10.1136/jnnp.56.9.993
46. Hodges LD, Nielsen T, Baken D. Physiological measures in participants with chronic fatigue syndrome, multiple sclerosis and healthy controls following repeated exercise: a pilot study. *Clin Physiol Funct Imaging.* (2018) 38:639–44. doi: 10.1111/cpf.12460
47. Ickmans K, Meeus M, De Kooning M, Lambrecht L, Pattyn N, Nijs J. Can recovery of peripheral muscle function predict cognitive task performance in chronic fatigue syndrome with and without fibromyalgia? *Phys Ther.* (2014) 94:511–22. doi: 10.2522/ptj.20130367
48. Inbar O, Dlin R, Rotstein A, Whipp BJ. Physiological responses to incremental exercise in patients with chronic fatigue syndrome. *Med Sci Sports Exerc.* (2001) 33:1463–70. doi: 10.1097/00005768-200109000-00007
49. Kent-Braun JA, Sharma KR, Weiner MW, Massie B, Miller RG. Central basis of muscle fatigue in chronic fatigue syndrome. *Neurology.* (1993) 43:125–31. doi: 10.1212/WNL.43.1_Part_1.125

50. Montague TJ, Marrie TJ, Klassen GA, Bewick, DJ, Horacek BM. Cardiac function at rest and with Exercise in the chronic fatigue syndrome. *Chest.* (1989) 95:779–84.
51. Mullis R, Campbell IT, Wearden AJ, Morriss RK, Pearson DJ. Prediction of peak oxygen uptake in chronic fatigue syndrome. *Br J Sports Med.* (1999) 33:352–6. doi: 10.1136/bjsm.33.5.352
52. Nagelkirk PR, Cook DB, Peckerman A, Kesil W, Sakowski T, Natelson BH, et al. Aerobic capacity of Gulf War veterans with chronic fatigue syndrome. *Mil Med.* (2003) 168:750–5. doi: 10.1093/milmed/168.9.750
53. Nijs J, Vanherberghen K, Duquet W, De Meirleir K. Chronic fatigue syndrome: lack of association between pain-related fear of movement and exercise capacity and disability. *Phys Ther.* (2004) 84:696–705. doi: 10.1093/ptj/84.8.696
54. Nijs J, De Meirleir K. Prediction of peak oxygen uptake in patients fulfilling the 1994 CDC criteria for chronic fatigue syndrome. *Clin Rehabil.* (2004) 18:785–92. doi: 10.1191/0269215504cr751oa
55. Nijs J, De Meirleir K, Wolfs S, Duquet W. Disability evaluation in chronic fatigue syndrome: associations between exercise capacity and activity limitations/participation restrictions. *Clin Rehabil.* (2004) 18:139–48. doi: 10.1191/0269215504cr708oa
56. Nijs J, Zwinnen K, Meeusen R, de Geus B, De Meirleir K. Comparison of two exercise testing protocols in patients with chronic fatigue syndrome. *J Rehabil Res Dev.* (2007) 44:553–9. doi: 10.1682/JRRD.2006.12.0153
57. Nijs J, Meeus M, McGregor NR, Meeusen R, de Schutter G, van Hoof E, et al. Chronic fatigue syndrome: exercise performance related to immune dysfunction. *Med Sci Sports Exerc.* (2005) 37:1647–54. doi: 10.1249/01.mss.0000181680.35503.ce
58. Nijs J, Demol S, Wallman K. Can submaximal exercise variables predict peak exercise performance in women with chronic fatigue syndrome? *Arch Med Res.* (2007) 38:350–3. doi: 10.1016/j.arcmed.2006.10.009
59. Nijs J, Van de Putte K, Louckx F, Truijen S, De Meirleir K. Exercise performance and chronic pain in chronic fatigue syndrome: the role of pain catastrophizing. *Pain Med.* (2008) 9:1164–72. doi: 10.1111/j.1526-4637.2007.00368.x
60. Pardaens K, Haagdorens L, Van Wambeke P, Van den Broeck A, Van Houdenhove B. How relevant are exercise capacity measures for evaluating treatment effects in chronic fatigue syndrome? Results from a prospective, multidisciplinary outcome study. *Clin Rehabil.* (2006) 20:56–66. doi: 10.1191/0269215506cr914oa
61. Riley MS, O'Brien CJ, McCluskey DR, Bell NP, Nicholls DP. Aerobic work capacity in patients with chronic fatigue syndrome. *BMJ.* (1990) 301:953–6. doi: 10.1136/bmj.301.6758.953
62. Robinson M, Gray SR, Watson MS, Kennedy G, Hill A, Belch JJ, et al. Plasma IL-6, its soluble receptors and F2-isoprostanes at rest and during exercise in chronic fatigue syndrome. *Scand J Med Sci Sports.* (2010) 20:282–90. doi: 10.1111/j.1600-0838.2009.00895.x
63. Shukla SK, Cook D, Meyer J, Vernon SD, Le T, Clevidence D, et al. Changes in gut and plasma microbiome following exercise challenge in myalgic encephalomyelitis/chronic fatigue syndrome (ME/CFS). *PLoS ONE.* (2015) 10:e0145453. doi: 10.1371/journal.pone.0145453
64. Sisto SA, LaManca J, Cordero DL, Bergen MT, Ellis SP, Drastal S, et al. Metabolic and cardiovascular effects of a progressive exercise test in patients with chronic fatigue syndrome. *Am J Med.* (1996) 100:634–40. doi: 10.1016/S0002-9343(96)00041-1
65. Vermeulen RC, Kurk RM, Visser FC, Sluiter W, Scholte HR. Patients with chronic fatigue syndrome performed worse than controls in a controlled repeated exercise study despite a normal oxidative phosphorylation capacity. *J Transl Med.* (2010) 8:93. doi: 10.1186/1479-5876-8-93
66. Vermeulen RC, Vermeulen van Eck IW. Decreased oxygen extraction during cardiopulmonary exercise test in patients with chronic fatigue syndrome. *J Transl Med.* (2014) 12:20. doi: 10.1186/1479-5876-12-20.
67. Katz BZ, Boas S, Shiraishi Y, Mears CJ, Taylor R. Exercise tolerance testing in a prospective cohort of adolescents with chronic fatigue syndrome and recovered controls following infectious mononucleosis. *J Pediatr.* (2010) 157:468–72, e461. doi: 10.1016/j.jpeds.2010.03.025
68. Broadbent S, Coutts R. Graded versus intermittent exercise effects on lymphocytes in chronic fatigue syndrome. *Med Sci Sports Exerc.* (2016) 48:1655–63. doi: 10.1249/MSS.0000000000000957
69. Weinstein AA, Drinkard BM, Diao G, Furst G, Dale JK, Straus SE, et al. Exploratory analysis of the relationships between aerobic capacity and self-reported fatigue in patients with rheumatoid arthritis, polymyositis, and chronic fatigue syndrome. *PM R.* (2009) 1:620–8. doi: 10.1016/j.pmrj.2009.04.007
70. Holmes GP, Kaplan JE, Gantz NM, Komaroff AL, Schonberger LB, Straus SE, et al. Chronic fatigue syndrome: a working case definition. *Ann Intern Med.* (1988) 108:387–9. doi: 10.7326/0003-4819-108-3-387
71. Dwyer J, Bybee R. Heart rate indices of the anaerobic threshold. *Med Sci Sports Exerc.* (1983) 15:72–6. doi: 10.1249/00005768-198315010-00013
72. Weltman A, Snead D, Seip R, Schurrer R, Weltman J, Rutt R, et al. Percentages of maximal heart rate, heart rate reserve and VO2max for determining endurance training intensity in male runners. *Int J Sports Med.* (1990) 11:218–22. doi: 10.1055/s-2007-1024795
73. Lee DK. Alternatives to P value: confidence interval and effect size. *Korean J Anesthesiol.* (2016) 69:555–62. doi: 10.4097/kjae.2016.69.6.555
74. Israel H, Richter RR. A guide to understanding meta-analysis. *J Orthop Sports Phys Ther.* (2011) 41:496–504. doi: 10.2519/jospt.2011.3333
75. Stevens S, Snell C, Stevens J, Keller B, VanNess JM. Cardiopulmonary exercise test methodology for assessing exertion intolerance in myalgic encephalomyelitis/chronic fatigue syndrome. *Front Pediatr.* (2018) 6:242. doi: 10.3389/fped.2018.00242
76. Rowell LB. *Human Cardiovascular Control.* London: Oxford University Press (1993).
77. Light KC, White AT, Tadler S, Iacob E, Light AR. Genetics and gene expression involving stress and distress pathways in fibromyalgia with and without comorbid chronic fatigue syndrome. *Pain Res Treat.* (2012) 2012:427869. doi: 10.1155/2012/427869
78. VanElzakker MB. Chronic fatigue syndrome from vagus nerve infection: a psychoneuroimmunological hypothesis. *Med Hypotheses.* (2013) 81:414–23. doi: 10.1016/j.mehy.2013.05.034
79. Tanaka M, Tajima S, Mizuno K, Ishii A, Konishi Y, Miike T, et al. Frontier studies on fatigue, autonomic nerve dysfunction, and sleep-rhythm disorder. *J Physiol Sci.* (2015) 65:483–98. doi: 10.1007/s12576-015-0399-y
80. Arroll MA. Allostatic overload in myalgic encephalomyelitis/chronic fatigue syndrome (ME/CFS). *Med Hypotheses.* (2013) 81:506–8. doi: 10.1016/j.mehy.2013.06.023.
81. Pagani M, Lucini D. Chronic fatigue syndrome: a hypothesis focusing on the autonomic nervous system. *Clin Sci (Lond).* (1999) 96:117–25.
82. Ratter J, Radlinger L, Lucas C. Several submaximal exercise tests are reliable, valid and acceptable in people with chronic pain, fibromyalgia or chronic fatigue: a systematic review. *J Physiother.* (2014) 60:144–50. doi: 10.1016/j.jphys.2014.06.011
83. Cook DB, Light AR, Light KC, Broderick G, Shields MR, Dougherty RJ, et al. Neural consequences of post-exertion malaise in myalgic encephalomyelitis/chronic fatigue syndrome. *Brain Behav Immun.* (2017) 62:87–99. doi: 10.1016/j.bbi.2017.02.009
84. Wasserman K, Stringer WW, Casaburi R, Koike A, Cooper CB. Determination of the anaerobic threshold by gas exchange: biochemical considerations, methodology and physiological effects. *Z Kardiol.* (1994) 83(Suppl. 3):1–12.
85. Ainsworth BE, Haskell WL, Herrmann SD, Meckes N, Bassett Jr DR, Tudor-Locke C, et al. *The Compendium of Physical Activities Tracking Guide.* Healthy Lifestyles Research Center; College of Nursing & Health Innovation; Arizona State University (2011). Available online at: https://sites.google.com/site/compendiumofphysicalactivities/home (Accessed July 18, 2018).

3

Hand Grip Strength as a Clinical Biomarker for ME/CFS and Disease Severity

Luis Carlos Nacul[1*], *Kathleen Mudie*[1], *Caroline C. Kingdon*[1*], *Taane G. Clark*[2] *and Eliana Mattos Lacerda*[1]

[1] *Department of Clinical Research, Faculty of Infectious and Tropical Diseases, International Centre for Evidence in Disability, London School of Hygiene and Tropical Medicine, London, United Kingdom,* [2] *Department of Infectious Disease Epidemiology, Faculty of Infectious and Tropical Diseases, Faculty of Epidemiology and Population Health, London School of Hygiene and Tropical Medicine, London, United Kingdom*

***Correspondence:**
Luis Carlos Nacul
luis.nacul@lshtm.ac.uk
Caroline C. Kingdon
caroline.kingdon@lshtm.ac.uk

Background: The diagnosis of myalgic encephalomyelitis (ME/CFS) in research and clinical practice has largely relied on clinical history, which can be subjective in nature. Clinical signs are often subtle, overlap with other conditions, and are not formally included as part of diagnostic workup. The characterization of clinical signs and biomarkers is needed for better diagnosis and classification of patients and to monitor treatment response. Hand grip strength (HGS) has been used as an objective measure of muscle strength and fatigue, which is a primary symptom of ME/CFS. We assessed the potential usefulness of HGS as a diagnostic marker in ME/CFS.

Methods: We compared HGS measurements from participants in the UK ME/CFS Biobank, with groups consisting of people with ME/CFS of differing severity ($n = 272$), healthy ($n = 136$), multiple sclerosis ($n = 76$) controls, and others with chronic fatigue not meeting the diagnosis of ME/CFS ($n = 37$). We correlated the maximum and minimum of, and differences between, 3 repeated HGS measurements with parameters of disease severity, including fatigue and pain analog scales, and physical and mental component summaries from the SF-36v2TM questionnaire across recruitment groups.

Results: HGS indicators were associated with having ME/CFS, with magnitudes of association stronger in severely affected than in mild/moderately affected patients. Compared with healthy controls, being severely affected was associated with a reduction in minimum HGS of 15.3 kg (95%CI 19.3–11.3; $p < 0.001$), while being mild/moderately affected was associated with a 10.5 kg (95%CI 13.2–7.8; $p < 0.001$) reduction. The association persisted after adjusting for age, sex and body mass index. ME/CFS cases also showed lower values of maximum HGS and significant drops in values from the first to second and third trials, compared to other study groups. There were significant correlations between HGS indicators and clinical parameters of disease severity, including fatigue analog scale (Spearman's Rho = −0.40, $p < 0.001$), pain analog scale (Rho = −0.38, $p < 0.001$), and physical component summary (Rho = 0.42, $p < 0.001$).

Discussion: HGS is markedly reduced in ME/CFS, particularly in patients with more severe disease, and may indicate muscle and fatigue related symptoms. HGS is a potential diagnostic tool in ME/CFS, and could also be used to enhance patient phenotyping and as an outcome measure following interventions

Keywords: ME/CFS, fatigue, biomarker, hand grip strength, severity, phenotyping

INTRODUCTION

Fatigue is common in the general population (1–3), and often accompanies infections and chronic disorders of the nervous, cardiovascular, respiratory, musculoskeletal, metabolic, and endocrine systems as well as mood disorders, such as depression and anxiety (4). It also commonly, and temporarily, affects healthy individuals in certain circumstances, such as following periods of excessive or prolonged physical or mental effort, or reduced periods of rest or of good quality sleep.

Myalgic Encephalomyelitis/Chronic Fatigue Syndrome (ME/CFS) presents with disabling symptoms lasting for at least 6 months and resulting in a substantial reduction in activity levels and quality of life (5–7). The etiology is unknown and there are no diagnostic biomarkers for the disease. Prevalence is difficult to determine, ranging from 0.1% to 0.7% (8). Among other symptoms, including post-exertional malaise, unrefreshing sleep, memory, and concentration problems, fatigue is the most recognizable and is considered a central symptom of ME/CFS.

Nevertheless, fatigue may be difficult to characterize and may be confounded by malaise, pain and other issues such as somnolence, dyspnea (difficulty with breathing) and muscle weakness. Patients may use several terms to describe it, such as tiredness, lack of energy or "brain fog," to represent the difficulty or inability in initiating activity (perception of generalized weakness) (9), reduced capacity in maintaining activity (easy fatigability), and difficulty with concentration, memory and emotional stability (mental fatigue) (10).

The measurement of fatigue in research studies has been subjective and has relied on questionnaires or scales. Symptoms may be exaggerated or underestimated by the individual, and they can vary according to cultural aspects and other factors, such as the presence of other symptoms and mood changes. For these reasons, objective measures of fatigue and disease status are highly desirable, both for diagnostic and classification purposes of people with ME/CFS.

Hand grip strength (HGS) is a reliable measurement of localized muscle strength and reflects the force derived from the combined contraction of extrinsic hand muscles. Originally developed for hand surgery to determine capacity after trauma or surgery, hand grip strength correlates well with other muscle function tests such as knee extension strength (11). Moreover, reduced HGS has been associated with morbidity and mortality, with low values associated with falls, disability, impaired health-related quality of life and prolonged length of stay in hospital (11–13). It has also shown to be strongly correlated with post-operative complications and has been reported as a predictor of loss of functional status and short-term survival in hospitalized patients (14, 15).

In this study, we assess the potential use of HGS parameters as objective measures of disease status and severity in ME/CFS, and correlate it with fatigue and pain severity and with physical and mental functioning.

METHODS

Study Design and Population

This was an analytical cross-sectional study using baseline data from participants in the UK ME/CFS Biobank (UKMEB). Participants included people with a medically confirmed ME/CFS diagnosis from the UK National Health Service (NHS) and assessed for compliance with study criteria, i.e., Centers for Disease Control (CDC-94) (6) and/or Canadian Consensus Criteria (CCC) (5); people with apparently normal function and no symptoms of fatigue nor any severe disease ("healthy controls" or "HC"); people with multiple sclerosis (MS) confirmed by an NHS neurologist ("MS cases"); and people with chronic fatigue not compliant with the study criteria ("CF/nonME").

Procedures for recruitment, selection, and diagnosis have been described previously (16). In summary, participants were recruited through NHS general practices (GPs) and specialist services. All potential UKMEB participants who were aged 18–60 years and gave informed consent were re-assessed by the research team at the recruitment stage for eligibility into the study, which included assessment for compliance with ME/CFS diagnostic criteria for this cohort of participants. The inclusion/exclusion criteria are summarized in **Table 1**. People with ME/CFS (PWME) were then further stratified by disease severity into two categories: mild/moderately affected (MEmm) if they are ambulatory, and severely affected (MEsa) if they are house- or bed-bound.

Ethical approval was granted by the London School of Hygiene & Tropical Medicine (LSHTM) Ethics Committee (ref. 6123), the National Research Ethics Committee (REC; ref. 11/LO/1760, IRAS ID: 77765), and the NHS Research Governance and Developments Offices (R&D), which oversee the recruitment of research participants from government health services.

Data Collection

Data collection ran from March 2012 to December 2015. The study protocol was identical for all participants, regardless of recruitment category.

HGS was quantified during the participant's clinical assessment and examination, by a team member (research

TABLE 1 | UKMEB inclusion and exclusion criteria.

Inclusion criteria	Exclusion criteria
ME/CFS cases: clinical diagnosis according to CDC-1994 and/or Canadian Consensus Criteria; diagnosis confirmed by research nurse upon completing baseline assessments CF/nonME: diagnosis of ME/CFS from clinician but does not fulfill study criteria upon completing baseline assessments Healthy controls: no past or present fatiguing and/or other major morbidity, such as cancer or coronary heart disease MS cases: confirmed diagnosis made previously by NHS neurologist, in compliance with the NICE guidelines	cases and controls: - recent use (in preceding 3 months) of drugs known to alter immune function, anti-viral medications, and vaccinations - history of acute and chronic infections, such as hepatitis B/C, tuberculosis, HIV, or other severe illness or severe mood disorders - pregnant women and those within 12 months post-partum and/or currently lactating

ME/CFS, Myalgic Encephalomyelitis/Chronic Fatigue Syndrome; CF/nonME, chronic fatigue not meeting study criteria for ME/CFS; MS, multiple sclerosis; CDC, Centers for Disease Control; NHS, National Health Services; NICE, National Institute for Health and Care Excellence.

nurse or doctor), using a simple precision instrument that offers a quantitative and objective measure of isometric muscular strength of the hand and forearm. We followed standard procedures using a Jamar Hydraulic Hand Dynamometer (model #5030J1–JA Corp) for that aim (17). Participants were seated with back, pelvis, and knees as close to 90 degrees as possible. The shoulder was abducted and neutrally rotated with the elbow flexed at 90 degrees, the forearm neutral, and the wrist held between 0 and 15 degrees of ulnar deviation. The dynamometer was presented vertically, in line with the forearm, to the participant's dominant hand. Grip size was adjusted for comfort (9, 18). Participants were then instructed to squeeze the hand grip as hard as they could, which took $\sim$ 3 s, in three successive trials with 30 s in between each. The entire procedure took $\sim$ 3 min to complete, including instructions.

The strength values were scored using force production in kilograms (0–90). HGS has been shown to have excellent test-retest reliability (intraclass correlations (ICC) 0.97–0.99) and intra-rater reliability (ICC 0.96–0.98) in healthy adults (19) and has been used in various diseases (20–22).

During the clinical assessment, alongside clinical parameters that included height and weight, measures of fatigue and pain intensity were recorded on fatigue (23) and pain (24) analog scales, respectively. The fatigue and pain analog scales are unidimensional measures of intensity and have been widely used in diverse adult populations, e.g., in rheumatic diseases, chronic hepatitis-C infection and systemic lupus (23–26). Each of them can be described as a continuous scale comprised of a horizontal line, 10 centimeters in length, and anchored by two vertical descriptors, one for each symptom extreme (no fatigue/pain and worst imaginable fatigue/pain). High scores, with a maximum of 10, indicate greater intensities of fatigue and pain. Fatigue and pain analog scales have been shown to exhibit good test-retest reliability ($r = 0.94$ for both) and to have high construct validity with 5-point verbal descriptive scales ($r = 71$ and $r = 0.78$, respectfully) (23, 24). Body mass index (BMI) in kg/m^2 was calculated using participants' height and weight.

In addition, participants completed an extended questionnaire, which includes the SF-36V2^{TM} questionnaire (27), the Fatigue Severity Scale (FSS) (28), and socio-demographic data, such as age and sex, among other variables. The SF-36v2^{TM} comprises of 36 questions providing information on functional status and well-being (29). The answers form eight distinct domains considering physical and mental functions, were summarized into physical (PCS) and mental (MCS) component summary scores. Low scores indicate reduced functional status and reduced mental vitality, respectively. The SF-36v2^{TM} is recognized as a reliable tool that has been used and validated across different populations, and has been used extensively in ME/CFS [L. a. (7, 30, 31)]. A full report of the development of this instrument has been published elsewhere (29). The FSS contains 9 items that relate to statements of fatigue, which are scored between 1 (strongly disagree) and 7 (strongly agree) by the participant. The total score is calculated by adding those attributed to each question, and varies from 9 to 63. Due to the strong correlation between FSS and the fatigue analog scales ($r = 0.8$, $p < 0.001$ in our sample), we opted to use the latter only in our analysis.

Statistical Analysis

Answers to the SF-36v2^{TM} questions were scored in health domains using the SF Health Outcomes^{TM} Scoring Software 4.5 (QualityMetric Inc., RI, United States) and are presented as "normalized" physical and mental summary scores." Data were analyzed using STATA^{TM} version 15.0 (StataCorp, TX, United States). The maximum and minimum (of three measurements) of HGS were obtained for each participating individual.

Descriptive characteristics were obtained for the whole study population, separated by category of recruitment. Histograms of HGS were visually inspected for shape of distributions. For categorical variables, total numbers and percentages were obtained. For continuous variables, means and standard deviations were provided for normally distributed variables and medians and inter-quartile ranges otherwise. Mean scores (and standard deviations) were calculated for the hand grip strength values. Chi-squared tests and ANOVA F-statistics were used in simple univariate analyses to compare categorical and continuous variables between recruitment categories (32).

To investigate whether HGS was associated with being a ME/CFS case, we plotted minimum and maximum HGS (HGS_{min} and HGS_{max}, respectively) against recruitment categories. Bivariate linear regression was used to further explore the associations with indicators of HGS entered into the model as a continuous score and healthy controls (HC) as the baseline comparator. We then adjusted for potential confounding by age, gender, and BMI in multivariate regression analyses.

To examine the change in HGS_{min} and HGS_{max} over the three successive measurements, we plotted their means at each time point within each recruitment category. Differences between HGS indicators (HGS_{max} and HGS_{min}) means at each time point were compared in the following way: time point 1–time point 2, time point 1–time point 3, and time point 2–time point 3.

As the difference between mean HGS at the second and third time points was not statistically different ($p = 0.21$) in the overall study population or in any of the study groups, the average of these two measurements was used for calculating the difference between the first and a subsequent measurement. Therefore, the difference between the first and the average of 2nd and 3rd values represented the overall drop or increase in HGS over subsequent trials, referred to as the HGS-difference (HGS_{diff}). Positive values represent a drop in values from the first to subsequent trials. Paired t-tests were used to determine whether the means were significantly different within recruitment categories.

To examine whether HGS was correlated with parameters of disease severity, Spearman's rank-order correlations were computed. A correlation matrix was obtained, and graphs produced. To further explore the association of disease severity parameters with indicators of HGS, multivariate regression analyses were performed adjusting for recruitment category, age, sex, and BMI.

RESULTS

The distributions of participant characteristics by recruitment category are shown in **Table 2**. Females were over-represented (72%) in the study. Mean age varied across study groups; HC (45.4 years; 95% Confidence Interval (CI) 43.4, 47.4) and CF/nonME (45.4 years; 95%CI 43.4, 47.4) were slightly younger and cases of MS were slightly older (52.5 years; 95%CI 50.6, 54.4). Mean BMI ranged from 24.3 (95%CI 23.0, 25.7) in MEsa to 26.4 (95% ci 25.3, 27.4) in MEmm.

The mean values for the fatigue analog scales were 7.4 (95%CI 7.0, 7.7) for MEsa and 6.7 (95%CI 6.4, 7.0) for MEmm. These values were significantly ($p < 0.0001$) higher than for HC (1.5; 95%CI 1.2, 1.8), CF/nonME (4.5; 95%CI 3.4, 5.5) and MS cases (5.4; 95%CI 4.7, 5.9). The pain analog scales were also significantly higher in ME/CFS cases ($P < 0.0001$); the mean values were: 5.3 (95%CI 4.6, 6.0) for Mesa, 4.9 (95%CI 4.6, 5.3) for MEmm, and 1.0 (95%CI 0.7, 1.2) for HC, with values for other groups in between these. The Physical Component Summary (PCS) in particular, and also Mental Component Summary (MCS) scores were much lower ($p < 0.001$) in MEsa, (19.0 PCS; 95%CI 17.7, 20.4 and 44.2 MCS; 95%CI 41.4, 46.9) and MEmm (31.0 PCS; 95%CI 30.0, 32.2 and 39.2 MCS; 95%CI 37.8, 40.6) compared with HC (57.0 PCS; 95%CI 56.2, 57.9 and 52.1 MCS; 95%CI 50.7, 53.5), CF/nonME (45.7 PCS; 95%CI 42.9, 48.6 and 43.7 MCS; 95%CI 40.6, 46.8) and MS cases (38.4 PCS; 95%CI 35.6, 41.2 and 46.1 MCS; 95%CI 43.6, 48.5), indicating reduced functional status and mental vitality among people with ME/CFS (**Table 2**).

When mean values of HGS were observed over time (i.e., over successive trials), no trend was seen within HC, MS cases, and CF/nonME (**Figure 1**). Among these recruitment categories, there was a slight (non-significant) drop in values between the first and second trials, which was typically followed by a slight increase in values from the second to the third trials. A similar trend was found for MEmm, except that the drop in values between the 1st and 2nd trials was more marked ($p < 0.01$). However, among MEsa, the mean HGS decreased markedly from first, to second ($P = 0.03$), and then again to the third time point ($P = 0.13$), whereas HGS for MEmm increased from second to third trial ($P = 0.19$).

TABLE 2 | Characteristics of the study population, separated by recruitment category.

Factors		Healthy Controls (*N* = 136)	MS cases (*N* = 76)	CF/nonME (*N* = 37)	MEmm (*N* = 216)	MEsa (*N* = 56)	*p*-value for difference b/n groups*
Sex N(%)	Females	84 (62.8)	59 (77.6)	24 (64.9)	166 (76.9)	43 (76.8)	0.02
Age	mean(SD)	45.4 (12.0)	52.5 (8.4)	45.4 (10.3)	47.1 (11.0)	45.9 (11.5)	0.0001
BMI	mean(SD)	24.9 (4.3)	26.3 (6.1)	24.7 (5.2)	26.4 (6.0)	24.3 (5.0)	0.04
hand grip1	mean(SD)	34.4 (13.9)	23.1 (11.8)	32.2 (15.5)	25.2 (11.9)	21.2 (9.7)	<0.0001
hand grip2	mean(SD)	33.9 (14.0)	22.5 (12.9)	31.4 (17.2)	23.5 (12.6)	19.2 (9.2)	<0.0001
hand grip3	mean(SD)	34.1 (14.2)	22.6 (12.7)	31.4 (18.1)	23.9 (12.4)	18.5 (9.2)	<0.0001
min hand grip	mean(SD)	32.0 (13.8)	20.3 (12.0)	29.0 (16.8)	21.6 (11.9)	16.7 (9.2)	<0.0001
max hand grip	mean(SD)	36.2 (14.1)	25.1 (12.4)	34.2 (16.8)	27.1 (12.2)	22.9 (9.2)	<0.0001
Fatigue Analog Scale	mean(SD)	1.5 (1.5)	5.3 (2.5)	4.5 (2.2)	6.7 (1.6)	7.4 (1.4)	<0.0001
Pain Analog Scale	mean(SD)	1.0 (1.5)	3.4 (2.7)	2.2 (2.0)	4.9 (2.5)	5.3 (2.7)	<0.0001
PCS	mean(SD)	57.0 (4.9)	38.4 (12.2)	45.7 (8.4)	31.0 (8.6)	19.0 (4.7)	<0.0001
MCS	mean(SD)	52.1 (8.1)	46.1 (10.8)	43.7 (9.0)	39.2 (9.9)	44.2 (9.9)	<0.0001

χ^2 for categorical variables; F-statistic for continuous variables. HC, healthy controls; MS, multiple sclerosis; CF/nonME, chronic fatigue not meeting study criteria for ME/CFS; MEmm, ME/CFS mild/moderately affected; MEsa, ME/CFS severely affected; BMI, body mass index; PCS, physical component summary; MCS, mental component summary; SD, standard deviation.

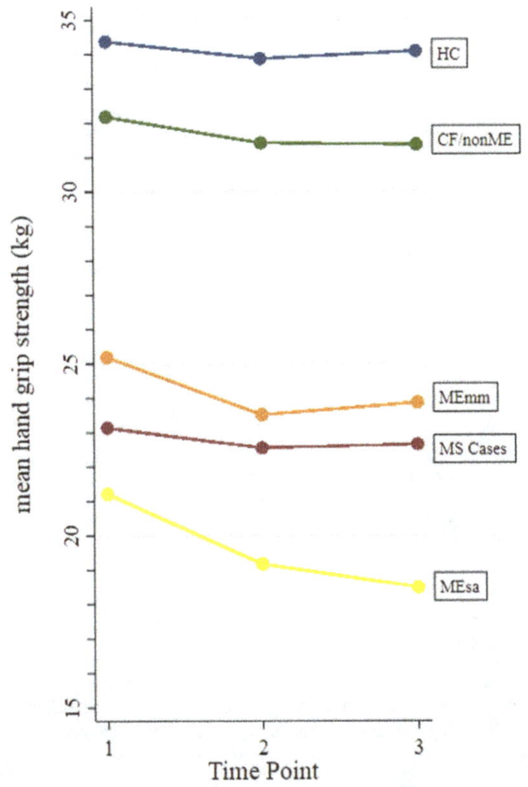

FIGURE 1 | Mean hand grip strength at each time point within each recruitment category. HC, healthy controls; MS, multiple sclerosis; CF/nonME, chronic fatigue not meeting study criteria for ME/CFS; MEmm, ME/CFS mild/moderately affected; MEsa, ME/CFS severely affected.

Associations of Hand Grip Strength Parameters With Being a ME/CFS Case (HGS_{max}, HGS_{min}, and HGS_{diff})

The mean of the HGS_{max} measurements was highest among HC (36.2 kg; 95%CI 33.8, 38.6) and lowest among MEsa (22.9 kg; 95%CI 20.4, 25.4) ($p < 0.0001$). The same was true for the average HGS_{min} measurements, with HC producing a mean of 32.0 kg (95%CI 30.7, 33.4) and MEsa,16.7 kg (95%CI 14.2, 19.2). Among HC, MS and CF/nonME cases, both the HGS_{max} and HGS_{min} values were similar (**Figure 2**).

Table 3 shows the difference between HGS parameters of various study groups and HCs, with negative values indicating values below that of HCs. Compared with HCs, the values of HG_{min} were on average 15.3 kg lower in MEsa (−15.3 Kg; 95%CI −19.3, −11.3), 11.8 kg lower in MS cases (−11.8 kg; 95%CI −15.3, −8.2), and 10.5 kg lower in MEmm cases (−10.5 kg; −13.2, −7.8). These differences were all statistically significant at $P < 0.001$. CF/nonME values were similar to that of HCs (−3.0; 95%CI −7.6, 1.5; $P = 0.19$). The same trend was found for HGS_{max} but was less pronounced. After adjusting for age, sex, and BMI, changes in mean HGS compared with HC were attenuated for all but CF/nonME. MEsa still showed the lowest HGS_{min} value (−10.2 kg; 95%CI −13.3, −7.1) compared with HC, however MS cases (−5.9 kg; 95%CI −8.8, −2.9) now showed similar values to CF/nonME cases (−5.5; 95%CI −10.0, −1.0).

The results for the HGS_{diff} are shown in **Table 4**. Overall, for all recruitment categories, there was a slight decrease in mean HGS_{diff} (1.07 kg; 95%CI 0.68, 1.47; $p < 0.001$). For HC (0.39 kg; 95%CI −0.20, 0.99 $p = 0.19$), MS cases (0.64; 95%CI −0.32, 1.60; $p = 0.19$), and CF/nonME (0.79; 95%CI −0.74, 2.32; $p = 0.30$), none of these differences were significant. However, for ME/CFS cases (both MEmm and MEsa), the HGS_{diff} were higher and statically significant ($P < 0.01$).

Correlations of Hand Grip Strength With Parameters of Disease Severity

Overall, HGS_{max} and HGS_{min} were low to moderately correlated with clinical parameters of disease severity, including fatigue and pain analog scales and PCS, but weakly correlated with MCS (**Supplementary Table 1**).

Results from bivariate and multivariate regression analyses for the association of HGS indicators and parameters of disease severity are presented in **Table 5**. For every one unit increase in kilograms of HGS_{min}, fatigue severity and pain severity analog scales decreased by 0.23 (95%CI −0.29, −0.17) and 1.47 (95%CI −1.86, −1.08), respectively. Alternatively, PCS increased by 0.33 kg (95%CI 0.26, 0.41) and MCS increased by 0.21 kg (95%CI 0.10, 0.32) for each unit increase in kilograms of HGS_{min}. The same can be seen for HGS_{max}, but less markedly. Adjustment for the variables age, sex, and BMI resulted in slightly weaker, but still significant, associations in all cases.

DISCUSSION

Concepts of Fatigue, Strength, Physical Functioning, and Their Measurement

The concept of fatigue is multidimensional and lacks a universally accepted definition. It may be central or peripheral in origin. Central fatigue refers to a state of less-than-optimal outputs from the brain, in particular, from cortical motor area to motor units where nervous fibers stimulate muscle fibers to produce contraction. In contrast, peripheral fatigue represents an impairment of the contractile function of skeletal muscle fibers and the inability of the muscle to produce force (33, 34).

In ME/CFS, fatigue is a key symptom, used for the diagnosis and the assessment of disease severity. However, there is no single descriptor that accurately defines it. It is usually assessed by direct questioning and reported presence of the symptom during diagnosis workup; symptom classifiers may include duration, frequency, persistence or recurrence, and intensity. When establishing compliance with diagnostic criteria, people may be asked, for example, how long they have experienced fatigue, and whether it is present for more than 50% of the time.

Questionnaires, such as the UKMEB symptoms assessment or clinical phenotyping questionnaires (16), or the DePaul Symptoms Questionnaire (35) have been used to establish the presence and severity of fatigue and other symptoms. The fatigue (23) and pain analog scales (24), which are used in this study,

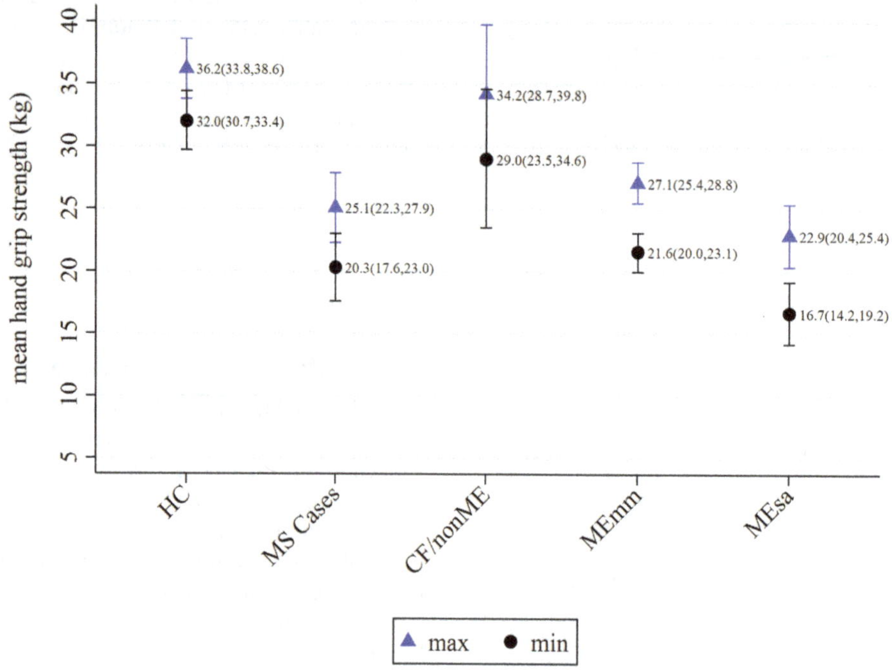

FIGURE 2 | Means of maximum and minimum hand grip strengths within recruitment categories, with 95% confidence intervals. HC, healthy controls; MS, multiple sclerosis; CF/nonME, chronic fatigue not meeting study criteria for ME/CFS; MEmm, ME/CFS mild/moderately affected; MEsa, ME/CFS severely affected.

TABLE 3 | Crude and adjusted associations of minimum and maximum hand grip strengths with recruitment categories, compared with healthy controls using ANOVA.

Factors	Crude		Adjusted*	
	Change in mean HGS kg (95%CI)	*p*-value**	Change in mean HGS kg (95%CI)	*p*-value**
HGS_{min}				
HC	0.0		0.0	
MS controls	−11.8 (−15.3, −8.2)	<0.001	−5.9 (−8.8, −2.9)	<0.001
CF/nonME	−3.0 (−7.6, 1.5)	0.19	−5.5 (−10.0, −1.0)	0.02
MEmm	−10.5 (−13.2, −7.8)	<0.001	−7.6 (−10.1, −5.1)	<0.001
MEsa	−15.3 (−19.3, −11.3)	<0.001	−10.2 (−13.3, −7.1)	<0.001
HGS_{max}				
HC	0.0		0.0	
MS controls	−11.0 (−14.7, −7.4)	<0.001	−5.3 (−8.2, −2.4)	<0.001
CF/nonME	−2.0 (−6.6, 2.7)	0.41	−4.3 (−8.8, 0.24)	0.06
MEmm	−9.1 (−11.8, −6.3)	<0.001	−6.1 (−8.6, −3.5)	<0.001
MEsa	−13.3 (−17.3, −9.2)	<0.001	−7.9 (−11.1, −4.8)	<0.001

**adjusted for sex, age, and BMI **t-statistic. HC, healthy controls; MS, multiple sclerosis; CF/nonME, chronic fatigue not meeting study criteria for ME/CFS; MEmm, ME/CFS mild/moderately affected; MEsa, ME/CFS severely affected; BMI, body mass index.*

are simple and widely used instruments to ascertain fatigue and pain severity; they do, however, rely on self-reporting. This undoubtedly carries some subjectivity and, although both internal validity and test-retest reliability have been shown to be high (24), it is more difficult to establish comparability in the way different individuals interpret and report on fatigue and its severity. This may be particularly problematic in the case of ME/CFS, where the experience of fatigue is usually both physical and mental–described as "lack of stamina or physical energy" and "brain fog and cognitive problems," respectively—and is closely associated with a range of other symptoms. Such symptoms may or may not be interpreted as part of the same symptom complex, which may include post-exertional malaise, pain, flu-like symptoms and unrefreshing sleep, to name a few associated symptoms. The pathological fatigue experienced by people with ME/CFS, which some refer to as "ME fatigue", to distinguish from fatigue or tiredness that represent everyday experience, may be very hard to express and quantify in objective terms.

TABLE 4 | Comparison of difference between hand grip strength at time point 1 and the average of hand grip strength at time points 2 and 3 within each recruitment category, using paired t-test.

Pairs	Paired Differences (hand grip 1-avg hand grip 2 and 3)			*p*-value
	Mean	95% CI Lower	95% CI Upper	
Overall	1.07	0.68	1.47	<0.001
HC	0.39	−0.20	0.99	0.19
MS cases	0.64	−0.32	1.60	0.19
CF/nonME	0.79	−0.74	2.32	0.30
MEmm	1.38	0.75	2.01	<0.0001
MEsa	2.38	0.54	4.22	0.01

HC, healthy controls; MS, multiple sclerosis; CF/nonME, chronic fatigue not meeting study criteria for ME/CFS; MEmm, ME/CFS mild/moderately affected; MEsa, ME/CFS severely affected.

TABLE 5 | Crude and adjusted associations of hand grip strength indicators with disease severity parameters.

Disease severity parameters	Crude		Adjusted*	
	Change in mean hand grip strength kg (95%CI)	p-value**	Change in mean hand grip strength kg (95%CI)	p-value**
HGS_{min}				
Fatigue analog scale	−0.23 (−0.29, −0.17)	<0.001	−0.14 (−0.20, −0.08)	<0.001
Pain analog scale	−1.47 (−1.86, −1.08)	<0.001	−0.93 (−0.17, −0.69)	<0.001
PCS	0.33 (0.26, 0.41)	<0.001	0.24 (0.17, 0.31)	<0.001
MCS	0.21 (0.10, 0.32)	<0.001	0.07 (0.01, 0.13)	0.02
HGS_{max}				
Fatigue analog scale	−0.20 (−0.26, −0.13)	<0.001	−0.13 (−0.19, −0.07)	<0.001
Pain analog scale	−1.29 (−1.68, −0.89)	<0.001	−0.84 (−1.07, −0.60)	<0.001
PCS	0.30 (0.22, 0.37)	<0.001	0.24 (0.18, 0.31)	<0.001
MCS	0.17 (0.06, 0.28)	<0.001	0.07 (0.01, 0.13)	0.03

*adjusted for recruitment category, age, sex, and BMI; **t-statistic. PCS, physical component summary; MCS, mental component summary; BMI, body mass index.

The experience of fatigue or of feeling ill (with ME/CFS) may also be measured indirectly through the impact on people's lives, such as on the ability of individuals to perform physical or mental tasks, including self-care or engaging in work, study and social activities. Some fatigue scales incorporate the impact of fatigue on functioning (28), but more generally, instruments that measure functionality or quality of life have been used to indicate the impact of the health status on individuals affected. The SF-36v2™ is one such well-validated and widely used instrument, and we used in our analyses the Physical and Mental Component Summaries derived from answers given by participants, as proxy measures for the impact of fatigue and disease on the life of individuals studied.

With the challenges involved in measuring fatigue, and more broadly disease severity in ME/CFS, the importance of an objective measurement cannot be overestimated, particularly one which could be used in research studies to aid diagnosis and clinical phenotyping. Assessments indicating levels of severity and impact could be used on a longitudinal basis to inform disease progress and, potentially, disease prognosis.

Hand Grip Strength as a Tool for Measuring Disease Status

Although the testing of HGS was originally created to evaluate patients undergoing hand surgery, this measurement has been shown to be associated with reduced muscle strength and decreased physical fitness more broadly (36). The latter is one of the strongest predictors of individual future health status, characterized by the ability to perform daily activities with vigor and without overdue fatigue. Physical fitness is an important predictor of mortality and morbidity for older and younger adults and teenagers, which can be applied in socially, economically and culturally diverse populations (36–39).

Reduced muscle strength and decreased hand grip have been associated with a few specific situations, such as muscle or nerve injury and malnutrition. More broadly, though, grip strength has been shown to be a simple, yet powerful indicator of overall physical health status and as a predictor of future disability, morbidity, health deterioration (40) and mortality (15), and to assess treatment in various diseases, such as chronic obstructive pulmonary disease (41) and rheumatoid arthritis (20, 42). HGS has also been used to predict cardiovascular risk in pre-diabetic and diabetic patients (38). Associations of poor HGS and future disability and mortality have been observed even among healthy subjects (43), suggesting it could perhaps be used as an early, though nonspecific, indicator of risk for health deterioration.

The underlying mechanisms explaining the association between grip strength and health status are poorly understood, except in cases where local factors such as upper limb muscle damage are in place. Nevertheless, there is sufficient evidence that HGS is a measurement of not only muscle strength, but also of overall physical health. However, unlike cardiorespiratory fitness testing, which demands special location and equipment, measurement of HGS is a simple and mobile tool; making them particularly useful for community-based health evaluations, especially for severe cases of ME/CFS, who normally are house-bound.

Summary of Results and Interpretation

Overall, patients with ME/CFS and MS had significant lower HGS values than HC. MS is the most common immune-mediated inflammatory demyelinating disease of the central nervous system. One of the most prominent features of MS is motor weakness. Therefore, it is expected people with MS to display lower HGS (44, 45). However, it is interesting that ME/CFS patients also had significantly lower HGS values compared to HC, even after controlling for age, sex, and BMI, with even mild cases showing lower HGS. People with ME/CFS are not malnourished and have preserved muscle tonus, suggesting that other than local factors related to the integrity of upper limb must be involved. We suggest these might relate to ongoing inflammation or disruption of signaling mechanisms between central nervous system and periphery, and it may also represent an overall measurement of "physical health and functioning."

Furthermore, HGS among people with ME/CFS significantly dropped in measured strength between the first and subsequent trials, when compared with HC. This effect was not observed in cases of MS nor in those with chronic fatigue which did not meet the criteria for ME/CFS. This finding may relate to early fatigability, where an already reduced ability to produce substantive muscle power in the first trial is further compromised in subsequent attempts. The understanding of the mechanisms behind the lack of rapid recovery in demonstrable muscle force produced between subsequent (hand grip) trials, may be the key to explaining the pathological nature of fatigability and post-exertional symptoms in people with ME/CFS. It is possible that disruptions in muscle energy metabolism or in the continuous production and release of energy by muscle cells, or in nervous system signaling could be involved, however, further experiments would be required for any conclusions to be made.

We have also shown that higher HGS was associated with lower fatigue and pain intensities and with higher functional status and mental vitality. The correlations were stronger for physical than mental component summaries of the SF-36v2^{TM}, suggesting a lesser role for lack of motivation as a single factor explaining poorer results in those with ME/CFS. Such significant correlations of HGS values and indicators of symptom severity and disease status provide further indications for the value of including of HGS as an objective test to enhance patient phenotyping in ME/CFS as part of clinical practice and in research.

Our results are in line with previous small studies, and reinforce the importance of HGS as part of the clinical assessment of people with ME/CFS (46). Patients meeting the CDC-94 criteria for ME/CFS (6) had previously shown significantly reduced HGS_{max} compared to non-fatigued individuals, with example values for right hand force of 31 Kg in ME/CFS vs. 42 Kg in healthy sedentary controls ($n = 8$ in each group) (47) and 24.3 Kg in ME/CFS vs. 35.8 Kg in healthy controls ($n = 30$ and 15 in CFS and controls, respectively) (48). However, no difference in values was found comparing PWME to those with major depression (48). HGS was also used to assess the effects of an exercise intervention among 11 women with ME/CFS meeting either CDC-1994 (6) or International Consensus Criteria [B. M. (49)], who showed a significant improvement in left hand HGS (from 20 to 26 Kg), but not in right hand HGS following the intervention (50), suggesting a role for HGS as an outcome measure in the evaluation of interventions. People with ME/CFS were also previously shown to have slower and incomplete recovery of HGS values following effort challenge, compared with non-fatigued (51, 52) and controls with MS (51). These studies included 48 and 10 ME/CFS cases, respectively.

Study Strengths and Limitations

The study included a relatively large number of participants with ME/CFS ($N = 272$), including different levels of severity, and used both healthy and diseased individuals for comparison groups. We used standardized methods for diagnosis and characterization of participants, which included rigorous procedures for selection, clinical assessment and phenotyping, according to the UK ME/CFS Biobank protocol (16). This was, however, an observational cross-sectional study, and the use of HGS as a diagnostic tool and the mechanisms by which variation in values reflect pathophysiology will require further studies. Similarly, validation of the study in individuals with a range of disease durations, including those with more recent disease as well as in different geographical locations and ethnicities, will be needed to widen the representativeness of the study to other populations and in patients at various disease stages. Furthermore, there are multiple types of MS, and by combining cases of MS all into one category, the results may have been diluted. However, this is not likely to have made a significant difference as differences in dynamic fatigability have been found when comparing MS and healthy controls but not when comparing types of MS (45).

CONCLUSIONS AND IMPLICATIONS

In this study, we investigated the potential use of HGS as an objective measure of disease status and severity in people with ME/CFS and assessed the correlation of HGS with fatigue/pain severity and physical/mental functioning. HGS was markedly reduced in people with ME/CFS, particularly in those who were severely affected. Furthermore, strength decreased with each successive measurement among people with ME/CFS, which suggests early fatigability, or that they tire more easily than healthy or diseased controls. The abnormal pattern of handgrip strength shown in ME/CFS cases give further indications of the distinct nature of ME/CFS and shed more light into the pathological nature of the fatigue symptom complex experienced by those with the disease. The exact mechanisms involved in reduced power and fatigability require further exploration. Nevertheless, the results shown here have practical implications in better defining a fatigue phenotype that help identify cases of ME/CFS and that can be used as an objective tool for diagnosis and measuring disease severity.

AUTHOR CONTRIBUTIONS

LN conceived, and with KM, CK, and EL, designed and conducted the study and acquired the data. LN and KM designed the analyses and interpreted the data. All authors contributed to drafting and to revising the manuscript critically for important intellectual content. All authors approved the final version of the manuscript to be published.

ACKNOWLEDGMENTS

We thank the UCL/RFH Biobank staff and the UK Primary Care Network for their contributions. We are grateful to the many people who have generously contributed to the biobank by donating their time, resources, and energy to participate in the study.

REFERENCES

1. Engberg I, Segerstedt J, Waller G, Wennberg P, Eliasson M. Fatigue in the general population- associations to age, sex, socioeconomic status, physical activity, sitting time and self-rated health: the northern Sweden MONICA study 2014. *BMC Public Health* (2017) 17:654. doi: 10.1186/s12889-017-4623-y
2. Skapinakis P, Lewis G, Mavreas V. Cross-cultural differences in the epidemiology of unexplained fatigue syndromes in primary care. *Br J Psychiatr.* (2003) 182:205–9. doi: 10.1192/bjp.182.3.205
3. Van'T Leven M, Zielhuis GA, Van Der Meer JW, Verbeek AL, Bleijenberg G. Fatigue and chronic fatigue syndrome-like complaints in the general population*. *Eur J Pub Health* (2010) 20:251–7. doi: 10.1093/eurpub/ckp113
4. Shepherd C, Chaudhuri A. *ME/CFS/PVFS: An Exploration of the Key Clinical Issues.* Gawcott: The ME Association (2013)
5. Carruthers BM, Jain AK, DeMeirleir KL, Peterson D, Klimas NG, Lerner AM, et al. Myalgic encephalomyelitis/chronic fatigue syndrome : clinical working case definition, diagnostic and treatment protocols. *J Chronic Fatigue Syndr.* (2003) 11:7–36. doi: 10.1300/J092v11n01

6. Fukuda K, Straus SE, Hickie I, Sharpe MC, Dobbins JG, Komaroff A. The chronic fatigue syndrome: a comprehensive approach to its definition and study. *Int Chronic Fatigue Syndr Study Group Ann Internal Med.* (1994) 121:953–9. doi: 10.7326/0003-4819-121-12-199412150-00009
7. Kingdon CC, Bowman EW, Curran H, Nacul L, Lacerda EM. Functional status and well-being in people with myalgic encephalomyelitis/chronic fatigue syndrome compared with people with multiple sclerosis and healthy controls. *Pharmacoecon Open* (2018) 1–12. doi: 10.1007/s41669-018-0071-6
8. Nacul L, Lacerda EM, Kingdon CC, Curran H, Bowman EW. How have selection bias and disease misclassification undermined the validity of myalgic encephalomyelitis/chronic fatigue syndrome (ME/CFS) studies? *J Health Psychol.* (2018) 1:359105317695803. doi: 10.1177/1359105317695803
9. Al Snih S, Markides KS, Ottenbacher KJ, Raji MA. Hand grip strength and incident ADL disability in elderly Mexican Americans over a seven-year period. *Aging Clin Exp Res.* (2004) 16:481–6. doi: 10.1007/BF03327406
10. Markowitz A, Rabow M. Palliative management of fatigue at the close of life: "It feels like my body is just worn out." *J Am Med Assoc.* (2007) 298:217. doi: 10.1001/jama.297.3.295
11. Norman K, Stobäus N, Smoliner C, Zocher D, Scheufele R, Valentini L, et al. Determinants of hand grip strength, knee extension strength and functional status in cancer patients. *Clin Nutri.* (2010) 29:586–91. doi: 10.1016/j.clnu.2010.02.007
12. Norman K, Stobäus N, Gonzalez MC, Schulzke JD, Pirlich M. Hand grip strength: outcome predictor and marker of nutritional status. *Clin Nutri.* (2011) 30:135–42. doi: 10.1016/j.clnu.2010.09.010
13. Postorino MC, Torti C, Carè I, Pisani V, Strazzulla A, Vaccaro V, et al. Is hand-grip another culprit for the risk of fractures in HIV-positive patients? *New Microbiologica* (2016) 39:71–4.
14. Angst F, Drerup S, Werle S, Herren DB, Simmen BR, Goldhahn J. Prediction of grip and key pinch strength in 978 healthy subjects. *BMC Musculoskel Dis.* (2010) 11:2–7. doi: 10.1186/1471-2474-11-94
15. Sayer AA, Kirkwood TBL. Grip strength and mortality: a biomarker of ageing? *Lancet* (2015) 386:226–7. doi: 10.1016/S0140-6736(14)62349-7
16. Lacerda EM, Bowman EW, Cliff JM, Kingdon CC, King EC, Lee JS, et al. The UK ME/CFS Biobank for biomedical research on Myalgic Encephalomyelitis/Chronic Fatigue Syndrome (ME/CFS) and multiple sclerosis. *Open J Bioresour.* (2017) 4:4. doi: 10.5334/ojb.28
17. Patterson, Medical. *Jamar Hydraulic Hand Dynamometer Owner's Manual.* (2018) Available online at: https://www.performancehealth.com/amfile/file/download/file_id/6971/product_id/27106/ (Accessed October 11, 2018).
18. Massy-Westropp NM, Gill TK, Taylor AW, Bohannon RW, Hill CL. Hand grip strength: age and gender stratified normative data in a population-based study. *BMC Res Notes* (2011) 4:127. doi: 10.1186/1756-0500-4-127
19. Lagerström C, Nordgren B, Lagerstrom C, Nordgren B. Methods for measuring maximal isometric grip strength during short and sustained contractions, including intra-rater reliability. *Upsala J Med Sci.* (1996) 101:273–85. doi: 10.3109/03009739609178926
20. Fraser A, Vallow J, Preston A, Cooper RG. Predicting "normal" grip strength for rheumatoid arthritis patients. *Rheumatology* (1999) 38:521–8. doi: 10.1093/rheumatology/38.6.521
21. Savva C, Mougiaris P, Xadjimichael C, Karagiannis C, Efstathiou M. Test-retest reliability of handgrip strength as an outcome measure in patients with symptoms of shoulder impingement syndrome. *J Manipulat Physiol Therapeut.* (2018) 41:252–7. doi: 10.1016/j.jmpt.2017.09.005
22. Yau K, Farragher JF, Kim SJ, Famure O, Jassal SV. A longitudinal study examining the change in functional independence over time in elderly individuals with a functioning kidney transplant. *Can J Kidney Health Dis.* (2018) 5:205435811877509. doi: 10.1177/2054358118775099
23. Hewlett S, Dures E, Almeida C. Measures of fatigue: Bristol Rheumatoid Arthritis Fatigue Multi-Dimensional Questionnaire (BRAF MDQ), Bristol Rheumatoid Arthritis Fatigue Numerical Rating Scales (BRAF NRS) for severity, effect, and coping, Chalder Fatigue Questionnaire (CFQ), Checklist. *Arthr Care Res.* (2011) 63(Suppl. 11):S263–86. doi: 10.1002/acr.20579
24. Hawker GA, Mian S, Kendzerska T, French M. Measures of adult pain: Visual Analog Scale for Pain (VAS Pain), Numeric Rating Scale for Pain (NRS Pain), McGill Pain Questionnaire (MPQ), Short-Form McGill Pain Questionnaire (SF-MPQ), Chronic Pain Grade Scale (CPGS), Short Form-36 Bodily Pain Scale SF. *Arthr Care Res.* (2011) 63:240–52. doi: 10.1002/acr.20543
25. Lai J, Beaumont J, Ogale S, Brunetta P, Cella D. Validation of the functional assessment of chronic illness therapy-fatigue scale in patients with moderately to severely active systemic lupus erythematosus, participating in a clinical trial. *J Rheumatol.* (2011) 38:672–9. doi: 10.3899/jrheum.100799
26. Rosa K, Fu M, Gilles L, Cerri K, Peeters M, Bubb J, et al. Validation of the fatigue severity scale in chronic hepatitis C. *Health Qual Life Outcomes* (2014) 12:1–12. doi: 10.1186/1477-7525-12-90
27. Ware J, Sherbourne C. *User's Manual for the SF-35v2 Health Survey.* 2nd ed. Lincoln, RI: QualityMetric Incorporated. (2007).
28. Krupp LB, LaRocca NG, Muir-Nash J, Steinberg AD. The fatigue severity scale: application to patients with multiple sclerosis and systemic lupus erythematosus. *Archiv Neurol.* (1989) 46:1121–3. doi: 10.1001/archneur.1989.00520460115022
29. Ware Jr JE, Kosinski MA, Bjorner JB, Turner-Bowker DM, Gandek B, Maruish ME. *User's Manual for the SF-36v2TM Health Survey.* Lincoln: QualityMetric Incorporated. (2007) 86–130.
30. Jason LA, Brown A, Clyne E, Bartgis L, Evans M, Brown M. Contrasting case definitions for chronic fatigue syndrome, myalgic encephalomyelitis/chronic fatigue syndrome and myalgic encephalomyeliti. *Evaluat Health Profess.* (2012) 35:280–304. doi: 10.1177/0163278711424281.Contrasting
31. National Institutes of Neurological Disorders and Stroke. *Myalgic Encephalomyelitis/Chronic Fatigue Syndrome Standards - NINDS Common Data Elements.* (2018) Available online at: https://www.commondataelements.ninds.nih.gov/MECFS.aspx#tab=Data_Standards (Accessed October 11, 2018).
32. Kirkwood BR, Sterne JA. *Essential Medical Statistics.* 2nd ed. Oxford, UK: Blackwell Publishing Company (2003).
33. Chaudhuri A, Behan PO. Fatigue and basal ganglia. *J Neurol Sci.* (2000) 179:34–42. doi: 10.1016/S0022-510X(00)00411-1
34. Gandevia S. Spinal and supraspinal factors in human muscle fatigue. *Physiol. Rev.* (2001) 81:1725–89. doi: 10.1152/physrev.2001.81.4.1725
35. Jason LA, So S, Brown AA, Sunnquist M, Evans M. Test–retest reliability of the DePaul symptom questionnaire. *Fatigue* (2015) 3:16–32. doi: 10.1080/21641846.2014.978110
36. Leong DP, Teo KK, Rangarajan S, Lopez-Jaramillo P, Avezum A, Orlandini A, et al. Prognostic value of grip strength: findings from the Prospective Urban Rural Epidemiology (PURE) study. *Lancet* (2015) 386:266–73. doi: 10.1016/S0140-6736(14)62000-6
37. Artero EG, Lee D, Lavie CJ, España-Romero V, Sui X, Church TS, et al. Effects of muscular strength on cardiovascular risk factors and prognosis. *J Cardiopulm Rehabil.* (2012) 32:351–8. doi: 10.1097/HCR.0b013e3182642688.Effects
38. Lopez-Jaramillo P, Cohen DD, Gómez-Arbeláez D, Bosch J, Dyal L, Yusuf S, et al. Association of handgrip strength to cardiovascular mortality in pre-diabetic and diabetic patients: a subanalysis of the ORIGIN trial. *Int J Cardiol.* (2014) 174:458–61. doi: 10.1016/j.ijcard.2014.04.013
39. Ruiz J, Sui X, Lobelo F, Morrow J, Jackson A, Sjostrom M, et al. Association between muscular strength and mortality in men: prospective cohort study. *BMJ* (2008) 337:92–5. doi: 10.1136/bmj.a439
40. Rantanen T, Guralnik JM, Foley D, Masaki K, Leveille S, Curb J, et al. Midlife hand grip strength as a predictor of old age disability. *Am Med Assoc.* (1999) 281:558–60. doi: 10.1001/jama.281.6.558
41. Swallow EB, Reyes D, Hopkinson NS, Man WDC, Porcher R, Cetti EJ, et al. Quadriceps strength predicts mortality in patients with moderate to severe chronic obstructive pulmonary disease. *Thorax* (2007) 62:115–20. doi: 10.1136/thx.2006.062026
42. Oken O, Batur G, Gunduz R, Yorhanzioglu R. Factors associated with functional disability in patients with rheumatoid arthritis. *Rheumatol Int.* (2008) 29:163–6. doi: 10.1007/s00296-008-0661-1
43. Gale CR, Martyn CN, Cooper C, Sayer AA. Grip strength, body composition, and mortality. *Int J Epidemiol.* (2007) 36:228–35. doi: 10.1093/ije/dyl224
44. Chen C, Kasven N, Karpatkin H, Sylvester A. Hand strength and perceived manual ability among patients with multiple sclerosis. *Arch Phys Med Rehabil.* (2007) 88:794–7. doi: 10.1016/j.apmr.2007.03.010
45. Severijns D, Lamers I, Kerkhofs L, Feys P. Hand grip fatigability in persons with multiple sclerosis according to hand dominance and disease progression. *J Rehabil. Med.* (2015) 47:154–60. doi: 10.2340/16501977-1897
46. Twisk FN. Accurate diagnosis of myalgic encephalomyelitis and chronic

syndrome and severe depressive illness. *Psychol Med.* (2000) 30:433–42. doi: 10.1017/S0033291799001816

49. Carruthers BM, Van de Sande MI, De Meirleir KL, Klimas NG, Broderick G, Mitchell T, et al. Myalgic encephalomyelitis: international consensus criteria. *J Int Med.* (2011) 270:327–38. doi: 10.1111/j.1365-2796.2011.02428.x
50. Broadbent S, Coetzee S, Beavers R. Effects of a short-term aquatic exercise intervention on symptoms and exercise capacity in individuals with chronic fatigue syndrome/myalgic encephalomyelitis: a pilot study. *Eur J Appl Physiol.* (2018) 118:1801–10. doi: 10.1007/s00421-018-3913-0
51. Meeus M, Ickmans K, Struyf F, Kos D, Lambrecht L, Willekens P, et al. What is in a name? Comparing diagnostic criteria for chronic fatigue syndrome with or without fibromyalgia. *Clin Rheumatol.* (2014) 33. doi: 10.1007/s10067-014-2793-x
52. Paul L, Wood L, Behan W, Maclaren W. Demonstration of delayed recovery from fatiguing exercise in chronic fatigue syndrome. *Eur J Neurol.* (1999) 6:63–9. doi: 10.1046/j.1468-1331.1999.610063.x

fatigue syndrome based upon objective test methods for characteristic symptoms. *World J Methodol.* (2015) 5:68. doi: 10.5662/wjm.v5.i2.68

47. Siemionow V, Fang Y, Calabrese L, Sahgal V, Yue GH. Altered central nervous system signal during motor performance in chronic fatigue syndrome. *Clin Neurophysiol.* (2004) 115:2372–81. doi: 10.1016/j.clinph.2004.05.012
48. Lawrie SM, MacHale SM, Cavanagh JT, O'Carroll RE, Goodwin GM. The difference in patterns of motor and cognitive function in chronic fatigue

4

Myalgic Encephalomyelitis/Chronic Fatigue Syndrome in the Era of the Human Microbiome: Persistent Pathogens Drive Chronic Symptoms by Interfering with Host Metabolism, Gene Expression and Immunity

Amy Proal and Trevor Marshall*

Autoimmunity Research Foundation, Thousand Oaks, CA, United States

***Correspondence:**
Amy Proal
amy.proal@gmail.com

The illness ME/CFS has been repeatedly tied to infectious agents such as Epstein Barr Virus. Expanding research on the human microbiome now allows ME/CFS-associated pathogens to be studied as interacting members of human microbiome communities. Humans harbor these vast ecosystems of bacteria, viruses and fungi in nearly all tissue and blood. Most well-studied inflammatory conditions are tied to dysbiosis or imbalance of the human microbiome. While gut microbiome dysbiosis has been identified in ME/CFS, microbes and viruses outside the gut can also contribute to the illness. Pathobionts, and their associated proteins/metabolites, often control human metabolism and gene expression in a manner that pushes the body toward a state of illness. Intracellular pathogens, including many associated with ME/CFS, drive microbiome dysbiosis by directly interfering with human transcription, translation, and DNA repair processes. Molecular mimicry between host and pathogen proteins/metabolites further complicates this interference. Other human pathogens disable mitochondria or dysregulate host nervous system signaling. Antibodies and/or clonal T cells identified in patients with ME/CFS are likely activated in response to these persistent microbiome pathogens. Different human pathogens have evolved similar survival mechanisms to disable the host immune response and host metabolic pathways. The metabolic dysfunction driven by these organisms can result in similar clusters of inflammatory symptoms. ME/CFS may be driven by this pathogen-induced dysfunction, with the nature of dysbiosis and symptom presentation varying based on a patient's unique infectious and environmental history. Under such conditions, patients would benefit from treatments that support the human immune system in an effort to reverse the infectious disease process.

Keywords: microbiome, dysbiosis, holobiont, pathobiont, autoantibody, ME/CFS, molecular mimicry, gut-brain axis

INTRODUCTION: ME/CFS ENTERS THE ERA OF THE HUMAN MICROBIOME

Toward the end of a career spent studying persistent bacteria in chronic disease, microbiologist Gerald Domingue wrote, "It is unwise to dismiss the pathogenic capacities of any microbe in a patient with a mysterious disease" (1). This thinking greatly applies to the illness ME/CFS. ME/CFS is characterized by neuroinflammation, severe fatigue, excessive post-exertional exhaustion, disturbed sleep, flu-like episodes, cognitive problems, sensory hypersensitivity, muscle and joint pain, headache, bowel symptoms, and severe impairment of daily functioning (2). Severely ill individuals are often wheelchair dependent, bedridden, and unable to perform basic tasks of work or daily living.

The history of ME/CFS strongly suggests that infectious agents play a central role in driving the disease process. These include early associations with Epstein Barr Virus (EBV)/Human Herpes Virus 6 (HHV6), the relapsing-remitting nature of ME/CFS symptoms and antibodies/"autoantibodies" detected in patients with the disease (3, 4). A number of ME/CFS outbreaks have also been reported, in which numerous people in the same geographical location developed the illness simultaneously (2). Indeed, many ME/CFS patients present with symptoms after suffering from a severe bacterial or viral infection. These infections often correlate with travel to a foreign country or exposure to pollutants or molds, suggesting that such pathogens take advantage of factors that compromise the host immune system.

Chronic inflammation is a hallmark of persistent infection. Reports of cytokine activation in ME/CFS clarify that the disease is associated with an inflammatory response (5). Montoya et al. (6) found ME/CFS cytokine activation increased with disease severity, suggesting patients may struggle with a growing infectious burden over time. Other ME/CFS research teams have identified various forms of mitochondrial dysfunction in patients with the illness (7). There are now dozens of well-characterized mechanisms by which bacteria and viruses dysregulate mitochondrial metabolism (8, 9).

Many research teams have searched for well-characterized single pathogens in patients with ME/CFS. These analyses often reveal elevated titers of IGG and IGM antibodies toward pathogens such as Epstein Barr Virus, Cytomegalovirus, Parvovirus 19 and *M. pneumonia* (2, 3, 10). Several teams have also attempted to identify a single novel pathogen that might drive the entire ME/CFS disease process. However, the discovery of the human microbiome now allows single microbes and viruses to be studied as members of complex communities. Humans harbor these vast ecosystems of bacteria, viruses and fungi in nearly all tissue and blood (11–14). Organisms in the microbiome continually interact with each other, and with the human genome, to regulate host metabolism and gene expression in both health and disease (15, 16).

A growing number of inflammatory disease states, including neurological conditions and cancers, are tied to dysbiosis or imbalance of these human microbiome communities (17–20). Gut microbiome dysbiosis has been identified in ME/CFS (21). This dysbiosis is characterized by changes in microbe species composition and/or diversity. Pathogens, or groups of pathogens, can promote dysbiosis by altering their gene expression in ways that promote virulence, immunosuppression and dysregulation of host genetic and metabolic pathways (22).

When seemingly disparate biomedical findings on ME/CFS are interpreted through the lens of these microbiome-based paradigms and platforms, a cohesive picture of the ME/CFS disease process emerges. ME/CFS may be driven by pathogen-induced dysfunction, with resulting microbiome dysbiosis varying based on a patient's unique infectious and environmental history. Under such conditions, patients would benefit from treatments that, like those now being developed for cancer, support the human immune system in an effort to reverse the inflammatory disease process.

THE HUMAN MICROBIOME PERSISTS THROUGHOUT THE BODY

In the USA, ME/CFS cases were first formally reported to the CDC in the 1980s (2). At the time, human microbes were typically only detected with culture-based laboratory methods. Then, around the year 2000, novel genome-based technologies began to revolutionize the field of microbiology (23, 24). These technologies identify microbes based on their DNA or RNA signatures rather than their ability to grow in the laboratory. The results of these genome-based analyses were remarkable: vast communities of microbes were identified in the human body that had been missed by the older culture-based techniques. These extensive ecosystems of bacteria, viruses, fungi, and archaea are collectively known as the human microbiome (25–27).

Today, so many novel microbes have been identified in *Homo sapiens* that our human cells are equivalent to or even outnumbered by those of our microbial inhabitants (28). The tens of millions of unique genes harbored by this microbiome dwarf the ~20,500 genes in the human genome (12, 29). For example, just one 2017 analysis of the human gut, skin, mouth, and vaginal microbiomes uncovered millions of previously unknown microbial genes (11). This has forced science to redefine the human condition. Humans are best described as holobionts, in which the microbial genomes and the human genome continually interact to regulate metabolism and immunity (15, 16).

Early human microbiome studies characterized microbial ecosystems in the gut and on mucosal surfaces. However, the microbiome has now been shown to extend to nearly every human body site. These include the lungs, the bladder, the placenta, the testes, and the uterus [(19, 30–33)]. Jakobsen et al. (35) found that previously sterile implants removed from joints, bones, pacemakers, and skulls of symptom-free patients were colonized by a range of bacterial and fungal organisms. Another study demonstrated the presence of novel tissue specific bacterial DNA profiles in a variety of mouse organs including the brain, heart, liver, muscle and adipose tissue (36).

Microbial communities also appear to persist in healthy human blood (37–39). A DNA virome was recently identified in healthy human blood (40). Another study reported both bacterial and fungal communities in the blood of healthy subjects. Analysis of these organisms was performed by microbial resuscitation of blood culturing and microscopy in addition to next generation DNA sequencing (41). Whittle et al. (42) recently characterized a human blood microbiome using a range of complementary molecular and classical molecular biology techniques. Another study identified a larger amount of bacterial rDNA in blood specimens from healthy individuals than in matched reagent controls (24).

Kowarsky et al. (14) detected over 3,000 previously unidentified viruses, bacteria, and fungi in human blood samples obtained from immunocompromised patients. The study almost doubled the total number of anelloviruses found in humans. In order to classify many of these organisms the team was forced to add new branches to the "tree of life." They concluded that the newly discovered microbes "may prove to be the cause of acute or chronic diseases that, to date, have unknown etiology."

The microbiome is inherited and evolves with the host. Babies are seeded in the womb, during birth, and after birth by extensive microbiome communities in the placenta, the vaginal canal, and breast milk, among other body sites (43, 44). Microbes/pathogens acquired from the external environment are further incorporated into the microbiome over time. For example, once acquired, Cytomegalovirus persists as a member of the microbiome—with a significant impact on host immunity. Brodin et al. (45) found that the lifelong need for the body to control CMV causes approximately 10% of all T cells in CMV+ individuals to be directed against the virus.

Immune cells and associated microbes can travel between the human body and brain via several newly discovered pathways that bypass the classical blood-brain barrier (46). Benias et al. (47) documented a previously uncharacterized fluid-filled lattice of collagen bundles that appears to connect all human tissues. This human interstitium drains directly into the lymph nodes. Two research teams have demonstrated the existence of a previously undiscovered meningeal lymphatic system (46, 48, 49). The network's fluid pathways connect the cerebrospinal fluid and cervical lymph nodes directly to the brain.

OUR UNDERSTANDING OF THE HUMAN MICROBIOME AND VIROME CONTINUES TO EVOLVE

While great progress has been made in characterizing the human microbiome, our understanding of the body's microbial ecosystems is still in its infancy. Metagenomic analyses of the microbiome in all body sites regularly identify species or strains of bacteria, archaea, fungi, and/or viruses not previously understood to persist in *Homo sapiens* (13). For example, just one study of the bladder microbiome identified 129 previously unidentified viruses in subjects' urine samples (50).

New strains of known microbes are also regularly identified. For example, as of August 2018, the NCBI database contains ~1,833 *Lactobacillus* genomes, with newly characterized *Lactobacillus* genomes added on a weekly basis (51). Successful identification of these known or novel human organisms hinges on the careful choice of technology and methodology used for detection purposes (26). While the majority of human microbiome studies center on bacteria, awareness of viruses, fungi, and archaea has increased in recent years (52). For example, Manuela et al. (53) found an almost 1:1 ratio of archaeal to bacterial 16S rRNA genes in human appendix and nose samples. Identification of this archaeome abundance and diversity required use of a very specific archaea-targeting methodology.

Viruses are the most abundant life forms on the planet and in the human body, but have been relatively hard to detect until very recently (54). Viruses that primarily infect bacteria, called bacteriophages, are particularly abundant in human microbiome communities. Nguyen et al. (55) estimate that ~31 billion bacteriophages traffic human tissue and blood on a daily basis. However, the human virome also harbors a plethora of human-associated viruses. Newberry et al. (56) are correct to assert that this human virome is understudied in ME/CFS.

Paez-Espino et al. (57) at the Joint Genome Institute have undertaken a large project called "Uncovering the Earth's Virome." The Project's goal is to better identify known and novel viruses in Earth's ecosystems including the human body. Viral identification requires the use of specific metagenomic tools, pipelines, and annotation platforms, with findings entered in the JGI IMG/VR Database (57). The Project is progressing at such a rapid pace that viral diversity in IMG/VR has more than tripled since August 2016 (58), (**Figure 1**). Nevertheless, the vast majority of the gene content (over 15 million genes in total) remains unknown or hypothetical.

We must subsequently consider the possibility that as-yet unidentified microorganisms may contribute to chronic inflammatory conditions like ME/CFS. Failure to do so would be akin to studying ~2% of the animals in the rainforest and arriving at firm conclusions about the entire ecosystem based on that information alone. Certain members of the human microbiome may also be difficult to detect based on their location and/or lifestyle. For example, Chen et al. (59) found that elevated cytokine expression in response to HSV-infected peripheral nerve ganglia persisted even when the virus entered a latent, non-replicating state.

While it is important to pursue identification of novel organisms in ME/CFS blood and tissue, ample data already exists on better-studied components of the microbiome. Microbial and viral survival strategies, virulence mechanisms and collective behaviors are also characterized by a high degree of functional redundancy (60, 61). We must accept the complexity inherent to the human microbiome and further study these common mechanisms of survival and persistence. We must examine microbe and viral activity, microbe and viral gene expression, and the myriad ways in which the proteins and metabolites created by

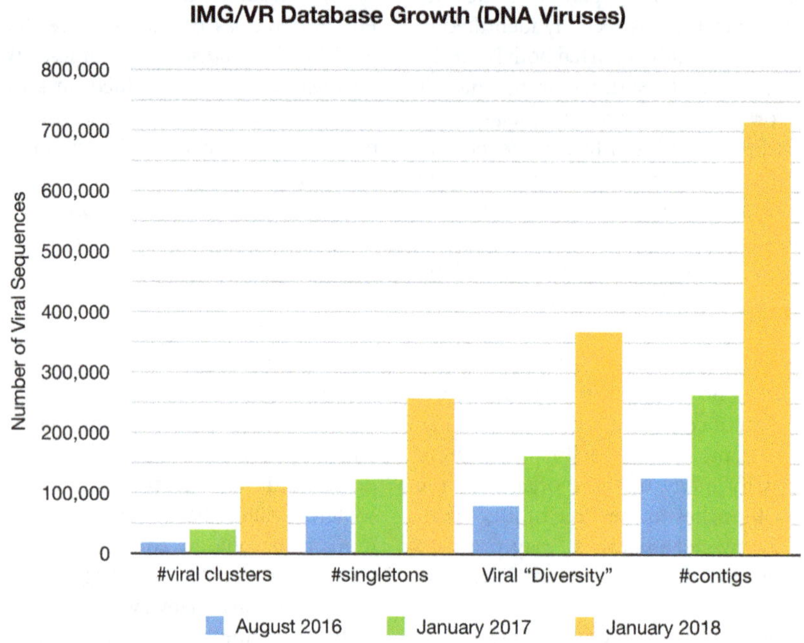

	#viral clusters	#singletons	Viral "Diversity"	#contigs
August 2016	18,470	61,682	80,152	125,842
January 2017	39,701	122,652	162,353	264,064
January 2018	109,968	257,267	367,235	715,672

FIGURE 1 | The IMG/VR database catalogs viruses in Earth's ecosystems including the human body. Viral diversity in IMG/VR has more than tripled since August 2016.

these organisms interact with the host immune system, the host genome, and each other.

THE HUMAN HOLOBIONT: MICROBES AND THEIR METABOLITES MODULATE THE ACTIVITY OF HUMAN PATHWAYS

The genes of our microbial inhabitants greatly outnumber the ~20,500 in the human genome. It follows that the majority of metabolites in *Homo sapiens* are produced or modified by the microbiome. Wikoff et al. (62) found a large effect of the gut microbiome on murine blood metabolites including antioxidants, toxins and amino acids. For example, production of the metabolite indole-3-propionic acid was completely dependent on the presence of gut microbes and could be established by colonization with the bacterium *Clostridium sporogenes*.

Many microbes, viruses and their corresponding proteins/metabolites directly modulate the activity of host metabolic, immune, and neurological pathways. In other words, the human holobiont is controlled by the human genome, our microbial/viral genomes and their respective metabolites working in tandem. A growing number of studies provide examples of this metabolic overlap. While many such studies have been conducted in mice, their general trends carry over to humans.

For example, ME/CFS is associated with natural killer (NK) cell abnormalities, including reduced natural killer cell activity (63). These findings must be interpreted to account for the fact that NK activity is modulated by the bacterial microbiome. One study found that bile acids modified by the gut microbiome impacted liver cell gene expression in a manner that controlled NK cell accumulation and anti-tumor activity (64). Similarly, a mixture of lactic acid bacteria from kefir increased the cytotoxicity of human NK KHYG-1 cells to human chronic leukemia cells and colorectal tumor cells (65). The microbiome and its metabolites also impact the activity of related immune cells. Rothhammer et al. (66) found that tryptophan created by the gut microbiome interacted with the AHR receptor on microglia/astrocytes. Subsequent changes in gene expression regulated communication between the two cell types.

Various forms of autonomic dysfunction are also common in ME/CFS (67, 68). It is subsequently important to consider that the microbiome may contribute to host blood pressure regulation. Pluznick et al. (69) found that gut microbiome-derived Short Chain Fatty Acids such as acetate and propionate travel to the kidneys and blood vessels. There they impacted activity of Olfr78 and Gpr41, two host receptors that control circulation and blood flow.

PATHOGENS AND THEIR PROTEINS/METABOLITES CAN DYSREGULATE HUMAN GENETIC AND METABOLIC PATHWAYS

Microbial modulation of host pathways can also drive inflammatory disease processes. Pathogens and their associated proteins/metabolites control human metabolism and gene expression in a manner that can push the holobiont toward a state of imbalance and illness. For example, Rizzo et al. (70) found that Human Herpes Viruses 6A/6B infected NK cells. This infection significantly modified expression of key host miRNAs and transcription factors. *Mycobacterium leprae* has been shown to alter human gene expression in a manner that allows it to hijack and reprogram adult Schwann cells to a stem-like state (71). In a murine model of diabetes, Liu et al. (72) found that eLtaS, a protein created by *S. aureus*, prevented insulin from correctly binding its target receptor. This inhibited the phosphorylation of downstream signaling proteins and caused the mice in the study to develop impaired glucose tolerance.

The ability of pathogens to interfere with host metabolism is tied to the dynamics of the communities in which they persist. Like organisms in any ecosystem, human microbes constantly interact, both directly and indirectly. The proteins and metabolites they create are also in continual interplay. Communities of microbes often exhibit synergistic interactions for improved nutrient acquisition, protection from host defenses, and survival in an inflammatory environment (73). These include biofilm formation and cooperative signaling via quorum sensing peptides. Humphries et al. (74) recently reported that biofilm bacteria can additionally communicate via ion channel-mediated electrical signaling.

Even viruses seldom act as single entities. Diversity and equilibrium of the bacterial microbiome is regulated by bacteriophage predator-prey dynamics (75). Pfeiffer and Virgin (27) found that enteric viral virulence is regulated by the activity of neighboring bacteria, fungi, and even helminths. These processes are called "transkingdom interactions." For example, human norovirus can bind carbohydrate histo-blood group antigens present on certain bacterial cells. This facilitates the ability of norovirus to infect human B cells (76).

MICROBIOME DYSBIOSIS

Interacting microbes may contribute to dysbiosis or imbalance of microbiome communities (77). This dysbiosis is characterized by substantial shifts in community structure and diversity. In many cases, pathogens proliferate to inhabit niches once occupied by more innocuous microbes.

Most well-studied inflammatory disease states are tied to some form of microbiome dysbiosis. These include psoriatic arthritis, systemic lupus erythematosus, type 1 and 2 diabetes, Parkinson's disease and a growing number of cancers (34, 78, 79). The gut microbiome can initiate and promote colorectal cancer at all stages of tumorigenesis by acting as an inducer of DNA damage, generating epigenetic changes, regulating cell growth, and modulating host immune responses (80). The breast tissue microbiome of women with breast cancer has been shown to differ substantially in composition, virulence and diversity from that of healthy controls (81). Species composition of the bronchoalveolar microbiome shifted toward a more pathogenic state in patients with sarcoidosis (82). Alterations in the enteric virome were reported prior to disease onset in children susceptible to developing type 1 diabetes (83).

Several research teams have tied ME/CFS to bacterial gut microbiome dysbiosis. Giloteaux et al. (21) found that gut microbiome bacterial diversity was decreased in ME/CFS subjects compared to heathy controls. The team also noted increases in certain bacterial species associated with either pro-inflammatory or anti-inflammatory activity. Nagy-Szakal et al. (84) also analyzed the ME/CFS gut microbiome. The study detected seven gut bacterial species whose relative abundance differed from that of control subjects and were strongly associated with ME/CFS.

While these findings are of interest, gut microbiome composition is additionally impacted by a host of environmental variables that cause large shifts in the region's microbial ecosystems. These include geographic location, food consumption, and even time of day (85). Many research teams studying inflammatory conditions have struggled to isolate and/or replicate disease-induced gut microbiome dysbiosis in the face of this "noise." For example, Frémont et al. (86) found that intestinal microbiome species composition differed between patients with ME/CFS and healthy controls. However, significant changes in intestinal microbiome composition were also identified between control subjects from Norway and controls subjects from Belgium. This variation was proposed to arise from differences in diet between the two cultures.

Studies of the ME/CFS blood microbiome may be less subject to this environment-induced variability. Furthermore, identification of microbial and/or viral communities in ME/CFS blood would allow for a broader picture of possible infectious and inflammatory processes. For example, Giloteaux et al. (21) found that ME/CFS subjects had higher levels of bacterial lipopolysaccharides (LPS), LPS-binding proteins and soluble CD14 in blood. The team suggested that these inflammatory markers may indicate translocation of gut bacteria into the blood. However, the markers could also reflect the presence of bacteria in the blood itself.

The blood microbiome can be characterized if the microbial DNA/RNA in samples is first separated from that derived from the human genome. Olde Loohuis et al. (87) used RNA sequencing of reads from whole blood to analyze microbial communities in the blood of almost 200 patients with three neurological conditions: bipolar disorder, schizophrenia, and amyoytrophic lateral sclerosis. The team identified a wide range of bacterial and archaeal phyla in subjects with all three disease states. They observed increased microbial diversity in schizophrenia subjects compared to the two other groups, and replicated the finding in an independent dataset. Stephen Quake's cell-free DNA shotgun sequencing technologies can also characterize bacterial communities in human blood, and can be additionally extended to identify viruses and fungi (14).

Communities of microbes and viruses may also persist in ME/CFS brain tissue. Readhead et al. (88) recently detected a range of persistent viruses in the Alzheimer's brain. These included herpesviruses, torque teno viruses, adenoviruses, and coronaviruses. The Alzheimer's brain has also been shown to harbor bacterial and fungal communities (89, 90). Branton et al. (91) identified hundreds of bacteria and bacteriophage-derived samples in brain tissue removed from patients with epilepsy, and in brain samples obtained from HIV/AIDS patients after autopsy.

In fact, studies of the virome provide significantly extended context on microbiome community dynamics and disease processes. This is because bacteriophages (phages) infect, and subsequently modulate the activity of the bacterial microbiome (75). For example, Duerkop et al. (92) characterized the intestinal virome in a model of T-cell-mediated murine colitis. The intestinal phage population changed in colitis, and transitioned from an ordered state to a stochastic dysbiosis. Phage populations that expanded during colitis were frequently connected to bacterial hosts that benefit from or are linked to intestinal inflammation. Tetz et al. (93) identified changes in the Parkinson's gut bacteriophage community. These included shifts in the phage/bacteria ratio of bacteria known to produce dopamine.

Species-level studies of the microbiome are also greatly enhanced by analyses that provide further context on disease activity. This is an important consideration because, in theory, the microbiome of a patient with ME/CFS could harbor the exact same microbial, viral and/or fungal species as that of a healthy subject. Yet many of these organisms could be *acting* very differently in patients with the disease. Species-level analyses of the ME/CFS microbiome must subsequently be accompanied by studies that characterize microbial and viral gene expression and/or metabolism.

COMPOSITION OF THE HUMAN PROTEOME AND METABOLOME REFLECT MICROBIOME AND ACTIVITY

Since many of the proteins and metabolites in the human holobiont are microbial in origin, composition of the ME/CFS proteome and metabolome change with microbiome species composition. Proteome and metabolome analyses additionally reflect microbiome activity. This is because microbes and viruses frequently alter their gene expression in ways that cause them to express different proteins and metabolites over time. The human genome and related epigenetic changes also contribute to the metabolic diversity, although the high level of redundancy between human and microbial metabolites can make the origin of these associations hard to pinpoint.

Schutzer et al. (94) demonstrated that the ME/CFS cerebrospinal proteome differs substantially from that of healthy controls (**Figure 2**). Indeed, 738 of 2,783 identified proteins (26.5%) were unique to patients with ME/CFS, providing strong evidence that ME/CFS is indeed characterized

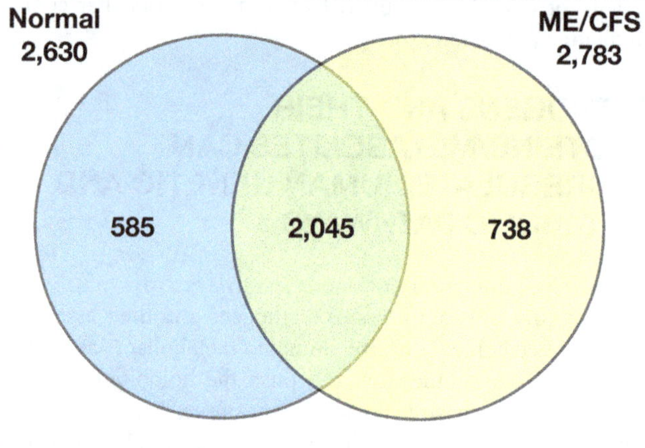

FIGURE 2 | Venn diagram of the qualitative distribution of proteins identified in cerebrospinal fluid from normal control subjects and ME/CFS subjects. Seven hundred and thirty eight of 2,783 identified proteins (26.5%) were unique to patients with ME/CFS. The numbers of proteins for each category separately is shown outside the circles (2,630 for normal controls, 2,783 for ME/CFS) (94).

by microbiome dysbiosis in tissue and blood. Composition of the blood metabolome has also been shown to shift in ME/CFS. One such study reported elevated plasma levels of choline, carnitine, and complex lipid metabolites in ME/CFS patients (84). Another analysis demonstrated a sustained hypo-metabolic response in patients with the disease (95). This dour-like state can be driven by exposure to adverse environmental conditions, as would be expected if the ME/CFS immune system struggles to manage microbiome dysbiosis and associated pathogens.

Studies of the metabolome are often conducted in an attempt to identify disease-specific biomarkers. However, the metabolome can also be screened for metabolites that directly induce or suppress biological function in patients with a given illness. These studies help dissociate cause from effect and allow for possible modulation of disease phenotype. For example, Johnson et al. (96) investigated the metabolic influence of microbial biofilms on colon cancer tissue and related cancer occurrence. They found that up-regulation of a biofilm-derived polyamide metabolite enhanced both biofilm formation and cancer growth.

MICROBES ACT DIFFERENTLY DEPENDING ON NEIGHBORING SPECIES AND IMMUNE STATUS

Studies of microbiome activity must account for the fact that pathogens detected in patients with ME/CFS are also regularly identified in healthy subjects or in patients with related inflammatory conditions. This is particularly true of studies that have searched for EBV, HHV6, Cytomegalovirus, and other viruses able to be identified by PCR and/or antibody testing in ME/CFS cohorts. This same trend is likely to hold for less-studied or unidentified human microbes and viruses. While these "overlapping" results are often viewed as problematic, they make sense in light of research that clarifies how differently microbes act depending on host immune status, neighboring species, and a wide range of other variables. For example, susceptibility to HIV infection has been shown to vary based on the species composition and activity of the bacterial vaginal microbiome (97).

Indeed, most human microbes are pathobionts: they can change their gene expression to act as pathogens under conditions of imbalance and immunosuppression (98–100). For example, *S. pneumoniae* can persist as a highly adapted commensal or a virulent pathogen depending on its ability to evade the host immune response (101). *S. aureus* causes a range of illnesses, from skin infections to life-threatening diseases such as endocarditis and meningitis. However, ~30% of the healthy human population harbors *S. aureus* as a member of the normal nasal microbiome (102). *S. aureus* virulence in these communities is determined by a number of factors, including the signaling and competitive strategies employed by neighboring microbes.

The same is true of *Escherichia coli (E. coli)*, which also persists in numerous forms. One study found that "commensal" *E. coli* could evolve into virulent clones in fewer than 500 generations (103). For most microbes, this evolution toward pathogenicity occurs via the acquisition of new genes or alteration of the current genome in a manner that induces gene loss (104). For example, loss of *mucA* increases the ability of *Pseudomonas aeruginosa* to evade phagocytosis and resist pulmonary clearance (105).

It should also be noted that every microbial species represents many different strains, each of which may vary in the set of genes it encodes or in the copy number of such genes. This intra-species variation endows each strain with distinct functional capacities, including differences in virulence, motility, nutrient utilization, and drug resistance (106). Greenblum et al. (106) identified extensive strain-level copy-number variation across species in metagenomic samples obtained from patients with irritable bowel syndrome. This was especially true of genes tied to specific community functions, including functions related to community lifestyle. Differences in gene copy-number also impacted adaptive functions linked to obesity. Yao et al. (107) found that deletion of a single Bacteriodes gene—and the bile salt hydrolase it expresses—altered host metabolism in a manner that impacted weight management, circadian rhythm and immunity.

A microbe or a virus' location can also influence its activity. For example, much of the human population harbors HHV-6. However, in Alzheimer's disease, HHV-6A was recently identified in human brain tissue (88). There, its activity was shown capable of regulating host molecular, clinical, and neuropathological networks in a manner that can contribute to inflammation and neuronal loss. VanElzakker (108) has proposed that HHV-6 may also infect the vagus nerve in ME/CFS, resulting in altered gut-brain axis signaling in patients with the illness.

The human immune system also plays a central role in determining microbe and viral activity. A robust immune response is often capable of controlling pathogen virulence. However, if pathogens overcome the immune response, or the immune system is suppressed by medications, chemicals, or other environmental factors, pathobionts are more likely to alter their gene expression in a manner that promotes disease.

PATHOBIONTS ALTER THEIR COLLECTIVE GENE EXPRESSION TO DRIVE DYSBIOSIS

Pathobionts can subvert the human immune response by collectively altering their gene expression. Yost et al. (100) performed an excellent gene ontology (GO) enrichment analysis of the oral microbiome during periodontal progression. Over the two-month study period, changes in the metagenome of non-progressing sites were minor. However, active sites that progressed to periodontitis were characterized by numerous functional genomic signatures. In fact, the team reported a complete rearrangement at the metagenome level between baseline sites that progressed to periodontitis and those that did not.

GO terms associated with processes including peptidoglycan biosynthesis and potassium transport were highly enriched at baseline sites that later progressed to periodontitis. Genes controlling ciliary motility and CRISPR-associated proteins were also active during initial stages of disease progression. At the breakdown point, active sites expressed genes associated with ferrous iron transport and response to oxidative stress. Progression to periodontitis was also correlated with increased expression of putative virulence factors associated with a range of bacterial species. Mycoplasma, bacteriophage, and eukaryotic viral activity were higher in progressing sites compared to baseline samples.

The team concluded that periodontitis progression is driven by the whole oral microbial community and not just a few select pathogens. In effect, under conditions of increasing inflammation and imbalance, the entire oral community appeared to *act together as a pathogen*. Indeed, groups of bacteria not generally considered pathogens upregulated a large number of the putative virulence factors in active sites. These included *Veillonella parvula*, a microbe almost always associated with dental health.

INTRACELLULAR PATHOGENS DRIVE MICROBIOME DYSBIOSIS

Community-wide shifts in microbiome virulence are often driven by dominant pathogens—organisms that become established as central components of the microbiome while suppressing commensal growth and activity (109). In other cases, keystone pathogens promote inflammation even when present as quantitatively minor members of the microbiome. For example, *P. gingivalis* often comprises just 0.01% of periodontal biofilms, yet drives destructive changes in host-microbe interplay by profoundly impairing the innate immune response (110).

Pathogens able to persist inside the cells of the immune system are uniquely positioned to drive inflammatory disease (111). Indeed, most well-characterized pathogens, including many connected to ME/CFS, are capable of intracellular persistence (112). By surviving in this fashion, they can directly

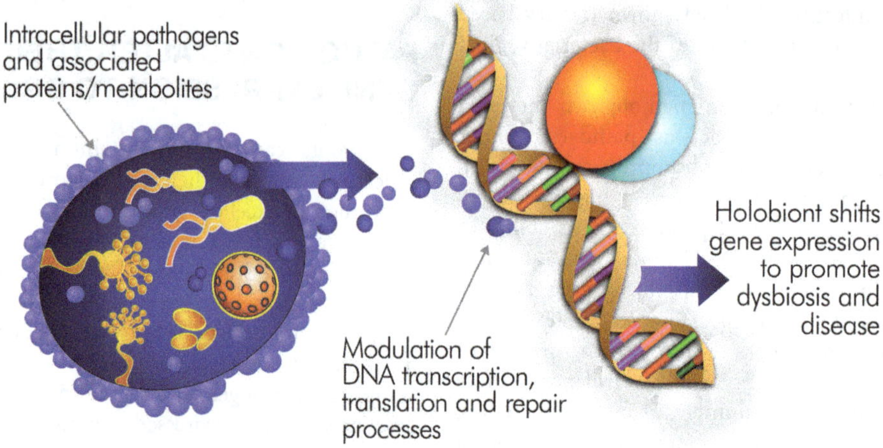

FIGURE 3 | Intracellular pathogens and the proteins/metabolites they express can directly interfere with human transcription, translation, and DNA repair processes.

interfere with human transcription, translation, and DNA repair processes (**Figure 3**). Pathogens in the cell cytoplasm may further dysregulate the epigenetic environment (113). For example, upon infecting a macrophage, *Mycobacterium tuberculosis* alters the expression of 463 human genes (114). *H. pylori* infection predisposes to genomic instability and DNA damage, including double strand breaks (115). EBV infection of B cells can also promote persistent damage to human DNA (116).

The thousands of metabolites and proteins expressed by intracellular pathogens also interact with the host genome, further modifying human gene expression in a manner that promotes disease. Even bacterial quorum sensing peptides can dysregulate human pathway activity. Wynendaele et al. (117) found that quorum sensing molecules created by gram-negative bacteria altered human gene expression in a manner that promoted *in vitro* angiogeneisis, tumor growth, and neovascularization in colon cancer.

Intracellular pathogens can also travel between cells via recently characterized tunneling nanotubules (TNTs) (118, 119). These cytoplasmic extensions of dendritic cells, glial cells and related human cells allow for the intracellular transfer of microRNAs, messenger RNAs, prions, viruses, and even whole organelles such as mitochondria (120, 121). For example, HIV-induced tunneling nanotubule formation appears to mediate approximately half of HIV virus spread among monocyte-derived macrophages (119).

MOLECULAR MIMICRY

Dysfunction driven by intracellular infection is compounded by the fact that microbial proteins and metabolites are often identical or similar in structure to those created by their human hosts. The molecular mimicry or sequence homology between these proteins and metabolites makes it increasingly difficult for the human holobiont to recognize "foreign" from "self."

For example, Altindis et al. (122) found that viruses carry sequences with significant homology to human insulin-like growth factors (VILPs). These VILPs can bind human and murine IGF-1 receptors *in vitro*, resulting in autophosphorylation and downstream signaling. *E. coli* harbors a large, diverse network of proteins that actively promote endogenous DNA damage in cells (123). However, at least 280 of these DNA-damaging proteins have human homologs that also promote DNA damage and mutagenesis in the human host.

Indeed, redundancy between human and microbial metabolites, proteins, and pathways is so great that the potential for molecular mimicry to contribute to host immune and metabolic dysfunction is semi-infinite. For example, viral vesicles and human extracellular vesicles (EVs) share considerable structural and functional similarity (124). These similarities are so extensive that it is difficult to distinguish EVs from (noninfectious) viruses.

DIFFERENT PATHOGENS EMPLOY COMMON SURVIVAL STRATEGIES

Many pathogens employ common survival mechanisms to persist in host cells, tissue and blood. The metabolic dysfunction driven by these different microbes and viruses can result in similar clusters of human inflammatory symptoms. The ability of various pathogens to dysregulate activity of the Vitamin D Nuclear Receptor (VDR) is an excellent example of how different microbes can drive similar disease processes. The VDR regulates expression of hundreds of human genes, many of which regulate inflammatory and malignant processes (125, 126). The receptor also controls signaling of TLR2 and several families of antimicrobial peptides including cathelicidin (LL-37) (127). Pathogens capable of slowing VDR activity can subsequently facilitate their survival by slowing the innate immune response.

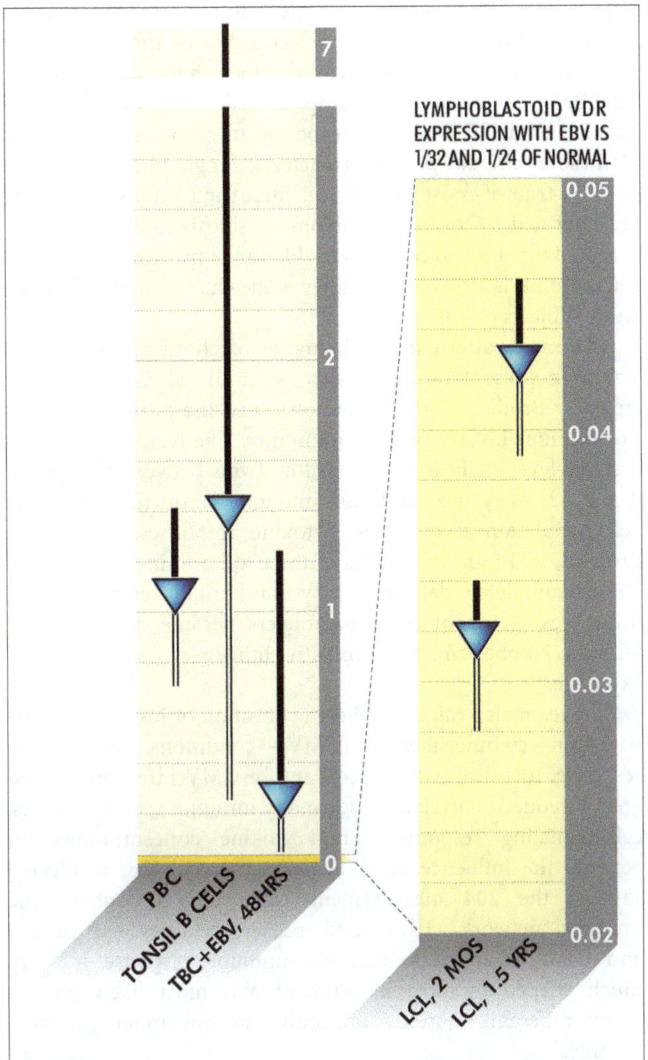

FIGURE 4 | VDR activity is downregulated as much as 20 times in Epstein Barr Virus-infected lymphoblastoid cell lines (128).

Pathogens frequently linked to ME/CFS or inflammatory disease have evolved to survive in this fashion. VDR activity is downregulated as much as 20 times in Epstein Barr Virus-infected lymphoblastoid cell lines (128) (**Figure 4**). HIV, *M. tuberculosis* Cytomegalovirus, *Borrelia burgdorferi* and *Mycobacterium leprae* additionally dysregulate VDR activity to various degrees (114, 129–132). The fungus Aspergillus fumigatus secretes a gliotoxin that significantly downregulates VDR expression (133). Because disabling the innate immune system via the VDR pathway is such a logical survival mechanism, other uncharacterized bacteria, viruses or fungi may have also evolved to dysregulate receptor activity.

It follows that ME/CFS patients with similar symptoms may not always test positive for the same mix of pathogens and/or communities of pathobionts. Similarly, composition of the ME/CFS microbiome, proteome and metabolome should be expected to differ somewhat from study to study. Instead of worrying about these inconsistencies, the ME/CFS research community should strive to better characterize even more common mechanisms of pathogen survival and persistence.

THE IMMUNE RESPONSE CHANGES IN RESPONSE TO PATHOGEN ACTIVITY

The ability of pathogens to disable the host immune response extends far beyond the VDR pathway. Pushalkar et al. (134) identified a distinct and abundant pancreatic microbiome associated with progressive pancreatic cancer. This dysbiotic microbiome drove oncogenesis by suppressing macrophage differentiation and T cell activity. Another study found that *Candida albicans*'s transition from extracellular to intracellular pathogen was accompanied by a coordinated, time-dependent shift in gene expression for both host and fungus (135). These gene expression changes led to a gradual decline in pro-inflammatory cytokine activation by the host immune system.

These findings shed light on a recent ME/CFS study. Hornig et al. (5) reported distinct alterations in plasma immune signatures—including prominent activation of both pro-and anti-inflammatory cytokines—early in the course of ME/CFS. However, these alterations were not observed in subjects with a longer duration of illness. There are a number of explanations for Hornig's observations. ME/CFS-associated pathogens may gradually alter their gene activity to persist in more latent, intracellular forms less recognized by the host immune system. Or, in early-stage ME/CFS, the immune system may actively attempt to target a growing infectious burden. Over time however, pathogens in the microbiome may disable the immune response to a point where "immune exhaustion" occurs (136, 137). Immunopathology and cytokine production would subsequently drop. The resulting disease state could be compared to a garden, in which healthy plants become progressively stifled by others, such as kudzu vine.

"ACUTE" PATHOGENS CAN SURVIVE IN PERSISTENT FORMS THAT DRIVE CHRONIC SYMPTOMS

Many research teams are studying how "acute" pathogens (i.e., well-characterized agents associated with known infectious diseases) can cause chronic symptoms by persisting in latent forms. These include Zika, *Borrelia burgdorferi*, influenza, and other well-characterized viruses and bacteria (138). Zika was shown capable of persisting in the cerebrospinal fluid (CSF) and lymph nodes of infected rhesus monkeys for months after the virus had been cleared from mucosal secretions, peripheral blood and urine (139). Viral persistence in both the lymph nodes and CSF was correlated with upregulation of genes involved in pro-inflammatory and anti-apoptotic pathways.

Tens of thousands of Ebola survivors have developed chronic symptoms months or years after initial infection (140). These "Post-Ebola Syndrome" symptoms include extreme fatigue, severe pain, eye problems, and a host of neurological issues. While the virus is hard to identify in the blood of such patients, Ebola has been detected in men's semen years after "recovery" (141). Another study found that, up to a month after initial infection, influenza viruses regulated the long-term expression of inflammatory and neuron/glia-specific genes in mice (142). This was associated with chronic neuroinflammation characterized by an increase in the number of activated microglia and impairment of spatial memory formation.

Persistent measles virus is associated with conditions such as Paget's disease, multiple sclerosis and Crohn's disease (143, 144). Measles virus RNA has been detected in blood, respiratory secretions, urine, and lymphoid tissue for weeks to months after clearance of the "acute" infection (145). Doi et al. (146) found that, *in vitro*, measles virus persistence correlated with viral transition from a lytic to non-lytic mode that allowed the virus to evade the host innate immune response.

Hundreds of studies demonstrate that acute bacterial pathogens can transition into latent forms that lack a classical cell wall (1). These persistent variants are referred to as L-form bacteria. Antibiotic use can induce persistent L-form growth. In fact, researchers create L-forms by deliberately culturing classical bacteria in conjunction with the beta-lactam antibiotics (147). One microarray analysis of L-form growth revealed up-regulation of genes shared in common with persister cells and biofilms (148). L-form bacteria have been implicated in dozens of chronic conditions including rheumatoid arthritis, multiple sclerosis and sarcoidosis (1, 149, 150).

A better understanding of these chronic sequelae would greatly benefit the ME/CFS community, since a similar chronic progression of symptoms is frequently documented in ME/CFS. At different points in history, ME/CFS has been called "Post-Polio Syndrome," "Chronic Mononucleosis Syndrome" and "Post-Viral Syndrome" due to the fact that chronic symptoms are often noted after acute infection with Polio Virus, Epstein Barr Virus, influenza or a range of other pathogens (151–153). Chia et al. (154) found that patients with acute enterovirus infection went on to develop a multitude of chronic symptoms consistent with an ME/CFS diagnosis. Years after the initial infection, enterovirus protein and RNA were still present in these patients' stomach biopsies.

It is clear that novel methodologies may be required to best identify pathogens in their latent forms. Pathogens that persist inside human immune cells and associated tunneling nanotubuoles have been particularly hard to detect. When persistent Zika virus was identified in rhesus monkeys, Zika-specific antibodies were not detected in the CSF, despite prolonged and robust responses in peripheral blood. This suggested an additional mechanism for viral persistence in certain "anotomic sanctuaries." Modern living has also increased the likelihood that "acute" infections may generate chronic sequelae. Before the advent of antibiotics, steroid medications and childhood vaccines, almost half of all children under the age of five died from acute infectious disease (45). Today, most individuals in first-world countries survive repeated acute infections over the course of decades.

UNIQUE INFECTIOUS HISTORY SHAPES ME/CFS DISEASE PROGRESSION

While certain dominant or keystone pathogens may be reliably identified in patients with ME/CFS, composition of the ME/CFS microbiome will likely differ between patients. Even in HIV/AIDS, where an easily detected virus dysregulates immunity, disease symptoms reflect a mix of those driven by HIV, and those driven by "co-infectious" agents able to take advantage of the immunocompromised host (155). No two patients with HIV/AIDS are expected to harbor the same mix of these additional persistent bacteria, fungi, and viruses. The same is true of most cancers, an increasing number of which are now tied to severe microbiome dysbiosis (34). It is widely accepted that no two cancers are alike, and any tumor-associated microbiome is expected to differ somewhat among individual study subjects (156).

This same pattern, in which unique infectious history impacts symptom presentation may also occur in ME/CFS. A recent study by Brodin et al. (45) demonstrated the profound impact of infectious history on host immunity. The team performed a systems-level analysis of 210 healthy twins between the ages of 8 and 82. They measured 204 immune parameters, including cell population frequencies, cytokine responses, and serum proteins, and found that 77% of these are dominated, and 58% almost completely determined, by non-heritable environmental influences. Many of these parameters became more variable with age, emphasizing the cumulative influence of environmental exposure.

The team also calculated how acquisition of just one chronic pathogen—cytomegalovirus (CMV)—conditions the immune response. Identical twins discordant for CMV infection showed greatly reduced correlations for many immune cell frequencies, cell signaling responses, and cytokine concentrations. In general, the influence of CMV was so broad that it affected 119 of the 204 measurements dispersed throughout the immune network. These and related findings led Brodin and team to conclude that the immune response is "very much shaped by the environment and most likely by the many different microbes an individual encounters in their lifetime."

COULD "SUCCESSIVE INFECTION CONTRIBUTE TO ME/CFS?"

The above suggests that ME/CFS may be driven by a process we have termed "successive infection." During successive infection, an "acute" infection or "initial immunosuppressive event" dysregulates the host immune system. This makes it easier for microbes to subvert the immune response by acting as polymicrobial entities. Pathobionts alter their gene expression to better promote community-wide virulence. Infected human cells fail to correctly express human metabolites in the presence of pathogen-generated proteins, metabolites, and enzymes. Dysfunction driven by molecular mimicry increases. Certain pathogens may infect mitochondria or central nervous system tissue. Intracellular pathogens slow the human immune response, causing the host to more easily acquire other infectious agents. This creates a snowball effect in which the microbiome becomes increasingly dysbiotic as the strength of the immune response weakens over time.

Eventually, the human host may present with symptoms characteristic of ME/CFS or a related inflammatory diagnosis. The unique symptoms any one patient develops are expected to vary based on the species, strain, virulence, and location of the pathogens driving dysbiosis, along with the myriad ways in which the metabolites and proteins created by these organisms cause dysfunction by interacting with those of the host.

Early childhood infections may predispose to dysbiosis at a later date (157). For example, measles depletes host B and T lymphocytes for up to 2–3 years after initial infection. This immunosuppression can reset previously acquired immunity and renders the host more susceptible to other pathogens (158). In other cases, a toxic environmental exposure, infection during surgery or the difficulty of enduring a traumatic event may weaken the immune response to a point where previously subclinical infections become active. ME/CFS outbreaks, in which numerous patients developed the illness at relatively the same time, may well represent this phenomenon at work.

The successive infectious process may even begin in the womb. Depending on the health of the parent, founding microbiome communities in the placenta, vagina and breast milk may already be dysbiotic. Cabrera-Rubio et al. (159) found that the breast milk microbiome of obese mothers tended to contain a different and less diverse bacterial community then that of normal-weight mothers. Pathogens in the placental microbiome can alter methylation of human DNA in a manner that may negatively impact the later life disease of premature babies (160).

Many aspects of modern living can additionally drive successive infection. Antibiotic use disrupts the ecology of the human microbiome (161). Antibiotic resistance genes from farm animals and produce are regularly transferred into the human food supply (162). Electromagnetic radiation has been shown to lower immunity (163). The immunosuppressive biologics and supplements often prescribed for inflammatory disease further allow pathobionts in the microbiome to proliferate. For example, Diaz et al. (164) found that the salivary bacteriome of patients taking immunosuppressive biologics was more permissive to the growth of oral opportunistic pathogens.

Modern society also exposes the average person to pathogens our recent ancestors were unlikely to encounter. International airports harbor pathogens from across the globe (165). Food products, and the microbes they contain, are frequently imported from foreign destinations (166). One study found a range of opportunistic pathogens enriched in showerhead biofilms (167). Numerous pathogens were identified in commonly smoked cigarettes (168). Many such pathogens are capable of persisting in human microbiome ecosystems, where the host may lack immunity toward their presence.

ME/CFS PATIENTS SHOULD BE STUDIED IN CONCERT WITH RELATED INFLAMMATORY CONDITIONS

ME/CFS is a spectrum disorder with a diagnostic criterion that includes a range of physical and neurological symptoms (2). If successive infection contributes to ME/CFS, this variability in symptom presentation is expected. Furthermore, factoring "unique infectious history" into the disease process helps explain why patients with ME/CFS often suffer from a multitude of symptoms not included in the official diagnostic criteria.

Because patients with ME/CFS suffer from such diverse symptoms, it has been argued that they should be grouped into separately studied "subgroups" (169). In some cases this makes sense. For example, studies that distinguish early-stage/late-stage ME/CFS patients may further elucidate how the immune response is modified by the microbiome over time. However, if successive infection contributes to ME/CFS, future research should also focus on better understanding the common pathogenesis shared by all subjects.

Indeed, successive infection may contribute to other conditions tied to microbiome dysbiosis, persistent infection, and adverse environmental exposure. ME/CFS should be studied in concert with these other conditions, which include Gulf War Syndrome, Ehlers-Danlos Syndrome, Chronic Lyme Disease, and fibromyalgia among others (170–174). The high levels of comorbidity and symptom overlap between patients with ME/CFS and these related inflammatory diagnoses strengthens this assumption.

"AUTOANTIBODIES" IN ME/CFS ARE LIKELY CREATED IN RESPONSE TO PERSISTENT PATHOGENS

A number of autoantibodies have been detected in patients with ME/CFS (4). This has led some research teams to postulate that ME/CFS should be regarded as an "autoimmune" disorder (175). However, the classical "theory of autoimmunity" is in the process of being re-evaluated (78, 176). Increasing evidence suggests that "autoantibodies" are actually created in response to chronic, persistent microbiome pathogens. Under such conditions molecular mimicry or structural homology between pathogen and host proteins can result in "collateral damage" toward human tissue. For example, Vojdani et al. (177) found that 25 different Alzheimer's-associated pathogens or their molecules could react with antibodies against amyloid beta via molecular mimicry or the binding of bacterial toxins to amyloid beta.

A growing body of research documents "autoantibody" production in response to a range of bacterial, viral and fungal pathogens/pathobionts. These pathogens are not short-term "triggers" but persist as members of complex microbiome communities. For example, "autoantibody" production was recently tied to microbiome pathobiont *Enterococcus gallinarum*. Manfredo et al. (178) detected *E. galinarum* in the mesenteric veins, lymph nodes, spleens and livers of mice made genetically prone to autoimmunity. In these mice, the bacterium initiated the production of "autoantibodies," inflammation and activated T cells. However, this "autoantibody" production stopped when *E. gallinarum's* growth was suppressed with the antibiotic vancomycin or with an intramuscular vaccine. In addition, *E. gallinarum*-specific DNA was recovered from liver biopsies of human autoimmune patients, and co-cultures with human hepatocytes replicated the murine findings.

Indeed, many pathogens can drive the activated or clonal T cell expansion often associated with "autoimmune" conditions. For example, Tuffs et al. (179) found that *S. aureus* endotoxins triggered uncontrolled activation of T cells. This led to a pro-inflammatory cytokine storm that accounted for both T cell activation and related inflammation.

THE GUT-BRAIN AXIS AND THE BRAIN MICROBIOME

Microbes and their metabolites control bidirectional signaling between the gut and the brain via pathways collectively known as the gut-brain axis (180). The gut-brain axis involves various afferent and efferent pathways including the vagus nerve, with signaling impacting neural, endocrine, and immune processes. The gut's enteric nervous system contains over 100 million neurons—more than in either the peripheral nervous system or spinal cord (181). It follows that gut microbiome dysbiosis may modulate brain activity. For example, Sampson et al. (79) transplanted fecal samples from patients with Parkinson's disease into germ-free mice. These mice, and not controls, exhibited physical symptoms associated with Parkinson's.

However, there is also growing evidence that humans may harbor a brain microbiome. Researchers at Harvard University are characterizing this ecosystem as part of the ongoing "Brain Microbiome Project." In what marks a major paradigm shift, multiple research teams have shown that both amyloid beta and prion protein (PrP) are potent antimicrobial peptides (182, 183). Amyloid beta exhibited antimicrobial activity against a range of common microorganisms with a potency equivalent to, and in some cases greater than, cathelicidin (LL-37) (184). These pathogens included *S. typhimurium*, *Candida albicans* and, more recently, a number of herpesviruses capable of persisting in the Alzheimer's brain (88, 185).

The findings strongly suggest that amyloid beta and PrP are not useless byproducts of abnormal brain catabolism. Rather, they appear to form a mediated response of the innate immune system toward infectious agents in brain tissue (186). A number of brain abnormalities have been reported in patents with ME/CFS (187). These findings must be interpreted in light of these novel infection-based paradigms and in concert with emerging data on the brain microbiome.

WHAT ABOUT THE HUMAN GENOME?

In a study of aortic aneurysms, Gottlieb et al. (188) reported that BAK1 SNP-containing alleles were detected in aortic tissue but not in blood samples from the same patients. More recently Ursini et al. (189) found that schizophrenia gene risk loci that interact with early-life complications are highly expressed in the placenta. However, these loci were differentially expressed in placentas from women who suffered complications during pregnancy. They were also differentially upregulated in placentae from male compared with female offspring.

These and related findings strongly suggest that the environment can select for human genome activity. For example, Harley et al. (190) found that in EBV infected cells, EBNA2 and its transcription factors modulated the activity of human genes associated with risk for multiple sclerosis, rheumatoid arthritis, type 1 diabetes and other conditions. In fact, nearly half of systemic lupus erythematosus risk loci were occupied by EBNA2 and co-clustering human transcription factors.

Studies of the human genome must also account for the full extent of microbial DNA and RNA in human tissue and blood. If a genomic assembler fails to account for this contamination, chances of a false positive single nucleotide polymorphism (SNP) increase significantly during analysis (191). Contamination with even a small amount of microbial DNA/RNA—just one or two base pairs of difference—is enough to cause significant statistical errors in this fashion.

IMMUNOSTIMULATION IN THE TREATMENT OF ME/CFS

If ME/CFS is driven by successive infection, treatments that support or activate the human immune system could improve microbiome health by allowing patients to better target persistent pathogens. Development of such therapies should be a priority for the ME/CFS research community. However, most immunostimulative treatments that target pathogens are characterized by immunopathology—a cascade of reactions in which inflammation, cytokine release and endotoxin release are generated as part of the immune system's response to microbial death (192–194). The death of intracellular pathogens is particularly difficult for the host to manage, as the body must deal with debris generated from apoptosis. Inflammation is also generated in response to bacterial cell wall components including the endotoxin lipopolysaccharide of Gram-negative strains (192). Luckily, immunopathology-generated symptoms are generally temporary in nature, and tend to subside as an increasing number of pathogens are eradicated.

Temporary immunopathology resulting from antimicrobial treatment has been documented for over a century, with symptoms varying depending on the nature of targeted pathogens. First referred to as the Jarisch–Herxheimer reaction, the phenomenon was originally observed during treatment of syphilis with mercury and penicillin (195, 196). The Jarisch-Herxheimer reaction/immunopathology has since been noted in a broad spectrum of chronic inflammatory conditions including tuberculosis and Brucellosis (197). Short-term immunopathology is also a central feature of acute infection. If a patient develops the flu, inflammatory symptoms increase as the immune system releases cytokines and chemokines in response to the infecting virus.

HIV/AIDS patients undergo a form of immunopathology called Immune Reconstitution Inflammatory Syndrome (IRIS) following treatment with Combination Antiretroviral Therapy (ART) (198). IRIS occurs as ART enables the host immune system to better target pathogens acquired during previous periods of

HIV-driven immunosuppression. A range of well-characterized pathogens have been linked to IRIS including the herpesviruses and *M. tuberculosis* (193). However, the inflammatory reaction is also noted in culture-negative patients, suggesting IRIS may also involve novel or uncharacterized pathogens (198).

Over the past decade, in concert with our clinical collaborators, we developed an immunostimulative therapy used to treat patients with a range of chronic inflammatory conditions (200). Treatment centers on the use of a putative VDR agonist in the form of olmesartan medoxomil, with the goal of reactivating components of innate immunity under VDR control. In 2013, we published a series of case histories demonstrating improvement in ME/CFS patients administered this treatment (199). However, all ME/CFS subjects administered the therapy experienced immunopathology and associated inflammatory symptom increases that lasted for many years. As a general trend, patients administered the treatment during earlier stages of disease experienced less immunopathology, emphasizing the need for immunostimulative therapies to be used in a predictive and even preventative fashion.

While some ME/CFS physicians may feel uneasy about the suffering induced by immunopathology, other research communities have become accustomed to treatments that cause temporary discomfort. Novel cancer immunotherapies also generate immunopathology by activating patient T cells. This allows the immune system to better target malignant tumors (194, 201). The resulting "cytokine release syndrome" leads to profound, temporary, symptom increases. However, these increased symptoms are considered acceptable, as patients who endure the reaction are more likely to enter a state of remission. Since many forms of cancer are tied to severe microbiome dysbiosis, at least part of the "cytokine release syndrome" may result from the death of persistent pathogens.

DISCUSSION

The history of ME/CFS strongly suggests that infectious agents play a central role in driving the disease process. However, the discovery of the human microbiome has revolutionized the manner in which persistent infection and chronic inflammation are understood and studied. Humans harbor extensive microbiome communities of bacteria, viruses, and fungi in nearly all tissue and blood. The hundreds of millions of unique genes harbored by this microbiome dwarf the ~20,500 in the human genome. Humans are best described as holobionts, in which these microbial genomes and the human genome continually interact to regulate host gene expression, metabolism and immunity.

Many inflammatory disease states, including neurological conditions and cancers, are tied to dysbiosis or imbalance of human microbiome communities in various body sites. While gut microbiome dysbiosis has already been identified in ME/CFS, distinct microbial and viral communities may additionally persist in ME/CFS blood and brain tissue. Possible identification of these microbiomes should be a priority for the ME/CFS research community, but analysis requires the use of very specific technologies and methodologies.

Pathogens and their associated proteins/metabolites control human metabolism and gene expression in a manner that can push the human holobiont toward a state of illness. Studies of microbiome dysbiosis in ME/CFS must consider this microbe and viral activity. Most human microbes can alter their gene expression to act as pathogens under conditions of imbalance and immunosuppression. This pathobiont behavior is further determined by the activity and virulence of neighboring microbes. Patients with ME/CFS may harbor many of the same microbes and viruses as heathy individuals, yet these pathobionts may act with increased virulence in patients with the illness.

Intracellular pathogens, including several associated with ME/CFS, have been shown to directly interfere with human transcription, translation, and DNA repair processes. Molecular mimicry between host and pathogen proteins/metabolites further exacerbates this interference. Interacting microbes can also drive disease by changing their collective gene expression. Other pathogens disable mitochondria, or may infect central nervous system tissue in ways that dysregulate signaling via the gut-brain axis. Antibodies and/or clonal T cells identified in patients with ME/CFS are likely activated in response to many of these persistent microbiome pathogens.

Different pathogens have evolved similar survival mechanisms to disable the host immune response and/or host metabolic pathways. The metabolic dysfunction driven by these different microbes can result in similar clusters of inflammatory symptoms. ME/CFS may be driven by this pathogen-induced dysfunction, with the nature of dysbiosis and symptom presentation varying based on a patient's unique infectious and environmental history. An initial infection or environmental exposure weakens the host immune system. This makes it easier for pathobionts to subvert the immune response and interfere with host gene expression and metabolism. A snowball effect begins, in which the microbiome becomes increasingly dysbiotic as the strength of the immune response weakens over time. The unique symptoms any one ME/CFS patient develops are expected to vary depending on the location, species, strain and virulence of the pathogens driving this dysbiosis. Thus, while certain dominant or keystone pathogens may be identified in ME/CFS, composition of the ME/CFS microbiome, metabolome, and proteome should be expected to differ somewhat among individual patients.

These common mechanisms suggest that ME/CFS is best studied in concert with other chronic conditions tied to microbiome dysbiosis, persistent infection and adverse environmental exposure. These include fibromyalgia and Gulf War Syndrome, but also conditions like Post-Ebola Syndrome in which severe chronic symptoms develop after infection with an "acute" infectious agent that is able to persist in latent forms.

Treatments that support or activate the human immune system could allow ME/CFS patients to improve microbiome health by better targeting pathogens over time. Like the novel immunotherapies being developed for cancers, these immunostimulative therapies would be expected to generate temporary immunopathology. Institutional reviewers hesitant to approve immunopathology-based therapies should consider that ME/CFS quality of life is typically very low, with patients demonstrating a substantial increase in mortality from suicide (202).

It often takes patients years to receive a diagnosis of ME/CFS. This delay wastes a valuable period during which the immune system is most responsive to immunostimulatory treatment. Patients treated during earlier stage disease are also less likely to experience severe or long-lasting immunopathology. This suggests that immunostimulative therapies should be administered in a predictive and even preventative fashion. In addition, interventions or treatments that might help patients better manage the byproducts of immunopathology (bacterial LPS etc.) should become a priority for the research community.

The overall success of ME/CFS research also hinges on the scientific community's willingness to embrace the concept of the human holobiont. In ME/CFS, the immune response, metabolism, central nervous system, and human gene expression are all linked by the activity of the microbiome and its associated proteins/metabolites. A greater focus on these interconnected systems is necessary, which will require increased collaboration between separate research teams.

AUTHOR CONTRIBUTIONS

AP drafted the manuscript, analyzed and interpreted data, and revised the manuscript for critically important intellectual content. TM drafted parts of the manuscript, analyzed/interpreted data and revised the manuscript for critically important intellectual content.

ACKNOWLEDGMENTS

The authors would like to acknowledge Michael Eason Kirkpatrick and Janet Raty for their help with graphic design. They also thank Sara Nicole Azevedo for her help with technical editing of the manuscript.

REFERENCES

1. Domingue GJSr, Woody HB. Bacterial persistence and expression of disease. *Clin Microbiol Rev.* (1997) 10:320–44.
2. Rowe PC, Underhill RA, Friedman KJ, Gurwitt A, Medow MS, Schwartz MS, et al. Myalgic encephalomyelitis/chronic fatigue syndrome diagnosis and management in young people: a primer. *Front Pediatr.* (2017) 5:121. doi: 10.3389/fped.2017.00121
3. Chapenko S, Krumina A, Logina I, Rasa S, Chistjakovs M, Sultanova M, et al. Association of active human herpesvirus-6,−7 and parvovirus b19 infection with clinical outcomes in patients with myalgic encephalomyelitis/chronic fatigue syndrome. *Adv Virol.* (2012) 2012:205085. doi: 10.1155/2012/205085
4. Loebel M, Grabowski P, Heidecke H, Bauer S, Hanitsch LG, Wittke K, et al. Antibodies to β adrenergic and muscarinic cholinergic receptors in patients with Chronic Fatigue Syndrome. *Brain Behav Immun.* (2016) 52:32–9. doi: 10.1016/j.bbi.2015.09.013
5. Hornig M, Montoya JG, Klimas NG, Levine S, Felsenstein D, Bateman L, et al. Distinct plasma immune signatures in ME/CFS are present early in the course of illness. *Sci Adv.* (2015) 1:e1400121. doi: 10.1126/sciadv.1400121
6. Montoya JG, Holmes TH, Anderson JN, Maecker HT, Rosenberg-Hasson Y, Valencia IJ, et al. Cytokine signature associated with disease severity in chronic fatigue syndrome patients. *Proc Natl Acad Sci.* (2017) 114:E7150–8. doi: 10.1073/pnas.1710519114
7. Myhill S, Booth NE, McLaren-Howard J. Chronic fatigue syndrome and mitochondrial dysfunction. *Int J Clin Exp Med.* (2009) 2:1–16.
8. Anand SK, Tikoo SK. Viruses as modulators of mitochondrial functions. *Adv Virol.* (2013) 2013:738794. doi: 10.1155/2013/738794
9. Jiang JH, Tong J, Gabriel K. Hijacking mitochondria: bacterial toxins that modulate mitochondrial function. *IUBMB Life.* (2012) 64:397–401. doi: 10.1002/iub.1021
10. Seishima M, Mizutani Y, Shibuya Y, Arakawa C. Chronic fatigue syndrome after human parvovirus B19 infection without persistent viremia. *Dermatology* (2008) 216:341–6. doi: 10.1159/000116723
11. Lloyd-Price J, Mahurkar A, Rahnavard G, Crabtree J, Orvis J, Hall AB, et al. Strains, functions and dynamics in the expanded Human Microbiome Project. *Nature* (2017) 550:61–6. doi: 10.1038/nature23889
12. Gilbert JA, Blaser MJ, Caporaso JG, Jansson JK, Lynch SV, Knight R, et al. Current understanding of the human microbiome. *Nat Med.* (2018) 24:392–400. doi: 10.1038/nm.4517
13. Huffnagle GB, Noverr MC. The emerging world of the fungal microbiome. *Trends Microbiol.* (2013) 21:334–41. doi: 10.1016/j.tim.2013.04.002
14. Kowarsky M, Camunas-Soler J, Kertesz M, De Vlaminck I, Koh W, Pan W, et al. Numerous uncharacterized and highly divergent microbes which colonize humans are revealed by circulating cell-free DNA. *Proc Natl Acad Sci USA.* (2017) 114:9623–8. doi: 10.1073/pnas.1707009114
15. Van de Guchte M, Blottière HM, Doré J. Humans as holobionts: implications for prevention and therapy. *Microbiome* (2018) 6:81. doi: 10.1186/s40168-018-0466-8
16. Postler TS, Ghosh S. Understanding the Holobiont: how microbial metabolites affect human health and shape the immune system. *Cell Metab.* (2017) 26:110–30. doi: 10.1016/j.cmet.2017.05.008
17. Rogers GB, Keating DJ, Young RL, Wong ML, Licinio J, Wesselingh S. From gut dysbiosis to altered brain function and mental illness: mechanisms and pathways. *Mol Psychiatry* (2016) 21:738–48. doi: 10.1038/mp.2016.50
18. Lerner A, Aminov R, Matthias T. Dysbiosis may trigger autoimmune diseases via inappropriate post-translational modification of host proteins. *Front Microbiol.* (2016) 7:84. doi: 10.3389/fmicb.2016.00084
19. Chen J, Domingue JC, Sears CL. Microbiota dysbiosis in select human cancers: evidence of association and causality. *Semin Immunol.* (2017) 32:25–34. doi: 10.1016/j.smim.2017.08.001
20. Kell DB, Pretorius E. No effects without causes: the iron dysregulation and dormant microbes hypothesis for chronic, inflammatory diseases. *Biol Rev Camb Philos Soc.* (2018) 93:1518–57. doi: 10.1111/brv.12407
21. Giloteaux L, Goodrich JK, Walters WA, Levine SM, Ley RE, Hanson MR, et al. Reduced diversity and altered composition of the gut microbiome in individuals with myalgic encephalomyelitis/chronic fatigue syndrome. *Microbiome* (2016) 4:30. doi: 10.1186/s40168-016-0171-4
22. Proal AD, Lindseth IA, Marshall TG. Microbe-microbe and host-microbe interactions drive microbiome dysbiosis and inflammatory processes. *Discov Med.* (2017) 23:51–60.
23. Turnbaugh PJ, Ley RE, Hamady M, Fraser-Liggett CM, Knight R, Gordon JI, et al. The human microbiome project. *Nature* (2007) 449:804–10. doi: 10.1038/nature06244
24. Nikkari S, McLaughlin IJ, Bi W, Dodge DE, Relman DA. Does blood of healthy subjects contain bacterial ribosomal DNA? *J Clin Microbiol.* (2001) 39:1956–9. doi: 10.1128/JCM.39.5.1956-1959.2001
25. Zou S, Caler L, Colombini-Hatch S, Glynn S, Srinivas P. Research on the human virome: where are we and what is next. *Microbiome* (2016) 4:32. doi: 10.1186/s40168-016-0177-y

26. Koskinen K, Pausan MR, Perras AK, Beck M, Bang C, Mora M. First insights into the diverse human archaeome: specific detection of archaea in the gastrointestinal tract, lung, and nose and on skin. *MBio* (2017) 8:e00824-17. doi: 10.1128/mBio.00824-17
27. Pfeiffer JK, Virgin HW. Viral immunity. transkingdom control of viral infection and immunity in the mammalian intestine. *Science* (2016) 351:aad5872. doi: 10.1126/science.aad587
28. Sleator RD. The human superorganism - of microbes and men. *Med Hypotheses* (2010) 74:214–5. doi: 10.1016/j.mehy.2009.08.047
29. Li J, Jia H, Cai X, Zhong H, Feng Q, Sunagawa S, et al. An integrated catalog of reference genes in the human gut microbiome. *Nat Biotechnol.* (2014) 32:834–41. doi: 10.1038/nbt.2942
30. O'Dwyer DN, Dickson RP, Moore BB. The lung microbiome, immunity, and the pathogenesis of chronic lung disease. *J Immunol.* (2016) 196:4839–47. doi: 10.4049/jimmunol.1600279
31. Aagaard K, Ma J, Antony KM, Ganu R, Petrosino J, Versalovic J. The placenta harbors a unique microbiome. *Sci Transl Med.* (2014) 6:237ra65. doi: 10.1126/scitranslmed.3008599
32. Kenny LC, Kell DB. Immunological tolerance, pregnancy, and preeclampsia: the roles of semen microbes and the father. *Front Med.* (2018) 4:239. doi: 10.3389/fmed.2017.00239
33. Thomas-White K, Forster SC, Kumar N, Van Kuiken M, Putonti C, Stares MD, et al. Culturing of female bladder bacteria reveals an interconnected urogenital microbiota. *Nat Commun.* (2018) 9:1557. doi: 10.1038/s41467-018-03968-5
34. Chen C, Song X, Wei W, Zhong H, Dai J, Lan Z, et al. The microbiota continuum along the female reproductive tract and its relation to uterine-related diseases. *Nat Commun.* (2017) 8:875. doi: 10.1038/s41467-017-00901-0
35. Jakobsen TH, Eickhardt SR, Gheorghe AG, Stenqvist C, Sønderholm M, Stavnsberg C, et al. Implants induce a new niche for microbiomes. *APMIS* (2018) 2018:2. doi: 10.1111/apm.12862
36. Lluch J, Servant F, Païssé S, Valle C, Valière S, Kuchly C, et al. The characterization of novel tissue microbiota using an optimized 16s metagenomic sequencing pipeline. *PLoS ONE* (2015) 10:e0142334. doi: 10.1371/journal.pone.0142334
37. Gosiewski T, Ludwig-Galezowska AH, Huminska K, Sroka-Oleksiak A, Radkowski P, Salamon D. Comprehensive detection and identification of bacterial DNA in the blood of patients with sepsis and healthy volunteers using next-generation sequencing method - the observation of DNAemia. *Eur J Clin Microbiol Infect Dis.* (2017) 36:329–36. doi: 10.1007/s10096-016-2805-7
38. Potgieter M, Bester J, Kell DB, Pretorius E. The dormant blood microbiome in chronic, inflammatory diseases. *FEMS Microbiol Rev.* (2015) 39:567–91. doi: 10.1093/femsre/fuv013
39. Païssé S, Valle C, Servant F, Courtney M, Burcelin R, Amar J, et al. Comprehensive description of blood microbiome from healthy donors assessed by 16S targeted metagenomic sequencing. *Transfusion* (2016) 56:1138–47. doi: 10.1111/trf.13477
40. Moustafa A, Xie C, Kirkness E, Biggs W, Wong E, Turpaz Y, et al. The blood DNA virome in 8,000 humans PLoS *Pathog.* (2017) 13:e1006292. doi: 10.1371/journal.ppat.1006292
41. Panaiotov S, Filevski G, Equestre M, Nikolova E, Kalfin R. Cultural isolation and characteristics of the blood microbiome of healthy individuals. *Adv Microbiol.* (2018) 8:406–21. doi: 10.3389/fcimb.2018.00005
42. Whittle E, Leonard MO, Harrison R, Gant TW, Tonge DP. Multi-Method characterisation of the human circulating microbiome. *bioRxiv* (2018). doi: 10.1101/359760
43. Nuriel-Ohayon M, Neuman H, Koren O. Microbial changes during pregnancy, birth, and infancy. *Front Microbiol.* (2016) 7:1031. doi: 10.3389/fmicb.2016.01031
44. Gomez-Gallego C, Garcia-Mantrana I, Salminen S, Collado MC. The human milk microbiome and factors influencing its composition and activity. *Semin Fetal Neonatal Med.* (2016) 21:400–5. doi: 10.1016/j.siny.2016.05.003
45. Brodin P, Jojic V, Gao T, Bhattacharya S, Angel CJ, Furman D, et al. Variation in the human immune system is largely driven by non-heritable influences. *Cell* (2015) 160:37–47. doi: 10.1016/j.cell.2014
46. Louveau A, Smirnov I, Keyes TJ, Eccles JD, Rouhani SJ, Peske JD, et al. Structural and functional features of central nervous system lymphatic vessels. *Nature* (2015) 523:337–41. doi: 10.1038/nature14432
47. Benias PC, Wells RG, Sackey-Aboagye B, Klavan H, Reidy J, Buonocore D, et al. Structure and distribution of an unrecognized interstitium in human tissues. *Sci Rep.* (2018) 8:4947. doi: 10.1038/s41598-018-23062-6
48. Aspelund A, Antila S, Proulx ST, Karlsen TV, Karaman S, Detmar M. A dural lymphatic vascular system that drains brain interstitial fluid and macromolecules. *J Exp Med.* (2015) 212:991–9. doi: 10.1084/jem.201 42290
49. Da Mesquita S, Louveau A, Vaccari A, Smirnov I, Cornelison RC, Kingsmore KM, et al. Functional aspects of meningeal lymphatics in ageing and Alzheimer's disease. *Nature* (2018) 25. doi: 10.1038/s41586-018-0368-8
50. Miller-Ensminger T, Garretto A, Brenner J, Thomas-White K, Zambom A, Wolfe AJ, et al. Bacteriophages of the urinary microbiome. *J Bacteriol.* (2018) 200:e00738-17. doi: 10.1128/JB.00738-17
51. Tatusova T, DiCuccio M, Badretdin A, Chetvernin V, Nawrocki EP, Zaslavsky L. NCBI prokaryotic genome annotation pipeline. *Nucleic Acids Res.* (2016) 44:6614–24. doi: 10.1093/nar/gkw569
52. Moissl-Eichinger C, Pausan M, Taffner J, Berg G, Bang C, Schmitz RA. Archaea are interactive components of complex microbiomes. *Trends Microbiol.* (2018) 26:70–85. doi: 10.1016/j.tim.2017.07.004
53. Manuela RP, Cintia C, Georg S, Holger T, Veronika S, Elisabeth S, et al. Measuring the archaeome: detection and quantification of archaea signatures in the human body. *bioRxiv* (2018) 30. doi: 10.1101/334748
54. Paez-Espino D, Eloe-Fadrosh EA, Pavlopoulos GA, Thomas AD, Huntemann M, Mikhailova N, et al. Uncovering Earth's virome. *Nature* (2016) 536:425–30. doi: 10.1038/nature19094
55. Nguyen S, Baker K, Padman BS, Patwa R, Dunstan RA, Weston TA, et al. Bacteriophage transcytosis provides a mechanism to cross epithelial cell layers. *MBio* (2017) 8:e01874-17. doi: 10.1128/mBio.01874-17
56. Newberry F, Hsieh SY, Wileman T, Carding SR. Does the microbiome and virome contribute to myalgic encephalomyelitis/chronic fatigue syndrome? *Clin Sci.* (2018) 132:523–42. doi: 10.1042/CS20171330
57. Paez-Espino D, Chen I, Palaniappan K, Ratner A, Chu K, Szeto E, et al. IMG/VR: a database of cultured and uncultured DNA Viruses and retroviruses. *Nucleic Acids Res.* (2017) 45:D457–65. doi: 10.1093/nar/gkw1030
58. Joint Genome Institute (2018). *IMG/VR Database Triples in Size.* Available online at: https://jgi.doe.gov/img-vr-vir
59. Chen SH, Garber D, Schaffer P, Knipe DM, Coen DM. Persistent elevated expression of cytokine transcripts in ganglia latently infected with herpes simplex virus in the absence of ganglionic replication or reactivation. *Virology* (2000) 278:207–16. doi: 10.1006/viro.2000.0643
60. Louca S, Polz M, Mazel F, Albright M, Huber J, O'Connor M, et al. Function and functional redundancy in microbial systems. *Nat Ecol Evol.* (2018) 2:936–43. doi: 10.1038/s41559-018-0519-1
61. Grzadziel J. Functional redundancy of soil microbiota – does more always mean better? *Polish J Soil Sci.* (2017) 50:1. doi: 10.17951/pjss/2017.50.1.75
62. Wikoff WR, Anfora A, Liu J, Schultz P, Lesley S, Peters E, et al. Metabolomics analysis reveals large effects of gut microflora on mammalian blood metabolites. *Proc Natl Acad Sci USA.* (2009) 106:3698–703. doi: 10.1073/pnas.0812874106
63. Brenu EW, Hardcastle S, Atkinson G, van Driel M, Kreijkamp-Kaspers S, Ashton K, et al. Natural killer cells in patients with severe chronic fatigue syndrome. *Auto Immun Highlights* (2013) 4:69–80. doi: 10.1007/s13317-013-0051-x
64. Ma C, Han M, Heinrich B, Fu Q, Zhang Q, Sandhu M, et al. Gut microbiome-mediated bile acid metabolism regulates liver cancer via NKT cells. *Science* (2018) 360:eaan5931. doi: 10.1126/science.aan5931
65. Yamane T, Sakamoto T, Nakagaki T, Nakano Y. Lactic acid bacteria from kefir increase cytotoxicity of natural killer cells to tumor cells. *Foods* (2018) 7:E48. doi: 10.3390/foods7040048
66. Rothhammer V, Mascanfroni I, Bunse L, Takenaka M, Kenison J, Mayo L, et al. Type I interferons and microbial metabolites of tryptophan modulate astrocyte activity and central nervous system inflammation via the aryl hydrocarbon receptor. *Nat Med.* (2016) 22:586–97. doi: 10.1038/nm.4106

67. Newton J, Okonkwo O, Sutcliffe K, Seth A, Shin J, Jones D. Symptoms of autonomic dysfunction in chronic fatigue syndrome. *QJM* (2007) 100:519–26. doi: 10.1093/qjmed/hcm057
68. Cambras T, Castro-Marrero J, Zaragoza M, Díez-Noguera A, Alegre J. Circadian rhythm abnormalities and autonomic dysfunction in patients with Chronic Fatigue Syndrome/Myalgic Encephalomyelitis. *PLoS ONE* (2018) 13:e0198106. doi: 10.1371/journal.pone.0198106
69. Pluznick J, Protzko R, Gevorgyan H, Peterlin Z, Sipos A, Han J, et al. Olfactory receptor responding to gut microbiota-derived signals plays a role in renin secretion and blood pressure regulation. *Proc Natl Acad Sci USA.* (2013) 110:4410–5. doi: 10.1073/pnas.1215927110
70. Rizzo R, Soffritti I, D'Accolti M, Bortolotti D, Di Luca D, Caselli E. Infection of NK cells modulates the expression of miRNAs and transcription factors potentially associated to impaired NK activity. *Front Microbiol.* (2017) 8:2143. doi: 10.3389/fmicb.2017.02143
71. Masaki T, Qu J, Cholewa-Waclaw J, Burr K, Raaum R, Rambukkana A. Reprogramming adult Schwann cells to stem cell-like cells by leprosy bacilli promotes dissemination of infection. *Cell* (2013) 152:51–67. doi: 10.1016/j.cell.2012.12.014
72. Liu Y, Liu F, Guan Z, Dong F, Cheng J, Gao Y. The extracellular domain of Staphylococcus aureus LtaS binds insulin and induces insulin resistance during infection. *Nat Microbiol.* (2018) 3:622–31. doi: 10.1038/s41564-018-0146-2
73. Irie Y, Parsek M. Quorum sensing and microbial biofilms. *Curr Top Microbiol Immunol.* (2008) 322:67–84.
74. Humphries J, Xiong L, Liu J, Prindle A, Yuan F, Arjes HA, et al. Species-independent attraction to biofilms through electrical signaling. *Cell* (2017) 168:200–209.e12. doi: 10.1016/j.cell.2016.12.014
75. De Sordi L, Lourenço M, Debarbieux L. "I will survive": a tale of bacteriophage-bacteria coevolution in the gut. *Gut Microbes* (2018) 18:1–18. doi: 10.1080/19490976.2018.1474322
76. Jones M, Watanabe M, Zhu S, Graves C, Keyes L, Grau K, et al. Enteric bacteria promote human and mouse norovirus infection of B cells. *Science* (2014) 346:755–9. doi: 10.1126/science.1257147
77. Petersen C, Round J. Defining dysbiosis and its influence on host immunity and disease. *Cell Microbiol.* (2014) 16:1024–33. doi: 10.1111/cmi.12308
78. Li B, Selmi C, Tang R, Gershwin M, Ma X. The microbiome and autoimmunity: a paradigm from the gut-liver axis. *Cell Mol Immunol.* (2018) 15:595–609. doi: 10.1038/cmi.2018.7
79. Sampson T, Debelius J, Thron T, Janssen S, Shastri G, Ilhan Z, et al. Gut microbiota regulate motor deficits and neuroinflammation in a model of Parkinson's Disease. *Cell* (2016) 167:1469–80.e12. doi: 10.1016/j.cell.2016
80. Wang X, Yang Y, Huycke M. Microbiome-driven carcinogenesis in colorectal cancer: models and mechanisms. *Free Radic Biol Med.* (2016) 105:3–15. doi: 10.1016/j.freeradbiomed.10.504
81. Urbaniak C, Gloor G, Brackstone M, Scott L, Tangney M, Reid G. The microbiota of breast tissue and its association with breast cancer. *Appl Environ Microbiol.* (2016) 82:5039–48. doi: 10.1128/AEM.01235-16
82. Zimmermann A, Knecht H, Häsler R, Zissel G, Gaede KI, Hofmann et al. Atopobium and Fusobacterium as novel candidates for sarcoidosis-associated microbiota. *Eur Respir J.* (2017) 50:1600746. doi: 10.1183/13993003.00746-2016
83. Zhao G, Vatanen T, Droit L, Park A, Kostic A, Poon T, et al. Intestinal virome changes precede autoimmunity in type I diabetes-susceptible children. *Proc Natl Acad Sci USA.* (2017) 114:E6166–75. doi: 10.1073/pnas.1706359114
84. Nagy-Szakal D, Williams BL, Mishra N, Che X, Lee B, Bateman L, et al. Fecal metagenomic profiles in subgroups of patients with myalgic encephalomyelitis/chronic fatigue syndrome. *Microbiome* (2017) 5:44. doi: 10.1186/s40168-017-0261-y
85. Caporaso J, Lauber C, Costello E, Berg-Lyons D, Gonzalez A, Stombaugh J, et al. Moving pictures of the human microbiome. *Genome Biol.* (2011) 12:R50. doi: 10.1186/gb-2011-12-5-r50
86. Frémont M, Coomans D, Massart S, De Meirleir K. High-throughput 16S rRNA gene sequencing reveals alterations of intestinal microbiota in myalgic encephalomyelitis/chronic fatigue syndrome patients. *Anaerobe* (2013) 22:50–6. doi: 10.1016/j.anaerobe.2013.06.002
87. Olde Loohuis L, Mangul S, Ori AP, Jospin G, Koslicki D, Yang HT, et al. Transcriptome analysis in whole blood reveals increased microbial diversity in schizophrenia. *Transl Psychiatry.* (2018) 8:96. doi: 10.1038/s41398-018-0107-9
88. Readhead B, Haure-Mirande J, Funk C, Richards M, Shannon P, Haroutunian V. Multiscale Analysis of independent Alzheimer's cohorts finds disruption of molecular, genetic, and clinical networks by human herpesvirus. *Neuron* (2018) 99:64–82.e7. doi: 10.1016/j.neuron.05.023
89. Pisa D, Alonso R, Rábano A, Rodal I, Carrasco L. Different brain regions are infected with fungi in Alzheimer's disease. *Sci Rep.* (2015) 5:15015. doi: 10.1038/srep15015
90. Alonso R, Pisa D, Fernández-Fernández A, Carrasco L. Infection of fungi and bacteria in brain tissue from elderly persons and patients with Alzheimer's disease. *Front Aging Neurosci.* (2018) 10:159. doi: 10.3389/fnagi.2018.00159
91. Branton WG, Ellestad KK, Maingat F, Wheatley BM, Rud E, Warren RL, et al. Brain microbial populations in HIV/AIDS: α-proteobacteria predominate independent of host immune status. *PLoS ONE* (2013) 8:e54673. doi: 10.1371/journal.pone.0054673
92. Duerkop BA, Kleiner M, Paez-Espino D, Zhu W, Bushnell B, Hassell B, et al. Murine colitis reveals a disease-associated bacteriophage community. *Nat Microbiol.* (2018) 23. doi: 10.1038/s41564-018-0210-y
93. Tetz G, Brown S, Hao Y, Tetz V. Parkinson's disease and bacteriophages as its overlooked contributors. *Sci Rep.* (2018) 8:10812. doi: 10.1038/s41598-018-29173-4
94. Schutzer SE, Angel T, Liu T, Schepmoes A, Clauss T, Adkins J, et al. Distinct cerebrospinal fluid proteomes differentiate post-treatment lyme disease from chronic fatigue syndrome. *PLoS ONE* (2011) 6:e17287. doi: 10.1371/journal.pone.001728
95. Naviaux RK, Naviaux JC, Li K, Bright AT, Alaynick WA, Wang L, et al. Metabolic features of chronic fatigue syndrome. *Proc Natl Acad Sci USA.* (2016) 113:E5472–80. doi: 10.1073/pnas.1607571113
96. Johnson CH, Dejea CM, Edler D, Hoang LT, Santidrian AF, Felding BH, et al. Metabolism links bacterial biofilms and colon carcinogenesis. *Cell Metab.* (2015) 21:891–7. doi: 10.1016/j.cmet.2015.04.011
97. Eastment MC, McClelland R. Vaginal microbiota and susceptibility to HIV. *AIDS.* (2018) 32:687–98. doi: 10.1097/QAD.0000000000001768
98. Chow J, Tang H, Mazmanian S. Pathobionts of the gastrointestinal microbiota and inflammatory disease. *Curr Opin Immunol.* (2011) 23:473–80. doi: 10.1016/j.coi.2011.07.010
99. Zechner E. Inflammatory disease caused by intestinal pathobionts. *Curr Opin Microbiol.* (2017) 35:64–9. doi: 10.1016/j.mib.2017.01.011
100. Yost S, Duran-Pinedo AE, Teles R, Krishnan K, Frias-Lopez J. Functional signatures of oral dysbiosis during periodontitis progression revealed by microbial metatranscriptome analysis. *Genome Med.* (2015) 7:27. doi: 10.1186/s13073-015-0153-3
101. Weiser J, Ferreira D, Paton J. Streptococcus pneumoniae: transmission, colonization and invasion. *Nat Rev Microbiol.* (2018) 16:355–67. doi: 10.1038/s41579-018-0001-8
102. Krismer B, Weidenmaier C, Zipperer A, Peschel A. The commensal lifestyle of Staphylococcus aureus and its interactions with the nasal microbiota. *Nat Rev Microbiol.* (2017) 15:675–87. doi: 10.1038/nrmicro.2017.104
103. Miskinyte M, Sousa A, Ramiro R, de Sousa J, Kotlinowski J, Caramalho I. The genetic basis of Escherichia coli pathoadaptation to macrophages. *PLoS Pathog.* (2013) 9:e1003802. doi: 10.1371/journal.ppat.1003802
104. Hottes A, Freddolino P, Khare A, Donnell Z, Liu J, Tavazoie S. Bacterial adaptation through loss of function. *PLoS Genet.* (2013) 9:e1003617. doi: 10.1371/journal.pgen.1003617
105. Cullen L, McClean S. Bacterial adaptation during chronic respiratory infections. *Pathogens* (2015) 4:66–89. doi: 10.3390/pathogens4010066
106. Greenblum S, Carr R, Borenstein E. Extensive strain-level copy-number variation across human gut microbiome species. *Cell* (2015) 160:583–94. doi: 10.1016/j.cell.2014.12.038
107. Yao L, Seaton S, Ndousse-Fetter S, Adhikari A, DiBenedetto N, Mina AI, et al. A selective gut bacterial bile salt hydrolase alters host metabolism. *Elife* (2018) 7:e37182. doi: 10.7554/eLife.37182

108. VanElzakker M. Chronic fatigue syndrome from vagus nerve infection: a psychoneuroimmunological hypothesis. *Med Hypotheses* (2013) 81:414–23. doi: 10.1016/j.mehy.2013.05.034
109. Hajishengallis G, Darveau R, Curtis M. The keystone-pathogen hypothesis. *Nat Rev Microbiol.* (2012) 10:717–25. doi: 10.1038/nrmicro2873
110. Hajishengallis G, Liang S, Payne M, Hashim A, Jotwani R, Eskan M. Low-abundance biofilm species orchestrates inflammatory periodontal disease through the commensal microbiota and complement. *Cell Host Microbe* (2011) 10:497–506. doi: 10.1016/j.chom.2011.10.006
111. Kell D, Potgieter M, Pretorius E. Individuality, phenotypic differentiation, dormancy and 'persistence' in culturable bacterial systems: commonalities shared by environmental, laboratory, and clinical microbiology. Version 2. *F1000Res.* (2015) 4:179. doi: 10.12688/f1000research.6709
112. Ercoli G, Fernandes V, Chung W, Wanford J, Thomson S, Bayliss C, et al. Intracellular replication of Streptococcus pneumoniae inside splenic macrophages serves as a reservoir for septicaemia. *Nat Microbiol.* (2018) 3:600–10. doi: 10.1038/s41564-018-0147-1
113. Indrio F, Martini S, Francavilla R, Corvaglia L, Cristofori F, Mastrolia S, et al. Epigenetic matters: the link between early nutrition, microbiome, and long-term health development. *Front Pediatr.* (2017) 5:178. doi: 10.3389/fped.2017.00178
114. Xu Y, Xie J, Li Y, Yue J, Chen J, Chunyu L, et al. Using a cDNA microarray to study cellular gene expression altered by Mycobacterium tuberculosis. *Chin Med J.* (2003) 116:1070–3.
115. Hanada K, Uchida T, Tsukamoto Y, Watada M, Yamaguchi N, Yamamoto K, et al. Helicobacter pylori infection introduces DNA double-strand breaks in host cells. *Infect Immun.* (2014) 82:4182–9. doi: 10.1128/IAI.02368-14
116. Hafez A, Luftig M. Characterization of the EBV-induced persistent DNA damage response. *Viruses.* (2017) 9:E366. doi: 10.3390/v9120366
117. Wynendaele E, Verbeke F, D'Hondt M, Hendrix A, Van De Wiele C, Burvenich C, et al. Crosstalk between the microbiome and cancer cells by quorum sensing peptides. *Peptides* (2015) 64:40–8. doi: 10.1016/j.peptides.2014.12.009
118. Rustom A, Saffrich R, Markovic I, Walther P, Gerdes H. Nanotubular highways for intercellular organelle transport. *Science.* (2004) 303:1007–10. doi: 10.1126/science.1093133
119. Hashimoto M, Bhuyan F, Hiyoshi M, Noyori O, Nasser H, Miyazaki M, et al. Potential role of the formation of tunneling nanotubes in HIV-1 spread in macrophages. *J Immunol.* (2016) 196:1832–41. doi: 10.4049/jimmunol.1500845
120. Zhu S, Victoria G, Marzo L, Ghosh R, Zurzolo C. Prion aggregates transfer through tunneling nanotubes in endocytic vesicles. *Prion* (2015) 9:125–35. doi: 10.1080/19336896.2015.1025189
121. Haimovich G, Ecker C, Dunagin M, Eggan E, Raj A, Gerst J, et al. Intercellular mRNA trafficking via membrane nanotube-like extensions in mammalian cells. *Proc Natl Acad Sci USA.* (2017) 114:E9873–82. doi: 10.1073/pnas.1706365114
122. Altindis E, Cai W, Sakaguchi M, Zhang F, GuoXiao W, Liu F, et al. Viral insulin-like peptides activate human insulin and IGF-1 receptor signaling: A paradigm shift for host-microbe interactions. *Proc Natl Acad Sci USA.* (2018) 115:2461–6. doi: 10.1073/pnas.1721117115
123. Xia J, Chiu L, Nehring RB, Bravo Nunez MA, Mei Q, Perez M. Bacteria-to-human protein networks reveal origins of endogenous DNA damage. *bioRxiv* (2018) 26. doi: 10.1101/354589
124. Nolte-'t Hoen E, Cremer T, Gallo R, Margolis L. Extracellular vesicles and viruses: Are they close relatives? *Proc Natl Acad Sci USA.* (2016) 113:9155–61. doi: 10.1073/pnas.1605146113
125. Wang T, Tavera-Mendoza L, Laperriere D, Libby E, MacLeod N, Nagai Y, et al. Large-scale *in silico* and microarray-based identification of direct 1,25-dihydroxyvitamin D3 target genes. *Mol Endocrinol.* (2005) 19:2685–95. doi: 10.1210/me.2005-0106
126. Wu S, Sun J. Vitamin D, vitamin D receptor, and macroautophagy in inflammation and infection. *Discov Med.* (2011) 11:325–35.
127. Meyer V, Saccone D, Tugizimana F, Asani F, Jeffery T, Bornman L. Methylation of the Vitamin D Receptor (VDR) gene, together with genetic variation, race, and environment influence the signaling efficacy of the toll-like receptor 2/1-VDR pathway. *Front Immunol.* (2017) 8:1048. doi: 10.3389/fimmu.2017.01048
128. Yenamandra S, Lundin A, Arulampalam V, Yurchenko M, Pettersson S, Klein G, et al. Expression profile of nuclear receptors upon Epstein – Barr virus induced B cell transformation. *Exp Oncol.* (2009) 31:92–6.
129. Nevado J, Tenbaum S, Castillo A, Sánchez-Pacheco A, Aranda A. Activation of the human immunodeficiency virus type I long terminal repeat by 1 alpha,25-dihydroxyvitamin D3. *J Mol Endocrinol.* (2007) 38:587–601. doi: 10.1677/JME-06-0065
130. Chan G, Bivins-Smith E, Smith M, Smith P, Yurochko A. Transcriptome analysis reveals human cytomegalovirus reprograms monocyte differentiation toward an M1 macrophage. *J Immunol.* (2008) 181:698–711.
131. Salazar J, Duhnam-Ems S, La Vake C, Cruz A, Moore M, Caimano M, et al. Activation of human monocytes by live Borrelia burgdorferi generates TLR2-dependent and -independent responses which include induction of IFN-beta. *PLoS Pathog* (2009) 5:e1000444. doi: 10.1371/journal.ppat.1000444
132. Liu PT, Wheelwright M, Teles R, Komisopoulou E, Edfeldt K, Ferguson B, et al. MicroRNA-21 targets the vitamin D-dependent antimicrobial pathway in leprosy. *Nat Med.* (2012) 18:267–73. doi: 10.1038/nm.2584
133. Coughlan C, Chotirmall S, Renwick J, Hassan T, Low T, Bergsson G, et al. The effect of Aspergillus fumigatus infection on vitamin D receptor expression in cystic fibrosis. *Am J Respir Crit Care Med.* (2012) 186:999–1007. doi: 10.1164/rccm.201203-0478OC
134. Pushalkar S, Hundeyin M, Daley D, Zambirinis C, Kurz E, Mishra A, et al. The pancreatic cancer microbiome promotes oncogenesis by induction of innate and adaptive immune suppression. *Cancer Discov.* (2018) 8:403–16. doi: 10.1158/2159-8290.CD-17-1134
135. Munoz JF, Delorey T., Ford CB, Li BY, Thompson DA, Rao RP, et al. Coordinated host-pathogen transcriptional dynamics revealed using sorted subpopulations and single, Candida albicans infected macrophages. *bioRxiv* (2018) 350322. doi: 10.1101/350322
136. McKinney EF, Lee JC, Jayne DR, Lyons PA, Smith KG. T-cell exhaustion, co-stimulation and clinical outcome in autoimmunity and infection. *Nature* (2015) 523:612–6. doi: 10.1038/nature14468
137. Sen DR, Kaminski J, Barnitz RA, Kurachi M, Gerdemann U, Yates KB, et al. The epigenetic landscape of T cell exhaustion. *Science* (2016) 354:1165–9. doi: 10.1126/science.aae0491
138. Cameron D. Proof that chronic lyme disease exists. *Interdiscip Perspect Infect Dis.* (2010) 2010:876450. doi: 10.1155/2010/876450
139. Aid M, Abbink P, Larocca R, Boyd M, Nityanandam R, Nanayakkara O, et al. Zika virus persistence in the central nervous system and lymph nodes of rhesus monkeys. *Cell* (2017) 169:610–20.e14. doi: 10.1016/j.cell.2017.04.008
140. Wilson H, Amo-Addae M, Kenu E, Ilesanmi O, Ameme D, Sackey S. post-ebola syndrome among ebola virus disease survivors in Montserrado County, Liberia. *Biomed Res Int.* (2016) 2018:1909410. doi: 10.1155/2018/1909410
141. Fischer W, Brown J, Wohl D, Loftis A, Tozay S, Reeves E, et al. Ebola virus ribonucleic acid detection in semen more than two years after resolution of acute ebola virus infection. *Open Forum Infect Dis.* (2017) 4:ofx155. doi: 10.1093/ofid/ofx155
142. Hosseini S, Wilk E, Michaelsen-Preusse K, Gerhauser I, Baumgärtner W, Geffers R, et al. Long-term neuroinflammation induced by influenza a virus infection and the impact on hippocampal neuron morphology and function. *J Neurosci.* (2018) 38:3060–80. doi: 10.1523/JNEUROSCI.1740-17.2018
143. Viola M, Scott C, Duffy P. Persistent measles virus infection *in vitro* and in man. *Arthritis Rheum.* (1978) 21(Suppl. 5):S47–51.
144. Wakefield A, Ekbom A, Dhillon A, Pittilo R, Pounder R. Crohn's disease: pathogenesis and persistent measles virus infection. *Gastroenterology* (1995) 108:911–6.
145. Griffin D, Lin W, Pan C. Measles virus, immune control, and persistence. *FEMS Microbiol Rev.* (2012) 36:649–62. doi: 10.1111/j.1574-6976.2012.00330.x
146. Doi T, Kwon H, Honda T, Sato H, Yoneda M, Kai C. Measles virus induces persistent infection by autoregulation of viral replication. *Sci Rep.* (2016) 6:37163. doi: 10.1038/srep37163
147. Casadesús J. Bacterial L-forms require peptidoglycan synthesis for cell division. *Bioessays* (2007) 29:1189–91. doi: 10.1002/bies.20680

148. Glover W, Yang Y, Zhang Y. Insights into the molecular basis of L-form formation and survival in Escherichia coli. *PLoS ONE* (2009) 4:e7316. doi: 10.1371/journal.pone.0007316
149. Markova N. L-form bacteria cohabitants in human blood: significance for health and diseases. *Discov Med.* (2017) 23:305–13.
150. Mattman LH.(2000). *Cell Wall Deficient Forms: Stealth Pathogens*. Boca Raton, FL: CRC Press.
151. Bruno R, Creange S, Frick N. Parallels between post-polio fatigue and chronic fatigue syndrome: a common pathophysiology? *Am J Med.* (1998) 105:66S−73S.
152. Straus SE. The chronic mononucleosis syndrome. *J Infect Dis.* (1988) 157:405–12.
153. Archer M. The post-viral syndrome: a review. *J R Coll Gen Pract.* (1987) 37:212–4.
154. Chia J, Chia A, Voeller M, Lee T, Chang R. Acute enterovirus infection followed by myalgic encephalomyelitis/chronic fatigue syndrome (ME/CFS) and viral persistence. *J Clin Pathol.* (2010) 63:165–8. doi: 10.1136/jcp.2009.070466
155. Chang C, Crane M, Zhou J, Mina M, Post J, Cameron B, et al. HIV and co-infections. *Immunol Rev.* (2013) 254:114–42. doi: 10.1111/imr.12063
156. Bedard P, Hansen A, Ratain M, Siu L. Tumour heterogeneity in the clinic. *Nature* (2013) 501:355–64. doi: 10.1038/nature12627
157. Proal A, Albert P, Marshall T. Autoimmune disease and the human metagenome. ed. Nelson KE. *Metagen Hum Body* (2010) 231–75. doi: 10.1007/978-1-4419-7089-3_12
158. Mina M, Metcalf C, de Swart R, Osterhaus A, Grenfell B. Long-term measles-induced immunomodulation increases overall childhood infectious disease mortality. *Science* (2015) 348:694–9. doi: 10.1126/science.aaa3662
159. Cabrera-Rubio R, Collado M, Laitinen K, Salminen S, Isolauri E, Mira A. The human milk microbiome changes over lactation and is shaped by maternal weight and mode of delivery. *Am J Clin Nutr.* (2012) 96:544–51. doi: 10.3945/ajcn.112.037382
160. Tomlinson MS, Bommarito PA, Martin EM, Smeester L, Fichorova RN, Onderdonk AB, et al. Microorganisms in the human placenta are associated with altered CpG methylation of immune and inflammation-related genes. *PLoS ONE* (2017) 12:e0188664. doi: 10.1371/journal.pone.0188664
161. Langdon A, Crook N, Dantas G. The effects of antibiotics on the microbiome throughout development and alternative approaches for therapeutic modulation.Genome *Med.* (2016) 8:39. doi: 10.1186/s13073-016-0294-z
162. Vignaroli C, Zandri G, Aquilanti L, Pasquaroli S, Biavasco F. Multidrug-resistant enterococci in animal meat and faeces and co-transfer of resistance from an Enterococcus durans to a human Enterococcus faecium. *Curr Microbiol.* (2011) 62:1438–47. doi: 10.1007/s00284-011-9880-x
163. Kolomytseva M, Gapeev A, Sadovnikov V, Chemeris N. Suppression of nonspecific resistance of the body under the effect of extremely high frequency electromagnetic radiation of low intensity. *Biofizika* (2002) 47:71–7.
164. Diaz P, Hong BY, Frias-Lopez J, Dupuy AK, Angeloni M, Abusleme L, et al. Transplantation-associated long-term immunosuppression promotes oral colonization by potentially opportunistic pathogens without impacting other members of the salivary bacteriome. *Clin Vaccine Immunol.* (2013) 20:920–30. doi: 10.1128/CVI.00734-12
165. Tatem AJ, Rogers DJ, Hay SI. Global transport networks and infectious disease spread. *Adv Parasitol.* (2006) 62:293–343. doi: 10.1016/S0065-308X(05)62009-X
166. Jansen W, Woudstra S, Müller A, Grabowski N, Schoo G, Gerulat B. The safety and quality of pork and poultry meat imports for the common European market received at border inspection post Hamburg Harbour between 2014 and 2015. *PLoS ONE* (2018) 13:e0192550. doi: 10.1371/journal.pone.0192550
167. Feazel LM, Baumgartner LK, Peterson KL, Frank DN, Harris JK, Pace NR. Opportunistic pathogens enriched in showerhead biofilms. *Proc Natl Acad Sci USA.* (2009) 106:16393–9. doi: 10.1073/pnas.0908446106
168. Sapkota AR, Berger S, Vogel TM. Human pathogens abundant in the bacterial metagenome of cigarettes. *Environ Health Perspect.* (2010) 118:351–6. doi: 10.1289/ehp.0901201
169. Twisk FN. The status of and future research into Myalgic Encephalomyelitis and Chronic Fatigue Syndrome: the need of accurate diagnosis, objective assessment, and acknowledging biological and clinical subgroups. *Front Physiol.* (2014) 5:109. doi: 10.3389/fphys.2014.00109
170. Lantos PM. Chronic Lyme disease. *Infect Dis Clin North Am.* (2015) 29:325–40. doi: 10.1016/j.idc.02.006
171. Halpin P, Williams MV, Klimas NG, Fletcher MA, Barnes Z, Ariza ME. Myalgic encephalomyelitis/chronic fatigue syndrome and gulf war illness patients exhibit increased humoral responses to the herpesviruses-encoded dUTPase: Implications in disease pathophysiology. *J Med Virol.* (2017) 89:1636–45. doi: 10.1002/jmv.24810
172. Hakim A, De Wandele I, O'Callaghan C, Pocinki A, Rowe P. Chronic fatigue in Ehlers-Danlos syndrome-Hypermobile type. *Am J Med Genet C Semin Med Genet.* (2017) 175:175–80. doi: 10.1002/ajmg.c.31542
173. Castro-Marrero J, Faro M, Aliste L, Sáez-Francàs N, Calvo N, Martínez-Martínez A. Comorbidity in chronic fatigue syndrome/myalgic encephalomyelitis: a nationwide population-based cohort study. *Psychosomatics* (2017) 58:533–43. doi: 10.1016/j.psym.2017.04.010
174. Treib J, Grauer MT, Haass A, Langenbach J, Holzer G, Woessner R. Chronic fatigue syndrome in patients with Lyme borreliosis. *Eur Neurol.* (2000) 43:107–9. doi: 10.1159/000008144
175. Blomberg J, Gottfries CG, Elfaitouri A, Rizwan M, Rosén A. Infection elicited autoimmunity and myalgic encephalomyelitis/chronic fatigue syndrome: an explanatory model. *Front Immunol.* (2018) 9:229. doi: 10.3389/fimmu.2018.00229
176. Proal AD, Marshall TG. Re-framing the theory of autoimmunity in the era of the microbiome: persistent pathogens, autoantibodies, and molecular mimicry. *Discov Med.* (2018) 25:299–308.
177. Vojdani A, Vojdani E, Saidara E, Kharrazian D. Reaction of amyloid-β peptide antibody with different infectious agents involved in alzheimer's disease. *J Alzheimers Dis.* (2018) 63:847–60. doi: 10.3233/JAD-170961
178. Manfredo V, Hiltensperger M, Kumar V, Zegarra-Ruiz D, Dehner C, Khan N. Translocation of a gut pathobiont drives autoimmunity in mice and humans. *Science* (2018) 359:1156–61. doi: 10.1126/science.aar7201
179. Tuffs SW, Haeryfar SM, McCormick JK. Manipulation of innate and adaptive immunity by staphylococcal superantigens. *Pathogens* (2018) 7:E53. doi: 10.3390/pathogens7020053
180. Carabotti M, Scirocco A, Maselli M, Severi C. The gut-brain axis: interactions between enteric microbiota, central and enteric nervous systems. *Ann Gastroenterol.* (2015) 28:203–9.
181. Mayer EA. Gut feelings: the emerging biology of gut-brain communication. *Nat Rev Neurosci.* (2011) 12:453–66. doi: 10.1038/nrn307
182. Soscia SJ, Kirby JE, Washicosky KJ, Tucker SM, Ingelsson M, Hyman B, et al. The Alzheimer's disease-associated amyloid beta-protein is an antimicrobial peptide. *PLoS ONE* (2010) 5:e9505. doi: 10.1371/journal.pone.0009505
183. Pasupuleti M, Roupe M, Rydengård V, Surewicz K, Surewicz WK, Chalupka A, et al. Antimicrobial activity of human prion protein is mediated by its N-terminal region. *PLoS ONE* (2009) 4:e7358. doi: 10.1371/journal.pone.0007358
184. Kumar DK, Choi SH, Washicosky KJ, Eimer WA, Tucker S, Ghofrani J, et al. Amyloid-β peptide protects against microbial infection in mouse and worm models of Alzheimer's disease. *Sci Transl Med.* (2016) 8:340ra72. doi: 10.1126/scitranslmed.aaf1059
185. Eimer WA, Vijaya Kumar DK, Navalpur Shanmugam NK, Rodriguez AS, Mitchell T, Washicosky KJ, et al. Alzheimer's disease-associated β-amyloid is rapidly seeded by herpesviridae to protect against brain infection. *Neuron* (2018) 99:56–63.e3. doi: 10.1016/j.neuron.2018.06.030
186. Itzhaki RF, Lathe R, Balin BJ, Ball MJ, Bearer EL, Braak H. Microbes and Alzheimer's disease. *J Alzheimers Dis.* (2016) 51:979–84. doi: 10.3233/JAD-160152
187. Zeineh MM, Kang J, Atlas SW, Raman MM, Reiss AL, Norris JL, et al. Right arcuate fasciculus abnormality in chronic fatigue syndrome. *Radiology* (2015) 274:517–26. doi: 10.1148/radiol.14141079
188. Gottlieb B, Chalifour LE, Mitmaker B, Sheiner N, Obrand D, Abraham C. BAK1 gene variation and abdominal aortic aneurysms. *Hum Mutat.* (2009) 30:1043–7. doi: 10.1002/humu.21046

189. Ursini G, Punzi G, Chen Q, Marenco S, Robinson J, Porcelli A, et al. Convergence of placenta biology and genetic risk for schizophrenia. *Nat Med.* (2018) 24:792–801. doi: 10.1038/s41591-018-0021-y
190. Harley JB, Chen X, Pujato M, Miller D, Maddox A, Forney C, et al. Transcription factors operate across disease loci, with EBNA2 implicated in autoimmunity. *Nat Genet.* (2018) 50:699–707. doi: 10.1038/s41588-018-0102-3
191. Proal AD, Albert PJ, Marshall TG. The human microbiome and autoimmunity. *Curr Opin Rheumatol.* (2013) 25:234–40. doi: 10.1097/BOR.0b013e32835cedbf
192. Kell DB, Pretorius E. On the translocation of bacteria and their lipopolysaccharides between blood and peripheral locations in chronic, inflammatory diseases: the central roles of LPS and LPS-induced cell death. *Integr Biol.* (2015) 7:1339–77. doi: 10.1039/c5ib00158g
193. Sharma SK, Soneja M. HIV & immune reconstitution inflammatory syndrome (IRIS). *Indian J Med Res.* (2011) 134:866–77. doi: 10.4103/0971-5916.92632
194. Maude S, Barrett D, Teachey DT, Grupp SA. Managing cytokine release syndrome associated with novel T cell-engaging therapies. *Cancer J.* (2014) 20:119–22. doi: 10.1097/PPO.0000000000000035
195. Arando M, Fernandez-Naval C, Mota-Foix M, Alvarez A, Armegol P, Barberá MJ, et al. The Jarisch-Herxheimer reaction in syphilis: could molecular typing help to understand it better? *J Eur Acad Dermatol Venereol.* (2018). 32:1791–5. doi: 10.1111/jdv.15078.
196. Farmer TW. Jarisch-herxheimer reaction in early syphilis. *JAMA* (1948) 138:480–5. doi: 10.1001/jama.1948.02900070012003
197. Meintjes G, Rabie H,., Wilkinson RJ, Cotton MF. Tuberculosis-associated immune reconstitution inflammatory syndrome and unmasking of tuberculosis by antiretroviral therapy. *Clin Chest Med.* (2009) 30:797–810. doi: 10.1016/j.ccm.2009.08.013
198. Müller M, Wandel S, Colebunders R, Attia S, Furrer H, Egger M. IeDEA Southern and Central Africa Immune reconstitution inflammatory syndrome in patients starting antiretroviral therapy for HIV infection: a systematic review and meta-analysis. *Lancet Infect Dis.* (2010) 10:251–61. doi: 10.1016/S1473-3099(10) 70026-8
199. Proal AD, Albert PJ, Marshall TG, Blaney GP, Lindseth IA. Immunostimulation in the treatment for chronic fatigue syndrome/myalgic encephalomyelitis. *Immunol Res.* (2013) 56:398–412. doi: 10.1007/s12026-013-8413-z
200. Proal AD, Albert PJ, Blaney GP, Lindseth IA, Benediktsson C, Marshall TG. Immunostimulation in the era of the metagenome. *Cell Mol Immunol.* (2011) 8:213–25. doi: 10.1038/cmi.2010.77
201. Shimabukuro-Vornhagen A, Gödel P, Subklewe M, Stemmler H, Schlößer H, Schlaak M. Cytokine release syndrome. *J Immunother Cancer* (2018) 6:56. doi: 10.1186/s40425-018-0343-9
202. Roberts E, Wessely S, Chalder T, Chang CK, Hotopf M. Mortality of people with chronic fatigue syndrome: a retrospective cohort study in England and Wales from the South London and Maudsley NHS Foundation Trust Biomedical Research Centre (SLaM BRC) Clinical Record Interactive Search (CRIS) Register. *Lancet* (2016) 387:1638–43. doi: 10.1016/S0140-6736(15) 01223-4

5

Impaired Health-Related Quality of Life in Adolescent Myalgic Encephalomyelitis/ Chronic Fatigue Syndrome: The Impact of Core Symptoms

*Maria Roma, Colleen L. Marden, Marissa A. K. Flaherty, Samantha E. Jasion, Erica M. Cranston and Peter C. Rowe**

Division of General Pediatrics and Adolescent Medicine, Department of Pediatrics, Johns Hopkins University School of Medicine, Baltimore, MD, United States

***Correspondence:**
Peter C. Rowe
prowe@jhmi.edu

Objective: The objectives of this study were to compare the health-related quality of life (HRQOL) of a North American population of adolescents and young adults with myalgic encephalomyelitis/chronic fatigue syndrome (ME/CFS) to (1) healthy controls (HC), (2) adolescents with ME/CFS in other countries, and (3) other forms of pediatric chronic illness, and (4) to examine the influence of the core illness symptoms in the Institute of Medicine (IOM) case definition on impaired HRQOL.

Study design: Cross-sectional study comparing individuals with ME/CFS referred to a tertiary care Chronic Fatigue clinic and HC. Eligible participants were age 10–30 years and met the Fukuda criteria for CFS. HC were eligible if they were age 10–30 years, with self-reported good, very good, or excellent general health. Pediatric HRQOL was measured using the PedsQL (Pediatric Quality of Life Inventory) and other validated instruments.

Results: We enrolled 55 consecutive ME/CFS patients (46 F) aged 10–23 years. From a pool of 69 potential HC we selected 55 with similar age and gender distribution for comparison. The total and subscale scores on the PedsQL and on all other measures of HRQOL indicated significantly worse function among those with ME/CFS (all $P < 0.001$). The self-reported frequency of post-exertional malaise (PEM) was significantly associated with the severity of impaired HRQOL ($P < 0.001$). Cognitive impairment had a weaker association with the PedsQL score ($P = 0.02$). Orthostatic intolerance was present in 96% of the ME/CFS population. Of the 55 who satisfied the Fukuda criteria, 47 (85%) also satisfied the IOM criteria for the diagnosis. Those meeting the IOM criteria had worse PedsQL total scores than those meeting just the Fukuda criteria ($P < 0.001$).

Conclusions: HRQOL was substantially lower in an ambulatory population of adolescents and young adults with ME/CFS than for healthy controls in North America, consistent with reports from other continents. HRQOL was also lower in ME/CFS than has been described in children with asthma, diabetes mellitus, epilepsy, eosinophilic gastroenteritis, and cystic fibrosis. The findings of this study lend further support to the inclusion of PEM, cognitive impairment, and orthostatic intolerance as core symptoms of pediatric ME/CFS.

Keywords: myalgic encephalomyelitis, chronic fatigue syndrome, health-related quality of life, orthostatic intolerance, post-exertional malaise

INTRODUCTION

Myalgic encephalomyelitis/chronic fatigue syndrome (ME/CFS) is a serious, complex, multisystem disorder (1, 2). Regardless of the criteria used to make the diagnosis, ME/CFS is characterized by a substantial impairment in previously tolerated levels of activity (1, 3–7). A relatively small number of studies have compared the health-related quality of life (HRQOL) in pediatric ME/CFS to that of healthy children. These studies have used different ME/CFS case definitions and different measures of overall function (8–11). In this study, we used data collected as part of the Johns Hopkins Pediatric CFS cohort study to compare the HRQOL in our population to healthy controls, to those with ME/CFS in European and Australian samples, and to published results in other pediatric chronic illnesses.

Most research on pediatric ME/CFS has been conducted using either a broad definition of CFS that requires the new onset of three or more months of disabling, unexplained fatigue, (4) or the International Chronic Fatigue Syndrome Study Group criteria for the illness, often termed the Fukuda criteria (3). The Fukuda criteria require at least 6 months of unexplained fatigue, together with the concurrent presence (for at least 6 months) of four of eight symptom criteria (unrefreshing sleep, self-reported impairment in short-term memory or concentration, sore throat, tender cervical or axillary lymph glands, muscle pain, multi-joint pain without joint swelling or redness, headaches of a new type, pattern, or severity, and post-exertional malaise [PEM] lasting more than 24 h). PEM refers to the exacerbation of fatigue but also other symptoms following increased physical or cognitive effort. Data from pediatric ME/CFS studies in the last 25 years have emphasized the frequency and clinical impact of PEM (12–14). In part to reflect the prevalence of PEM in clinical samples, revised expert consensus definitions for the illness have regarded PEM as an essential symptom without which ME/CFS should not be diagnosed (1, 5–7). In the most recent of the case definitions, a committee of the United States Institute of Medicine (IOM) conducted a review of the evidence on major ME/CFS symptoms and manifestations. The committee proposed that the main criteria for the diagnosis should be (1) a substantial reduction or impairment in the ability to engage in pre-illness levels of activity, persisting for more than 6 months and accompanied by new-onset fatigue, (2) post-exertional malaise, (3) unrefreshing sleep, and either (4a) cognitive impairment or (4b) orthostatic intolerance. The IOM committee recommended that the diagnosis of ME/CFS be questioned if these features were not present at least half the time and with at least moderate severity (1).

Operationalizing the IOM criteria requires further work, especially in pediatrics, as children might not be aware that certain symptoms are abnormal, and might not be able to attribute a specific grade of severity to each individual symptom. Because only one pediatric study thus far has examined the IOM criteria in detail (15), two additional objectives of the current investigation were to determine the proportion of study participants who met the Fukuda criteria alone vs. the Fukuda and IOM criteria, and to examine the relationship between overall impairment in HRQOL and the specific core criteria in the IOM definition.

METHODS

Participants

Consecutive individuals with ME/CFS were included if they had been referred to the Johns Hopkins Children's Center Chronic Fatigue Clinic between October 2008 and December 2012, were age 10–30 years, and satisfied the 1994 International Chronic Fatigue Syndrome Study Group criteria (3). Participants with ME/CFS entered the study with the expectation that they would be followed and treated clinically for 2 years. Individuals with primary depression who were referred by psychiatrists for evaluation of chronic fatigue were excluded, but those who had developed depression sometime after the onset of ME/CFS were included.

A pool of controls was recruited simultaneously with ME/CFS patients during the course of 4 years. Healthy controls (HC) in the same age range were eligible if they reported good, very good, or excellent general health. HC were recruited using information sheets and posted notices in the same pediatric specialty clinic area that houses the Chronic Fatigue Clinic. The majority of recruited controls consisted of the healthy offspring of health professionals employed at Johns Hopkins Children's Center, the friends of those children, and healthy family members and friends of the ME/CFS participants.

Both cases and controls were excluded if they had conditions or treatments expected to interfere with range of motion measurement, which was a separate focus of the study, as described elsewhere (16, 17). Controls were excluded if they had a self-reported condition often associated with chronic fatigue including ME/CFS, postural tachycardia syndrome (POTS), neurally mediated hypotension (NMH), fibromyalgia, recurrent syncope, or other chronic health conditions that can contribute to fatigue. We excluded controls with major depression as measured by a T-score >65 on the Child Depression Inventory (18, 19) or a score >13 on the Beck Depression Inventory (20, 21). The study was approved by the Institutional Review Board of the Johns Hopkins Medical Institutes. Written, informed consent was obtained from participants or their parents as appropriate.

Study Measures

Participants completed the following questionnaires about their general health at study entry:

1. Pediatric Quality of Life Inventory (PedsQL): The PedsQL is a brief, 23-item, multidimensional child self-report instrument for measuring HRQOL (22). The 23-item assessment examines how much of a problem the child has experienced in the past month with health and activities, feelings, ability to get along with others (which includes social relations, and stamina), and school functioning (cognition, attendance). Responses to each item range from 0 (never) to 4 (almost always). Raw scores are transformed to total scores that range from 0 to 100, with higher scores indicating better quality of life. Five subscales within the PedsQL address physical, emotional, social, school, and psychosocial functioning. The questionnaire is available in age-appropriate formats (Child Report for ages 8–12, Teen Report for 13–18, or Young Adult for 18–24 years). This instrument is reliable, valid and commonly used in pediatric ME/CFS and other pediatric chronic illness populations (10, 11, 23, 24).
2. Functional Disability Inventory (FDI): This one-page, 15-item self-report instrument for children and adolescents asks whether in the past 2 weeks respondents had any physical trouble or difficulty doing specific activities, such as walking up stairs, being at school all day, walking the length of a football field, or going shopping (25). Responses are scored as: 0 = no trouble, 1 = a little trouble, 2 = some trouble, 3 = a lot of trouble, 4 = impossible. The total score ranges from zero (no difficulty with any activity) to 60 (all activities impossible). The FDI has good reliability and validity. It has been used to study a variety of pediatric health problems, including chronic pain and ME/CFS (8, 26, 27).
3. Wood Mental Fatigue Inventory (WMFI): This questionnaire asks subjects to rate the frequency of nine mental fatigue symptoms in the past month on a Likert scale ranging from not at all (0) to very much (4). Higher scores indicate worse cognitive difficulty (28). This measure has been shown to discriminate effectively between ME/CFS patients who are ill and ME/CFS patients who have recovered (29), to correlate with overall well-being in adolescents and adults with ME/CFS (30), and to correlate with the degree of reported brain fog among those with postural tachycardia syndrome (31).
4. Child Depression Inventory (CDI): This 27 item, self-administered instrument measures the mood of the respondent over the preceding 2 weeks (18). The measure assesses behavioral and cognitive signs of depression, applicable to pediatric populations aged 7–17 years. Scores on the 27 items are ranked from 0 (best) to 2 (worst). T-scores of 65 or higher are considered clinically significant (19).
5. Beck Depression Inventory II (BDI): This self-administered, 21-item scale of depression has been validated in adolescents age 13 and older (20). Respondents rank the severity of individual symptoms of depression (including sadness, loss of pleasures, guilty feelings, self-dislike, indecisiveness, loss of energy, concentration difficulty, and fatigue) on a 0–3 scale. Scores of 14–19, 20–28, and 29–63 indicate mild, moderate, and severe depression, respectively (21).
6. PedsQL Multidimensional Fatigue Scale (MFS): This brief, one-page questionnaire measures how much of a problem individuals have had with specific tasks that reflect general fatigue, sleep and rest, and cognitive fatigue, and total fatigue over the preceding month (32). The questionnaire is valid for patients aged 13–18, as well as for college-aged populations (33). Responses on the 18 items range from 0, never a problem, to 4, almost always a problem. As with the PedsQL, the MFS raw scores are transformed to a 0 to 100 scale, with higher scores indicating less fatigue.
7. ME/CFS Symptom Assessment: All participants responded to a study questionnaire that assessed the frequency of Fukuda criteria CFS symptoms as well as lightheadedness in the 2 weeks before study enrollment. Possible responses for the frequency of lightheadedness, fatigue, body aches, joint aches, headaches, or trouble thinking, remembering, or concentrating, were: (a) all day long, every day, (b) several times a day, every day, (c) once or twice a day, every day, (d) several times a week, but not every day, (e) once or twice a week, (f) I haven't had [this symptom]. For the frequency of sore throats and tender glands, possible responses were: (a) every day, (b) more than 5 days but not every day, (c) a few days (2–5), (d) once, or (e) I have not had [this symptom]. For post-exertional malaise (PEM), we focused on physical activity as the trigger, and asked: "In the last 2 weeks, after mild exercise how often have you felt prolonged fatigue or a feeling of illness that lasts longer than 24 h?" Possible responses were (a) 4 or more times, (b) 2 to 3 times, (c) once, (d) never. For unrefreshing sleep, we asked, "In the last 2 weeks, upon awakening after a night's sleep how frequently have you felt refreshed?" Possible responses included (a) all of the time, (b) most of the time, (c) some of the time, (d) none of the time.

Other Measurement Criteria

Onset of ME/CFS

We categorized the type of onset for ME/CFS as abrupt, abrupt on gradual, or gradual. We deemed the onset abrupt if the symptoms emerged over several days in conjunction with an apparent infectious illness or other acute event, abrupt on gradual if individuals had a gradual onset of symptoms together with a marked exacerbation in association with an apparent infectious illness or other acute event, and gradual if there had been no abrupt or acute change at the onset of symptoms.

Measurement of IOM Criteria

To operationalize the IOM criterion for a substantial reduction or impairment in the ability to engage in pre-illness levels of activity, we used a frequency of fatigue occurring at least several days per week, and either a PedsQL total score or an FDI score that was >2 SD worse than the mean reported by HC in this study. To operationalize PEM, we used a self-reported frequency of at least once over 2 weeks for prolonged fatigue or the feeling of illness after mild exercise. Unrefreshing sleep had to be present most or all of the time. Cognitive impairment was measured as a self-reported frequency of difficulty thinking, remembering, or concentrating of several times per week or more, or a score on the WMFI or MFS cognitive subscale of >2 SD worse than the mean reported by HC.

Orthostatic intolerance was considered present if (a) self-reported lightheadedness occurred at least several times per week, (b) there was a history of recurrent syncope in the presence of a structurally normal heart, considered consistent with NMH (34) or (c) previous upright tilt testing or a passive standing testing (performed in patients not being treated with medications for orthostatic intolerance) had confirmed the presence of NMH or POTS. Among individuals not previously diagnosed with or under treatment for orthostatic intolerance, we conducted further orthostatic testing using a passive standing test, methods for the performance of which along with study definitions for POTS and NMH are described elsewhere (35).

Statistical Analysis

We compared the demographic and HRQOL measures between ME/CFS patients and healthy controls using independent samples *t*-tests or Chi-square tests and Fisher's exact tests depending on the type and distribution of the data. Responses on the symptom frequency questions for PEM, lightheadedness, and difficulty thinking and concentrating were trichotomized based on distributions that made clinical sense and created subgroups adequate for statistical comparison. We then compared these trichotomized symptom frequencies to the PedsQL total score or the FDI using one-way ANOVA; any significant differences between groups were then explored further using the *post-hoc* Bonferroni test. Statistical analyses were conducted using IBM Statistics SPSS version 25 (IBM Statistics, New York) and illustrations were prepared using GraphPad Prism version 7.00 for Windows (GraphPad Software, La Jolla, California, USA, www.graphpad.com). The analysis involved multiple comparisons, but not all comparisons were independent. To reduce the probability of a type I error, we considered a $P < 0.01$ as significant.

RESULTS

Study Population

Fifty-five consecutive participants who met the 1994 Fukuda criteria for ME/CFS (age range, 10–23 years) were included in this study. Over the study period, we recruited 69 HC. From that group, a research assistant blinded to the quality of life data selected 55 controls who were similar in age and gender to the ME/CFS patients. As shown in **Table 1**, 95% of the ME/CFS participants were white, and 84% female. Individuals with ME/CFS had been symptomatic for a median of 2 years before entry to the study (range, 7 months to 10 years). All were ambulatory; no participant was primarily bed-bound.

Twenty-five had developed ME/CFS symptoms abruptly in association with an apparent infectious illness or other acute event. An additional eight had an abrupt increase in the intensity of symptoms against a background of gradual development of some ME/CFS symptoms, while 22 had a gradual onset.

TABLE 1 | Demographic and clinical characteristics of the study participants.

	ME/CFS (*n* = 55)	HC (*n* = 55)	P
DEMOGRAPHIC VARIABLES			
Age, mean (SD)	16.5 (2.1)	17.1 (3.0)	0.25
Gender			1
Male	9	9	
Female	46	46	
Racial group			0.23
White	52	51	
American Indian	2	0	
Asian/Pacific Islander	1	2	
Other	0	2	
Hispanic			
No	55	52	
Yes	0	3	
TYPE OF ME/CFS ONSET (*n* = 55)			
Abrupt	25		
Gradual	22		
Abrupt on gradual	8		

Prevalence of Fukuda Features

Using cut-points that were closest to symptoms being present at least half the time, **Table 2** shows the rank order of the prevalence of Fukuda criteria symptoms for the 55 with ME/CFS and the 55 HC. As expected, those with ME/CFS had greater self-reported prevalence of all symptoms compared to HC. Of note, those with ME/CFS were most likely to report fatigue, unrefreshing sleep, PEM, and cognitive impairment, and were least likely to report sore throat, joint aches, and tender glands. Among controls, 15–20% endorsed unrefreshing sleep, body and joint pain, lightheadedness, and headaches several times per week.

HRQOL Comparisons Between ME/CFS Participants and Healthy Controls

Of the 55 with ME/CFS, 21 (38%) had changed from regular schooling due to their symptoms: seven (13%) had switched from full-time to part-time schooling, and 14 (25%) had received home tutoring. **Figure 1** shows that the PedsQL total and subscale scores were significantly lower for those with ME/CFS than for healthy individuals (all $P < 0.001$). As displayed in **Table 3**, the scores on all other measures showed significantly worse HRQOL for those with ME/CFS than for healthy controls ($P < 0.001$).

The study design excluded controls if they met criteria for depression, invalidating comparisons with the ME/CFS group. Of those with ME/CFS, 54/55 completed the BDI, the mean (SD) score for which was 15.3 (7.6). Forty-three percent had scores <14, 31% had scores from 14 to 19, 20% had scores from 20 to 28, and 6% had scores of 29 or higher. One child who was too young to complete the BDI had a normal CDI score. There was a significant negative correlation of the BDI with the PedsQL total score ($r = -0.68$; $P < 0.001$). Seven of the 46 (15%) who completed the CDI had T-scores in the clinically significant range of ≥ 65.

TABLE 2 | Comparison of self-reported frequency of Fukuda criteria symptoms in the preceding 2 weeks.

	ME/CFS (n = 55)(%)	HC (n = 55)(%)	P
FUKUDA CRITERIA			
Fatigue (several times/week or more)	100	5	<0.001
Unrefreshing sleep (most/all of the time)	98	18	<0.001
Post-exertional malaise (at least once in 2 weeks)	95	7	<0.001
Cognitive impairment (at least several times/week)	82	2	<0.001
Headache (several times/week or more)	77	18	<0.001
Body pain (several times/week or more)	69	20	<0.001
Sore throat (at least once/week)	51	7	<0.001
Joint aches (several times/week or more)	44	20	0.01
Tender glands (at least once/week)	40	2	<0.001

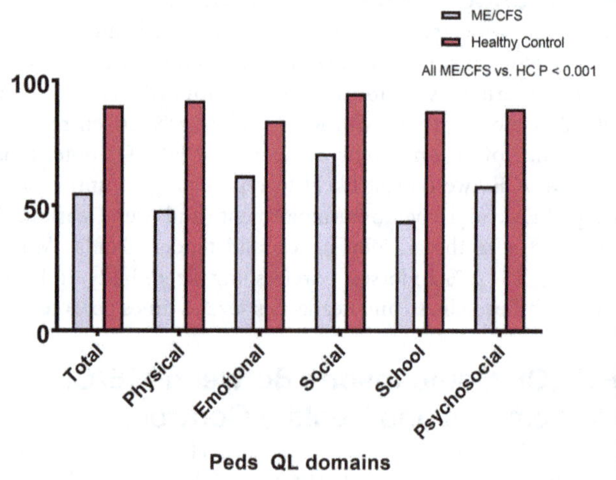

FIGURE 1 | PedsQL total and subscale scores for those with ME/CFS and healthy controls.

HRQOL Comparisons With Other Pediatric ME/CFS Studies

Table 4 illustrates the scores for the ME/CFS participants and HC from other studies that use the PedsQL to measure HRQOL in this illness. The PedsQL total score was slightly lower for the study populations from Norway and Australia than for our cohort. The relative pattern of subscale results was similar for those with ME/CFS participants in all studies, identifying relatively lower results for school function, and physical function than for social or emotional function.

The mean *(SD)* FDI score in this study was 21 (10), which was similar to the means of 24.0 (9.2) and 23.1 (9.2) for the 60 Norwegian ME/CFS adolescents in each group randomized to clonidine or placebo, respectively (27). Among 68 HC in that study, the mean FDI score was 1.6 (3.1). These results were also similar to the mean score of 24 in a sample of 20 with ME/CFS reported from the UK (8).

TABLE 3 | HRQOL comparisons for the FDI, MFS, and WMFI scales.

	ME/CFS *(n = 55)*	HC *(n = 55)*	*P*-value
FDI	21 (10)	2 (3)	<0.001
MFS			
Fatigue total	40 (18)	85 (12)	<0.001
Fatigue cognitive	52 (24)	89 (13)	<0.001
Fatigue sleep	34 (18)	77 (15)	<0.001
Fatigue general	34 (19)	89 (12)	<0.001
WMFI	14 (9)	2 (3)	<0.001

HC, healthy controls; FDI, Functional Disability Inventory; MFS, PedsQL Multidimensional Fatigue Scale; WMFI, Wood Mental Fatigue Inventory.

TABLE 4 | Comparison of PedsQL total and subscale scores with other pediatric ME/CFS studies.

	Roma ME/CFS *(n = 55)*	Winger* ME/CFS *(n = 120)*	Knight‡ ME/CFS *(n = 42)*	Roma HC *(n = 55)*	Winger HC *(n = 39)*
Total PedsQL	55 (15)	49 (13)	49 (15)	90 (10)	93 (8)
Physical	48 (17)	37 (17)	42 (23)	92 (9)	96 (8)
Emotional	62 (22)	60 (18)	57 (21)	84 (17)	88 (14)
Social	71 (20)	70 (15)	66 (18)	95 (9)	98 (4)
School	44 (20)	36 (19)	31 (17)	88 (12)	88 (14)
Psychosocial	58 (17)	57 (15)	51 (14)	89 (12)	91 (10)

**Data from Winger et al. (10).*
‡Data from Knight et al. (11).

Relationship of PEM, Cognitive Impairment, and Lightheadedness to HRQOL

To further investigate the interaction between the proposed core ME/CFS criteria and HRQOL, we examined whether greater frequencies of PEM, cognitive impairment, and lightheadedness were associated with worse scores on the various measures. **Figure 2A** shows that those reporting more frequent PEM in the preceding 2 weeks had significantly lower scores on the PedsQL (ANOVA F score = 10.73; $P = 0.0001$). *Post-hoc* comparisons using the Bonferroni test indicated that PedsQL scores were lower in those reporting PEM at least four times in 2 weeks than those reporting PEM 0-1 time ($P < 0.001$) or 2–3 times ($P = 0.001$), but not significantly different between those reporting PEM 2–3 times and 0–1 time ($P = 0.78$).

A significant association was also present for the relationship between the frequency of PEM in the past 2 weeks and scores on the FDI (**Figure 2B**) (ANOVA F score = 26.1; $P < 0.0001$). *Post-hoc* comparisons using the Bonferroni test indicated that

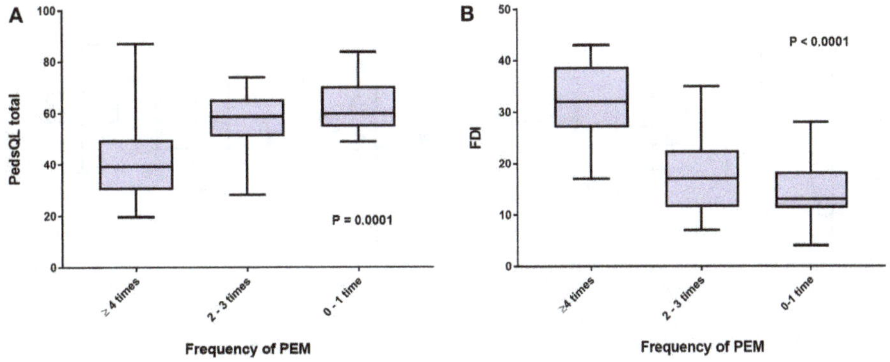

FIGURE 2 | HRQOL measured by **(A)**, Peds QL total score, and **(B)**, FDI, according to self-reported frequency of post-exertional malaise (PEM) in the preceding 2 weeks.

FDI score was lower in those reporting PEM at least four times in 2 weeks than those reporting PEM 0–1 time ($P < 0.001$) or 2–3 times ($P < 0.001$), but not significantly different between those reporting PEM 2–3 times and 0–1 time ($P = 0.18$).

As shown in **Figure 3A**, the relationship of cognitive impairment with the PedsQL total score was weaker (ANOVA F score = 4.55; $P = 0.02$), as was the relation between the frequency of lightheadedness and the PedsQL total score (**Figure 3B**; ANOVA F score = 2.72; $P = 0.08$).

Measuring the IOM Criteria

Table 5 shows the prevalence of impaired function, unrefreshing sleep, PEM, cognitive impairment, and orthostatic intolerance according to the methods we used for operationalizing the IOM criteria. Along with self-reported frequency of unrefreshing sleep, PEM, and the other core symptoms, we defined a substantial impairment in function as a questionnaire score that was 2 SD worse than the mean of healthy controls for the PedsQL (scores of 70 or below) or the FDI (scores of eight or higher). To supplement the self-reported frequency of trouble thinking and concentrating, we also used score of 2 SD worse than the mean for healthy controls on the WMFI (scores >8) or the MFS (scores of <63).

Of those with ME/CFS, 82% reported a frequency of cognitive impairment (difficulty thinking and concentrating) of at least several times per week vs. just 2% of healthy controls. Combining the self-reported symptom frequency with a WMFI or MFS cognitive subscale >2 SD worse than the mean for healthy controls identified six additional ME/CFS participants and five additional controls as meeting the criteria for trouble thinking and concentrating. As expected, there was a strong negative correlation between the WMFI scores and the cognitive subscale of the PedsQL MFS ($r = -0.90$; $P < 0.001$).

Lightheadedness at least several times per week was endorsed by 42/55 (76%) of those with ME/CFS. Four others who reported lightheadedness 1–2 times per week or less met other criteria for orthostatic intolerance: two had been diagnosed with NMH before study entry and were being treated with fludrocortisone at the time of the symptom questionnaire, and two others had a history of recurrent syncope in the presence of a structurally normal heart and were being treated with an increased intake of sodium and fluids at the time of questionnaire completion. Among the nine remaining participants with ME/CFS whose questionnaire responses indicated a frequency of lightheadedness of 1–2 times per week or less, one adolescent reported a discrepant history during the clinical interview, describing a daily "head rush" (identical to lightheadedness) with postural changes. She was therefore re-classified. Thus, 84% met the study criteria for orthostatic intolerance using the criteria of

TABLE 5 | Prevalence of Institute of Medicine ME/CFS criteria.

	ME/CFS ($n = 55$)(%)	HC ($n = 55$)(%)	P
1. Substantially impaired function			
Fatigue (several times/week or more)	100	5	<0.001
FDI or PedsQL >2 SD worse than mean scores for HC*	96	7	
2. Unrefreshing sleep (most/all of the time)	98	18	<0.001
3. Post-exertional malaise (at least once in 2 weeks)	95	7	<0.001
4.a. Cognitive impairment			
Trouble thinking and concentrating (several times/week or more)	82	2	<0.001
Symptom frequency plus WMFI or MFS cognitive subscale > 2 SD worse than mean for HC*	93	11	
4.b. Orthostatic intolerance			
LH (several times/week or more)	76	15	<0.001
LH frequency plus pre-study diagnosis/treatment of OI	84	15	<0.001

**P-values not computed because of the >2SD method of operationalizing the criterion. HC, healthy controls; FDI, Functional Disability Inventory; PedsQL, Pediatric Quality of Life Inventory; WMFI, Wood Mental Fatigue Inventory; MFS, PedsQL Multidimensional Fatigue Scale; LH, lightheadedness; OI, orthostatic intolerance.*

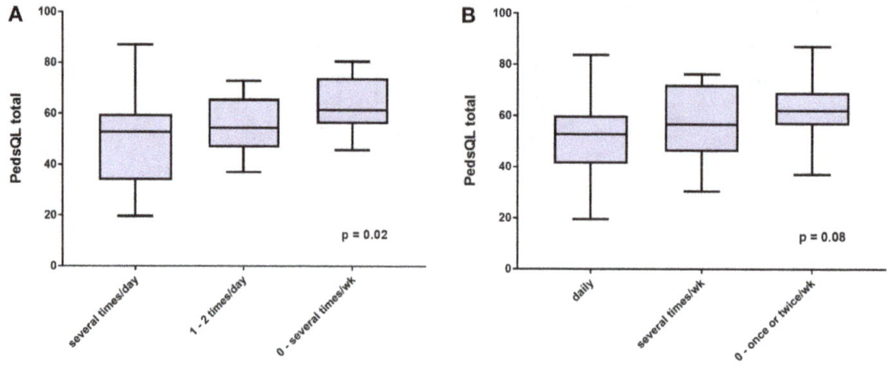

FIGURE 3 | HRQOL measured by PedsQL total score according to **(A)**, self-reported frequency of trouble thinking and concentrating, and **(B)**, self-reported frequency of lightheadedness, both in the preceding 2 weeks.

frequent lightheadedness and a prior diagnosis or treatment of orthostatic intolerance.

The remaining eight participants underwent a 10 min passive standing test; four were receiving no vasoactive medications at the time of testing, and four were being treated with one or more medications that had some potential to affect the HR and BP responses to orthostatic testing (amitriptyline for headaches [$n = 1$], stimulant medications for attention deficit disorder [$n = 1$], selective serotonin or serotonin/norepinephrine reuptake inhibitors for anxiety or low mood [$n = 2$], and oral contraceptives [$n = 1$]). Of the four medication-naïve participants, two developed POTS during the 10-min standing test, each with a 50 beat per min increase in HR while upright, and a third became presyncopal at the 6-min point of upright posture, consistent with NMH. All four had worsening or provocation of their typical chronic orthostatic or ME/CFS symptoms during the period of standing (most commonly increased fatigue, lightheadedness, and warmth). Of the four who were being treated with vasoactive medications, three developed POTS and increased symptoms, and the fourth reported increased orthostatic symptoms only during the passive standing test. In all, 96% had evidence of orthostatic intolerance if those who developed POTS or NMH during the standing test were added.

Proportion Satisfying the IOM Criteria

Forty-seven of the 55 participants (85%) who met the Fukuda criteria also satisfied the IOM criteria. Although all who met the Fukuda criteria reported fatigue several times per week or more, and all had some reduction of their pre-illness activity levels, when we applied the formal study criteria for a substantial reduction, two participants did not have a PedsQL or FDI score more than 2 SD below the mean of the healthy controls. A third participant reported refreshing sleep most of the time. Three further individuals did not endorse PEM. Two additional participants met all other criteria except for cognitive impairment or the study criteria for orthostatic intolerance. These eight who satisfied the Fukuda criteria but not the IOM criteria had significantly better scores than the 47 who met both the Fukuda and the IOM criteria on the PedsQL [70 (7) vs. 53 (15), $P <$ 0.001], and on the MFS [59 (15) vs. 36 (17), $P = 0.001$]. There were marginally non-significant differences on the FDI [13 (7) vs. 22 (10), P = 0.01], the WMFI [8 (7) vs. 15 (9), $P = 0.03$], and the BDI [10 (6) vs. 16 (7); $P = 0.03$].

DISCUSSION

HRQOL in ME/CFS

The results of this study provide further confirmation of earlier reports that adolescents and young adults with ME/CFS have a significantly lower HRQOL than their healthy peers. The mean PedsQL total score in this North American population is similar to the results reported by Knight et al. in Australia using the Fukuda criteria and by Winger et al. in Norway using a broad case definition (10, 11). The scores on the FDI were also similar to findings from the large study of 120 adolescents in Norway (27) and a small study of 20 in the United Kingdom (8), both of which employed a broad case definition. Although the participants in our study had slightly better overall function as measured by the total PedsQL scores at enrollment, there was a consistency in the distribution of PedsQL subscale scores across the three studies using that measure: all reported less impairment in the social and emotional domains of the PedsQL, and greater impairment in the domains measuring physical function and school function. The low scores on HRQOL confirm the findings of Kennedy et al. using the Child Health Questionnaire to assess 25 UK children who met the Fukuda criteria. In that study, scores on limitations due to physical health problems were lower than scores reporting limitations due to emotional or behavioral difficulties (9).

One objective of the study was to situate the HRQOL results for those with ME/CFS within the context of other chronic pediatric health conditions. The PedsQL has been used to measure overall function in many chronic pediatric illnesses, allowing comparison across diagnoses (23, 24). The mean (SD) PedsQL total score for those with ME/CFS in our study [55 (16)] was lower than the reported scores for North American children with cystic fibrosis [80 (14)], eosinophilic gastrointestinal disorder [68 (14)], epilepsy [76 (14)], type 1 diabetes [74 (16)], sickle cell disease [70 (18)], and renal transplants [75 (15)] (24), and comparable to pediatric fibromyalgia [56 (16)] and diplegic cerebral palsy [54 (13)] (23). One methodological caveat is that the PedsQL scores were not obtained at the same point of treatment for all chronic conditions, so direct statistical comparisons would be misleading. Treatment of ME/CFS had been initiated in only some of our patients at the time of administration of the PedsQL, whereas clinical samples of patients in the other studies likely would have included individuals at different stages of the usual treatment of their conditions, therefore resulting in higher scores than at the outset of treatment. Nonetheless, even without incorporating the scores of severely impaired ME/CFS patients, who were unable to participate in clinic-based studies, the lower scores of the ME/CFS participants emphasize the profound degree of interference of the illness with normal activities in childhood.

A novel finding of this study is the correlation of impairment in HRQOL with the frequency of PEM, at least for an ambulatory population with ME/CFS. Prior investigations of the importance of PEM had compared its frequency in those with ME/CFS to healthy controls, but, surprisingly, to the best of our knowledge, no study had examined the association of PEM with the severity of impairment or HRQOL, or with the severity of specific symptoms. Such comparisons would be important as a test of whether PEM is a critical symptom that should be accounted for in illness definitions. In our study, as the frequency of PEM increased, the mean PedsQL score fell and the mean FDI score increased, consistent with a significant association of PEM with worse overall function. This relationship might not be expected to obtain for those who are bedbound, as they might be too ill to engage in much physical activity or might electively restrict their activities to avoid provoking this symptom. Although a limitation of our assessment of PEM was that we only asked about PEM induced by mild physical activity, the responses to this single question identified PEM in 95% of the study population. Future studies will need to examine the added yield of questions about PEM following varying degrees of cognitive, orthostatic, or neuromuscular stress (36–38).

Implications for Measuring Orthostatic Intolerance

An important aspect of the study methodology was that we included a comprehensive evaluation of orthostatic intolerance, incorporating the self-reported frequency of lightheadedness as well as a detailed clinical history and, where necessary, orthostatic testing. Although significantly more ME/CFS participants described lightheadedness several times per week or more compared to healthy controls [76 vs. 15%, $P < 0.001$], the prevalence of orthostatic intolerance increased to 84% when a history of recurrent syncope or prior positive orthostatic testing was included. A further 12% developed POTS or NMH in response to a 10-min passive standing test in clinic, all of whom reported provocation of their usual ME/CFS symptoms when standing. There is as yet no consensus on which of these criteria should be considered valid for confirming orthostatic intolerance. Among the caveats about orthostatic testing that need to be considered are that (1) the response to head-up tilt table testing can be abnormal in otherwise healthy individuals, some of whom develop hypotension or syncope during the procedure (30, 39), (2) as the current HR criteria for POTS are defined, approximately 5% of healthy adolescents would have at least a 40 bpm increase in heart rate during 10 min upright (39), some of whom might endorse chronic lightheadedness in daily life. We are unsure how many healthy individuals would develop increased orthostatic symptoms during a 10-min passive standing test, although the available data from tilt testing suggests this would be infrequent. Singer et al. reported that 8/106 (8%) of healthy controls developed orthostatic symptoms during a 10 min head-up tilt test, none of whom had a history of syncope or orthostatic symptoms (39). Moreover, chronic fatigue was reported by only 5% of the healthy controls in our study. Because healthy controls have a low prevalence of chronic orthostatic symptoms in daily life, and a low prevalence of orthostatic symptoms provoked during upright tilt, we would assume a similarly low rate of provocation of orthostatic symptoms in healthy adolescents during passive standing tests. These caveats notwithstanding, our results illustrate the potential for the prevalence of orthostatic intolerance to be underestimated if it is only measured by self-reported lightheadedness. Other questions that ask about orthostatic provocation of fatigue, PEM, difficulty thinking and concentrating, headache, pain, nausea, and warmth deserve further study to determine whether they add to the yield of lightheadedness as a reflection of orthostatic intolerance in ME/CFS. Taken together, the findings from this study provide further support for the inclusion of orthostatic intolerance in the case definition of ME/CFS, as was recommended in the IOM report.

Implications for ME/CFS Case Definitions

Our study findings have several implications for case definitions of pediatric ME/CFS. First, although the 1994 Fukuda criteria for CFS had included post-exertional malaise (PEM) as one of eight symptom criteria, four of which were needed to meet the illness definition, individuals could satisfy the Fukuda criteria without experiencing PEM. Subsequent ME/CFS case series have shown that PEM is described by 71–96% of adolescents with ME/CFS (12–14). The data from our study showing a significant correlation of PEM with overall HRQOL impairment provide further support for the inclusion of PEM in pediatric case definitions for the disorder.

Second, because the Fukuda criteria were published in 1994, and modern attention was only drawn to orthostatic intolerance as a common co-morbid problem in 1995 (30, 40), the Fukuda criteria did not mention lightheadedness as a qualifying diagnostic feature. While orthostatic intolerance is mentioned more explicitly in subsequent case definitions, the Canadian Consensus Criteria (CCC) did not require orthostatic intolerance to be present in order to satisfy the diagnosis in either adults or children (5, 6). The CCC require that individuals report one symptom from among two of the following three categories: autonomic, neuroendocrine, and immune manifestations. It would thus be possible to meet the CCC ME/CFS definition with "recurrent feelings of feverishness and cold extremities" (neuroendocrine) and "sore throat" (immune), without having lightheadedness or objective evidence of orthostatic intolerance. To qualify as having ME/CFS by meeting such vague and non-specific symptom criteria could lead to inclusion of conditions other than ME/CFS in studies. It remains to be seen whether the other qualifying criteria for the pediatric CCC (fatigue for at least 3 months, unrefreshing sleep, pain, and neurocognitive manifestations) capture the main features of the illness well-enough to make the inclusion of the CCC autonomic/neuroendocrine/immune criteria irrelevant, raising the question of whether the diagnostic criteria could be further simplified.

Second, the international ME criteria list orthostatic intolerance as one manifestation under the rubric of "energy production/transportation impairments." While impaired energy production could be a cause of orthostatic intolerance, impaired energy production is more likely to be a consequence of orthostatic intolerance, directly related to reduced blood flow, and reduced oxygen delivery to tissues. The international ME criteria require only one symptom or feature from among four categories that include cardiovascular, respiratory, loss of thermostatic stability, or intolerance of extremes of temperature. An individual could thus satisfy the ME criteria with intolerance of cold temperature and sweating episodes, without clear evidence of orthostatic intolerance. Given the high prevalence of orthostatic intolerance in pediatric ME/CFS, our data suggest that this symptom requires greater emphasis than it received in the CCC and ME criteria, at least for pediatric case definitions.

Third, the desire for clinicians to have a sensitive case definition that will identify the largest number of individuals (who might then benefit from treatment) conflicts with the desire for researchers to have a more specific, restrictive case definition that identifies those with more profound impairment and ostensibly a more "pure" form of the illness (1). This dilemma is complicated by the lack of scientific clarity regarding whether ME/CFS is a single, unitary condition, or a disorder that encompasses several overlapping conditions with multiple causes. Debates about these issues are unlikely to be resolved until a gold standard diagnostic test is developed. In the current study, the Fukuda criteria identified a slightly larger group than the IOM criteria. Those who met both the Fukuda and the IOM criteria had more severe impairment than those who met the Fukuda criteria alone. Our study proportion meeting the IOM criteria differs substantially from the proportion reported by Asprusten et al. In contrast to the 85% meeting IOM criteria in our study, only 45/114 (39%) of their participants who met the broad definition of pediatric CFS (3 months of unexplained fatigue that interfered with normal school attendance) satisfied the IOM criteria (15). The IOM positive and negative groups in the Asprusten study did not differ on baseline measures except for the depressive symptoms scores on the Mood and Feelings Questionnaire. The FDI and Peds QL scores for the IOM positive and negative groups were not reported; scores on both questionnaires for the overall group were comparable to our study results. Given the similarity in overall HRQOL in participants enrolled in each study, the magnitude of the difference in the prevalence of IOM-positive participants in our study and the Asprusten study is unlikely to be due to chance. Rather, the large difference in proportions meeting the IOM criteria suggest that variability in the methods for operationalizing the IOM definition were responsible for the differences. Our operational definition of PEM required that it occur at least once over 2 weeks, which was reported by only 7% of HC. We assumed that some patients might be restricting their activity sufficiently to avoid provoking PEM, and reasoned that a single episode of prolonged PEM confirmed the presence of that symptom. This might have resulted in a less restrictive criterion for PEM than in the Asprusten study, which required the endorsement of four separate questions on the symptom, illustrating the potential for marked variability in outcomes to result from differences in the way in which disease criteria are operationalized.

Fourth, as the level of functional impairment increased in our participants with ME/CFS, so did the scores on the Beck Depression Inventory. There was a strong negative correlation between the Peds QL and the BDI scores. This result is influenced by the ascertainment in the BDI of several somatic symptoms that would be consistent with ME/CFS. Even among individuals who are free of self-reproach, anhedonia, and depressed mood, respondents could score a up to 15 points on the BDI for items related to indecisiveness, concentration difficulty (cognitive impairment), loss of energy, changes in sleeping pattern, and tiredness or fatigue (fatigue, impaired function), all of which would be expected to be common in adolescents with ME/CFS. We did not measure the independent influence of ME/CFS and mood disorders on HRQOL, but other pediatric investigators have done so. In their population of adolescents with ME/CFS, Winger and colleagues found higher rates of depressed mood using the Mood and Feelings Questionnaire (10). Higher levels of depressive symptoms were associated with lower quality of life in both ME/CFS patients *and* healthy controls, but both depressive symptoms and having ME/CFS were independently associated with worse HRQOL (10). The BDI and other depression questionnaires can be helpful clinically to identify those with greater reporting of self-reproach, guilt, and lack of self-worth—all symptoms that would warrant a greater focus on the individual's affective response to chronic illness. However, the questionnaires cannot distinguish whether the depression preceded or was a secondary reaction to being chronically ill with ME/CFS. Other measures of depressed mood that rely less on overlapping somatic symptoms of ME/CFS deserve further attention in pediatric ME/CFS research, as has been suggested in the adult ME/CFS population (41). The Hospital Anxiety and Depression Scale, as used by other ME/CFS groups (11, 42) might demonstrate less co-linearity and be more appropriate for determining whether there is a true correlation of disease severity and affective state.

LIMITATIONS

This study had several limitations. Because patients were evaluated at a tertiary care center, participants might not be representative of the entire population with pediatric ME/CFS. Our study population would have excluded those at the severe end of the spectrum who were bed-bound and unable to attend frequent clinic visits. Inclusion of bed-bound individuals would have had the effect of further lowering the HRQOL scores. Conversely, we included some with mild ME/CFS who did not meet the more stringent IOM criteria for the illness, although all had some limitation in their overall ability to engage in pre-illness activities. The 2-year median duration of illness and the intensity of the pre-study treatment trials may have affected the scores of HRQOL measurements.

We cannot exclude the possibility of selection and referral biases. For example, our group's interest in orthostatic intolerance might have resulted in a greater referral of individuals suspected of having orthostatic intolerance; 33% had been tested for that diagnosis at enrollment. For the remainder, the clinical history clarified that most were unaware of the relationship of orthostatic intolerance to ME/CFS, and were not aware of the clinical features of POTS and NMH. Other studies that use the same ascertainment methods for orthostatic intolerance will be needed to confirm our results.

The use of a cut-off that was more than two SD worse than the mean scores for HC as the definition of substantial impairment in general function or of cognitive impairment is relatively conservative. Further study will be needed to determine whether this excludes too many who might meet ME/CFS disease criteria using other methods of operationalizing the illness, such as less stringent cut-points of 1.5 SD from the control means.

CONCLUSION

The current study confirms a marked impairment in HRQOL in North American adolescents and young adults compared to healthy controls. The HRQOL data were similar to those reported in European and Australian pediatric ME/CFS populations, regardless of which case definition is used. All studies of adolescents report substantially worse function than have been reported for children with other common chronic health impairments. Our study identified a strong correlation of overall HRQOL with the frequency of PEM as well as a >90% prevalence of cognitive impairment and orthostatic intolerance. Individuals who met both the IOM and Fukuda criteria for the diagnosis had worse HRQOL than those who met the Fukuda criteria alone. The data from this study lend further support to the inclusion of PEM, cognitive impairment, and orthostatic intolerance as core features of pediatric ME/CFS, and should help inform future discussions regarding a pediatric case definition.

AUTHOR CONTRIBUTIONS

CM and PR designed the study. CM maintained the study database. SJ, MF, EC, and CM contributed to data entry. MR wrote the first draft of the manuscript. All authors contributed to manuscript revision, read and approved of the final manuscript, and data analysis.

ACKNOWLEDGMENTS

We thank the many patients and healthy volunteers who made this study possible. PR is supported by the Sunshine Natural Well-being Foundation Professorship. We thank Drs. C. (Linda) M. C. van Campen, and Frans C. Visser of the Stichting CardioZorg, Hoofddorp, The Netherlands, for their helpful comments on the manuscript.

REFERENCES

1. Institute of Medicine. *Committee on the Diagnostic Criteria for Myalgic Encephalomyelitis/Chronic Fatigue Syndrome. Beyond Myalgic Encephalomyelitis/Chronic Fatigue Syndrome: Redefining an Illness*. Washington, DC: The National Academies Press (2015).
2. Unger ER, Lin JM, Brimmer DJ, Lapp CW, Komaroff AL, Nath A, et al. CDC Grand Rounds: chronic fatigue syndrome–advancing research and clinical education. *MMWR* (2016) 65:1434–8. doi: 10.15585/mmwr.mm655051a4
3. Fukuda K, Straus SE, Hickie I, Sharpe M, Dobbins JG, Komaroff A, et al. Chronic fatigue syndrome: a comprehensive approach to its definition and study. *Ann Int Med.* (1994) 121:953–9. doi: 10.7326/0003-4819-121-12-199412150-00009
4. Royal College of Paediatrics and Child Health. *Evidence Based Guideline for the Management of CFS/ME (Chronic Fatigue Syndrome/Myalgic Encephalopathy) in Children and Young People*. London: Royal College of Paediatrics and Child Health (2004).
5. Carruthers BM, Jain AK, De Meirleir KL, Peterson DL, Klimas NG, Lerner AM, et al. Myalgic encephalomyelitis/chronic fatigue syndrome: clinical working case definition. *J Chronic Fatigue Synd.* (2003) 11:7–115. doi: 10.1300/J092v11n01_02
6. Jason LA, Bell DS, Rowe K, Van Hoof ELS, Jordan K, Lapp C, et al. A pediatric case definition for myalgic encephalomyelitis and chronic fatigue syndrome. *J Chronic Fatigue Synd.* (2006) 13:1–44. doi: 10.1300/J092v13n02_01
7. Carruthers BM, Van de Sande MI, De Meirleir KL, Klimas NG, Broderick G, Mitchell T, et al. Myalgic encephalomyelitis: international consensus criteria. *J Int Med.* (2011) 270:327–38. doi: 10.1111/j.1365-2796.2011.02428.x
8. Garralda ME, Rangel L. Impairment and coping in children and adolescents with chronic fatigue syndrome: a comparative study with other paediatric disorders. *J Child Psychol Psychiatry* (2004) 45:543–52. doi: 10.1111/j.1469-7610.2004.00244.x
9. Kennedy G, Underwood C, Belch JJ. Physical and functional impact of chronic fatigue syndrome/myalgic encephalomyelitis in childhood. *Pediatrics* (2010) 125:e1324–30. doi: 10.1542/peds.2009-2644
10. Winger A, Kvarstein G, Wyller VB, Ekstedt M, Sulheim D, Fagermoen E, et al. Health related quality of life in adolescents with chronic fatigue syndrome: a cross sectional study. *Health Q Life Outcomes* (2015) 13:e1–9. doi: 10.1186/s12955-015-0288-3
11. Knight SJ, Harvey A, Hennel S, Lubitz L, Rowe K, Reveley C, et al. Measuring quality of life and fatigue in adolescents with chronic fatigue syndrome: estimates of feasibility, internal consistency, and parent-adolescent agreement of the PedsQL™. *Fatig Biomed Health Behav.* (2015) 3:220–34. doi: 10.1080/21641846.2015.1090816
12. Davies S, Crawley E. Chronic fatigue syndrome in children aged 11 years old and younger. *Arch Dis Child.* (2008) 93:419–22. doi: 10.1136/adc.2007.126649
13. Knight S, Harvey A, Lubitz L, Rowe K, Reveley C, Veit F, et al. Paediatric chronic fatigue syndrome: complex presentations and protracted time to diagnosis. *J Paediatrics Child Health* (2013) 49:919–24. doi: 10.1111/jpc.12425
14. Nijhof SL, Maijer K, Bleijenberg G, Uiterwaal, C. S. P.M, Kimpen JLL, van de Putte EM. Adolescent chronic fatigue syndrome: prevalence, incidence, and morbidity. *Pediatrics* (2011) 127:e1169–75. doi: 10.1542/peds.2010-1147

15. Asprusten TT, Sulheim D, Fagermoen E, Winger A, Skovlund E, Wyller VB. Systemic exertion intolerance disease diagnostic criteria applied on an adolescent chronic fatigue syndrome cohort: evaluation of subgroup differences and prognostic utility. *BMJ Paediatr Open* (2018) 2:e000233. doi: 10.1136/bmjpo-2017-000233
16. Rowe PC, Marden CL, Flaherty M, Jasion SE, Cranston EM, Johns AS, et al. Impaired range of motion of limbs and spine in chronic fatigue syndrome. *J Pediatr.* (2014) 165:360–6. doi: 10.1016/j.jpeds.2014.04.051
17. Rowe PC, Marden CL, Flaherty MAK, Jasion SE, Cranston EM, Fontaine KR, et al. Two-year follow-up of impaired range of motion in chronic fatigue syndrome. *J Pediatr.* (2018) 200:249–53. doi: 10.1016/j.jpeds.2018.05.012
18. Kovacs M. The children's depression inventory (CDI). *Psychopharmacol Bull.* (1985) 21:995–8.
19. Kovacs M. *Children's Depression Inventory (CDI): Technical manual update.* North Tonawanda, NY: Multi-Health Systems (2003).
20. Beck AT, Ward CH, Mendelson M, Mock J, Erbaugh J. An inventory for measuring depression. *Arch Gen Psychiatry* (1961) 4:53–63. doi: 10.1001/archpsyc.1961.01710120031004
21. Beck AT, Steer RA, Brown GK. *BDI-II Manual.* San Antonio, TX: Harcourt Brace and Co (1996).
22. Varni JW, Seid M, Rode CA. The PedsQLTM: measurement model for the pediatric quality of life inventory. *Med Care* (1999) 37:126–39. doi: 10.1097/00005650-199902000-00003
23. Varni JW, Seid M, Kurtin PS. PedsQL 4.0: reliability and validity of the pediatric quality of life inventory version 4.0 generic core scales in healthy and patient populations. *Med Care* (2001) 39:800–12. doi: 10.1097/00005650-200108000-00006
24. Ingerski LM, Modi AC, Hood KK, Pai AL, Zeller M, Piazza-Waggoner C, et al. Health-related quality of life across pediatric chronic conditions. *J Pediatr.* (2010) 156:639–44. doi: 10.1016/j.jpeds.2009.11.008
25. Walker LS, Greene JW. The functional disability inventory: measuring a neglected dimension of child health status. *J Pediatr Psychol.* (1991) 16:39–58. doi: 10.1093/jpepsy/16.1.39
26. Claar RL, Walker LS. Functional properties of pediatric pain patients: psychometric properties of the functional disability inventory. *Pain* (2006) 121:77–84. doi: 10.1016/j.pain.2005.12.002
27. Sulheim DE, Fagermoen E, Winger A, Andersen AM, Godang K, Muller F, et al. Disease mechanisms and clonidine treatment in adolescent chronic fatigue syndrome: a combined cross-sectional and randomized clinical trial. *JAMA Pediatr.* (2014) 168:351–60. doi: 10.1001/jamapediatrics.2013.4647
28. Bentall RP, Wood GC, Marrinan T, Deans C, Edwards RHT. A brief mental fatigue questionnaire. *Br J Clin Psychol.* (1993) 32:375–9. doi: 10.1111/j.2044-8260.1993.tb01070.x
29. Wood GC, Bentall RP, Gopfert M, Edwards RHT. A comparative assessment of patients with chronic fatigue syndrome and muscle disease. *Psychol Med.* (1991) 21:619–28. doi: 10.1017/S0033291700 02225X
30. Bou-Holaigah I, Rowe PC, Kan J, Calkins H. Relationship between neurally mediated hypotension and the chronic fatigue syndrome. *JAMA* (1995) 274:961–7. doi: 10.1001/jama.1995.035301200 53041
31. Ross AJ, Medow MS, Rowe PC, Stewart JM. What is brain fog? An evaluation of the symptom in postural tachycardia syndrome. *Clin Auton Res.* (2013) 23:305–11. doi: 10.1007/s10286-013-0212-z
32. Varni JW, Burwinkle TM, Katz ER, Meeske K, Dickinson P. The PedsQL^{TM} in pediatric cancer: reliability and validity of the pediatric quality of life inventory^{TM} generic core scales, multidimensional fatigue scale, and cancer module. *Cancer.* (2002) 94:2090–106. doi: 10.1002/cncr. 10428
33. Varni JW, Limbers CA. The PedsQL^{TM} multidimensional fatigue scale in young adults: feasibility, reliability and validity in a University student population. *Q Life Res.* (2008) 17:105–14. doi: 10.1007/s11136-007-9282-5
34. Strickberger SA, Benson DW, Biaggioni I, Callans DJ, Cohen MI, Ellenbogen KA, et al. AHA/ACCF scientific statement on the evaluation of syncope. *J Am Coll Cardiol.* (2006) 47:473–84. doi: 10.1016/j.jacc.2005.12. 019
35. Roma M, Marden CL, Rowe PC. Passive standing tests for the office diagnosis of postural tachycardia syndrome: new methodological considerations. *Fatigue Biomed Health Behav.* (2018) 6:179–92. doi: 10.1080/21641846.2018.1512836
36. Cockshell SJ, Mathias JL. Cognitive functioning in people with chronic fatigue syndrome: a comparison between subjective and objective measures. *Neuropsychology* (2014) 28:394–405. doi: 10.1037/neu00 00025
37. Ocon AJ, Messer ZR, Medow MS, Stewart JM. Increasing orthostatic stress impairs neurocognitive functioning in chronic fatigue syndrome with postural tachycardia syndrome. *Clin Sci.* (2012) 122:227–38. doi: 10.1042/CS20 110241
38. Rowe PC, Fontaine KR, Lauver M, Jasion SE, Marden CL, Moni M, et al. Neuromuscular strain increases symptom intensity in chronic fatigue syndrome. *PLoS ONE* (2016) 11:e0159386. doi: 10.1371/journal.pone. 0159386
39. Singer W, Sletten DM, Opfer-Gehrking TL, Brands CK, Fischer PR, Low PA. Postural tachycardia in children and adolescents: what is abnormal? *J Pediatr.* (2012) 160:222–6. doi: 10.1016/j.jpeds.2011.08.054
40. Rowe PC, Bou-Holaigah I, Kan JS, Calkins H. Is neurally mediated hypotension an unrecognised cause of chronic fatigue? *Lancet* (1995) 345:623–4. doi: 10.1016/S0140-6736(95)90525-1
41. Brown M, Kaplan C, Jason L. Factor analysis of the beck depression inventory-II with patients with chronic fatigue syndrome. *J Health Psychol.* (2011) 17:799–808. doi: 10.1177/1359105311424470
42. Crawley E, Sterne JAC. Association between school absence and physical function in paediatric chronic fatigue syndrome/myalgic encephalopathy. *Arch Dis Child.* (2009) 94:752–6. doi: 10.1136/adc.2008.14 3537

6

Advances in ME/CFS: Past, Present and Future

*Kenneth J. Friedman**

Retired, Plantation, FL, United States

Correspondence:
Kenneth J. Friedman
kenneth.j.friedman@gmail.com

The forerunner of what is today termed myalgic encephalomyelitis/chronic fatigue syndrome (ME/CFS) was described by the U.S. Public Health Service in 1934. At the present time, we still do not know its cause and/or how to detect it by routine clinical laboratory tests. In consequence, the pathological nature of ME/CFS has been overlooked and the disease has been stigmatized by being mislabeled as psychosomatic or somatoform illness. Such misperceptions of the disease have led to insufficient research exploration of the disease and minimal to absent patient care. A 2015 Institute of Medicine report on the illness declared ME/CFS a disease affecting up to 2.5 million Americans and chastised the U.S. government for doing little to research the disease and to support its patients. Clinicians who currently treat this disease declare it to be more devastating than HIV/AIDS. A comparison of the histories of the two diseases, an examination of the current status of the two diseases, and a listing of the accomplishments that would be needed for ME/CFS to achieve the same level of treatment and care as currently experienced by patients with HIV/AIDS is provided.

Keywords: ME/CFS, HIV/AIDS, HISTORY, comparison, patient care, research

INTRODUCTION

Myalgic Encephalomyelitis/Chronic Fatigue Syndrome (ME/CFS) is a stigmatized, multisystem, complex, chronic disease that potentially affects up to 2.5 million Americans (1). Initially described in the United States in 1934 (2), it has alternatively been mischaracterized as hysteria (3), psychosomatic (4), and psychological illness (5).

The characterization of ME/CFS as a psychosomatic illness has led to a proliferation of literature describing cognitive behavioral therapy (CBT) and graded exercise therapy (GET) as non-physiological approaches to treat the illness. Patients have claimed harm from these therapies, but the pro-CBT literature alleges otherwise. Recently, literature disputing the benefits of CBT and GET has emerged (6), and the decision has been reached to withdraw some of the CBT and GET studies (7).

Many members of the healthcare community and the public are dismissive of ME/CFS as a disease (8) and, therefore, according to criteria published by the U.S. Institute of Medicine (now the National Academy of Medicine), ME/CFS qualifies as a stigmatized illness (9). Such illnesses are difficult to treat because of healthcare provider dismissive attitudes (10) and the lack of community support for patients (11). Compounding these difficulties for ME/CFS patients is the failure to find consistent abnormalities in routine, clinical laboratory tests which can confirm a ME/CFS diagnosis. Without the availability of an accepted, laboratory, diagnostic test indicating the presence of a unique infectious agent, metabolic or organ system abnormality, there is reluctance to believe that ME/CFS is a pathophysiological illness. In consequence, the search for the etiological agent or agents of ME/CFS, specific treatments for its relief, medications or a vaccine specific for the disease have been hampered. Without such knowledge and tools, physicians and other healthcare providers receive little healthcare provider education about the disease. Knowing the previous struggles for research and treatment, and the current status of patient care for a disease which similarly suffered from stigmatization, unknown disease etiology, and no known treatment, but has progressed much further in a shorter amount of time, helps clarify what can be achieved for ME/CFS in the future.

Our current understanding of ME/CFS is that it is a complex, chronic, debilitating, physical disease characterized by post-exertional malaise, severe, and debilitating fatigue, cognitive problems, sleep dysfunction, pain, and immune, autonomic, neurological, endocrine, and gastrointestinal symptoms (12). The severity of symptoms varies from day-to-day within the patient, and varies among patients. Severity of disease is graded from patients being mildly affected, through moderately affected, to the severely affected. The severely affected are either house- or bedbound, may be unable to move, speak or tolerate light (13). Post-exertional malaise (PEM) is considered one of the key symptoms of ME/CFS and is defined as the exacerbation of the patient's symptoms following minimal physical or mental activity, occurring hours, days, or weeks after the triggering activity, and lasting for disproportionately long lengths of time (days, weeks, or months).

Diagnosis of ME/CFS is difficult. Without the availability of a diagnostic test, several sets of diagnostic criteria have been proposed. Fukuda et al. (14) has been the most popular, but it must be remembered that it was proposed as, and is, a research case definition never intended for clinical diagnosis. The recent Institute of Medicine report (1) proposes simplified criteria which have not been widely embraced. Without a disease specific test or biomarker, there is no choice but to base diagnosis on the symptoms reported by the patient. Some symptoms are considered mandatory for the diagnosis, whereas others are considered supportive. There is a reluctance to diagnose adults with ME/CFS until they have been ill for at least 6 months and their co-morbidities have been addressed. For children and adolescents, and for humanitarian reasons, the length of time of required illness prior to receiving a ME/CFS diagnosis has been shortened to 3 months (15), but the treating physician should use his/her own discretion.

Treatment of ME/CFS has been difficult. The availability of treatment and therapeutic approach varies among countries. Some countries lack awareness of ME/CFS (16), others subscribe to ME/CFS as treatable by changing the way the patient thinks and behaves through a CBT approach (17, 18), while some have embraced ME/CFS being an organic disease in practice (19) but fail to reach all patients and caregivers in need (20). Recently, O'Leary (21) has put forward the argument that despite a previous, long-term, professional consensus that CFS be classified as a psychosomatic illness, the insistence of globally respected health authorities that ME/CFS be treated as a serious, biological disease (1) raises ethical concerns as to whether efforts to continue treating ME/CFS as a mental disorder (in the U.K.) should continue.

While HIV/AIDS was far more devastating than ME/CFS when what was to be called AIDS was first reported, it no longer is. At this point in time it is comparable or less severe than ME/CFS for the majority of patients as witnessed by the following two quotes from physicians who treat both: (1) "In my experience, *(ME/CFS) is one of the most disabling diseases that I care for, far exceeding HIV disease except for the terminal stages."*—Dr. Daniel Peterson (22). (2) *I split my clinical time between the two illnesses, and I can tell you if I had to choose between the two illnesses (in 2009) I would rather have H.I.V. But C.F.S., which impacts a million people in the United States alone, has had a small fraction of the research dollars directed toward it."*—Dr. Nancy Klimas, AIDS and CFS researcher and clinician, University of Miami (23).

THE PAST

It has been over 80 years since the first literature-documented outbreak of ME/CFS in the United States in 1934 (2). Yet, this illness remains poorly characterized and there is no defined course of treatment. In contrast, the time span from the first description of HIV/AIDS to the development of treatment with Federal Drug Administration (FDA)-approved drugs was less than a decade (24). Attempts to classify ME/CFS have been misleading. The majority of ME/CFS cases have been classified as, "sporadic," despite the infectious origin of most cases: Hickie et al. (25) report that 6 % of Epstein Barr Virus, Ross River Virus and Q fever patients develop ME/CFS, with the severity of viral infection being the best predictor of contracting ME/CFS. In 1955, McEvedy and Beard (3) labeled a cluster outbreak of the illness as "mass hysteria," and the *New York Times* cheekily renamed the illness, "Yuppie Flu," mischaracterizing the illness as exclusively affecting young and upcoming professionals (26). To the contrary, research shows that ME/CFS affects all socioeconomic groups of the American population, with socioeconomically disadvantaged populations perhaps being more greatly affected (27).

Mischaracterization of ME/CFS has led to inappropriate and, for some, harmful treatment options (28). Characterization of ME/CFS as a psychosomatic illness has led to the belief that cognitive behavioral therapy (CBT) and graded exercise therapy (GET) are therapeutic if not curative (6). The publications demonstrating the therapeutic and potentially curative values of CBT and GET have now been challenged (18). Attempts to correct the literature are currently underway (29). When a child has ME/CFS, the parent or parents may be accused of Munchausen's Syndrome By Proxy (MSBP). In some cases, these children have been removed from the home leading to increased severity of illness (30).

Some of the professional scientists who have pursued ME/CFS have jeopardized their careers and livelihood (31). Medical school clinicians have been told to stop seeing ME/CFS patients because they require too much of a clinician's time, and, if they do not stop, they will need to work elsewhere. Researchers have been told that ME/CFS research will not be considered for their promotions, and if they are not promoted, they will need to leave the institution. Medical educators have been told that ME/CFS educational activities are not, "professional," and those activities are banned from the workplace. While the NIH State of Knowledge ME/CFS Workshop, held in 2011, exposed and documented these problems (31), there has been no documentation of NIH objecting to any of these practices. NIH could withhold or limit funding to institutions which discourage or do not permit medical research and patient care for diseases that are of importance to the NIH. Not even the American Association of University Professors (AAUP), which claims academic freedom as its core mission (32), has objected to academic, institutional bans on ME/CFS research, clinical care, and educational activities.

The Guardian summarized the history of inquiry into ME/CFS this way: "... *for much of the past three decades, CFS has been treated as the proverbial skeleton in the closet of the medical world. Potential researchers have been scared off by the stigma associated with the disease, and government funding has been non-existent". "When I was a medical student in the '90s, we were instructed that CFS patients could not be seen in our clinic," Montoya recalls. "And a letter was sent out to those patients telling them not to come"* (33).

The U.S. government's support of ME/CFS research and patient care has been less than stated and not commensurate with the burden of the disease. When the U.S. Congress allocated funds for a Centers for Disease Control and Prevention (CDC) investigation of ME/CFS, the Director of the Chronic Fatigue Syndrome (CFS) Program (CFS is the former name of ME/CFS), Dr. William C. Reeves, filed a whistleblower complaint against the agency, alleging that millions of dollars committed to CFS research had actually been spent on other activities (34). But, it took a request from Sen. Harry Reid, D-NV to the General Accounting Office (GAO) to obtain a report (35). The GAO report stated that about one-third of the funds had been spent on non-CFS-related activities (36). Publicly exposed, the CDC agreed to restore the misappropriated funds and to institute measures which would prevent recurrences (37). According to the U.S. Government General Accounting Office (38): " *at CDC, the lengthy and uncertain process for allocating CFS funds to the branch responsible for most of the CFS work has resulted in delays in undertaking particular projects; ... further, CDC's redirection of funds has resulted in reductions in CFS resources that have impeded the agency's CFS research...coordination between CDC and NIH and their use of input from external researchers and patient advocates in developing agency research programs have been limited.*"

From the mid-1990's until this year, there have been signs of increased interest of the federal government in ME/CFS: In 1997, the Chronic Fatigue Syndrome Coordinating Committee, composed of researchers, clinicians and patient advocates, was formed and tasked with advising the U.S. Secretary of Health and Human Services on matters related to ME/CFS (39). In 2003, the Coordinating Committee was replaced by the Chronic Fatigue Syndrome Advisory Committee (CFSAC) (40). In 2006, then Director of the CDC Julie Gerberding launched a, "Spark Awareness," campaign for ME/CFS which included a ME/CFS public awareness campaign, and the distribution of a *CFS Toolkit for Health Care Professionals* to aid in the diagnosis and treatment of ME/CFS (41). However, despite those efforts, the recent studies of Tidmore et al. (42) and Sunnquist et al. (43) have shown that definitive care of persons with ME/CFS in the United States is still lacking.

In 2014, the Department of Health and Human Services issued a $1 million contract to the Institute of Medicine (IOM) for a report (44) on specific aspects of ME/CFS. The IOM Report (1) finds the federal response to ME/CFS deficient. In response to that report, both the National Institutes of Health (NIH) and the CDC promised to modify and enhance their ME/CFS programs, and to correct the deficiencies identified in the IOM report. A long-term plan or commitment which addresses all of the concerns raised in the IOM report has yet to be announced. Wadman (45) reported in *Science* magazine that NIH spending for ME/CFS would double, and NIH would solicit proposals for basic and clinical research centers. The CDC is revising and creating new educational materials for its ME/CFS web pages. The revised pages are pledged to reflect the content and recommendations of both the IOM report and the CDC's ME/CFS stakeholders' meeting held in September, 2016 (46).

While these are indications of improved attitudes toward ME/CFS in two key agencies of the U.S. federal government, there remain indications that the federal government has not fully embraced or accepted ME/CFS for the pathophysiological disease that it is: By its own admission, the NIH intramural, Clinical Center study of ME/CFS and an NIH-sponsored Pathways to Prevention meeting (47) were prompted by the 2015 IOM report. The recommendations of the Chronic Fatigue Syndrome Advisory Committee from its first research recommendation in 2004 to the date of publication of the IOM report were apparently insufficient to motivate the NIH to increase ME/CFS extramural funding or establish an intramural clinical program. An increase in research funding was attained subsequent to the IOM report (48). However, until 1999, NIH implied that ME/CFS is a women's disease (which it is not) by running its ME/CFS programs out of the Office of Research on Women's Health (49). A recent study finds 35 to 40 percent of adults diagnosed with ME/CFS are men (50) This fall, the Secretary of Health and Human Services decided to not renew the charter of the Chronic Fatigue Syndrome Advisory Committee stating the goals of the Advisory Committee had been achieved (51).

The U.S. government allocates far fewer research dollars for ME/CFS than it does for other chronic diseases of commensurate severity. For example, the estimated 2018 research expenditure for HIV/AIDS in the United States is $2.2 billion (52). With an estimated 1.1 million HIV/AIDS patients living in the U.S (53), the research expenditure per patient is $2,000. If the IOM report is correct, there may be more than double the number of ME/CFS patients living in the U.S. The ME/CFS research expenditure for FY 2017 was $13,967,704 (54), resulting in $5.58 spent per patient. The federal government spends 357 times more on HIV/AIDS research than on ME/CFS. The IOM report states, "*The committee was struck by the relative paucity of research on ME/CFS conducted to date...*" (1).

The federal government allocates more resources for orphan diseases—diseases that affect <200,000 U.S. citizens—than it does for ME/CFS. The NIH orphan diseases program provides services which include a centralized database, liaison services, consortia funding and a contact registry (55). None of these services are provided for ME/CFS by any federal agency.

THE PRESENT

ME/CFS is a worldwide disease. The reported prevalence of ME/CFS varies in different parts of the world. Son (56) searched prevalence studies in the literature and found prevalence studies from 13 countries. Within-country prevalence ranged from 0.0004 percent in Australia to 3.6 percent in the United States. Adolescent prevalence ranged from 0.9 percent in the United Kingdom to 0.11 in the Netherlands.

ME/CFS may affect up to 2.5 million Americans (1). An estimated 25 percent of ME/CFS patients have severe ME/CFS, i.e., are either house- or bed-bound at some point in their lives (57). ME/CFS patients need more care than patients with many other illnesses (1). Yet, there are regions in the United States where they do not receive any specialized, medical care (43). There is no laboratory test or diagnostic marker for ME/CFS (58). There is not one FDA-approved drug for the treatment of ME/CFS (59). In contrast, there are approximately 40 FDA approved drugs for the treatment of HIV/AIDS (60). And there is obviously no cure for ME/CFS (59).

Three recent documents, authored by the federal government itself, suggest the need for increased federal participation in the ME/CFS Agenda: (a) the Institute of Medicine Report (1), (b) the NIH Pathways to Prevention Report (61), and (c) the NIH State of Knowledge Workshop Report (62). In addition to documenting the discrimination experienced by ME/CFS patients, the clinicians who treat them, and the researchers who study their illness, the NIH State of Knowledge Workshop Report also identified a need for more interdisciplinary research, more researchers, and translational research, defined as starting at the bedside, going to the laboratory bench, and back to the patient again (63).

There are other reasons to increase federal support for ME/CFS research and patient care: (1) The federal government has an obligation to provide fair opportunity to all persons and eliminate impediments to fair opportunity: "*No persons should be denied social benefits on the basis of underserved disadvantageous properties*" (64). This concept of "fair opportunity" has led to calls to eliminate health disparities (65, 66).

(2) The federal government has an obligation to treat ME/CFS patients because they constitute a medically underserved population. ME/CFS patients qualify as a medically underserved population by virtue of geographic and financial barriers to care (42). Both Tidmore et al. (42) and Sunnquist et al. (43) found: (a) areas of the United States in which there are no ME/CFS specialized care providers, (b) areas in which there are an inadequate number of specialized care providers, (c) areas in which there are an inadequate number of knowledgeable primary care providers, and (d) a national lack of educational opportunities for physicians and medical students to obtain the didactic and clinical experience necessary to diagnose and to treat ME/CFS.

(3) The U.S. government has the ability to initiate a national, federal, healthcare program for an identified, disabled, patient population within the United States, a population that otherwise lacks equal access to healthcare and, therefore, represents a medically underserved population (67). These arguments were part of the justification for establishing multiple Centers of Excellence for ME/CFS in the United States, presented at the Chronic Fatigue Syndrome Advisory Committee meeting held May 17-18, 2016 and incorporated into recommendations submitted to the Office of the Secretary of Health of the United States (68). Currently, there is not one, federally sponsored or supported ME/CFS clinic in the United States.

The IOM report (1) held the promise of being a watershed moment for ME/CFS: A prestigious, independent, scientific body declared ME/CFS a disease, and the government response to it, inadequate. Thus, far, the responses of both the NIH and the CDC are not commensurate with the severity of the disease nor the number of people affected: Were the federal government to address the current needs of the ME/CFS community, it would need to provide ME/CFS funding commensurate to that of other diseases of similar severity that impact a similar number of patients (as, for example, HIV/AIDS). There would need to be commensurate numbers of treatment centers staffed by physicians capable of providing definitive care.

It has been 3 years since the publication of the 2015 IOM report. Were the IOM report to have had impact, there would be an increase in ME/CFS research, and an increase in public awareness of ME/CFS subsequent to the publication of the report. Such desired increases are not apparent in an examination of the number of research articles published per year in the scientific literature or in the number of articles published per year in the lay literature before and after the 2015 IOM report. These conclusions were reached by determining the number of ME/CFS citations per year in the scientific and lay literature before and after the IOM report. To ascertain the number of articles in the scientific literature, *PubMed* was queried searching article titles for any of the terms used as names for ME/CFS (myalgic encephalomyelitis, chronic fatigue syndrome, ME/CFS, CFS/ME, CFS, SEID, systemic exertion intolerance disease). Results are shown in **Table 1**.

To determine if the IOM report had impact on public awareness, the lay literature was similarly searched utilizing two databases: *Proquest U.S. Newstream* and *EBSCO's Academic Search Premier. Newstream* is described as a database covering newspapers, news websites, blogs, and many national and regional titles. *Academic Search* is described as an interdisciplinary database of newspapers, magazines and journals. The results of querying these two databases are shown in **Table 2**.

The hoped for increases in research publications and/or public awareness as expressed as increases in number of articles in the scientific or lay literature, subsequent to the publication of the IOM report, have not occurred 3 years after the publication of this report.

TABLE 1 | ME/CFS publications/year in the scientific literature.

Year	# of ME/CFS articles published
2010	204
2011	213
2012	153
2013	195
2014	158
2015	205
2016	197
2017	199
2018 to 12/1	178

TABLE 2 | ME/CFS publications/year in the lay literature.

Year	Newstream articles/Year	EBSCO Premier articles/Year
2010	328	252
2011	402	311
2012	253	227
2013	202	211
2014	257	171
2015	249	229
2016	182	191
2017	250	218
2018	166 (to 11/29/18)	141 (to 11/29/18

THE FUTURE

The goals of ME/CFS researchers, healthcare providers, and patients are the same as the goals of others confronting different chronic, debilitating disease: the availability of palliative if not curative treatment, an understanding of the etiology of the disease, development of therapeutic agents specific for the disease, and the development of a vaccine or some other preventative measures. The IOM report (1) concludes that progress in these areas has been disappointingly slow. That opinion is supported by comparing the progress made in the research, treatment and prevention of ME/CFS to that of HIV/AIDS.

At the current time, a comparison between treatment and care of HIV/AIDS patients and ME/CFS patients is reasonable. Both are chronic conditions, with immunological underpinnings. However, whereas HIV (human immunodeficiency virus) has been identified as the cause of AIDS (69), several viruses (e.g., Epstein-Barr, Ross River, and Coxiella burnetti) are associated with the onset of ME/CFS (70). And there are reports of non-viral, physiological abnormalities which may trigger or contribute to the symptoms of ME/CFS (71). It is therefore possible that identifying the causative agent or agents for ME/CFS may take longer than the time needed to discover the AIDS virus. But whereas the HIV/AIDS virus was discovered within a decade, it has been more than eight decades since the description of ME/CFS, and the causative agent or agents have yet to be identified. In the United States, the latest CDC estimate of HIV/AIDS patients suggests that there may be twice as many ME/CFS patients [2.5 million estimated in the IOM report (1)] as HIV/AIDS patients [estimated to be 1.1 million patients by the (72)].

While HIV/AIDS was far more devastating than ME/CFS when the disease was first described, it no longer is. At this point in time it is comparable or less severe than ME/CFS for the majority of patients as attested to by Drs. Peterson and Klimas - two physicians who are well experienced in the treatment of both (22, 23).

At the onset of the AIDS epidemic, the diagnosis of AIDS was a death sentence (73). Today, a 20-year-old, infected with HIV, if appropriately treated, is expected to live into his/her 70's (74). AIDS advocacy (the AIDS Movement) was able to bring U.S. federal spending for AIDS to $3 billion/year, stimulate the development and distribution of 33 drugs in 7 seven different categories for the treatment of AIDS, and transform AIDS from a death sentence to a chronic, treatable condition (75). Many of those gains for HIV/AIDS patients continue today (76).

The accomplishments of the AIDS Community are enviable. From the first report of what would be named HIV/AIDS on June 5, 1981 (77):

- a Congressional Hearing on AIDS was held in <1 year's time.
- $5 million was given to the CDC for surveillance and $10 million given to the NIH for research <6 months later.
- A clinic dedicated to the treatment of AIDS patients opened approximately 1.5 years after the first reporting.
- The World Health Organization held its first AIDS meeting and began global surveillance for HIV/AIDS <3 years after the first reporting.
- The cause of HIV/AIDS was announced by the National Cancer Institute 3 years after the first reporting.
- The first, specific therapeutic drug (antiretroviral agent) was approved 6 years after the first case report of AIDS.
- The Surgeon General mailed 107 million copies of a booklet, "Understanding AIDS," to American households 7 years after the first case report.
- The Food and Drug Administration (FDA) permitted the importation of unapproved drugs for the treatment of HIV/AIDS 7 years after the first case report.
- The United Nations (UN) and World Health Organization (WHO) supported World AIDS Day 7 years after the first case report.
- Health Resources and Services Administration (HRSA) awarded HIV planning grants for, "systems of care," 7 years after the first case report.

All this was accomplished by a living HIV/AIDS population in the United States of under 100,000 patients (78).

Despite HIV/AIDS currently being considered a manageable disease, the proposed U.S. HIV/AIDS budget for 2018 was $32 billion of which 85 % ($20.7 billion) was for domestic care and treatment programs, 9% ($3.1 billion) for domestic care and housing assistance, 7 % ($2.2 billion) for domestic research, and 2 % ($0.7 billion) for domestic prevention (52). There are no domestic care, treatment, prevention, or housing programs for ME/CFS patients. For ME/CFS, a disease estimated to have more than double the number of patients, and with a quality of life judged to be as or more diminished than that of HIV/AIDS, the disparity in patient care and patient benefits is unsettling.

AIDS patients were identified in 1981 and the virus causing AIDS was identified in 1984 (79). NIH expenditure for AIDS research for the period of 1981–1984 was $132,881,000 [calculated from Table 4.2, (80)]. Knowing that AIDS is caused by a single virus, whereas multiple viruses and other triggers precipitate ME/CFS, the research expenditure likely needed to determine the etiology of ME/CFS will be equal to or greater than the research expenditure required to determine the causal agent of AIDS. The federal government and the patient community need to be aware of the probable cost of identifying the causal agent or agents of ME/CFS.

The accomplishments for and by the HIV/AIDS Community, while attributed to HIV/AIDS "activism," (81) make it clear that the U.S. government could have done and still can do much more for ME/CFS. The accomplishments for and by the HIV/AIDS Community may suggest goals for the ME/CFS Community. A lack of parity of research and benefits is logically and ethically difficult to justify.

With the non-renewal of the Chronic Fatigue Syndrome Advisory Committee charter by the U.S. Secretary of Health (82), there is no formal venue in which the inequalities of ME/CFS research and treatment of ME/CFS patients can be addressed. But, knowing what has not worked for the ME/CFS Community in the past, and knowing what has worked for others who have suffered similar disparities in disease-specific healthcare and medical research, may prove helpful to the severely underserved ME/CFS Community.

AUTHOR'S NOTE

"Advances in ME/CFS Research and Clinical Care: Past, Present and Future" is a Perspective article written to be the first article appearing in "Advances in ME/CFS Research and Clinical Care," the invited, themed issue of Frontiers in Pediatrics of which I serve as Guest Editor. The purpose of the article is to provide the reader with background knowledge helpful for better appreciating the subsequent articles in the journal issue. Although what we currently call ME/CFS was described by the forerunner of the Centers for Disease Control and Prevention (in the United States) in the 1930's, it has been mischaracterized until 2015, when the Institute of Medicine declared the symptoms of the syndrome so severe, and the research supporting pathophysiological underpinnings of the syndrome sufficiently substantial, to declare the illness a disease.

The history of ME/CFS up to the publication of the IOM report is quite similar to the history of HIV/AIDS which was first identified in the early 1980's. However, the path or time to acceptance of HIV/AIDS as a "real" disease, and the development of drugs and treatment for it, have been far shorter.

A comparison of the two diseases is, therefore, inevitable, logical and useful.

AUTHOR CONTRIBUTIONS

The author confirms being the sole contributor of this work and has approved it for publication.

ACKNOWLEDGMENTS

The author acknowledges feedback from several colleagues during the preparation of this work.

REFERENCES

1. Institute of Medicine. *Beyond Myalgic Encephalomyelitis/Chronic Fatigue Syndrome: Redefining an Illness.* Washington, DC: The National Academies Press (2015).
2. Gilliam AG. *Epidemiological Study on an Epidemic, Diagnosed as Poliomyelitis, Occurring Among the Personnel of Los Angeles County General Hospital during the summer of 1934.* Washington, DC: United States Government Printing Office United States Treasury Department Public Health Service Public Health Bulletin (1938).
3. McEvedy C, Beard A. Royal Free epidemic of 1955: a reconsideration. *Br Med J.* (1970) 1:7–11.
4. Neu D, Mairesse O, Montana X, Gilson M, Corazza F, Lefevre N, et al. Dimensions of pure chronic fatigue: psychophysical, cognitive and biological correlates in the chronic fatigue syndrome. *Eur J Appl Physiol.* (2014) 114:1841–51. doi: 10.1007/s00421-014-2910-1
5. O'Sullivan S. *Is It All in Your Head?: True Stories of Imaginary Illness.* London: Chatto and Windus (2015).
6. Twisk NM. CBT/GET is ineffective and potentially harmful. ME/CFS patients seem to die considerably younger. *BMJ.* (2010) 340:738. doi: 10.1136/bmj.c738
7. Rehmeyer J, Tuller D. *Opinion: Getting It Wrong On Chronic Fatigue Syndrome.* The New York Times. (2017). Available online at: https://www.nytimes.com/2017/03/18/opinion/sunday/getting-it-wrong-on-chronic-fatigue-syndrome.html?_r=2 (accessed March 9, 2019).
8. Shepherd C. *It's Time for Doctors to Apologise to Their ME Patients.* The Telegraph. (2015). Available online at: http://www.telegraph.co.uk/news/health/12033810/Its-time-for-doctors-to-apologise-to-their-ME-patients.html (accessed July 28, 2017).
9. National Academies of Sciences Engineering and Medicine [US]. *Ending Discrimination Against People with Mental and Substance Use Disorders: The Evidence for Stigma Change.* Washington, DC: The National Academies Press (2016).
10. Bink AB. *Stigma and Discrimination in Behavioral and Physical Healthcare Settings. Commissioned Paper for the Committee on the Science of Changing Behavioral Health Social Norms.* Illinois Institute of Technology. (2015) Available online at: http://sites.nationalacademies.org/cs/groups/dbassesite/documents/webpage/dbasse_170041.pdf (accessed July 28, 2017).
11. Centers for Disease Control and Prevention [US]. *Attitudes Toward Mental Illness — 35 States, District of Columbia, and Puerto Rico, 2007.* Morbidity and Mortality Weekly Report (2010). Available online at: https://www.cdc.gov/mmwr/preview/mmwrhtml/mm5920a3.htm) (accessed July 28, 2017).
12. Friedberg F, Bateman L, Bested A, Davenport T, Friedman K, Gurwitt A, et al. ME/CFS: *A Primer for Clinical Practioners.* Chicago, IL: IACFS/ME (2014). Available online at: https://iacfsme.org/portals/0/pdf/Primer_Post_2014_conference.pdf (accessed March 10, 2019).
13. Pheby D, Saffron L. Risk factors for severe ME/CFS. *Biology and Medicine* (2009)1:50–74.
14. Fukuda K, Straus SE, Hickie I, Sharpe MC, Dobbins JG, Komaroff A. The chronic fatigue syndrome: a comprehensive approach to its definition and

study. International Chronic Fatigue Syndrome Study Group. *Ann Intern Med.* (1994) 121:953–9.

15. NICE. *National Institute for Health and Clinical Excellence. Chronic fatigue syndrome/myalgic encephalomyelitis (or encephalopathy): Diagnosis and management of CFS/ME in adults and children.* London (2007).
16. Cho H, Menezes P, Hotopf M, Bhugra D, Wessely S. Comparative epidemiology of chronic fatigue syndrome in Brazilian and British primary care: Prevalence and recognition. *Br J Psychiatry.* (2009) 194:117–22. doi: 10.1192/bjp.bp.108.051813
17. National Health Service. *NHS Choices: Chronic Fatigue Syndrome.* (2018). Available online at: https://www.nhs.uk/conditions/chronic-fatigue-syndrome-cfs/treatment/ (accessed March 9, 2019).
18. Friedberg F. Cognitive behavioral therapy: why is it so vilified in the chronic fatigue syndrome community? *Fatigue Biomed Health Behav.* (2016) 4:127–31. doi: 10.1080/21641846.2016.1200884
19. Tuominen P. *ME/CFS – Chronic Fatigue Syndrome.* 1177 The Healthcare Guide's Editorial Staff. (2016). Available online at: https://translate.google.com/translate?sl=svandtl=enandu=https%3A%2F%2Fwww.1177.se%2FFakta-och-rad%2FSjukdomar%2FMECFS%2F (accessed March 9, 2019).
20. Bergdahl A, Hallsenius L. *Now the Police Say: Here's What Happened to the Family in Bjarred.* News24. (2018). Avaialble online at: https://translate.google.com/translate?hl=andsl=svandtl=enandu=https%3A%2F%2Fnyheter24.se%2Fnyheter%2Finrikes%2F919530-efter-polisens-presskonferens-har-ar-vad-som-hande-familjen-i-bjarred (accessed March 9, 2019).
21. O'Leary D. Ethical classification of ME/CFS in the United Kingdom. *Bioethics.* (2019) 00:1-7. doi: 10.1111/bioe.12559
22. Peterson D. (1995) *Introduction to Research and Clinical Conference.* Fort Lauderdale, FL: JCFS.
23. New York Times Blog. (2009). Available online at: https://consults.blogs.nytimes.com/2009/10/15/readers-ask-a-virus-linked-to-chronic-fatigue-syndrome (accessed December 12, 2018).
24. Kaiser Family Foundation. *Global HIV/AIDS Timeline.* (2018). Avaialble online at: https://www.kff.org/global-health-policy/timeline/global-hivaids-timeline/ (accessed December 12, 2018).
25. Hickie I, Davenport T, Wakefield D, Vollmer-Conna U, Cameron B, Vernon, S, et al. Post-infective and chronic fatigue syndromes precipitated by viral and non-viral pathogens: prospective cohort study. *Br Med J.* (2006) 333:575. doi: 10.1136/bmj.38933.585764.AE
26. Boffey PM. *Fatigue 'Virus' Has Experts More Baffled and Skeptical Than Ever.* New York Times. (1987). Available online at: https://www.nytimes.com/1987/07/28/science/fatigue-virus-has-experts-more-baffled-and-skeptical-than-ever.html?pagewanted=all (accessed December 11, 2018).
27. Kamaldeep SB, Dinos S, Ashby D, Nasroo J, Wessely S, White PD. Chronic fatigue syndrome in an ethnically diverse population: the influence of psychosocial adversity and physical inactivity. *BMC Med.* (2011) 9:26. doi: 10.1186/1741-7015-9-26
28. Jason LA, Taylor RR, Kennedy C, Jordan K, Song S, Johnson DE, et al. Chronic fatigue syndrome: sociodemographic subtypes in a community-based sample. *Eval Health Prof.* (2000) 23:243–63. doi: 10.1177/01632780022034598
29. Tuller D. *Virology Blog 19 October 2018. Trial By Error: Cochrane Decides To Withdraw Flawed Exercise Review.* (2018). Avaialble online at: http://www.virology.ws/2018/10/19/trial-by-error-cochrane-decides-to-withdraw-flawed-exercise-review/ (accessed December 9, 2018).
30. Bell DS. Munchausen's syndrome by proxy, factitious disorders in children and myalgic encephalomyelitis/chronic fatigue syndrome. *IACFS/ME Newsletter attachment.* (2015). Avaialble online at: http://iacfsme.org/PDFS/2015DecNewsletter/Attachment-1-Dec-2015-Bell-Munchausen-s-Syndrome-b.aspx (accessed July 28, 2017).
31. Friedman K. *Elephants In The Room, N.I.H. State of Knowledge Workshop On ME/CFS.* (2011). Avaialble online at: http://immunedysfunction.org/images/Elephants%20in%20the%20Room%20As%20Delivered.pdf (accessed July 28, 2017).
32. American Association of University Professors [US]. *Our Programs: Protecting Our Freedom.* (2018). Avaialble online at: https://www.aaup.org/our-work/protecting-academic-freedom (accessed July 28, 2017).
33. Cox D. Is chronic fatigue syndrome finally being taken seriously? *The Guardian. Health and Well Being.* (2016). Avaialble online at: https://www.theguardian.com/lifeandstyle/2016/apr/04/chronic-fatigue-syndrome-cfs-taken-seriously (accessed December 12, 2018).
34. Stephens J, Strauss V. *Retaliation Alleged at CDC.* The Washington Post (1999).
35. Las Vegas Sun (1998) *Monday, Oct. 5, Reid Asks GAO to Investigate Whether CDC Lied to Congress.* Available online at: https://lasvegassun.com/news/1998/oct/05/reid-asks-gao-to-investigate-whether-cdc-lied-to-c/ (accessed July 28, 2017).
36. General Accounting Office [US]. *Report to the Honorable Harry Reid, U.S. Senate Chronic Fatigue Syndrome CDC and NIH Research Activities Are Diverse, but Agency Coordination Is Limited.* GAO/HES-00-98 (2000b) Available online at: http://www.gao.gov/new.items/he00098.pdf (accessed July 28, 2017).
37. Reuters Limited. *GAO Criticizes CDC, NIH Handling of Chronic Fatigue Research.* (2000). Avaialble online at: http://www.ncf-net.org/library/GAOCriticizesCDC.htm (accessed July 28, 2018).
38. General Accounting Office. *Chronic Fatigue Syndrome. CDC and NIH Research Activities Are Diverse, but Agency Coordination Is Limited.* (2000). Available online at: https://www.gao.gov/assets/240/230415.pdf (accessed December 13, 2018).
39. Centers for Disease Control and Prevention [US]. *Centers for Disease Control and Prevention National Center for Infectious Diseases.* Chronic Fatigue Syndrome Coordinating Committee 1997 – 1999 (1997). Available online at: http://www.cfids-me.org/cfscc/members9799.html (accessed July 28, 2017).
40. US Department of Health and Human Services *Chronic Fatigue Syndrome Advisory Committee Home Meetings.* (2014). Available online at: http://wayback.archive-it.org/3919/20140324192802/http://www.hhs.gov/advcomcfs/meetings/index.html (accessed *July* 28, 2017).
41. Collins S. *Solve CFS Spring/Summer 2009: Public Awareness By The Numbers. Solve ME/CFS Initiative.* (2009). Available online at: https://issuu.com/solvemecfsinitiative/docs/springsummer2009 (accessed December 10, 2018).
42. Tidmore TM, Jason LA, Chapo-Kroger L, So S, Brown A, Silverman MC. Lack of knowledgeable healthcare access for patients with neuro-endocrine-immune diseases. *Front. Clin. Med.* (2015) 2:46–54.
43. Sunnquist M, Nicholson L, Jason LA, Friedman KJ. Access to medical care for individuals with myalgic encephalomyelitis and chronic fatigue syndrome: a call for centers of excellence. *Mod Clin Med Res.* (2017) 1:28–35. doi: 10.22606/mcmr.2017.11005
44. Assistant Secretary of Health US. *Department of Health and Human Services. FAQs on an HHS Contract With the IOM to Recommend Clinical Diagnostic Criteria for ME/CFS.* (2016). Available online at: https://www.hhs.gov/ash/advisory-committees/cfsac/notices/faqs-on-an-hhs-contract-with-the-iom-to-recommend-clinical-diagnostic-criteria-for-me-cfs/index.html (accessed December 9, 2018).
45. Wadman M. NIH to double funding for chronic fatigue syndrome, but patient distrust remains. *Science Magazine.* (2016). Available online at: http://www.sciencemag.org/news/2016/11/nih-double-funding-chronic-fatigue-syndrome-patient-distrust-remains (accessed July 28, 2017).
46. Belay E. *CDC Report to the HHS CFS Advisory Committee.* (2016). Avaialble online at: https://www.hhs.gov/sites/default/files/cfsac-cdc-national-center-report-presentation-jan2017.pdf (accessed July 28, 2017).
47. National Institutes of Health Office of Communication News Release [US]. *NIH Takes Action to Bolster Research on Myaglic Encephalomyeltis/Chronic Fatigue Syndrome.* (2015). Available online at: https://www.nih.gov/news-events/news-releases/nih-takes-action-bolster-research-myalgic-encephalomyelitis/chronic-fatigue-syndrome (accessed December 9, 2018).
48. National Institutes of Health News Release [US]. *NIH Announces Centers for Myalgic Encephalomyelitis/Chronic Fatigue Syndrome Research. Collaborative Projects Will Advance Research and Knowledge About Debilitating Disease.* (2017). Avaialble online at: https://www.nih.gov/news-events/news-releases/nih-announces-centers-myalgic-encephalomyelitis-chronic-fatigue-syndrome-research (accessed December 10, 2018).
49. National Institutes of Health News Release [US]. *NIH Announces Awards in Chronic Fatigue Syndrome Research.* (2006). Available online at: https://www.nih.gov/news-events/news-releases/nih-announces-awards-chronic-fatigue-syndrome-research (accessed November 29, 2018).

50. Valdez A, Hancock E, Adebayo S, Kiernicki D, Proskauer, D, Attewell J, et al. (2019) Estimating prevalence, demographics, and costs of ME/CFS using large scale medical claims data and machine learning. *Front. Pediatric.* 6:412. doi: 10.3389/fped.2018.00412
51. Office of the Assistant Secretary for Health HHS gov [US]. *Chronic Fatigue Syndrome Advisory Committee (CFSAC) The Charter for the Chronic Fatigue Syndrome Advisory Committee expired on September 5, 2018.* (2018). Available online at: https://www.hhs.gov/ash/advisory-committees/cfsac/index.html (accessed December 10, 2018).
52. Kaiser Family Foundation. *U.S. Federal Funding for HIV/AIDS; Trends Over Time.* (2017) Available onlinhe at: https://www.kff.org/global-health-policy/fact-sheet/u-s-federal-funding-for-hivaids-trends-over-time/ (accessed December 10, 2018).
53. AmFAR. *Statistics: United States.* The Foundation for AIDS Research. (2018) Available online at: https://www.amfar.org/about-hiv-and-aids/facts-and-stats/statistics--united-states/ (accessed December 10, 2018).
54. Spotila J. *Occupy M.E. Post of March 20, 2018.* 2017 NIH Spending on ME/CFS Research. (2018). Available online at: http://occupyme.net/2018/03/20/2017-nih-spending-on-mecfs-research/ (accessed December 11, 2018).
55. Rare Clinical Diseases Research Network. *Bridging the Gap between Rare Diseases and Research.* (2017). Available online at: https://www.rarediseasesnetwork.org/about/index.htm (accessed July 28, 2017).
56. Son GS. Review of the prevalence of chronic fatigue worldwide. *J Kor Orient Med.* (2012) 33:25–32.
57. Pendergrast T, Brown A, Sunnquist M, Jantke R, Newton JL, Strand EB, et al. (2016). Housebound versus nonhousebound patients with myalgic encephalomyelitis and chronic fatigue syndrome. *Chronic Illn.* 12:292–307. doi: 10.1177/1742395316644770
58. Scheibenbogen C, Freitag H, Blanco J, Capelli E, Lacerda E, Authier J, et al. The European ME/CFS Biomarker Landscape project an initiative of the European network EUROMENE. *J Transl Med.* (2017) 15:162. doi: 10.1186/s12967-017-1263-z
59. Centers for Disease Control and Prevention [US]. *Myalgic Encephalomyelitis/Chronic Fatigue Syndrome Treatment.* (2018). Available online at: https://www.cdc.gov/me-cfs/treatment/index.html (accessed December 11, 2018).
60. AIDSinfo. *FDA-approved HIV Medicines.* (2018). Available online at: https://aidsinfo.nih.gov/understanding-hiv-aids/fact-sheets/21/58/fda-approved-hiv-medicines (accessed December 13, 2018).
61. National Institutes of Health [US]. *Pathways to Prevention (P2P). Advancing the Research on Myalgic Encephalomyelitis/Chronic Fatigue Syndrome (ME/CFS).* (2014). Available online at: https://prevention.nih.gov/programs-events/pathways-to-prevention/workshops/me-cfs/workshop-resources#finalreport (accessed July 28, 2017).
62. National Institutes of Health [US]. *State of Knowledge Workshop. Myalgic Encephalomyelitis/Chronic Fatigue Syndrome (ME/CFS) Research.* (2011). Available online at: http://www.meassociation.org.uk/wp-content/uploads/2011/08/SoK-Workshop-Report-508-compliant-8-5-11.pdf (accessed July 28, 2017).
63. Rubio DM, Schoenbaum EE, Lee LS, Schteingart DE, Marantz PR, Anderson KE, et al. Defining translational research: implications for training. *Acad Med.* (2010) 85:470–475. doi: 10.1097/ACM.0b013e3181ccd618
64. Beauchamp L, Childress JF. *Principles of Biomedical Ethics.* 5th ed. New York, NY: University Press (2001).
65. Centers For Disease Control and Prevention. *Healthy People 2010.* (2011). Available online at: https://www.cdc.gov/nchs/healthy_people/hp2010.htm (accessed December 11, 2018).
66. Kass NE. Public health ethics: from foundations and frameworks to justice and global public health. *J Law Med Ethics.* (2004) 32:232–42. doi: 10.1111/j.1748-720X.2004.tb00470.x
67. Vanderbilt AA, Dail MD. Jaberi P. Reducing health disparities in underserved communities via interprofessional collaboration across health care professions. *J Multidiscip Healthc.* (2015) 8:205–8. doi: 10.2147/JMDH.S74129
68. Kaplan G. *COE's Recommendations. Creating Centers of Excellence for ME/CFS.* (2016). Available online at: https://www.hhs.gov/ash/advisory-committees/cfsac/recommendations/2016-05-17/coe-recommendations/index.html (accessed December 11, 2018).
69. HIV.gov. *What are HIV and AIDS.* (2017). Available online at: https://www.hiv.gov/hiv-basics/overview/about-hiv-and-aids/what-are-hiv-and-aids (accessed *March* 9, 2019).
70. Centers for Disease Control and Prevention [US]. *Myalgic Encephalomyelitis/Chronic Fatigue Syndrome. Possible Causes.* (2018c). Available online at: https://www.cdc.gov/me-cfs/about/possible-causes.html (accessed March 9, 2019).
71. WebMD. *What is Chronic Fatigue Syndrome?.* (2019). Available online at: https://www.webmd.com/chronic-fatigue-syndrome/what-is-chronic-fatigue-syndrome#2 (accessed March 9, 2019).
72. Centers for Disease Control and Prevention [US]. *HIV Surveillance Report. Statistics Overview HIV Prevalence Estimate.* (2018b). Available online at: https://www.cdc.gov/hiv/statistics/overview/index.html (accessed December 11, 2018).
73. Park A. *HIV Used to be a Death Sentence. Here's What's Changed In 35 Years.* Time (2016). Available online at: http://time.com/4585537/world-aids-day-hiv/ (accessed December 11, 2018).
74. Healthline Red. HIV Then and Now. *HIV by the Numbers: Facts, Statistics, and You.* (2018). Available online at: https://www.healthline.com/health/hiv-aids/facts-statistics-infographic?utm_medium=emailandutm_source=email-shareandutm_campaign=social-sharebar-referred-desktop (accessed December 13, 2018).
75. Abbott F. ACT UP and the AIDS Crisis. *Digital Public Library of America.* (2016). Available online at: http://dp.la/primary-source-sets/act-up-and-the-aids-crisis (accessed December 11, 2018).
76. Preidt R. *HIV Life Expectancy Nears Normal With Treatment.* (2017). Available online at: https://www.webmd.com/hiv-aids/news/20170510/life-expectancy-with-hiv-nears-normal-with-treatment#1 (accessed December 14, 2018).
77. Centers for Disease Control and Prevention [US]. Pneumocystis Pneumonia. Morbidity and Mortality Weekly Report. Los Angeles. Available online at: https://www.cdc.gov/mmwr/preview/mmwrhtml/mm5021a1.htm (accessed December 11, 2018).
78. AIDS.gov A Timeline of HIV/AIDS (2018). Available online at: https://www.hiv.gov/sites/default/files/aidsgov-timeline.pdf (accessed December 11, 2018).
79. Gallo R, Montagnier L. The discovery of HIV as the cause of AIDS. *N Engl J Med.* (2003) 349:2283–5. doi: 10.1056/NEJMp038194
80. Institute of Medicine. *Institute of Medicine (US) Committee to Study the AIDS Research Program of the National Institutes of Health.* Washington, DC: National Academies Press (1991). Available online at: https://www.ncbi.nlm.nih.gov/books/NBK234084/ (accessed March 10, 2019).
81. Act Up. *Act Up Accomplishments – 1987–2012.* (2018) Available online at: https://actupny.com/actions/ (accessed December 12, 2018).
82. HHS Gov [US]. *Chronic Fatigue Syndrome Advisory Committee (CFSAC).* (2018). Available online at: https://www.hhs.gov/ash/advisory-committees/cfsac/index.html (accessed December 11, 2018).

7

Epstein-Barr Virus Induced Gene-2 Upregulation Identifies a Particular Subtype of Chronic Fatigue Syndrome/ Myalgic Encephalomyelitis

*Jonathan R. Kerr**

Department of Microbiology, West Suffolk Hospital Foundation Trust, Bury St Edmunds, United Kingdom

Correspondence:
Jonathan R. Kerr
jonathan@ssl-mail.com

Chronic Fatigue Syndrome/Myalgic Encephalomyelitis (CFS/ME) is a chronic multisystem disease characterized by a variety of symptoms, and exhibits various features of an autoimmune-like disease. Subtypes are well recognized but to date are difficult to identify objectively. The disease may be triggered by infection with a variety of micro-organisms, including Epstein-Barr virus (EBV). A subset of CFS/ME patients exhibit up regulation of EBV virus induced gene 2 (*EBI2*) mRNA in peripheral blood mononuclear cells (PBMC), and these patients appear to have a more severe disease phenotype and lower levels of EBNA1 IgG. *EBI2* is induced by EBV infection and has been found to be upregulated in a variety of autoimmune diseases. *EBI2* is a critical gene in immunity and central nervous system function; it is a negative regulator of the innate immune response in monocytes. Its heterogeneous expression in CFS/ME could explain the variable occurrence of a variety of immune and neurological abnormalities which are encountered in patients with CFS/ME. The *EBI2* subtype occurred in 38–55% CFS/ME patients in our studies. Further work is required to confirm the role of EBV and of *EBI2* and its oxysterol ligands in CFS/ME, and to identify the most practical means to identify patients of the EBI subtype. There are two *EBI2* antagonists currently in development, and these may hold promise in the treatment of CFS/ME patients of the EBI subtype.

Keywords: Chronic Fatigue Syndrome, Myalgic Encephalomyelitis, Epstein-Barr virus, Epstein-Barr virus induced gene 2, autoimmune, microarray, real-time polymerase chain reaction

INTRODUCTION

Chronic Fatigue Syndrome/Myalgic Encephalomyelitis (CFS/ME) is a chronic multisystem disease characterized by at least 6 months of fatigue and a variety of other symptoms, including headache, sore throat, muscle pain, joint pain, muscle weakness, post-exertional malaise, sleep abnormalities, and secondary anxiety and depression (1). It is most likely that heterogeneity in CFS/ME is the reason that although there have been many immune and other abnormalities found in patients, none are universal and so there are currently no biomarkers of CFS/ME *per se*. This is used as evidence against a biological pathogenesis of the disease, however, the most plausible explanation is that CFS/ME is a heterogeneous autoimmune-like disease with a variety of subtypes, a phenomenon typical of autoimmune disease.

Particular problems are, first, that the CFS/ME is unique as a chronic autoimmune-like disease, in that there is no objective means to confirm the diagnosis. Secondly, there are a variety of names and diagnostic criteria some of which do not exclude major depression, as is required by the CDC criteria (1) and Canadian criteria (2). Thirdly, there has been a push to combine biological and unrelated psychological approaches in CFS/ME research. Of course, psychological aspects must be included, but only in terms of what we know is relevant to current knowledge of CFS/ME. Namely, that psychological stress can trigger the disease, and that anxiety and depression are secondary phenomena in CFS/ME (1, 2).

By analogy to autoimmune diseases, psychological aspects are known to be almost universal, for example, anxiety in ulcerative colitis, rheumatoid arthritis, psoriasis, asthma, etc. And the anxiety is believed to underlie relapses and flare-ups which may precipitate hospital admission and use of immune-modifying treatments in a variety of autoimmune diseases.

In this paper, I will review the heterogeneity of CFS/ME, its clinical presentation and triggering factors including Epstein-Barr Virus (EBV) reactivation, CFS/ME as an autoimmune-like disease, Epstein-Barr virus induced (EBI) gene 2 (*EBI2*) dysregulation in CFS/ME, the "EBI subtype" and the future possibility for therapeutic pharmacological EBI2 antagonism in CFS/ME patients.

HETEROGENEITY OF CFS/ME

Heterogeneity among CFS/ME patients is well recognized. There are clear differences in type of onset (sudden vs. gradual), duration of illness, and different types of illness (predominant pain, predominant flu-like illness, predominant neurological type illness, etc.). In a comparative review of systemic and neurological symptoms in 12 outbreaks of CFS/ME, epidemic neuromyasthenia and ME, marked heterogeneity in the range of neurological symptoms was observed (3), and outbreaks could be grouped into four levels of increasing neurological involvement. Janal et al. (4) subtyped CFS/ME patients according to "minor" symptoms, and identified three subtypes; neurological, musculoskeletal, and infectious. Extreme scores in one or more of these factors accounted for 66% of the sample. Depression and anxiety were not more prevalent in any particular subtype. Jason et al. (5) analyzed data from 18,675 CFS/ME patients and found strong evidence for the existence of a variety of subtypes based on sociodemographic status and disability. Jason et al. (6) have outlined the importance of subtyping of CFS/ME patients, both for the study of pathogenesis and for response to available treatments. These authors identified CFS/ME subtypes based on level of disability, viral, immune, neuroendocrine, neurological, autonomic, and genetic aspects. Proper identification and study of CFS/ME subtypes has been hampered by the lack of concensus as to how to diagnose the disease.

CFS/ME AS A CHRONIC FLU-LIKE ILLNESS TRIGGERED BY VIRUS INFECTION

At its most simple, CFS/ME can be considered to be a chronic flu-like illness triggered by virus infection, and that the symptoms of CFS/ME are those of a resulting flu-like illness (fatigue, impairment in short term memory or concentration, sore throat, muscle pain, joint pain without swelling or redness, headaches, unrefreshing sleep, and post-exertional malaise) (7). Psychological symptoms (anxiety and depression) are common during flu-like illnesses, and are secondary in otherwise healthy persons. There is a biological basis for such secondary psychological symptoms in that circulating proinflammatory cytokines result in activation of glial cells in the brain and secretion of proinflammatory cytokines by these cells, causing the symptoms of depression, lethargy and anxiety (8). We are all familiar with such short term illness and its symptoms, including the secondary psychological symptoms. We are familiar with the sickness behavior we exhibit during these short term illnesses. For example, we prefer to go to bed early rather than stay out late (8). The principal difference between a short term flu-like illness secondary to virus infection, and CFS/ME, is the duration, severity and the global effect on the lives of patients. In the case of CFS/ME, generally 6 months of symptoms are required (1), while a short term flu-like illness would typically last <2 weeks.

PSYCHOLOGICAL STRESS IS KEY TO VIRUS TRANSMISSION, INFECTION, AND CFS/ME

For any given virus infection, outcomes vary according to many factors. However, for the purposes of CFS/ME, the key factor is psychological stress. It has been shown for a variety of viruses that psychological stress is necessary for successful virus transmission from one person to another (9). Furthermore, it has been shown that psychological stress is necessary for symptoms to develop after successful transmission, as opposed to asymptomatic infection (9). It is well known that psychological stress is key in the reactivation of herpes viruses, and this precedes the recurrence of cold sores (herpes simplex virus) (10), shingles (varicella-zoster virus) (11), and Epstein-Barr virus (EBV) (12, 13). Psychological stress has been shown to be important in triggering a large proportion of cases of CFS/ME, and this fits perfectly with a viral pathogenesis. Psychological stress is universal and is expected under various circumstances, for example, student examinations, loss of a parent or partner, etc.

IMPORTANT MICROBIAL TRIGGERS OF CFS/ME

Micro-organisms which have been documented to trigger CFS/ME include EBV, enteroviruses, cytomegalovirus (CMV), human herpesvirus-6 (HHV-6), human parvovirus B19, hepatitis

TABLE 1 | Microbial infections which have been shown to trigger CFS/ME.

Micro-organism (virus or bacterium)	Microbial persistence after the acute phase*	Treatment	References
Enteroviruses	No	Interferons α, γ	(14–19)
Epstein-Barr virus (EBV)	Yes	Valacyclovir, Valgancyclovir	(20–25)
Cytomegalovirus (CMV)	Yes	Cidofovir, Human normal immunoglobulin (IVIG)	(18)
Human herpes virus-6	Yes	Cidofovir	(18, 26, 27)
Parvovirus B19	Yes	IVIG	(28–31)
Hepatitis C	Yes	Interferon / ribavirin	(18)
Chlamydia pneumoniae	No	Tetracycline, clarithromycin	(18, 32)
Coxiella burnetii	Yes	Tetracyclines	(33)

**The majority of those micro-organisms important in triggering CFS/ME have been shown to persist following the acute phase.*

C, *Chlamydia pneumonia,* and *Coxiella burnetii* (**Table 1**). EBV is known to infect 90% humans, the majority of which become infected in childhood due to transmission in oral secretions. Following acute infection, EBV persists life-long. It is not clear what percentage of CFS/ME patients are infected with EBV, but in one UK study, it was 90% (34). It is recognized that for each microbial trigger of CFS/ME, that there are a variety of possible clinical outcomes of acute infection, including CFS/ME. It is also recognized, that of those patients who suffered an acute microbial infection which led to development of CFS/ME, there are a number of possible resulting CFS/ME phenotypes, and that this varies depending on other, as yet unknown factors. Therefore, of those patients who developed CFS/ME following parvovirus B19 infection, for example, some will have a CFS/ME phenotype with predominant musculoskeletal pain, while others will have less predominant pain, and more problems with sleep, memory, and concentration, for example. Therefore, there is a lack of correlation between the particular microbial or other trigger and the resulting CFS/ME phenotype.

CFS/ME EXHIBITS FEATURES OF AN AUTOIMMUNE DISEASE

A variety of features suggest that CFS/ME may be an autoimmune-like disease. CFS/ME may be triggered by virus infection, and its course characterized by a typical "viral" flu-like illness (7). These observations have led to the recognition that the immune response plays a large and significant role in the pathogenesis of the disease. There are striking similarities between CFS/ME and various autoimmune diseases, for example, Multiple Sclerosis (MS). And, the existence of subtypes of CFS/ME is a further parallel to autoimmune diseases, in which subtypes are well recognized. There are various examples of subtypes of autoimmune diseases exhibiting specific pathogenetic mechanisms, such that particular subtypes of particular autoimmune diseases may be amenable to specific treatments while other subtypes of the same autoimmune disease are not. Studies have demonstrated a variety of immune abnormalities in CFS/ME patients (**Table 2**), many of which are also found in patients with autoimmune disease. A variety of autoantibodies have been demonstrated in serum of CFS/ME patients including those against nuclear and membrane structures, neurotransmitters and their receptors, cytoplasmic intermediate filaments, EBV dUTPase, and neoepitopes resulting from oxidative or nitrosative damage (53). There is considerable co-morbidity of CFS/ME with other immune or autoimmune diseases, including fibromyalgia (30–77%), postural orthostatic tachycardia syndrome (POTS) (11–40%), Hashimoto's thyroiditis (17–20%), and a family history of an autoimmune disease (18–41%) (53). We have also found upregulated EBI2 mRNA expression in a subset of CFS/ME patients which also occurs in autoimmune diseases (see below).

Two clinical trials of monoclonal anti-CD20 antibody, rituximab, in CFS/ME patients demonstrate partial or complete benefit in 60%, and in some of these the remission was sustained. This treatment, in both trials, exhibited a delayed onset of response of ~4 months, suggesting that benefit was not directly mediated by CD20 depletion, but by plasma cell depletion followed by washout of short-lived autoantibodies (54, 55).

EBV REACTIVATION IS A MODEL FOR PSYCHOLOGICAL STRESS AND TRIGGERING OF CFS/ME

Acute EBV infection has been shown to be an important virus trigger of CFS/ME (20–22). Study of acute EBV infection in medical students shows that EBV preferentially reactivates during the psychologically stressful time of examinations as compared with other less stressful periods of the academic year (56). This has also been shown for military recruits in training at examination times (57). This reactivation is also paralleled by changes in a large variety of immune markers of cellular immunity which are important in the long-term control and suppression of replication of persistent and asymptomatic EBV in the normal person (12, 13). These studies elegantly document the importance of the balance between persistent EBV and cellular immune system competency which can be disrupted by psychological stress, leading to reactivation and replication of EBV, and subsequent manifestation of symptoms of EBV infection, which if the stress is maintained, can become prolonged and lead to CFS/ME and other diseases, such as nasopharyngeal cancer and post-transplant lymphoproliferative disorder (PTLD) (58). The various types of stress that can adversely affect the efficacy of the cellular immune response include marital stress (59), student examination stress (56), attachment anxiety or fear of abandonment and rejection (60),

TABLE 2 | Various immunological abnormalities which have been reported in CFS/ME patients.

Positive study findings in CFS	Negative study findings	References	
		Positive findings	Negative findings
Significant increase in B cells expressing CD20 and CD21	No difference in B cells between CFS and Normals	(35, 36)	(37, 38)
An increase in CD8+/HLADR+ and CD8+/CD38+ T cells	No difference in CD8+/HLADR+ and CD8+/CD38+ T cells	(35, 36)	(38)
Increased T cell differentiation	No increased T cell differentiation	(39)	(38)
NK cell dysfunction		(40)	
Reduction in CD3-/CD16+ and CD57+/CD56+ NK cells with an expansion of the CD8+/CD56+ and CD16-/CD56+ NK subsets and total circulating B cells		(36)	
Deficiency in NKH.1+ T3 cell numbers and decreased NK cell function in patients with CFS who had evidence of EBV reactivation		(41)	
Deficiency in cellular immunity with reduced cytotoxicity of NK cells with increased NK numbers		(35)	
Total NK numbers normal, with decreased NK cell activity as compared to normal (CFS family)		(42, 43)	
Decreased antibody-mediated cellular cytotoxicity (ADCC)		(43)	
Th2 profile of CD4 helper T cell responsiveness		(44–46)	
Reduced TGF1 mRNA expression		(47)	
Increased neutrophil apoptosis		(48)	
Deficiency of IgG1 in 2 CFS patients		(49)	
Deficiency of IgG1 and IgG3 in CFS compared with healthy sedentary controls. IgG1 and IgG3 were even lower in CFS with concurrent axis-I depression as compared with CFS itself		(50)	
Deficiency of IgG1, IgG3, and IgG4		(51)	
Deficiency of IgG3		(52)	

loneliness (61), etc. But physical stress by itself does not have this effect (62).

Psychological stress triggers release of glucocorticoids which activate EBV lytic infection through the upregulation of the immediate early BZLF1 gene expression (63). The cause of the pro-inflammatory state with EBV reactivation is the EBV-encoded deoxyuridine triphosphate nucleotidohydrolase (dUTPase) which modulates innate immunity in human primary monocyte-derived macrophages through toll-like receptor (TLR)-2 signaling leading to NF-κB activation and the production of pro-inflammatory cytokines. EBV dUTPase induces sickness responses in mice (64). Restraint stress (unavoidable stress which causes autonomic and behavioral changes) results in impairment of learning and memory which is due to expression of EBV dUTPase (65).

CFS/ME patients exhibit prolonged raised antibody titers against EBV dUTPase and EBV DNApol which are neutralizing, and may be used to identify CFS patients in which their disease pathogenesis is due to ongoing EBV reactivation (66). However, global screening of serum antibody responses to an EBV peptide array in serum of CFS/ME patients compared with controls revealed strikingly similar patterns (67).

EPSTEIN-BARR VIRUS (EBV) INDUCED GENE 2 (*EBI2*)

Epstein-Barr Virus (EBV) induced gene 2 (*EBI2*) is a G-Protein Coupled Receptor (GPCR), also known as GPR183, which was originally identified as the main induced gene in Burkitt's Lymphoma cells upon infection with EBV (68). *EBI2* has been found to be highly expressed in peripheral blood mononuclear cells (PBMC) (B, T, NK, monocytes, and granulocytes) during EBV reactivation (68–70), is a regulator of B cell partitioning in tissues of the lymphoid system and is critical for T-cell mediated antibody responses (71–74) and inflammation (71, 72, 75). *EBI2* has also been found in dendritic cells and monocytes (76). *EBI2* is activated by oxysterols and pertussis toxin-sensitive heterotrimeric G proteins, resulting in decreased cyclic AMP, mobilization of calcium and activation of the extracellular signal related kinase (ERK) pathway (69, 77). High affinity *EBI2* agonists are the oxysterol, 7α 25-dihydroxycholesterol (7α25HC) and related compounds (78, 79). Activation of *EBI2* with 7α25HC results in a wide range of functional responses including cell migration and calcium mobilization (78, 79). 7α25HC is synthesized from cholesterol

(80). Other oxysterols also activate EBI2 but with lower potency (78).

EBI2 also plays an important role in the central nervous system (69). Astrocytes are the macrophages of the brain and protect it against invading pathogens and astrocyte abnormalities are implicated in multiple sclerosis (MS), Parkinsons Disease (PD), Amyotrophic Lateral Sclerosis (ALS), and Alzheimer Disease (AD). Oligodendrocytes are the main cells involved in myelination of nerve fibers of the brain and are implicated in leukodystrophies and leukoencephalopathies. Cholesterol is a crucial component of myelin and cholesterol deficiency results in motor symptoms (81). Abnormal levels of oxysterols have been found in AD, MS and Experimental Allergic Encephalomyelitis (EAE). Mutations in CYP7B1 gene have been demonstrated in Spastic Paraplegia Gene 5 (SPG5) and lead to lesions of upper motor neurones, periventricular areas and subcortical white matter (82, 83). Brain cholesterol is synthesized in the brain as it can't traverse the blood brain barrier (BBB) (84, 85). The cholesterol metabolite, 24(S)-hydroxycholesterol (24(S)HC) is a brain-specific oxysterol which is thought to be synthesized exclusively in the brain and secreted into the circulation via the BBB to maintain steady levels of brain cholesterol (85). Circulating 24(S)HC is believed to be a biomarker for brain cholesterol homeostasis and neurodegenerative disease (MS, PD, AD) (85–87). Oxysterols also have detrimental effects on myelin and oligodendrocyte viability (88, 89).

Dysregulation of *EBI2* expression has been demonstrated in EBV infection (68, 69, 73, 74, 76), melanoma metastasis, lymphoblastic leukemia, glioblastoma, bone cancer metastasis, systemic lupus erythematous, chronic rhino sinusitis with nasal polyps, Type 1 Diabetes (69), and CFS/ME (90) (see below). Aberrant oxysterol signaling has been demonstrated in Multiple Sclerosis, Experimental Allergic Encephalomyelitis (EAE), Alzheimer's disease, Parkinsons Disease, Motor Neurone Disease, Cerebrotendinous Xanthomatosis, Hereditary spastic paraplegia type 5 (SPG5), Huntingdon Disease, Age related macular degeneration, atherosclerosis, Inflammatory bowel disease, and osteoporosis (69). *EBI2* regulates several genes, important in monocyte function, which are important in the pathogenesis of glioblastoma multiforme and Type 1 Diabetes Mellitus. Knock down of the *EBI2* gene in rat monocytes, results in upregulated IRF7 expression. As IRF7 is a critical regulator of the type 1 interferon response, this suggests that *EBI2* is a negative regulator of the innate immune response in macrophages (91). However, the precise role played by *EBI2* in EBV infection remains to be clarified (68, 69).

EXPRESSION OF EBI2 IN CFS/ME

We have previously found that CFS/ME patients exhibit significantly upregulated expression of *EBI2* in PBMC as compared with normal controls, in gene expression arrays and reverse-transcriptase polymerase chain reaction (RT-PCR) confirmation assays (90). *EBI2* mRNA (NM_004951) expression was found to be significantly upregulated by a factor of 1.3 in microarray experiments using PBMC from 25 CFS patients vs. 50 normal human controls matched 2:1. This upregulation was confirmed using RT-PCR in 55 CFS/ME patients vs. 75 normal human controls at a fold difference of 3.44 ($P = 0.0012$) using ABI assay number Hs00270639_s1 (90). In this study, *EBI2* was found to be unregulated in 55% CFS/ME patients, one of whom was a 26 year old woman whose CFS/ME had been triggered by laboratory documented EBV infection 10 years prior (90). All those with raised expression of EBI2 were also positive for serum anti-VCA IgG.

Microarray experiments identified 88 human genes which were upregulated in CFS/ME, and the RT-PCR expression data on these 88 human genes in 52 CFS patients was then clustered and this identified seven gene expression subtypes. These gene expression derived subtypes differed significantly in measures of clinical symptomatology and neurocognitive functioning (90). Of these 88 human genes which were differentially expressed in CFS patients, they could be divided into two groups each with 44 genes, one group of which showed quite predictable up regulation across most CFS/ME patients and in the other group, the expression was much more variable. *EBI2* was one of those which was more variably upregulated in PBMC of CFS/ME patients. This is illustrated in **Figure 1**, in which 12 of 31 (38%) patients exhibited *EBI2* up regulation as compared with none of 40 normal controls.

Although it was known in 2008 that *EBI2* was upregulated in PBMC of CFS/ME patients (90), the significance was not understood at the time as little was known about the gene and its function. However, with the recent identification of *EBI2* as a critical regulator of the immune response with importance for a variety of autoimmune diseases and cancer, its significance in the pathogenesis of CFS/ME has been recognized.

POSSIBLE LINK BETWEEN *EBI2* EXPRESSION, EBV LATENCY, AND CLINICAL SEVERITY IN CFS/ME

As part of a separate study of microbial infections in CFS/ME, we analyzed EBV antibody markers in 117 CFS/ME patients which had been grouped into eight subtypes (A-H) based on clustering of RT-PCR expression data for 88 CFS/ME-associated genes (34). These 117 CFS/ME patients included 55 CFS/ME patients who had been included in the previous study (90), 56 CFS/ME patients who had not previously been studied and six whose disease had been triggered by acute Q fever (QFS) (34). The CFS/ME patients exhibited 90% EBV seropositivity which is to be expected (34).

Subtype D was the most interesting in terms of EBV infection markers and clinical phenotype (34). Subtype D consisted only of females and had the most severe clinical phenotype, with the lowest functional level on SF-36 scoring (physical role, vitality, general health, bodily pain, and total score) and a high frequency of muscle pain and sleep problems (**Figures 2A,B**). *EBI2* was expressed at the highest level in PBMC of subtype D patients [fold difference (CFSME/Normal), 14.93] as compared with the other subtypes [Mean fold difference (CFSME/Normal), 3.004] (34).

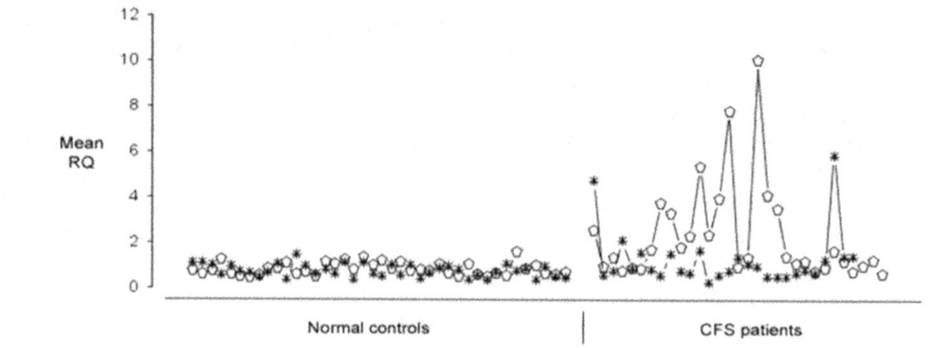

FIGURE 1 | Expression of Epstein-Barr Virus (EBV) induced gene 2 (*EBI2*) (open ellipse) and Neuropathy Target Esterase (NTE) (asterisk) genes in 40 healthy blood donors (shown on the **Left**) and 31 Chronic Fatigue Syndrome/Myalgic Encephalomyelitis (CFS/ME) patients (shown on the **Right**). Upregulated *EBI2* mRNA expression was demonstrated in 12 of 31 CFS/ME patients, and in none of the controls.

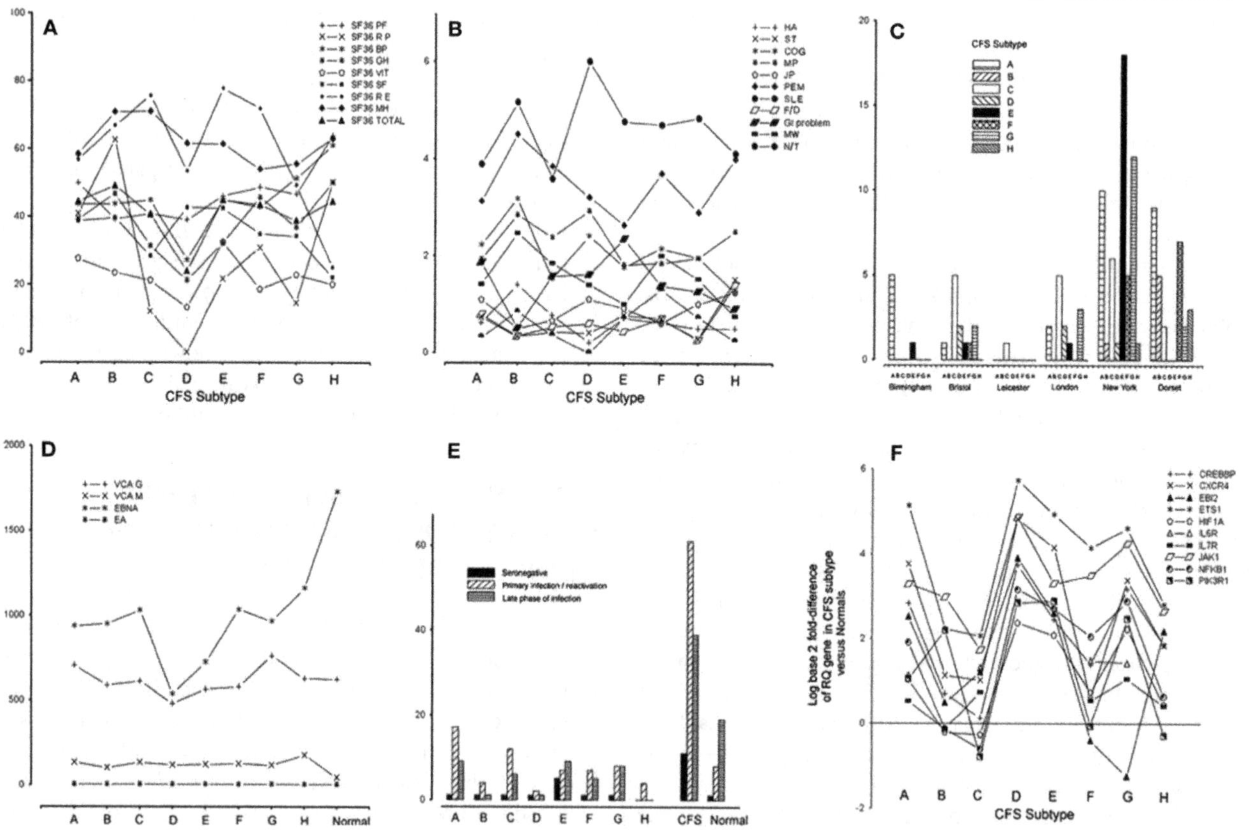

FIGURE 2 | (A) Medical Outcomes Survey Short Form-36 (SF36) domain and total scores for each chronic fatigue syndrome/myalgic encephalomyelitis (CFS/ME) subtype: physical function (PF), physical role (RP), bodily pain (BP), general health (GH), vitality (VIT), social functioning (SF), emotional role (RE), mental health (MH), and total score (Total). **(B)** Scores indicating occurrence and severity of 11 clinical symptoms for each CFS/ME subtype: headache (HA), sore throat (ST), swollen glands (GLA), cognitive defect (COG), muscle pain (MP), joint pain (JP), muscle weakness (MW), post-exertional malaise (PEM), sleep problems (SLE), fainting/dizziness (F/D), gastrointestinal complaints (GI), numbness/tingling (N/T), spatial span (SSP), verbal recognition memory (VRM). **(C)** Histogram showing the numbers of CFS/ME patients of each subtype occurring in each of the six geographical locations. **(D)** Epstein-Barr virus (EBV) antibody titers [viral capsid antigen (VCA) IgM, VCA IgG, early antigen (EA) IgG, Epstein-Barr nuclear antigen (EBNA) IgG] in each CFS/ME subtype and the normal comparison group. **(E)** Distribution of categories of EBV serostatus (seronegative, primary/re-activation, late phase of infection) in the CFS/ME subtypes, A-H, in CFS/ME (all subtypes combined) and in normal controls. **(F)** Log (base 2) of fold-difference values of 10 human genes known to be important in EBV infection, in eight CFS subtypes (A-H). Reproduced from **Figure 1** of reference no. 34 with permission from BMJ Publishing Group Ltd.

There were no discernible differences in EBV antibody markers [viral capsid antigen (VCA) IgM and IgG, early antigen (EA) IgG, and Epstein-Barr nuclear antigen (EBNA) IgG] between subtypes, except that in Subtype D, CFS/ME patients had a markedly reduced titer of EBNA IgG (**Figure 2D**).

Epstein-Barr virus nuclear antigen 1 gene (*EBNA1*) is important in establishing and maintaining the altered state that cells undergo during EBV infection, and is the only EBV protein found in all EBV-associated malignancies. *EBNA1* has a glycine-alanine repeat which stabilizes the protein, prevents its breakdown, impairs antigen processing, and MHC class I-restricted antigen presentation, resulting in inhibition of the CD8-restricted cytotoxic T lymphocyte response against EBV infected cells, thus favoring latency (92). The finding that CFS/ME patients of subtype D with *EBI2* mRNA upregulation had lower titers of EBNA IgG than the other subtypes (**Figure 2D**), supports the idea that subtype D is associated with a higher prevalence of EBV latency, as lytic infection is required to expose this antigen to circulating lymphocytes, a necessary step in developing serum EBNA IgG positivity.

In one study, it was shown that in 10% CFS/ME patients, EBNA IgG titers were low or absent (93). Multicolor flow cytometry revealed that the frequencies of EBNA-1-specific triple TNF-α/IFN-γ/IL-2 producing CD4(+) and CD8(+) T-cell subsets were significantly diminished in CFS/ME patients (93).

Within the CFS/ME-associated gene signature of 88 human genes, 12 had recognized associations with EBV infection. One of these was *EBI2*, as discussed, and the others were *NFKB1*, *EGR1*, *ETS1*, *GABPA*, *CREBBP*, *CXCR4*, *HIF1A*, *JAK1*, *IL6R*, *IL7R*, and *PIK3R1*. Striking associations were found for these 12 genes across subtypes, and subtype D had the highest levels of all of them in PBMC (**Figure 2F**).

HETEROGENEOUS *EBI2* UPREGULATION MAY CONTRIBUTE TO THE VARIABILITY OF IMMUNE AND NEUROLOGICAL ABNORMALITIES IN CFS/ME

The following have been variably been found in CFS/ME patients; increase in the number of circulating B lymphocytes, increase in activated T lymphocytes, reduction in NK cell numbers and/or function, deficiency in antibody-mediated cellular cytotoxicity (ADCC), Th2 profile of helper T cell responsiveness, reduced TGF1 expression, increased neutrophil apoptosis, and deficiencies in particular IgG subsets (**Table 2**). During the normal humoral immune response, activated B cells upregulate *EBI2* which mediates their journey to the outer follicle where they interact with T helper cells. After CD40 engagement, *EBI2* expression results in cells moving away from the B-T boundary toward the outer and inner areas of the follicle (73), differentiation into plasmablasts, and mounting of a rapid antibody response. Some B cells move to the central follicle, differentiate into germinal center B cells, to later exhibit antibody affinity maturation (71-75). A higher than normal expression of *EBI2* could result in both increased numbers of B cells in the circulation, and in reduced T cell help and therefore deficiencies in particular IgG subsets, and reduced antibody affinity maturation. EBV reactivation is associated with expansion of differentiated and activated CD4 and CD8 T lymphocytes and later with decline in these cells as exhaustion takes over (94), and so the timing of EBV infection in CFS/ME will affect research studies on immune abnormalities. NK cells are important in defense during the early stages of primary EBV infection (94). Innate immune control of lytic EBV infection by early differentiated NK cells was found to attenuate infectious mononucleosis (IM) (95). It has been proposed that NK cells are important in the long-term control of EBV (96), which may account for the variable findings related to NK numbers and function in CFS/ME, as not all CFS/ME patients will have EBV reactivation at the time of sampling.

Abnormalities in white matter, gray matter and in cerebral perfusion have been found in CFS/ME patients, and these occur in a similar presentation to those of MS patients. Both CFS/ME and MS patients have reduced cerebral perfusion, gray matter reduction and white matter hyper intensities, although individual patients are variably affected (97). As *EBI2* expression and oxysterol dysregulation have been linked with the pathogenesis of MS (69), and as MS is characterized by a relapsing and remitting course, in which subtypes exist and in which *EBI2* is variably upregulated in some of these, it is logical to suggest that heterogeneous *EBI2* expression may similarly play a role in the neurological abnormalities found in CFS/ME.

Although we know that there are a variety of immune abnormalities which occur with regularity in CFS/ME patients, these do not occur invariably, and none can be used as a marker for the presence of the disease. However, the upregulation of *EBI2* in a subset of CFS/ME patients may contribute to this phenomenon.

EBI2 MODULATORS

EBI2 is a key receptor in B, T and dendritic cells, modulating the T and B cell response to blood borne antigens (76). As *EBI2* and/or its oxysterol ligands are upregulated in B cell malignancies and autoimmune diseases (Type 1 Diabetes, rheumatoid arthritis, systemic lupus erythematosus, and multiple sclerosis), two *EBI2* modulators are being developed. GSK682753A is a small molecule, potent EBI2 antagonist which blocks 7a25HC stimulation of the *EBI2* receptor in a recombinant system (98). NIBR189 is a potent selective antagonist of *EBI2*, which has been developed in paradigms relevant to cardiovascular disease (99).

LIMITATIONS OF THE HYPOTHESIS THAT EBI2 UPREGULATION IS IMPORTANT IN A SUBSET OF CFS/ME PATIENTS

The raw data underpinning the present review were generated by only one research group. Therefore, it would be important that these findings are replicated in additional CFS/ME patients and normal controls by independent research groups.

Elevated levels of antibodies to EBV VCA, EA, and DNase have been reported to occur in CFS/ME patients (20, 21, 66, 100–105) albeit inconsistently (106–108). However, it is important to understand that EBV antibody markers may associate with CFS/ME, but this does not prove that EBV has triggered the disease in those particular cases. The seroprevalence of EBV in the general population and in CFS/ME patients is ~90%. And the proportion of CFS/ME patients with EBI2 upregulation was found to be between 38 and 55% CFS/ME patients, all of whom had IgG to EBV VCA. For a disease in which a variety of microbial triggers are recognized, our findings are consistent with the hypothesis that upregulation of EBI2 is important in the pathogenesis of disease in a subset of CFS/ME patients. However, this hypothesis remains wholly unproven and it is not understood what factors, in addition to EBV infection, are required for upregulation of EBI2 in an individual patient.

Although EBI2 was found to be the most upregulated gene in EBV-infected Burkitt lymphoma cells (68) and has been shown to be important in a variety of autoimmune diseases and cancers, the particular role of EBI2 in the pathogenesis of EBV infection still remains to be elucidated. Therefore, the possible pathogenetic role of EBI2 upregulation in CFS/ME patients remains speculative at present.

CONCLUSION

CFS/ME is a heterogeneous disease which is frequently triggered by virus infection, including EBV. Subtypes are well recognized but to date are difficult to identify objectively. Evidence is presented to document that a subset of CFS/ME patients exhibit up regulation of *EBI2* mRNA in PBMC. *EBI2* is a gene which is induced by EBV infection and which has been found to be upregulated in a variety of autoimmune diseases. EBI2 is a critical gene in immunity and central nervous system function; it is a negative regulator of the innate immune response in monocytes. Its heterogeneous expression in CFS/ME may indicate an ongoing host response to EBV reactivation and on this basis, could explain the heterogeneous occurrence of many of the immune and neurological abnormalities reported in CFS/ME patients. The EBI subtype may account for 38–55% CFS/ME patients. *EBI2* antagonists may hold promise for the treatment of CFS/ME patients of the EBI subtype. Further work is required to confirm the role of EBV and of *EBI2* and its oxysterol ligands in CFS/ME, and to identify the most practical means to identify patients of the EBI subtype.

AUTHOR CONTRIBUTIONS

JK conceived the idea for this review, collated the data, and wrote the paper, without assistance from any other person.

REFERENCES

1. Fukuda K, Straus SE, Hickie I, Sharpe MC, Dobbins JG, Komaroff A. The chronic fatigue syndrome: a comprehensive approach to its definition and study. International Chronic Fatigue Syndrome Study Group. *Ann Intern Med.* (1994) 121:953–9. doi: 10.7326/0003-4819-121-12-199412150-00009
2. Carruthers BM, van de Sande MI, De Meirleir KL, Klimas NG, Broderick G, Mitchell T, et al. Myalgic encephalomyelitis: international consensus criteria. *J Intern Med.* (2011) 270:327–38. doi: 10.1111/j.1365-2796.2011.02428.x
3. Briggs NC, Levine PH. A comparative review of systemic and neurological symptomatology in 12 outbreaks collectively described as chronic fatigue syndrome, epidemic neuromyasthenia, and myalgic encephalomyelitis. *Clin Infect Dis.* (1994) 18(Suppl. 1):S32–42. doi: 10.1093/clinids/18.Supplement_1.S32
4. Janal MN, Ciccone DS, Natelson BH. Sub-typing CFS patients on the basis of "minor" symptoms. *Biol Psychol.* (2006) 73:124–31. doi: 10.1016/j.biopsycho.2006.01.003
5. Jason LA, Taylor RR, Kennedy CL, Jordan KM, Song S, Johnson D, et al. Chronic fatigue syndrome: symptom subtypes in a community based sample. *Women Health.* (2003) 37:1–13. doi: 10.1300/J013v37n01_01
6. Jason LA, Corradi K, Torres-Harding S, Taylor RR, King C. Chronic fatigue syndrome: the need for subtypes. *Neuropsychol Rev.* (2005) 15:29–58. doi: 10.1007/s11065-005-3588-2
7. Devanur LD, Kerr JR. Chronic fatigue syndrome. *J Clin Virol.* (2006) 37:139–50. doi: 10.1016/j.jcv.2006.08.013
8. Dantzer R. Cytokine, sickness behavior, and depression. *Neurol Clin.* (2006) 24:441–60. doi: 10.1016/j.ncl.2006.03.003
9. Cohen S, Tyrrell DA, Smith AP. Psychological stress and susceptibility to the common cold. *N Engl J Med.* (1991) 325:606–12. doi: 10.1056/NEJM199108293250903
10. Padgett DA, Sheridan JF, Dorne J, Berntson GG, Candelora J, Glaser R. Social stress and the reactivation of latent herpes simplex virus type 1. *Proc Natl Acad Sci USA.* (1998) 95:7231–5. doi: 10.1073/pnas.95.12.7231
11. Kim CK, Choi YM, Bae E, Jue MS, So HS, Hwang ES. Reduced NK cell IFN-γ secretion and psychological stress are independently associated with herpes zoster. *PLoS ONE.* (2018) 13:e0193299. doi: 10.1371/journal.pone.0193299
12. Glaser R, Rice J, Sheridan J, Fertel R, Stout J, Speicher C, et al. Stress-related immune suppression: health implications. *Brain Behav Immun.* (1987) 1:7–20. doi: 10.1016/0889-1591(87)90002-X
13. Glaser R, Pearson GR, Jones JF, Hillhouse J, Kennedy S, Mao HY, et al. Stress-related activation of Epstein-Barr virus. *Brain Behav Immun.* (1991) 5:219–32. doi: 10.1016/0889-1591(91)90018-6
14. Yousef GE, Bell EJ, Mann GF, Murugesan V, Smith DG, McCartney RA, et al. Chronic enterovirus infection in patients with postviral fatigue syndrome. *Lancet.* (1988) 1:146–50. doi: 10.1016/S0140-6736(88)92722-5
15. Gow JW, Behan WM, Clements GB, Woodall C, Riding M, Behan PO. Enteroviral RNA sequences detected by polymerase chain reaction in muscle of patients with postviral fatigue syndrome. *BMJ.* (1991) 302:692–6. doi: 10.1136/bmj.302.6778.692
16. Clements GB, McGarry F, Nairn C, Galbraith DN. Detection of enterovirus-specific RNA in serum: the relationship to chronic fatigue. *J Med Virol.* (1995) 45:156–61. doi: 10.1002/jmv.1890450208
17. Chia JK. The role of enterovirus in chronic fatigue syndrome. *J Clin Pathol.* (2005) 58:1126–32. doi: 10.1136/jcp.2004.020255
18. Chia JK, Chia A. Diverse etiologies for chronic fatigue syndrome. *Clin Infect Dis.* (2003) 36:671–2. doi: 10.1086/367666
19. Lane RJ, Soteriou BA, Zhang H, Archard LC. Enterovirus related metabolic myopathy: a postviral fatigue syndrome. *J Neurol Neurosurg Psychiatry.* (2003) 74:1382–6. doi: 10.1136/jnnp.74.10.1382

20. Jones JF. Epstein-Barr virus and the chronic fatigue syndrome: a short review. *Microbiol Sci.* (1988) 5:366–9.
21. Straus SE, Tosato G, Armstrong G, Lawley T, Preble OT, Henle W, et al. Persisting illness and fatigue in adults with evidence of Epstein-Barr virus infection. *Ann Intern Med.* (1985) 102:7–16. doi: 10.7326/0003-4819-102-1-7
22. White PD, Thomas JM, Kangro HO, Bruce-Jones WD, Amess J, Crawford DH, et al. Predictions and associations of fatigue syndromes and mood disorders that occur after infectious mononucleosis. *Lancet.* (2001) 358:1946–54. doi: 10.1016/S0140-6736(01)06961-6
23. Lerner AM, Beqaj SH, Deeter RG, Dworkin HJ, Zervos M, Chang CH, et al. A 6-month trial of valacyclovir in the Epstein-Barr virus subset of chronic fatigue syndrome: improvement in left ventricular function. *Drugs Today.* (2002) 38:549–61. doi: 10.1358/dot.2002.38.8.820095
24. Montoya JG, Kogelnik AM, Bhangoo M, Lunn MR, Flamand L, Merrihew LE, et al. Randomized clinical trial to evaluate the efficacy and safety of valganciclovir in a subset of patients with chronic fatigue syndrome. *J Med Virol.* (2013) 85:2101–9. doi: 10.1002/jmv.23713
25. Watt T, Oberfoell S, Balise R, Lunn MR, Kar AK, Merrihew L, et al. Response to valganciclovir in chronic fatigue syndrome patients with human herpesvirus 6 and Epstein-Barr virus IgG antibody titers. *J Med Virol.* (2012) 84:1967–74. doi: 10.1002/jmv.23411
26. Ablashi DV, Eastman HB, Owen CB, Roman MM, Friedman J, Zabriskie JB, et al. Frequent HHV-6 reactivation in multiple sclerosis (MS) and chronic fatigue syndrome (CFS) patients. *J Clin Virol.* (2000) 16:179–91. doi: 10.1016/S1386-6532(99)00079-7
27. Nicolson GL, Gan R, Haier J. Multiple co-infections (*Mycoplasma*, *Chlamydia*, human herpes virus-6) in blood of chronic fatigue syndrome patients: association with signs and symptoms. *APMIS.* (2003) 111:557–66. doi: 10.1034/j.1600-0463.2003.1110504.x
28. Jacobson SK, Daly JS, Thorne GM, McIntosh K. Chronic parvovirus B19 infection resulting in chronic fatigue syndrome: case history and review. *Clin Infect Dis.* (1997) 24:1048–51. doi: 10.1086/513627
29. Kerr JR, Barah F, Mattey DL, Laing I, Hopkins SJ, Hutchinson IV, et al. Circulating tumour necrosis factor-alpha and interferon-gamma are detectable during acute and convalescent parvovirus B19 infection and are associated with prolonged and chronic fatigue. *J Gen Virol.* (2001) 82:3011–9. doi: 10.1099/0022-1317-82-12-3011
30. Kerr JR, Bracewell J, Laing I, Mattey DL, Bernstein RM, Bruce IN, et al. Chronic fatigue syndrome and arthralgia following parvovirus B19 infection. *J Rheumatol.* (2002) 29:595–602.
31. Kerr JR, Cunniffe VS, Kelleher P, Bernstein RM, Bruce IN. Successful intravenous immunoglobulin therapy in 3 cases of parvovirus B19-associated chronic fatigue syndrome. *Clin Infect Dis.* (2003) 36:e100–6. doi: 10.1086/374666
32. Chia JK, Chia LY. Chronic *Chlamydia pneumoniae* infection: a treatable cause of chronic fatigue syndrome. *Clin Infect Dis.* (1999) 29:452–3. doi: 10.1086/520239
33. Arashima Y, Kato K, Komiya T, Kumasaka K, Matsukawa Y, Murakami M, et al. Improvement of chronic nonspecific symptoms by long-term minocycline treatment in Japanese patients with *Coxiella burnetii* infection considered to have post-Q fever fatigue syndrome. *Intern Med.* (2004) 43:49–54. doi: 10.2169/internalmedicine.43.49
34. Zhang L, Gough J, Christmas D, Mattey DL, Richards SC, Main J, et al. Microbial infections in eight genomic subtypes of chronic fatigue syndrome/myalgic encephalomyelitis. *J Clin Pathol.* (2010) 63:156–64. doi: 10.1136/jcp.2009.072561
35. Klimas NG, Salvato FR, Morgan R, Fletcher MA. Immunologic abnormalities in chronic fatigue syndrome. *J Clin Microbiol.* (1990) 28:1403–10.
36. Tirelli U, Marotta G, Improta S, Pinto A. Immunological abnormalities in patients with chronic fatigue syndrome. *Scand J Immunol.* (1994) 40:601–8. doi: 10.1111/j.1365-3083.1994.tb03511.x
37. Robertson MJ, Schacterle RS, Mackin GA, Wilson SN, Bloomingdale KL, Ritz J, et al. Lymphocyte subset differences in patients with chronic fatigue syndrome, multiple sclerosis and major depression. *Clin Exp Immunol.* (2005) 141:326–32. doi: 10.1111/j.1365-2249.2005.02833.x
38. Sabath DE, Barcy S, Koelle DM, Zeh J, Ashton S, Buchwald D. Cellular immunity in monozygotic twins discordant for chronic fatigue syndrome. *J Infect Dis.* (2002) 185:828–32. doi: 10.1086/339194
39. Straus SE, Fritz S, Dale JK, Gould B, Strober W. Lymphocyte phenotype and function in the chronic fatigue syndrome. *J Clin Immunol.* (1993) 13:30–40. doi: 10.1007/BF00920633
40. Whiteside TL, Friberg D. Natural killer cells and natural killer cell activ- ity in chronic fatigue syndrome. *Am J Med.* (1998) 105:27–34S. doi: 10.1016/S0002-9343(98)00155-7
41. Caligiuri M, Murray C, Buchwald D, Levine H, Cheney P, Peterson D, et al. Phenotypic and functional deficiency of natural killer cells in patients with chronic fatigue syndrome. *J Immunol.* (1987) 139:3306–13.
42. Levine PH, Whiteside TL, Friberg D, Bryant J, Colclough G, Herberman RB. Dysfunction of natural killer activity in a family with chronic fatigue syndrome. *Clin Immunol Immunopathol.* (1998) 88:96–104. doi: 10.1006/clin.1998.4554
43. Aoki T, Miyakoshi H, Usuda Y, Herberman RB. Low NK syndrome and its relationship to chronic fatigue syndrome. *Clin Immunol Immunopathol.* (1993) 69:253–65. doi: 10.1006/clin.1993.1178
44. Visser J, Blauw B, Hinloopen B, Brommer E, de Kloet ER, Kluft C, et al. CD4 T lymphocytes from patients with chronic fatigue syndrome have decreased interferon-gamma production and increased sensitivity to dexamethasone. *J Infect Dis.* (1998) 177:451–4. doi: 10.1086/517373
45. Skowera A, Cleare A, Blair D, Bevis L, Wessely SC, Peakman M. High levels of type 2 cytokine-producing cells in chronic fatigue syndrome. *Clin Exp Immunol.* (2004) 135:294–302. doi: 10.1111/j.1365-2249.2004.02354.x
46. Hanson SJ, Gause W, Natelson B. Detection of immunologically significant factors for chronic fatigue syndrome using neural-network classifiers. *Clin Diagn Lab Immunol.* (2001) 8:658–62. doi: 10.1128/CDLI.8.3.658-662.2001
47. Tomoda A, Joudoi T, Rabab el-M, Matsumoto T, Park TH, Miike T. Cytokine production and modulation: comparison of patients with chronic fatigue syndrome and normal controls. *Psychiatry Res.* (2005) 134:101–4. doi: 10.1016/j.psychres.2005.01.002
48. Kennedy G, Spence V, Underwood C, Belch JJ. Increased neutrophil apoptosis in chronic fatigue syndrome. *J Clin Pathol.* (2004) 57:891–3. doi: 10.1136/jcp.2003.015511
49. Read R, Spickett G, Harvey J, Edwards AJ, Larson HE. IgG1 subclass deficiency in patients with chronic fatigue syndrome. *Lancet.* (1988) 1:241–2. doi: 10.1016/S0140-6736(88)91091-4
50. Natelson BH, Haghighi MH, Ponzio NM. Evidence for the presence of immune dysfunction in chronic fatigue syndrome. *Clin Diagn Lab Immunol.* (2002) 9:747–52. doi: 10.1128/CDLI.9.4.747-752.2002
51. Komaroff AL, Geiger AM, Wormsely S. IgG subclass deficiencies in chronic fatigue syndrome. *Lancet.* (1988) 1:1288–9. doi: 10.1016/S0140-6736(88)92109-5
52. Linde A, Hammarstrom L, Smith CI. IgG subclass deficiency and chronic fatigue syndrome. *Lancet.* (1988) 1:885–6. doi: 10.1016/S0140-6736(88)91633-9
53. Sotzny F, Blanco J, Capelli E, Castro-Marrero J, Steiner S, Murovska M, et al. European network on ME/CFS (EUROMENE). Myalgic encephalomyelitis/chronic fatigue syndrome - evidence for an autoimmune disease. *Autoimmun Rev.* (2018) 17:601–9. doi: 10.1016/j.autrev.2018.01.009
54. Fluge O, Bruland O, Risa K, Storstein A, Kristoffersen EK, Sapkota D, et al. Benefit from B- lymphocyte depletion using the anti-CD20 antibody rituximab in chronic fatigue syndrome. A double-blind and placebo-controlled study. *PLoS ONE.* (2011) 6:e26358. doi: 10.1371/journal.pone.0026358
55. Fluge O, Risa K, Lunde S, Alme K, Rekeland IG, Sapkota D, et al. B-lymphocyte depletion in Myalgic encephalopathy/chronic fatigue syndrome. An open-label phase II study with rituximab maintenance treatment. *PLoS ONE.* (2015) 10:e0129898. doi: 10.1371/journal.pone.0129898
56. Glaser R, Pearl DK, Kiecolt-Glaser JK, Malarkey WB. Plasma cortisol levels and reactivation of latent Epstein-Barr virus in response to examination stress. *Psychoneuroendocrinology.* (1994) 19:765–72. doi: 10.1016/0306-4530(94)90023-X
57. Glaser R, Friedman SB, Smyth J, Ader R, Bijur P, Brunell P, et al. The differential impact of training stress and final examination stress on herpesvirus latency at the United States Military Academy at West Point. *Brain Behav Immun.* (1999) 13:240–51. doi: 10.1006/brbi.1999.0566
58. Li H, Liu S, Hu J, Luo X, Li N, M Bode A, et al. Epstein-Barr virus lytic reactivation regulation and its pathogenic role in carcinogenesis. *Int J Biol Sci.* (2016) 12:1309–18. doi: 10.7150/ijbs.16564

59. Jaremka LM, Glaser R, Malarkey WB, Kiecolt-Glaser JK. Marital distress prospectively predicts poorer cellular immune function. *Psychoneuroendocrinology.* (2013) 38:2713–9. doi: 10.1016/j.psyneuen.2013.06.031
60. Fagundes CP, Jaremka LM, Glaser R, Alfano CM, Povoski SP, Lipari AM, et al. Attachment anxiety is related to Epstein-Barr virus latency. *Brain Behav Immun.* (2014) 41:232–8. doi: 10.1016/j.bbi.2014.04.002
61. Glaser R, Kiecolt-Glaser JK, Speicher CE, Holliday JE. Stress, loneliness, and changes in herpesvirus latency. *J Behav Med.* (1985) 8:249–60. doi: 10.1007/BF00870312
62. Aubrecht TG, Weil ZM, Abi Salloum B, Ariza ME, Williams M, Reader B, et al. Chronic physical stress does not interact with Epstein-Barr Virus (EBV)-encoded dutpase to alter the sickness response. *J Behav Brain Sci.* (2015) 5:513–23. doi: 10.4236/jbbs.2015.511049
63. Yang EV, Webster Marketon JI, Chen M, Lo KW, Kim SJ, Glaser R. Glucocorticoids activate Epstein Barr virus lytic replication through the upregulation of immediate early BZLF1 gene expression. *Brain Behav Immun.* (2010) 24:1089–96. doi: 10.1016/j.bbi.2010.04.013
64. Padgett DA, Hotchkiss AK, Pyter LM, Nelson RJ, Yang E, Yeh PE, et al. Epstein-Barr virus-encoded dUTPase modulates immune function and induces sickness behavior in mice. *J Med Virol.* (2004) 74:442–8. doi: 10.1002/jmv.20196
65. Aubrecht TG, Weil ZM, Ariza ME, Williams M, Reader BF, Glaser R, et al. Epstein-Barr virus (EBV)-encoded dUTPase and chronic restraint induce impaired learning and memory and sickness responses. *Physiol Behav.* (2014) 137:18–24. doi: 10.1016/j.physbeh.2014.07.001
66. Lerner AM, Ariza ME, Williams M, Jason L, Beqaj S, Fitzgerald JT, et al. Antibody to Epstein-Barr virus deoxyuridine triphosphate nucleotidohydrolase and deoxyribonucleotide polymerase in a chronic fatigue syndrome subset. *PLoS ONE.* (2012) 7:e47891. doi: 10.1371/journal.pone.0047891
67. Loebel M, Eckey M, Sotzny F, Hahn E, Bauer S, Grabowski P, et al. Serological profiling of the EBV immune response in Chronic Fatigue Syndrome using a peptide microarray. *PLoS ONE.* (2017) 12:e0179124. doi: 10.1371/journal.pone.0179124
68. Birkenbach M, Josefsen K, Yalamanchili R, Lenoir G, Kieff E. Epstein-Barr virus-induced genes: first lymphocyte-specific G protein-coupled peptide receptors. *J Virol.* (1993) 67:2209–20.
69. Rutkowska A, Dev KK, Sailer AW. The role of the Oxysterol/EBI2 pathway in the immune and central nervous systems. *Curr Drug Targets.* (2016) 17:1851–60. doi: 10.2174/1389450117666160217123042
70. Benned-Jensen T, Norn C, Laurent S, Madsen CM, Larsen HM, Arfelt KN, et al. Molecular characterization of oxysterol binding to the Epstein-Barr virus-induced gene 2 (GPR183). *J Biol Chem.* (2012) 287:35470–83. doi: 10.1074/jbc.M112.387894
71. Gatto D, Paus D, Basten A, Mackay CR, Brink R. Guidance of B cells by the orphan G protein-coupled receptor EBI2 shapes humoral immune responses. *Immunity.* (2009) 31:259–69. doi: 10.1016/j.immuni.2009.06.016
72. Gatto D, Wood K, Brink R. EBI2 operates independently of but in cooperation with CXCR5 and CCR7 to direct B cell migration and organization in follicles and the germinal center. *J Immunol.* (2011) 187:4621–8. doi: 10.4049/jimmunol.1101542
73. Kelly LM, Pereira JP, Yi T, Xu Y, Cyster JG. EBI2 guides serial movements of activated B cells and ligand activity is detectable in lymphoid and nonlymphoid tissues. *J Immunol.* (2011) 187:3026–32. doi: 10.4049/jimmunol.1101262
74. Pereira JP, Xu Y, Cyster JG. A role for S1P and S1P1 in immature-B cell egress from mouse bone marrow. *PLoS ONE.* (2010) 5:e9277. doi: 10.1371/journal.pone.0009277
75. Pereira JP, Kelly LM, Xu Y, Cyster JG. EBI2 mediates B cell segregation between the outer and centre follicle. *Nature.* (2009) 460:1122–6. doi: 10.1038/nature08226
76. Sun S, Liu C. 7α, 25-dihydroxycholesterol-mediated activation of EBI2 in immune regulation and diseases. *Front Pharmacol.* (2015) 6:60. doi: 10.3389/fphar.2015.00060
77. Hannedouche S, Zhang J, Yi T, Shen W, Nguyen D, Pereira JP, et al. Oxysterols direct immune cell migration via EBI2. *Nature.* (2011) 475:524–7. doi: 10.1038/nature10280
78. Liu C, Yang XV, Wu J, Kuei C, Mani NS, Zhang L, et al. Oxysterols direct B-cell migration through EBI2. *Nature.* (2011) 475:519–23. doi: 10.1038/nature10226
79. Yi T, Wang X, Kelly LM, An J, Xu Y, Sailer AW, et al. Oxysterol gradient generation by lymphoid stromal cells guides activated B cell movement during humoral responses. *Immunity.* (2012) 37:535–48. doi: 10.1016/j.immuni.2012.06.015
80. Saher G, Brügger B, Lappe-Siefke C, Möbius W, Tozawa R, Wehr MC, et al. High cholesterol level is essential for myelin membrane growth. *Nat Neurosci.* (2005) 8:468–75. doi: 10.1038/nn1426
81. Schüle R, Schöls L. Genetics of hereditary spastic paraplegias. *Semin Neurol.* (2011) 31:484–93. doi: 10.1055/s-0031-1299787
82. Biancheri R, Ciccolella M, Rossi A, Tessa A, Cassandrini D, Minetti C, et al. White matter lesions in spastic paraplegia with mutations in SPG5/CYP7B1. *Neuromuscul Disord.* (2009) 19:62–5. doi: 10.1016/j.nmd.2008.10.009
83. Leoni V, Caccia C. Oxysterols as biomarkers in neurodegenerative diseases. *Chem Phys Lipids.* (2011) 164:515–24. doi: 10.1016/j.chemphyslip.2011.04.002
84. Björkhem I, Meaney S. Brain cholesterol: long secret life behind a barrier. *Arterioscler Thromb Vasc Biol.* (2004) 24:806–15. doi: 10.1161/01.ATV.0000120374.59826.1b
85. Lütjohann D, Papassotiropoulos A, Björkhem I, Locatelli S, Bagli M, Oehring RD, et al. Plasma 24S-hydroxycholesterol (cerebrosterol) is increased in Alzheimer and vascular demented patients. *J Lipid Res.* (2000) 41:195–8.
86. Leoni V, Masterman T, Diczfalusy U, De Luca G, Hillert J, Björkhem I. Changes in human plasma levels of the brain specific oxysterol 24S-hydroxycholesterol during progression of multiple sclerosis. *Neurosci Lett.* (2002) 331:163–6. doi: 10.1016/S0304-3940(02)00887-X
87. Makoukji J, Shackleford G, Meffre D, Grenier J, Liere P, Lobaccaro JM, et al. Interplay between LXR and Wnt/β-catenin signaling in the negative regulation of peripheral myelin genes by oxysterols. *J Neurosci.* (2011) 31:9620–9. doi: 10.1523/JNEUROSCI.0761-11.2011
88. Trousson A, Bernard S, Petit PX, Liere P, Pianos A, El Hadri K, et al. 25-hydroxycholesterol provokes oligodendrocyte cell line apoptosis and stimuates the secreted phospholipase A2 type IIA via LXR beta and PXR. *J Neurochem.* (2009) 109:945–58. doi: 10.1111/j.1471-4159.2009.06009.x
89. Moog C, Luu B, Beck JP, Italiano L, Bischoff P. Studies on the immunosuppressive properties of 7,25-dihydroxycholesterol-I. Reduction of interleukin production by treated lymphocytes. *Int J Immunopharmacol.* (1988) 10:511–8. doi: 10.1016/0192-0561(88)90067-7
90. Kerr JR, Petty R, Burke B, Gough J, Fear D, Sinclair LI, et al. Gene expression subtypes in patients with chronic fatigue syndrome/myalgic encephalomyelitis. *J Infect Dis.* (2008) 197:1171–84. doi: 10.1086/533453
91. Heinig M, Petretto E, Wallace C, Bottolo L, Rotival M, Lu H, et al. A trans-acting locus regulates an anti-viral expression network and type 1 diabetes risk. *Nature.* (2010) 467:460–4. doi: 10.1038/nature09386
92. Frappier L. Contributions of Epstein-Barr nuclear antigen 1 (EBNA1) to cell immortalization and survival. *Viruses.* (2012) 4:1537–47. doi: 10.3390/v4091537
93. Loebel M, Strohschein K, Giannini C, Koelsch U, Bauer S, Doebis C, et al. Deficient EBV-specific B- and T-cell response in patients with chronic fatigue syndrome. *PLoS ONE.* (2014) 9:e85387. doi: 10.1371/journal.pone.0085387
94. Pender MP, Csurhes PA, Burrows JM, Burrows SR. Defective T-cell control of Epstein-Barr virus infection in multiple sclerosis. *Clin Transl Immunol.* (2017) 6:e126. doi: 10.1038/cti.2016.87
95. Chijioke O, Landtwing V, Münz C. NK cell influence on the outcome of primary Epstein-Barr virus infection. *Front Immunol.* (2016) 7:323. doi: 10.3389/fimmu.2016.00323
96. Münz C. Epstein-Barr virus-specific immune control by innate lymphocytes. *Front Immunol.* (2017) 8:1658. doi: 10.3389/fimmu.2017.01658
97. Morris G, Berk M, Puri BK. A comparison of neuroimaging abnormalities in multiple sclerosis, major depression and chronic fatigue syndrome (Myalgic Encephalomyelitis): is there a common cause? *Mol Neurobiol.* (2018) 55:3592–609. doi: 10.1007/s12035-017-0598-z
98. Benned-Jensen T, Madsen CM, Arfelt KN, Smethurts C, Blanchard A, Jepras R, et al. Small molecule antagonism of oxysterol-induced Epstein-Barr virus induced gene 2 (EBI2) activation. *FEBS Open Bio.* (2013) 3:156–60. doi: 10.1016/j.fob.2013.02.003

99. Gessier F, Preuss I, Yin H, Rosenkilde MM, Laurent S, Endres R, et al. Identification and characterization of small molecule modulators of the Epstein-Barr virus-induced gene 2 (EBI2) receptor. *J Med Chem.* (2014) 57:3358–68. doi: 10.1021/jm4019355
100. Buchwald D, Sullivan JL, Komaroff AL. Frequency of 'chronic active Epstein-Barr virus infection' in a general medical practice. *JAMA.* (1987) 257:2303–7.
101. Hellinger WC, Smith TF, Van Scoy RE, Spitzer PG, Forgacs P, Edson RS. Chronic fatigue syndrome and the diagnostic utility of antibody to Epstein-Barr virus early antigen. *JAMA.* (1988) 260:971–3. doi: 10.1001/jama.1988.03410070099036
102. Holmes GP, Kaplan JE, Stewart JA, Hunt B, Pinsky PF, Schonberger LB. A cluster of patients with a chronic mononucleosis-like syndrome. Is Epstein-Barr virus the cause? *JAMA.* (1987) 257:2297–302. doi: 10.1001/jama.1987.03390170053027
103. Lerner AM, Beqaj SH, Deeter RG, Fitzgerald JT. IgM serum antibodies to Epstein-Barr virus are uniquely present in a subset of patients with the chronic fatigue syndrome. *In Vivo.* (2004) 18:101–6.
104. Sairenji T, Yamanishi K, Tachibana Y, Bertoni G, Kurata T. Antibody responses to Epstein-Barr virus, human herpesvirus 6 and human herpesvirus 7 in patients with chronic fatigue syndrome. *Intervirology.* (1995) 38:269–73. doi: 10.1159/000150450
105. Kawai K, Kawai A. Studies on the relationship between chronic fatigue syndrome and Epstein-Barr virus in Japan. *Intern Med.* (1992) 31:313–8. doi: 10.2169/internalmedicine.31.313
106. Cameron B, Flamand L, Juwana H, Middeldorp J, Naing Z, Rawlinson W, et al. Serological and virological investigation of the role of the herpesviruses EBV, CMV and HHV-6 in post-infective fatigue syndrome. *J Med Virol.* (2010) 82:1684–8. doi: 10.1002/jmv.21873
107. Wallace HL II, Natelson B, Gause W, Hay J. Human herpesviruses in chronic fatigue syndrome. *Clin Diagn Lab Immunol.* (1999) 6:216–23.
108. Whelton CL, Salit I, Moldofsky H. Sleep, Epstein-Barr virus infection, musculoskeletal pain, and depressive symptoms in chronic fatigue syndrome. *J Rheumatol.* (1992) 19:939–43.

8

Endometriosis as a Comorbid Condition in Chronic Fatigue Syndrome (CFS): Secondary Analysis of Data from a CFS Case-Control Study

Roumiana S. Boneva [1*†], *Jin-Mann S. Lin* [1], *Friedrich Wieser* [2†], *Urs M. Nater* [3†], *Beate Ditzen* [3†], *Robert N. Taylor* [2†] *and Elizabeth R. Unger* [1]

[1] *Division of High-Consequence Pathogens and Pathology, National Center for Emerging and Zoonotic Infectious Diseases, Centers for Disease Control and Prevention, Atlanta, GA, United States,* [2] *Department of Gynecology and Obstetrics, Emory University School of Medicine, Atlanta, GA, United States,* [3] *Department of Psychiatry and Behavioral Sciences, Emory University School of Medicine, Atlanta, GA, United States*

Correspondence:
Roumiana S. Boneva
rboneva@cdc.gov

Background: Endometriosis (EM) is a recognized co-morbid condition in women with chronic fatigue syndrome (CFS). This analysis evaluates the impact of EM on the health of women with CFS by comparing selected health characteristics and laboratory parameters in women with CFS with and without EM (CFS+EM and CFS-only).

Methods: This secondary analysis included all 36 women with CFS from a cross-sectional study of CFS in Wichita, KS, conducted between 2002 and 2003. The health characteristics and laboratory parameters of interest included functioning, fatigue, CFS-related symptoms, gynecologic history, routine laboratory parameters, inflammatory markers, cortisol levels, allostatic load, and sleep parameters (overnight polysomnography). We used parametric or non-parametric tests to compare group differences in the selected health characteristics and laboratory parameters. For examining the association between EM and variables of interest, logistic regression models were performed and odds ratios (OR) with 95% confidence intervals (CI) were reported for the magnitude of associations. Statistical significance was set at 0.05 (two-sided).

Results: The mean age of this study sample was 50.9 years. Of women with CFS, 36.1% reported having EM. Age and body mass index (BMI) did not differ between CFS+EM and CFS-only groups. When examining the impact of EM, compared to women with CFS-only, women with both CFS and EM were more likely to report chronic pelvic pain [OR = 9.00 (95% CI, 1.47–55.25)] and hysterectomy [OR = 10.3 (1.82–58.39)], had more CFS symptoms (6.8 ± 0.3 vs. 5.5 ± 0.3, $p = 0.02$), younger mean age at menopause onset (36.4 ± 3.0 vs. 47.0 ± 2.7 years, $p = 0.03$), higher mean number of obstructive apnea episodes per hour (20.3 vs. 4.4, $p = 0.05$) and reported more negative life events (15.8 vs. 4.4, $p = 0.05$). Other parameters did not differ significantly between the two groups.

Conclusions: We found more than a third of women with CFS reported endometriosis as a comorbid condition. The endometriosis comorbidity was associated with chronic pelvic pain, earlier menopause, hysterectomy, and more CFS-related symptoms. However, endometriosis in women with CFS did not appear to further impact functioning, fatigue, inflammatory markers, or other laboratory parameters. Further investigations including younger women are warranted.

Keywords: endometriosis, chronic fatigue syndrome, chronic pelvic pain, menopause, hysterectomy, sleep, cortisol, inflammatory markers

INTRODUCTION

Chronic fatigue syndrome (CFS), also referred to as myalgic encephalomyelitis (ME) or ME/CFS, is a serious chronic condition characterized by significant impairment in activity levels due to profound fatigue, worsening symptoms after seemingly minimal physical, or mental exertion, sleep problems, as well as difficulties with memory and concentration or orthostatic intolerance (1). Patients with ME/CFS also frequently experience chronic joint and muscle pain. Conditions with chronic pain as a major symptom, such as ME/CFS, endometriosis (EM), fibromyalgia, interstitial cystitis/bladder pain, irritable bowel syndrome, temporomandibular joint syndrome, and chronic migraines, have been termed chronic overlapping pain conditions. There is evidence that persons with one of these conditions are more likely to have another one as a co-morbidity (2, 3). We conducted this analysis to examine the functional impact of EM as a co-morbid condition in women with CFS.

We focused on EM as a comorbidity for several reasons. EM is an estrogen dependent inflammatory disease, which affects 5–10% of women of reproductive age (4, 5); 0.5 to 5% of fertile women and 24–40% of infertile women (6–8). In a survey of women with EM, about 20% reported one or more co-morbidities such as CFS, autoimmune diseases, migraine, and other chronic pain syndromes (9). That survey estimated that, compared to women in the general population, those with EM were eight times more likely to have CFS. Similarly, among women with CFS, EM is a common comorbidity. In a study of CFS that focused on reproductive history risk factors, 19% of women with CFS reported EM whereas only 8% of women without CFS reported EM (10). Reports also show that CFS and EM share a variety of abnormalities and "risk factors." Changes in daily cortisol secretion have been reported in persons with EM (11, 12) as well as in those with CFS (13). Stress has been implicated in the pathogenesis of EM and its symptoms (9, 14, 15) as well as in chronic pain syndromes, such as fibromyalgia and CFS (16, 17). Allostatic load, a measure of life-long-stress, has been shown to be higher in women with CFS (18).

Abbreviations: ALI, allostatic load index; BMI, body mass index [kg/m2]; CFS, chronic fatigue syndrome; CFS+EM, CFS with endometriosis; CFS-only, CFS without endometriosis; CRP, C-reactive protein; CTQ, childhood trauma questionnaire; DTS, Davidson trauma scale; EM, Endometriosis; GLM, Generalized Linear Model; IL-6, interleukin 6; LES, life experiences survey; MFI-20, Multiple fatigue inventory; PSS, perceived stress scale; SF-36, a 36-item short-form of the Medical Outcomes Survey questionnaire; OSA, obstructive sleep apnea; SDS, self-rating depression scale; STAI, state-trait anxiety inventory; TNF, tumor necrosis factor.

In this report, we sought to examine the impact of EM on CFS. More specifically, we compare women with CFS and EM (termed "CFS+EM") and women with CFS only (termed "CFS-only") in regard to health and function scores, fatigue scores, number of CFS symptoms, select variables from the gynecological history, psychosocial and stress variables, and select laboratory parameters.

METHODS

Data Source and Study Sample

Data were derived from participants in a 2-day in-hospital case-control study (the source study) of CFS conducted between 2002 and 2003. Participants were previously identified in the Wichita (Kansas, USA) 4-year longitudinal population-based surveillance study of CFS (18). The source study adhered to U.S. Department of Health and Human Services human experimentation guidelines and received Institutional Review Board approval from CDC and Abt associates. All participants gave written informed consent. Demographic data were collected during a computer assisted telephone interview and confirmed at the clinic. Participants underwent a comprehensive in-hospital clinical evaluation over 2 days. The study used the operationalized 1994 CFS case definition (19, 20). Participants who had medical or psychiatric conditions that could explain their symptoms were excluded from the CFS classification. In the source study, 43 persons were diagnosed as having CFS (18, 20); 36 of them were women and were all included in this secondary analysis. Body mass index (BMI) was calculated from height and weight measured at the clinic at the time of physical exam: BMI = weight [kg]/ height^2 [m^2].

Patient-Reported Outcomes

We assessed functional health and well-being with the Medical Outcomes Survey short form-36 version 2 (SF-36 v2) (21, 22) and fatigue with the 20-item multi-dimensional fatigue inventory (MFI-20) (23). We used the CDC Symptom Inventory (CDC-SI) to evaluate the presence, frequency, and severity/intensity of all CFS case-defining symptoms, with SI score calculated as the product of the frequency and intensity/severity of symptoms (24–26). The higher the scores of MFI-20 and CDC-SI scales, the worse the fatigue/symptom severity; in contrast–lower SF-36 scores reflect worse functional health.

We collected data on gynecologic conditions and surgeries using a previously described short, structured gynecologic history questionnaire (27). The questionnaire included questions relating to endometriosis ("Have you ever suffered from endometriosis?"), chronic pelvic pain ("In the past 6 months have you experienced lower abdominal or pelvic pain that is unrelated to your menstrual periods?") and menopause (menopausal yes or no; if yes, age their periods stopped). Women were also asked whether they had had their uterus and/or ovaries removed.

We assessed stress with the Short Form of the Childhood Trauma Questionnaire (CTQ) for severity of different types of childhood trauma (28), the Perceived Stress Scale (PSS) (29) for an index of chronic stress or strain, and coping with these stresses, and the Life Experiences Survey (LES) (30) for acute and chronic life stresses. We used the self-administered Spielberger State-Trait Anxiety Inventory (STAI) to measures core symptoms of anxiety as a general trait and as a current state based on responses to 40 items (31). We used the Self Rating Depression Scale (SDS), a 20-item questionnaire, to measure core symptoms of depression on a 4-point Likert scale (32). Subjects were screened for posttraumatic stress disorder (PTSD) based on the self-administered Davidson Trauma Scale (DTS) (33).

Sleep Study

Polysomnography parameters were derived from the overnight polysomnography recordings performed during the second in-clinic night and aggregate results for CFS cases and controls along with detailed methods have been previously reported (34, 35). In brief, polysomnography was performed in the period 10:00 p.m. (when lights were turned out) until 7:00 a.m. the next day. We used data from women with CFS (with or without EM) and included variables of total sleep time, respiratory disturbance index (RDI) scores, snore index, obstructive sleep apnea (OSA) scores, sleep efficiency, and wake time.

Laboratory Tests of Biological Specimens

Sample collection and testing have been described (36). Complete blood counts (CBC), routine blood chemistry, serum cortisol, catecholamines, and inflammatory markers (C-reactive protein [CRP], the pro-inflammatory cytokines interleukin 6 [IL-6], and tumor necrosis factor alpha [TNF-α]) were measured from fasting blood samples obtained at 7:00 a.m. In addition to serum cortisol, 24 h urinary cortisol was also measured.

Allostatic Load Index (ALI)

Allostatic load is the body's cumulative "wear and tear" due to repeated cycles of adaptation to stress (37) and could be measured by a composite score called allostatic load index (ALI). This index included 11 components representing metabolic and cardiovascular parameters, inflammatory response parameters, hypothalamus-pituitary-adrenal axis activity parameters, and measures of sympathetic nervous system (SNS) activity. Aggregate data on allostatic load for all the CFS cases and their controls have been previously reported (38).

In this report, comparisons of health parameters focus on women with "CFS+EM" vs. women with "CFS-only." Data on controls with endometriosis ("EM-only") and controls without EM are available in the appended material (which includes tables with results across four groups: "CFS+EM," "CFS-only," "Controls with EM," and "Controls without EM"). We present some of those data in the main text when relevant.

Statistical Analyses

We used the Chi-square (or Fisher's exact test, when indicated) to examine the independence of categorical variables and analysis of variance to test mean differences between the two groups. Mean and Standard Error of Mean (SEM) were used to summarize the results. Cortisol values were log-transformed to obtain normal or near-normal data distribution. Where applicable, non-parametric tests were used for comparing non-normally distributed continuous variables. In addition, we used logistic regression to calculate odds ratios (OR) with 95% confidence intervals (CI) as a measure of association between selected health characteristics and study group. For variables known to be associated with BMI, we calculated respectively adjusted ORs. Statistical significance was set at $p < 0.05$.

RESULTS

The demographic data for women included in this analysis are presented in **Table 1**. The women's mean (SEM) age was 51.1 (1.0) years, median—52.5 years, range 27–69 years (with 61% being 50 or older). Ninety four percent were white, 72.6% were employed, 55.9% had a household income of over $40,000 and over two-thirds had more than high school education (**Table 1**). Endometriosis was reported significantly more frequently by the CFS group—36% (13 of 36) than by the well, non-fatigued controls—17% (8 of 48), $p = 0.04$ (see **Tables 1S, 2S**).

TABLE 1 | Demographic characteristic for the sample of 36 women with chronic fatigue syndrome (CFS cases) in the case-control study of chronic fatigue syndrome, Wichita, USA, 2002–2003.

Variable \ Group	All CFS (n = 36)
Mean age (SEM)	50.9 (1.5)
Age Group	
18–29	1 (2.8%)
30–39	4 (11.1%)
40–49	10 (27.8%)
50 and older	21 (58.3%)
Race	
White	32 (88.9%)
Other (Black and Native American)	4 (11.1%)
Education	
High school graduate(c)	14 (38.9%)
Associate degree, some college, or college degree	22 (61.1%)
Income ($/Year)	
=<20,000	11 (30.6%)
20,000–40,000	13 (36.1%)
Over 40,000	9 (25.0%)
Missing	3 (12.5%)

All values are numbers and (%) except for age, which is shown as mean.
SEM, standard error of the mean.
(c), includes one participant who had some high school education but no diploma.

TABLE 2 | Comparison of select characteristics in women with CFS by subgroup—with and without endometriosis comorbidity.

Variable \ Group	All CFS (n = 36)	CFS+EM (n = 13)	CFS-only (n = 23)	p
Age	50.9 (1.5)	54.0 (1.8)	49.1 (2.1)	0.39
BMI	29.5 (0.7)	28.6 (1.0)	30.0 (1.0)	0.29
Mean duration of CFS illness (years)	17.0 (2.7)	16.8 (3.3)	17.1 (2.3)	0.93
Onset of CFS illness[(a)]				0.73
Sudden, *n (%)*	6 (16.7%)	2 (15.4%)	4 (17.4%)	
Gradual, *n (%)*	29 (80.6%)	11 (84.6%)	18 (78.3%)	
Missing, *n (%)*	1 (2.7%)	–	1 (4.3%)	
Presence of post-exertional malaise				0.28
Yes, *n (%)*	30 (83.3%)	12 (92.3%)	18 (78.3%)	
No, *n (%)*	6 (16.7%)	1 (7.7%)	5 (21.7%)	
SF-36 Subscales (Range 0–100)[(b)]				
General health	51.6 (3.5)	53.9 (5.7)	50.3 (4.6)	0.64
Mental health	66.0 (3.3)	68.6 (6.5)	64.5 (3.6)	0.55
Physical functioning	50.4 (3.6)	46.9 (5.4)	52.4 (4.7)	0.47
Role emotional	55.6 (7.0)	64.1 (11.6)	50.7 (8.9)	0.37
Role physical	18.8 (5.0)	11.5 (7.8)	22.8 (6.5)	0.29
Social functioning	49.0 (3.9)	49.0 (7.9)	48.9 (4.2)	0.99
Vitality	17.8 (2.1)	19.6 (4.0)	16.7 (2.3)	0.51
Bodily pain	40.1 (2.7)	37.0 (3.8)	41.8 (3.7)	0.40
MFI-20 Subscales (Range 4–20)[(c)]				
General fatigue	17.7 (0.3)	17.1 (0.4)	17.9 (0.4)	0.74
Physical fatigue	14.4 (0.5)	13.8 (0.9)	14.7 (0.6)	0.44
Mental fatigue	14.1 (0.7)	12.8 (1.2)	14.9 (0.8)	0.17
Reduced activity	14.8 (0.6)	14.5 (0.8)	15.0 (0.8)	0.67
Reduced motivation	12.3 (0.7)	12.2 (1.1)	12.3 (0.9)	0.98
CDC Symptom Inventory				
Number of CFS symptoms	5.9 (0.2)	6.8 (0.3)	5.5 (0.3)	0.02
Symptom Inventory Score	46.0 (3.4)	51.4 (5.7)	43.0 (4.3)	0.24
Gynecologic Variables				
Pelvic pain[(d)], *n* (%)	8 (22.2%)	6 (46.2%)	2 (8.7%)	0.02
Hysterectomy, *n* (%)	19 (52.8%)	11 (84.6%)	8 (34.8%)	<0.01
Postmenopausal, *n* (%)	25 (69.4%)	12 (92.3%)	13 (56.5%)	0.03
Mean age at menopause onset	41.7 (2.3) (n = 20)	36.4 (3.0) (n = 10)	47.0 (2.7) (n = 10)	0.03
Hysterectomy in the subset of post-menopausal women only, *n* (%)	19/25 (76%)	11/12 (91.7%)	8/13 (61.5%)	0.16

CFS, chronic fatigue syndrome; EM, endometriosis; CFS+EM, women who had CFS and endometriosis; CFS-only, women who had CFS but not endometriosis
Values are shown as mean (SEM, standard error of the mean) or number (percentage), n (%).
[(a)] *One missing response in the CFS-only group.*
[(b)] *Lower score indicates worse health status/more disability.*
[(c)] *Higher score indicates more fatigue.*
[(d)] *Non-menstrual, chronic pelvic or lower abdominal pain.*

The "CFS+EM" and "CFS-only" subgroups did not differ significantly in mean age or mean BMI (**Table 2**). In both subgroups most women reported gradual onset of CFS and there was no significant difference in mean duration of the CFS illness (~17 years) (**Table 2**). Women with CFS+EM reported post-exertional malaise more frequently (92.3%) than women with CFS-only (78.3%) but this difference was not statistically significant. There were no significant differences in the means of the SF-36 subscale scores and the MFI-20 scores (**Table 2**). However, compared to CFS-only, the CFS+EM group had a significantly greater number of CFS symptoms from the symptom inventory (SI): 6.8 ± 0.3 (mean ± SEM) vs. 5.5 ± 0.3, $p = 0.02$; the total CFS SI score was also higher (51.4 ± 5.7 vs. 43.0 ± 4.3) but not significantly different, $p = 0.30$.

Gynecologic Characteristics (Table 2)

Non-menstrual, chronic pelvic, or lower abdominal pain was reported significantly more frequently by women with CFS+EM (46.2%) than the CFS-only group (8.7%), $p = 0.02$; OR = 9.00 (95% CI, 1.47–55.25). Compared to CFS-only, women with

CFS+EM were 9 times as likely to be menopausal, OR = 9.23 (1.02–83.33), BMI adjusted OR = 10.79 (1.13–103.11). Notably, among menopausal women, the mean age at menopause onset in the CFS+EM group was 36.4 ± 3.0 years—a decade earlier than in the CFS-only group (47.0 ± 2.7), $p = 0.03$. Hysterectomy rates were significantly higher in the CFS+EM group than the CFS-only group (84.6 vs. 34.8%), OR = 10.31 (95% CI, 1.82–58.39), BMI adjusted OR = 16.13 (2.30–113.23), $p = 0.005$. Of the 36 women with CFS, 8 (22%) reported pelvic pain, 75% of whom also reported endometriosis (**Table 2S**).

Psychometric Characteristics (Table 3)

The mean scores for negative life events were significantly higher in women with CFS+EM than in the CFS-only group (15.8 vs. 7.1, $p = 0.049$); the total Life Events Score (LES) was also higher in CFS+EM (19.0 vs. 12.3) but not significantly different. All other scores were similar in the two groups.

Laboratory Parameters (Table 4)

Blood counts and blood chemistry were all within normal limits but the CFS+EM group had slightly higher hemoglobin and hematocrit than the CFS-only group, $p \leq 0.05$. Inflammatory markers—CRP, IL-6, and TNF-alpha—were not elevated in either subgroup, and TNF-alpha was lower in CFS+EM group than in the CFS group. Serum cortisol, 24-h urinary cortisol, and salivary cortisol levels (appended material) did not differ significantly.

Sleep Study: Polysomnography Parameters (Table 5)

The total sleep time per night was about 20 min shorter in the CFS+EM group than in the CFS-only group (394 ± 15.8 vs. 414.7 ± 9.0), $p = 0.30$. The CFS+EM had higher mean scores for OSA episodes (20.3 ± 11.3 events/h, i.e., within the moderate severity range) than the CFS-only group (4.0 ± 2.3), $p = 0.12$ by Kruskal-Wallis test, $p = 0.05$ after adjusting for BMI. The other sleep parameters did not differ between the two groups.

TABLE 3 | Comparisons of psychometric variables in women with CFS by subgroup—with and without endometriosis.

Variables	CFS+EM (*n* = 13)	CFS-only (*n* = 23)	*p*
	Mean (SEM)		
CTQ Scores			
Emotional abuse	10.8 (1.4)	10.9 (1.4)	0.95
Physical abuse	8.1 (1.2)	7.8 (0.7)	0.85
Sexual abuse	7.5 (0.7)	8.9 (1.4)	0.47
Emotional neglect	12.0 (1.5)	11.7 (1.3)	0.90
Physical neglect	7.9 (1.0)	6.6 (0.5)	0.18
Total CTQ score	46.3 (4.7)	46.0 (4.5)	0.97
PSS Score (total)	16.4 (2.1)	17.7 (1.4)	0.58
LES			
Positive events	3.2 (1.1)	5.2 (1.2)	0.28
Negative events*	15.8 (5.6)	7.1 (1.5)	0.05
Overall LES change	19.0 (5.8)	12.3 (2.1)	0.20
SDS index	54.5 (2.0)	55.4 (1.9)	0.77
STAI			
Trait	41.1 (3.1)	43.3 (2.3)	0.58
State	38.2 (12.3)	37.7 (2.3)	0.90
DTS Score (total)	29.1 (7.5)	30.1 (4.8)	0.90

*CTQ, childhood trauma questionnaire; PSS, perceived stress scale; LES, life experiences survey, *Negative events are presented in absolute value; SDS, self-rating depression scale; STAI, state-trait anxiety inventory; DTS, Davidson trauma scale.*

DISCUSSION

In this study, which used a convenience sample from a population-based study of CFS in Wichita, KS, we confirmed a significantly higher prevalence of EM in women with CFS (36%) than in controls without CFS (17%). In this middle-aged group of women with CFS, comorbid endometriosis was associated with a higher number of CFS symptoms, higher prevalence of chronic pelvic pain, higher rates of hysterectomy and menopause and, most notably, with a decade-earlier menopause onset than in women with CFS-only. However, the endometriosis comorbidity in women with CFS was not associated with significantly worse functioning (SF-36 subscales), fatigue (MFI subscales), or laboratory parameters. As a group, women with CFS and EM reported, on average, one more CFS case-defining symptom and had a higher composite symptom inventory score than women with CFS-only. A higher proportion of women with CFS+EM reported post-exertional malaise. Although the latter two differences were not statistically significant, they may be clinically relevant and may reflect a health impact not otherwise captured by instruments such as SF-36 or MFI-20.

Gynecologic Characteristics

Nearly half (46.2%) of the women with CFS+EM reported chronic pelvic or abdominal pain unrelated to menstrual periods; this is similar to the frequency reported in other studies of EM (39, 40). However, it is unlikely that active EM could explain this pain in our study as only one of the 13 women in the CFS+EM group was not menopausal and 85% of the women had undergone hysterectomy. It may reflect increased pain sensitivity that has been observed in women with chronic pelvic pain (41). The CFS+EM group had a very early mean age at menopause—36 years. This early menopause was probably surgically induced as 85% of the women with CFS+EM reported hysterectomy. A large study of younger US women with EM (mean age 36 years) found that 20% had already undergone oophorectomy and/or hysterectomy (39). Our findings are also similar to the findings from a study in women with fibromyalgia, which found that women with hysterectomy reported more pain and more symptoms than women with fibromyalgia who had not had hysterectomy (42). It is also possible that some patients with chronic pelvic pain who had never undergone surgical intervention may have had endometriosis, which was otherwise undiagnosed. However, only two of the 23 women with "CFS-only" reported chronic pelvic pain. In this case, we might have underestimated the already strong association between chronic pelvic pain and "CFS + EM." Many of the women in this study

TABLE 4 | Comparisons of mean values for selected laboratory parameters and allostatic load index in women with CFS, by subgroup—with and without endometriosis comorbidity.

Parameter	CFS+EM (*n* = 13)	CFS-only (*n* = 23)	*p*
Hemoglobin	13.8 (0.2)	13.3 (0.1)	0.04
Hematocrit	40.6 (0.6)	39.3 (0.4)	0.05
Red blood cells	4.5 (0.1)	4.5 (0.0)	0.63
WBC	7.5 (0.6)	7.3 (0.3)	0.74
Granulocytes	4.3 (0.4)	4.1 (0.3)	0.76
Lymphocytes	2.4 (0.3)	2.4 (0.2)	0.94
Protein			
Total protein	7.4 (0.1)	7.3 (0.1)	0.65
Albumin	3.7 (0.1)	3.6 (0.0)	0.28
Electrolytes			
Sodium	140.1 (0.5)	139.6 (0.4)	0.50
Potassium	3.8 (0.1)	3.9 (0.1)	0.58
Calcium	9.0 (0.1)	9.0 (0.1)	0.96
Alkaline phosphatase	92.5 (6.0)	99.4 (7.8)	0.55
Carbon dioxide	27.0 (0.3)	26.1 (0.5)	0.25
Anion gap	9.8 (0.4)	9.8 (0.4)	0.92
Select inflammatory markers			
High sensitivity CRP	4.5 (1.2)	5.2 (0.9)[a]	0.46*
Interleukin-6 (IL-6)	2.3 (0.3)	2.7 (0.3)[a]	0.34*
TNF-alpha	2.1 (0.1)	3.1 (0.4)[a]	0.02*
Cortisol			
Mean serum free cortisol	19.9 (1.3)	17.1 (1.3)	0.12*
Urinary free cortisol/24 h	20.2 (3.5)	17.6 (2.6)	0.53
Allostatic index score	2.9 (0.5)[b]	3.0 (0.4)[c]	0.86

CFS, chronic fatigue syndrome; EM, endometriosis; CFS+EM, women who had CFS and endometriosis; CFS-only, women who had CFS but not endometriosis; CRP, C-reactive protein; IL-6, interleukin 6; TNF, tumor necrosis factor.
[a]Values available for 20 subjects.
[b]Values available for 8 subjects.
[c]Values available for 14 subjects.
**Kruskal-Wallis test.*

were menopausal, which is a limitation of the study as we cannot answer the question whether the enhanced symptomatology in women with "CFS+EM" is due to active endometriosis, residual effect of endometriosis, or is completely unrelated.

Sleep Parameters

Sleep problems are one of the main symptoms in CFS (19, 43). In our study women with CFS+EM had a mean of 20.3 obstructive sleep apnea events per hour, which places them in the clinical category of moderately severe obstructive sleep apnea (defined as 15–30 events/h), while the CFS-only group had fewer than 5 events/h. The prevalence of obstructive sleep apnea in women is very low prior to menopause but increases sharply after that (44). The CFS+EM group had been in menopause for a mean of ~18 years (while the CFS-only group had been in menopause for a mean of 2 years). Thus, the higher OSA scores in the CFS+EM group may be a corollary of both the earlier onset and higher

TABLE 5 | Sleep characteristics of the women with chronic fatigue syndrome, by subgroup—with and without endometriosis.

Sleep variable	CFS+EM (*n* = 13)	CFS-only (*n* = 23)	*p* (*BMI adjusted*)
	Mean (SEM)[a]		
Total sleep time (minutes)	394.5 (15.8)	414.7 (9.0)	0.30
Respiratory disturbance index	8.2 (3.1)	6.5 (2.3)	0.31 (0.16*)
Obstructive apnea (episodes per hour)	20.3 (11.3)	4.4 (2.3)	0.05 (0.12*)
Snore index	6.5 (3.3)	7.1 (1.7)	0.70
Latency to sleep onset (minutes)	22.8 (6.4)	20.7 (4.3)	0.90
Mean sleep latency (minutes)	10.5 (1.4)	8.9 (1.1)	0.49
Rapid eye movement (REM) sleep (as a proportion of total sleep time)	0.21 (0.0)	0.24 (0.0)	0.45
Sleep efficiency (as a proportion of total sleep time)	0.9 (0.0)	0.9 (0.0)	0.41
Wake (as a proportion of total sleep time)	0.1 (0.0)	0.1 (0.0)	0.41

CFS+EM, chronic fatigue syndrome and endometriosis comorbidity; CFS-only, chronic fatigue syndrome without endometriosis.
**Kruskal–Wallis test (cannot be adjusted for BMI)*
[a]Means are the estimated mean values obtained with BMI included in the generalized linear model.

prevalence of menopause compared with women in the CFS-only group, but it is not likely to be an effect of obesity as women with CFS+EM had slightly lower BMI (mean 28.6 ± 1.0) than those with CFS only (30.0 ± 1.0) and we also adjusted for BMI in the model. The 20 min/night shorter sleep duration in women with CFS+EM (395 min/night) was not statistically different from that in women with CFS-only (414 min/night) but compared to the average 480 min (8 h) considered normal/optimal for adults, the mean sleep duration of the CFS+EM group was 85 min/night shorter (66 min per night for the CFS-only group). Compared to what would be optimal per week, the CFS+EM group appears to accumulate a weekly sleep deficit of more than 9 h (and CFS-only group—a weekly deficit of over 7 h)—that is, they are missing the equivalent of one night of sleep per week.

Laboratory Parameters

In this cross-sectional study, endometriosis comorbidity in CFS did not affect negatively the studied laboratory parameters. Higher levels of inflammatory markers such as TNF-alpha have been reported in women with EM (45). In our study inflammatory markers were not higher in the CFS group and, on the contrary, TNF-alpha was even lower. Some authors have found higher levels of serum cortisol in infertile women suffering from advanced endometriosis (46) but in our study sample of middle-aged women endometriosis comorbidity was not associated with significant differences in cortisol levels in serum, or 24-h urinary cortisol excretion. It should be noted, however, that most women in our study were middle-aged, postmenopausal and thus older than the premenopausal women included in other studies of inflammatory markers and cortisol levels in endometriosis.

Psychological Variables

Although previous studies indicate that childhood stress may be linked to chronic pain syndromes such as fibromyalgia and chronic fatigue syndrome (16, 17), we did not find differences between the two groups in relation to stress experienced during childhood. Further, the groups did not differ in perceived stress during the past month, and there were no differences in indices of psychological well-being, such as depression, anxiety, or posttraumatic stress. We may thus conclude that women with CFS and endometriosis are not in worse mental health than those with CFS only, although they do report having experienced more negative life events.

Study's Strengths and Limitations

Although this study is based on a relatively small, convenience sample, its major strength is that the original study of fatiguing illness was derived from the general population of a defined geographic area and that, during the 2-day clinical evaluation, participants underwent comprehensive clinical, and laboratory evaluation to rule out conditions not compatible with a CFS diagnosis. The availability of data from the structured gynecologic history questionnaire made it possible to conduct this secondary analysis and evaluate the health impact of endometriosis on CFS. Limitations of the study include: the small proportion of women younger than 40 years (the full impact of EM might not be noted as most women were post-menopausal and EM was likely to be "inactive"), recruitment from a single geographic area (Wichita, KS), and lack of racial/ethnic diversity (94% Caucasian women) limiting generalizability of our findings. In addition, the design of the source study did not include review of medical records to confirm self-reported endometriosis and determine method of diagnosis. However, previous studies show that self-reported endometriosis has fairly good predictive ability for diagnostic confirmation in medical records (47) and a high positive predictive value of self-reported gynecologic conditions and surgeries (48). Another limitation of the study is that we did not have information on comorbidities such as irritable bowel syndrome and interstitial cystitis, which play a role in chronic pelvic pain, and we could not control for these conditions in the analyses. In interpreting the study findings it should be kept in mind that data came from a convenience sample—the source study was not specifically designed to evaluate the effects of endometriosis on health in women with CFS, and used a research case definition (19) that does not require the presence of post-exertional malaise as currently recommended by the 2015 Institute of Medicine report for the clinical diagnosis of ME/CFS (1). Further, the mean age of women in this sample was ~51 years and our findings may not be applicable to younger age groups or generalizable to U.S. women outside this community.

CONCLUSIONS

Our study found that patients with CFS and comorbid EM have more CFS symptoms, higher prevalence of chronic pelvic/lower abdominal pain, higher rates of hysterectomy, and significantly earlier onset of menopause than women with only CFS. We did not identify significant differences in functioning, fatigue scores, or inflammatory markers to be associated with comorbid EM. However, the full impact of EM might not be noted in our sample as most women were post-menopausal and EM was likely to be "inactive." Further studies that include younger and more racially/ethnically diverse women are warranted.

ETHICS STATEMENT

The source study adhered to U.S. Department of Health and Human Services human experimentation guidelines and received Institutional Review Board approval from CDC and Abt associates. All participants gave written informed consent.

AUTHOR CONTRIBUTIONS

RB performed the final analysis, interpreted results, and wrote the manuscript. FW, UN, and RB wrote an earlier version (with a different focus) for which UN, FW, RB, JML, RT, and BD all contributed to the earlier analysis and content. All authors have critically read earlier versions of the manuscript and contributed content. EU has critically read and edited previous and current version and made suggestions for its final focus. All authors have read and approved the final version of the manuscript. All authors have contributed to this manuscript.

ACKNOWLEDGMENTS

The authors wish to acknowledge Elizabeth Maloney, M.S., Dr.P.H., and William C. Reeves, M.D., M.Sc., for their critical review of earlier versions of this manuscript.

REFERENCES

1. IOM (Institute of Medicine). *Beyond Myalgic Encephalomyelitis/Chronic Fatigue Syndrome: Redefining An Illness*. Washington, DC: The National Academies Press (2015).
2. Warren JW, Langenberg P, Clauw DJ. The number of existing functional somatic syndromes (FSSs) is an important risk factor for new, different FSSs. *J Psychosom Res*. (2013) 74:12–7. doi: 10.1016/j.jpsychores.2012.09.002
3. IOM (Institute of Medicine). *Relieving Pain in America: A Blueprint for Transforming Prevention, Care, Education, and Research*. Washington, DC: The National Academies Press (2011).
4. Burney RO, Giudice LC. Pathogenesis and pathophysiology of endometriosis. *Fertil Steril*. (2012) 98:511–9. doi: 10.1016/j.fertnstert.2012.06.029
5. Bulun SE. Endometriosis. *N Engl J Med*. (2009) 360:268–79. doi: 10.1056/NEJMra0804690
6. Ozkan S, Murk W, Arici A. Endometriosis and infertility: epidemiology and evidence-based treatments. *Ann NY Acad Sci*. (2008) 1127:92–100. doi: 10.1196/annals.1434.007
7. Eskenazi B, Warner ML. Epidemiology of endometriosis. *Obstet Gynecol Clin North Am*. (1997) 24:235–58. doi: 10.1016/S0889-8545(05)70302-8
8. Houston DE, Noller KL, Melton LJ, Selwyn BJ, Hardy RJ. Incidence of pelvic endometriosis in Rochester, Minnesota, 1970–1979. *Am J Epidemiol*. (1987) 125:959–69. doi: 10.1093/oxfordjournals.aje.a114634
9. Sinaii N, Cleary SD, Ballweg ML, Nieman LK, Stratton P. High rates of autoimmune and endocrine disorders, fibromyalgia, chronic fatigue syndrome and atopic diseases among women with endometriosis: a survey analysis. *Hum Reprod*. (2002) 17:2715–24. doi: 10.1093/humrep/17.10.2715
10. Harlow BL, Signorello LB, Hall JE, Dailey C, Komaroff AL. Reproductive correlates of chronic fatigue syndrome. *Am J Med*. (1998) 105:94S–99S. doi: 10.1016/S0002-9343(98)00173-9
11. Siedentopf F, Tariverdian N, Rucke M, Kentenich H, Arck PC. Immune status, psychosocial distress and reduced quality of life in infertile patients with endometriosis. *Am J Reprod Immunol*. (2008) 60:449–61. doi: 10.1111/j.1600-0897.2008.00644.x
12. Tariverdian N, Theoharides TC, Siedentopf F, Gutierrez G, Jeschke U, Rabinovich GA, et al. Neuroendocrine-immune disequilibrium and endometriosis: an interdisciplinary approach. *Semin Immunopathol*. (2007) 29:193–210. doi: 10.1007/s00281-007-0077-0
13. Nater UM, Maloney E, Boneva RS, Gurbaxani BM, Lin JM, Jones JF, et al. Attenuated morning salivary cortisol concentrations in a population-based study of persons with chronic fatigue syndrome and well controls. *J Clin Endocrinol Metab*. (2008) 93:703–9. doi: 10.1210/jc.2007-1747
14. Heim C, Ehlert U, Hanker JP, Hellhammer DH. Abuse-related posttraumatic stress disorder and alterations of the hypothalamic-pituitary-adrenal axis in women with chronic pelvic pain. *Psychosom Med*. (1998) 60:309–18. doi: 10.1097/00006842-199805000-00017
15. Harrison V, Rowan K, Mathias J. Stress reactivity and family relationships in the development and treatment of endometriosis. *Fertil Steril*. (2005) 83:857–64. doi: 10.1016/j.fertnstert.2004.10.033
16. Heim C, Ehlert U, Hanker JP, Hellhammer DH. Psychological and endocrine correlates of chronic pelvic pain associated with adhesions. *J Psychosom Obstet Gynaecol*. (1999) 20:11–20. doi: 10.3109/01674829909075572
17. Heim C, Nater UM, Maloney E, Boneva R, Jones JF, Reeves WC. Childhood trauma and risk for chronic fatigue syndrome: association with neuroendocrine dysfunction. *Arch Gen Psychiatry*. (2009) 66:72–80. doi: 10.1001/archgenpsychiatry.2008.508
18. *Wichita Clinical Study Data Access*. Available online at: https://www.cdc.gov/me-cfs/programs/wichita-data-access.html (accessed November 9, 2017).
19. Fukuda K, Straus SE, Hickie I, Sharpe MC, Dobbins JG, Komaroff A. The chronic fatigue syndrome: a comprehensive approach to its definition and study. International Chronic Fatigue Syndrome Study Group. *Ann Intern Med*. (1994) 121:953–9. doi: 10.7326/0003-4819-121-12-199412150-00009
20. Reeves WC, Wagner D, Nisenbaum R, Jones JF, Gurbaxani B, Solomon L, et al. Chronic fatigue syndrome—a clinically empirical approach to its definition and study. *BMC Med*. (2005) 3:19. doi: 10.1186/1741-7015-3-19
21. Ware JE Jr, Sherbourne CD. The MOS 36-item short-form health survey (SF-36). I. Conceptual framework and item selection. *Med Care*. (1992) 30:473–83. doi: 10.1097/00005650-199206000-00002
22. Ware JE Jr. SF-36 health survey update. *Spine*. (2000) 25:3130–9. doi: 10.1097/00007632-200012150-00008
23. Smets EM, Garssen B, Bonke B, De Haes JC. The Multidimensional Fatigue Inventory (MFI) psychometric qualities of an instrument to assess fatigue. *J Psychosom Res*. (1995) 39:315–25. doi: 10.1016/0022-3999(94)00125-O
24. *CDC Symptom Inventory*. Available online at: https://www.cdc.gov/me-cfs/pdfs/wichita-data-access/symptom-inventory-doc.pdf (accessed November 9, 2017).
25. *CDC Symptom Inventory Scoring Algorithm*. Available online at: https://www.cdc.gov/me-cfs/pdfs/wichita-data-access/si-scoring-algorithm.pdf (accessed 9 November 9, 2017).
26. Wagner D, Nisenbaum R, Heim C, Jones JF, Unger ER, Reeves WC. Psychometric properties of the CDC Symptom Inventory for assessment of chronic fatigue syndrome. *Popul Health Metr*. (2005) 3:8. doi: 10.1186/1478-7954-3-8
27. Boneva RS, Maloney EM, Lin JM, Jones JF, Wieser F, Nater UM, et al. Gynecological history in chronic fatigue syndrome: a population-based case-control study. *J Womens Health*. (2011) 20:21–8. doi: 10.1089/jwh.2009.1900
28. Bernstein DP, Fink L. *Childhood Trauma Questionnaire: A Retrospective Self-Report Manual*. San Antonio, TX: The Psychological Corporation (1998).
29. Cohen S, Kamarck T, Memslstein R. A global measure of perceived stress. *J Health Soc Beh*. (1983) 24:385–96. doi: 10.2307/2136404
30. Sarason IG, Johnson JH, Siegel JM. Assessing the impact of life changes: development of the Life Experiences Survey. *J Consult Clin Psychol*. (1978) 46:932–46. doi: 10.1037/0022-006X.46.5.932
31. Spielberger CD. *Manual for the State-Trait Anxiety Inventory (STAI)*. Palo Alto, CA: Consulting Psychologists Press (1983).
32. Zung WWK. A self-rating depression scale. *Arch Gen Psychiatry*. (1965) 12:371–9. doi: 10.1001/archpsyc.1965.01720310065008
33. Davidson JR, Book SW, Colket JT, Tupler LA, Roth S, David D, et al. Assessment of a new self-rating scale for post-traumatic stress disorder. *Psychol Med*. (1997) 27:153–60. doi: 10.1017/S0033291796004229
34. Reeves WC, Heim C, Maloney EM, Youngblood LS, Unger ER, Decker MJ, et al. Sleep characteristics of persons with chronic fatigue syndrome and non-fatigued controls: results from a population-based study. *BMC Neurol*. (2006) 16:41. doi: 10.1186/1471-2377-6-41
35. Decker MJ, Tabassum H, Lin JMS, Reeves WC. Electroencephalographic correlates of chronic fatigue syndrome. *Behav Brain Funct*. (2009) 5:43. doi: 10.1186/1744-9081-5-43
36. Vernon SD, Reeves WC. The challenge of integrating disparate high-content data: epidemiologic, clinical, and laboratory data collected during an in-hospital study of chronic fatigue syndrome. *Pharmacogenomics*. (2006) 7:345–54. doi: 10.2217/14622416.7.3.345
37. McEwen BS, Stellar E. Stress and the individual. Mechanisms leading to disease. *Arch Intern Med*. (1993) 153:2093–101. doi: 10.1001/archinte.1993.00410180039004
38. Maloney EM, Gurbaxani BM, Jones JF, Coelho LdS, Pennachin C, Goertzel BN. Chronic fatigue syndrome and high allostatic load. *Pharmacogenomics*. (2006) 7:467–73. doi: 10.2217/14622416.7.3.467
39. Sinaii N, Cleary SD, Younes N, Ballweg ML, Stratton P. Treatment utilization for endometriosis symptoms: a cross-sectional survey study of lifetime experience. *Fertil Steril*. (2007) 87:1277–86. doi: 10.1016/j.fertnstert.2006.11.051
40. Tirlapur SA, Kuhrt K, Chaliha C, Ball E, Meads C, Khan KS. The "evil twin syndrome" in chronic pelvic pain: a systematic review of prevalence studies of bladder pain syndrome and endometriosis. *Int J Surg*. (2013) 11:233–7. doi: 10.1016/j.ijsu.2013.02.003
41. Nasr-Esfahani M, Jarrell J. Cotton-tipped applicator test: validity and reliability in chronic pelvic pain. *Am J Obstet Gynecol*. (2013) 208:52.e1–5. doi: 10.1016/j.ajog.2012.11.005
42. Vincent A, Whipple MO, Luedtke CA, Oh TH, Sood R, Smith RL, et al. Pain and other symptom severity in women with fibromyalgia and a previous hysterectomy. *J Pain Res*. (2011) 4:325–9. doi: 10.2147/JPR.S25490
43. Carruthers BM, Jain AK, De Meirleir KL, Peterson DL, Klimas NG, Lerner AM, et al. Myalgic encephalomyelitis/chronic fatigue syndrome: clinical working case definition, diagnostic and treatment protocols. *J Chronic Fatig Syndr*. (2003) 11:7–116. doi: 10.1300/J092v11n01_02

44. Eichling PS, Sahni J. Menopause related sleep disorders. *J Clin Sleep Med.* (2005) 1:291–300. Available online at: http://jcsm.aasm.org/articles/010312.pdf
45. Bedaiwy MA, Falcone T, Sharma RK, Goldberg JM, Attaran M, Nelson DR, et al. Prediction of endometriosis with serum and peritoneal fluid markers: a prospective controlled trial. *Hum Reprod.* (2002) 17:426–31. doi: 10.1093/humrep/17.2.426
46. Lima AP, Moura MD, Rosa e Silva AA. Prolactin and cortisol levels in women with endometriosis. *Braz J Med Biol Res.* (2006) 39:1121–7. doi: 10.1590/S0100-879X2006000800015
47. Saha R, Marions L, Tornvall P. Validity of self-reported endometriosis and endometriosis-related questions in a Swedish female twin cohort. *Fertil Steril.* (2017) 107:174–8. doi: 10.1016/j.fertnstert.2016.09.038
48. Phips AI, Buist SM. Validation of self-reported history of hysterectomy and oophorectomy among women in an integrated group practice setting. *Menopause.* (2009) 16:576–81. doi: 10.1097/gme.0b013e31818ffe28

Disclaimer: The findings and conclusions in this report are those of the authors and do not necessarily represent the official position of the Centers for Disease Control and Prevention.

9

Meeting the Educational Needs of Young, ME/CFS Patients: Role of the Treating Physician

*Faith R. Newton**

Department of Education, Delaware State University, Dover, DE, United States

Keywords: myalgic encephalomyelitis/chronic fatigue syndrome (ME/CFS), ME/CFS, chronic fatigue syndrome, educating students with ME/CFS, schools and ME/CFS, education and ME/CFS, classroom accommodations and ME/CFS, academic success and ME/CFS

***Correspondence:**
Faith R. Newton
fnewton@desu.edu

INTRODUCTION

Myalgic Encephalomyelitis/Chronic Fatigue Syndrome (ME/CFS) is a disabling, chronic disease characterized by the body's inability to produce sufficient energy for normal everyday activities. Children with ME/CFS experience debilitating fatigue referred to as post-exertional malaise (PEM) after minimal mental or physical exertion which is not relieved by sleep. It can significantly reduce the ability of the child to take part in personal, educational, or social activities and can compromise executive function, and can result in a moderate to severe disability. As many as 1% of school-age children suffer from this disease in varying degrees of severity, and ME/CFS has been shown to negatively impact school attendance, participation, connectedness, and academic performance (1). Some studies suggest that ME/CFS may be the major cause of extended school absences (2).

Whereas, the literature supplying practice-based guidance for other chronic conditions affecting children in school, such as Autism and Attention Deficit Hyperactivity Disorder (ADHD) will be found in educational journals, very little guidance for students with ME/CFS appears in the clinical medicine literature. Although school nurses are beginning to play a larger role in supporting these children, physicians or healthcare providers retain primary responsibility of informing the school system of the needed adjustments for the young ME/CFS patient to succeed in the school environment.

This article argues that the physician has a much broader responsibility to provide diagnostic, symptomatic, and treatment information about ME/CFS than they would with other conditions such as Autism or ADHD that qualify students for special services. For students with ME/CFS, the physician's letter required in the school's evaluation process is a critical resource to advise and guide education professionals regarding appropriate student placement, classroom support, and instructional accommodations or modifications. The specifics of what should be included in a model physician's letter are included.

PAUCITY OF ME/CFS EDUCATIONAL PUBLICATIONS IN COMPARISON TO OTHER DISEASES AFFECTING SCHOOL PERFORMANCE

A comparison of available popular and professional literature generally available to educators regarding ME/CFS and the corpus of materials available on Autism and ADHD is instructive. All three conditions impact millions of schoolchildren: ADHD (6.1%), Autism (4.5%), ME/CFS (1%) (3, 4). There are copious practice-based resources available to educators providing services to students suffering from ADHD and Autism. A recent search for popular and professional education resources on Amazon for ADHD returned over 1,000 hits; a similar search for Autism generated 4,000 results. An examination of the titles indicated that, while the quality of the content varies, over 80% of the items were relevant to the topic of educational practices that support students with these conditions.

For ME/CFS, the situation is very different: Even by using multiple terminology references ("CFS" vs. "ME/CFS" vs. "Chronic Fatigue Syndrome," etc.) and not using specific terms to narrow the results to pediatric ME/CFS, the total number of distinct Amazon returns was only thirty-two in a search performed on October 22, 2018. Of these, 28 proved to be search artifacts; they were non-related items offered by the search engine based on erroneous application of the search terms. Of the four valid results, all were either very general, treated education only as a minor subset of the topic, or included ME/CFS as one of a number of diseases given superficial coverage. Where the easily accessible literature on ADHD and Autism returned hundreds of workbooks, teacher guides, and reference materials for school psychologists, such materials were completely absent for pediatric ME/CFS.

Google searches regarding educational support for the three conditions returned similar results in a search performed on October 22, 2019. While relatively detailed, practitioner-oriented materials for ADHD and Autism are abundant, the best search returns for ME/CFS involve basic checklists about the signs, symptoms, and potential impact of the disease, to which a small number of skeletal bullet points about educational support may or may not be appended.

Conversely, there is a rich, clinical literature regarding ME/CFS in professional medical sources, with a small but significant percentage directly relevant to educational support. A Google Scholar search on October 22, 2018, for peer-reviewed articles, case studies, technical notes, short communications, and reviews on ME/CFS since 2014 currently returns over 18,600 hits; when redundant and erroneous responses are filtered, the number remains high. Nearly 12,000 items (3,000/year) on this disease have been published over the past 4 years, and about 120 (1%) have potential direct applicability to educational support for children suffering from pediatric ME/CFS. The nature of the publications, however, suggests limited availability to education professionals, who are unlikely to be pouring over the pages of *BMC Pediatrics; Brain, Behavior, and Immunity; Current Rheumatology Reports; European Journal of Pediatrics; Frontiers in Pediatrics; Physiotherapy;* or the *Journal of Rehabilitation Medicine.*

ME/CFS EDUCATION-RELATED FINDINGS IN CLINICAL MEDICAL LITERATURE

Clinicians who remain current in the literature relating to ME/CFS are privy to significant findings that, if known by professional educators, would enhance their ability to enable students suffering from this disease to better achieve academic success. The first general statistical study of school function among students with ME/CFS that extends beyond merely examining attendance and considers the broader impact of the disease on participation, academic performance, and socialization has only recently appeared in *Frontiers in Pediatrics* (1).

Understanding the role of cognitive dysfunction and compromised executive function in school-age children with ME/CFS is essential for teachers attempting to modify lessons and assignments. This knowledge is needed to develop effective instructional strategies that will allow ME/CFS students to succeed. While such resources exist in the clinical medical literature, that information has yet to appear in professional education publications. A summary review of cognitive disfunction caused by ME/CFS appeared in *Current Rheumatology Reports* (5); a comprehensive survey of cognitive/neurological consequences of post-exertional malaise was published in *Brain, Behavior and Immunity* (6), as well as a more directly applicable study of ME/CFS's impacts on cognitive functioning in adolescents in the *European Journal of Pediatrics* (7).

The import of these articles often extends beyond providing teachers a better understanding of the disease and its symptoms. Information contained in these articles can be used directly in assessments for specials services or even in the classroom. *The American Journal of Occupational Therapy* (8) recently published a study that assists teachers in understanding the potential and limitations of students with ME/CFS symptoms. Information contained in these articles, when combined with work illuminating the attention processes of these students in *Behavior, Research and Therapy* (9), comes very close to providing a guide for teachers in mitigating important facets of compromised executive functioning in the classroom. A study in *Physiotherapy* (10) documents the association between ME/CFS pain, comorbidity with other diseases like Fybromyalgia, and cognitive performance. Specific strategies for applying this type of information in schools has appeared in the pages of *Fatigue* (11) and are only beginning to penetrate related literature such as *Journal of School Health* (12).

Journal titles have been mentioned here to make the point that this kind of educationally relevant clinical information has not yet significantly penetrated the mainstream of professional education literature, and is likely to be both unknown and unavailable to school psychologists, guidance counselors, administrators, nurses, and teachers. This situation is beginning to change: Both the Centers for Disease Control and Prevention (13) and the Open Medicine Foundation (14) maintain and update fact sheets on ME/CFS for education professionals, while practice-based articles have begun appearing in publications like *NASN School Nurse* (15). However, there are few professional educators publishing such practice-based material based on current clinical findings, and the bulk of existing material remains relatively inaccessible to educators.

THE ROLE OF THE PHYSICIAN IN SUPPORTING EDUCATORS

Despite international differences in law and policy, the role of physicians in assisting their school-age patients with disability or disease in gaining access to special services has traditionally centered on documenting for the school the diagnosis, severity, treatment, and prognosis for their patients. Often this occurs through a physician's letter (16). Professional educators then convene in various committees or work groups to address the issue of adapting curriculum, classroom instruction, and other aspects of delivering education based on the student's specific challenges. In most cases, the physician is not an integral part of these groups, though she or he may sometimes be consulted for additional information.

The physician's letter is the most effective document for effecting the needed special services required by students with ME/CFS, because it contains the critical information about the student's condition and limitations. The letter generally remains a permanent part of the student's record during the development of instructional modifications, unlike oral communications or even emails.

COMPONENTS OF AN EFFECTIVE PHYSICIAN'S LETTER REGARDING ME/CFS

Providing a diagnosis of ME/CFS is generally not a sufficient guide for educators, because the disease itself is not well-understood, and because ME/CFS is inherently highly variable in severity and symptoms. Physicians need to explain the nature of the disease and the effect of the disease on the individual in question. Here, as in subsequent sections of the letter, references with URL links are exceptionally helpful to educators.

The explanation will normally need to be from 1 to 3 paragraphs in length, and at a minimum cover the following if present in the patient: debilitating fatigue and malaise after minimal exertion; the unpredictability of the severity and length of fatigue; loss of mental/physical stamina with post-exertional malaise; lack of cognitive focus ("brain fog"); orthostatic intolerance; difficulty regulating body temperature; non-refreshing sleep; and myofascial, joint, or abdominal pain. For reference, two of the most useful short summaries of ME/CFS written in language accessible to educators can be found in the Open Medicine Foundation (14) and Centers for Disease Control and Prevention (3) Fact Sheet.

Beyond the general inclusion of diagnosis, severity, treatment, and prognosis, the letter should include extended sections on specific symptoms that will manifest in the classroom, affect school work in general, and recommend changes to the instructional program (either in terms of curriculum, assignments, attendance, or schedule).

With regard to symptoms, more detail is almost always better than less. School officials need to know, for example, that attendance issues and inability to complete a full day's schedule are likely to be chronic issues that, at best, will be slowly responsive to treatment. This notifies and allows them to plan for shortened schedules, consider the deployment of tutors to the homes of chronically absent students, or use educational services over the entire calendar year. Classroom teachers need to be informed that these children will be easily distractible; have difficulty completing sequential tasks or multi-tasking without special support; may demonstrate slower processing speed and difficulty recalling words; and will not be able to "push through" their fatigue to finish assignments. Teachers also need to be aware that one of the cognitive hallmarks of ME/CFS is often the student's inability to self-monitor or self-regulate his or her own fatigue levels.

Detailed recommendations tend to be problematic for physicians, many of whom may be reluctant to impose their views across professional disciplines, while the vocabularies used by the two profession are different. The latter can be an exceptionally high hurdle, as educational terms are often quite different from clinical medical terminology, and have specific procedural and legal connotations. In the United States, for example, the terms "accommodation" and "modification," when applied to a school setting, are not by any means synonymous, and imply significantly different levels of legal protections for the student and organizational accountability for the school.

However, most educators are open to receiving as much relevant clinical information as possible about a disease they may not have encountered, and about which there is little practice-oriented material. Direct communication, either by email or telephone, with the school psychologist or educational diagnostician who is heading the school's study group for the student will often provide more clarity for the physician regarding what would be helpful in the physician's letter if experience is lacking. The school nurse can provide a critical bridge between the clinician and educators, and is well positioned to become the child's chief medical advocate in the school. Parents can also often provide useful information, although care should be taken to consider the difference between their perspective and that of teachers and school officials.

The most consistently effective method of providing recommendations is to match symptoms directly to recommendations. If symptoms of slow processing speed and limited stamina are present, recommendations of additional time to complete assignments, no penalties for late assignments, and perhaps even a significantly reduced workload provide useful direction. When a patient has demonstrated sensitivity to temperature changes in his or her environment, it is useful to spell out precisely how this should impact the choice of classrooms. If a student needs consistent hydration, there should be an explicit recommendation that any policies against bringing drinks into a classroom should be waived.

It is especially important to address issues of prolonged and unpredictable absences; inability to complete a full school day, or inability to complete homework with specific recommendations. Here the physician should not feel required to go into extreme detail, but to include recommendations about modifying daily schedules, reducing course loads where appropriate, or waiving consequences associated with normal attendance polices (especially the need for multiple doctor's notes for absences). Physicians should also address prognosis; along with unpredictably, educators often do not understand that this disease has a reported recovery rate of 60% by 5 years and by 12 years of ~88% (16).

Finally, it is always useful, as mentioned above, to include references to relevant clinical materials that may assist the school in charting an effective educational course for a student suffering from ME/CFS. Items referenced in this article are a good place to start, but physicians treating pediatric ME/CFS cases should make every effort to stay abreast of new publications that may assist educators.

A sample physician's letter may be found in Rowe (16); while obviously less detailed than that which would be generated in a real clinical case, it follows the general guidelines provided above, and can be used by any physician as a starting point for composition.

CONSIDERATIONS OF TIME AND EFFORT ON THE PART OF PHYSICIANS

The clinician involvement recommended here is obviously much more laborious than usual for dealing with children suffering from diseases like Autism or ADHD. These demands will also fall more heavily on pediatricians and other clinicians who treat children with ME/CFS, but whose practice is not specifically focused on this disease. As a disease that is diagnosed by exclusion, and with no known cause, ME/CFS is not a psychological illness, however, though depression and anxiety can occur as it does in other chronic illnesses (14).

In terms of patient outcome, the time spent by the physician in assisting the young patient retain educational achievement is time well spent. For patients and their families, dealing with school-related issues consumes far more time and energy on a daily basis than managing medications or any other ME/CFS-abating procedure. From a psychological and motivational standpoint, these families often equate an inability to achieve success in school with long-term negative impacts on their child. Even if the child responds to treatment after months or years, and achieves partial remission of symptoms, the lost semesters at school and the opportunities to complete an education and thereby become a potentially self-sustaining adult, can make dealing with this disease appear daunting. The additional hour expended by the physician in the thoughtful preparation of his or her letter to the school can improve motivation and reduce stress, while simultaneously increasing the chances of successful clinical and educational outcomes for this child.

AUTHOR CONTRIBUTIONS

The author confirms being the sole contributor of this work and has approved it for publication.

REFERENCES

1. Knight SJ, Politis J, Garnham C, Scheinberg A, Tollit MA. School functioning in adolescents with Chronic Fatigue Syndrome. *Front Pediatr.* (2018) 6:302. doi: 10.3389/fped.2018.00302/full
2. Smith R. *Chronic Fatigue Syndrome is 'Major' Cause of School Absence: Research.* Telegraph (2011). Available online at: https://www.telegraph.co.uk/news/health/news/8950705/Chronic-fatigue-syndrome-is-major-cause-of-school-absence-research.html (accessed October 31, 2018).
3. Center for Disease Control and Prevention. *Attention-Deficit/Hyperactivity Disorder (ADHD).* (2018). Available online at: https://www.cdc.gov/ncbddd/adhd/data.html (accessed October 31, 2018).
4. Waugh I. *The Prevalence of Autism (Including Asperger Syndrome) in School Age Children in Northern Ireland 2018.* Department of Health Northern Ireland Information & Analysis Directorate (2018). Available online at: https://www.health-ni.gov.uk/sites/default/files/publications/health/asd-children-ni-2018.pdf (accessed October 29, 2018).
5. Cvejic E, Birch RC, Vollmer-Conna U. Cognitive dysfunction in Chronic Fatigue Syndrome: a review of recent evidence. *Curr Rheumatol Rep.* (2016) 18:24. doi: 10.1007/s11926-016-0577-9
6. Cook DB, Light AR, Light KC, Broderick G, Shields MR, Dougherty RJ, et al. Neural consequences of post-exertion malaise in Myalgic Encephalomyelitis/Chronic Fatigue Syndrome. *Brain Behav Immunity.* (2017) 62:87–99. doi: 10.1016/j.bbi.2017.02.009
7. Nijhof LN, Nijhof SL, Bleijenberg G, Stellato RK, Kimpen JL, Hulshoff Pol HE, et al. The impact of Chronic Fatigue Syndrome on cognitive functioning in adults. *Eur J Pediatr.* (2016) 175:245–52. doi: 10.1007/s00431-015-2626-1
8. Kos D, Van Eupen I, Meirte J, Van Cauwenbergh D, Moorkens G, Meeus M, et al. Activity pacing self-management in Chronic Fatigue Syndrome: a randomized controlled trial. *Am J Occupat Ther.* (2015) 69:6905290020. doi: 10.5014/ajot.2015.016287
9. Hou R, Moss-Morris R, Risdale A, Lynch J, Jeeveratnam P, Bradley BP, et al. Attention processes in Chronic Fatigue Syndrome: attentional bias for health-related threat and the role of attentional control. *Behav Res Theor.* (2014) 52:9–16. doi: 10.1016/j.brat.2013.10.005
10. Ickmans K, Meeus M, De Kooning M, Lambrecht L, Pattyn N, Nijs J. Associations between cognitive performance and pain in Chronic Fatigue Syndrome: comorbidity with fibromyalgia does matter. *Physiotherapy.* (2015) 101:e635–6. doi: 10.1016/j.physio.2015.03.3465
11. Newton F. Improving academic success for students with myalgic encephalomyelitis/chronic fatigue syndrome. *Fatigue Biomed Health Behav.* (2015) 3:97–103. doi: 10.1080/21641846.2015.1004831
12. Tollit M, Politis J, Knight S. Measuring school functioning in students with Chronic Fatigue Syndrome: a systematic review. *J Sch Heath.* (2018) 88:74–89. doi: 10.1111/josh.12580
13. Center for Disease Control and Prevention. *Myalgic Encephalomyelitis/Chronic Fatigue Syndrome.* (2017). Available online at: https://www.cdc.gov/me-cfs/me-cfs-children/factsheet-educational-professional.html (accessed October 31, 2018).
14. Newton F. *Tools to Help Children with Chronic Fatigue Syndrome.* Open Medicine Foundation (2017). Available online at: https://www.healthrising.org/forums/resources/tools-to-help-children-with-chronic-fatigue-syndrome-me-cfs-succeed.451/ (accessed October 31, 2018).
15. Friedman KJ, Mattey B, Newton F. School nurses can improve the lives of students with Myalgic/Encephalomyelitis/Chronic Fatigue Syndrome. *NASN Sch Nurse.* (2018) 33:372–9. doi: 10.1177/1942602X18795299
16. Rowe PC, Underhill RA, Friedman KJ, Gurwitt A, Medow MS, Schwartz MS, et al. Myalgic Encephalomyelitis/ Chronic Fatigue Syndrome Diagnosis and management in Young people: a primer. *Front Pediatr.* (2017) 5:121. doi: 10.3389/fped.2017.00121

10

Blood Volume Status in ME/CFS Correlates with the Presence or Absence of Orthostatic Symptoms

C. (Linda) M. C. van Campen [1]*, Peter C. Rowe [2] and Frans C. Visser [1]

[1] Stichting Cardiozorg, Hoofddorp, Netherlands, [2] Department of Pediatrics, Johns Hopkins University School of Medicine, Baltimore, MD, United States

Correspondence:
C. (Linda) M. C. van Campen
info@stichtingcardiozorg.nl

Introduction: Conflicting data have been published on the reduction of circulating blood volume in adults with Myalgic encephalomyelitis/chronic fatigue syndrome (ME/CFS). The aim of the present study was to compare blood volumes based on the presence or absence of orthostatic symptoms.

Methods and results: Twenty consecutive adults with ME/CFS participated in the study. All underwent dual isotope blood volume measurement and were evaluated for a clinical suspicion of orthostatic intolerance (OI). The mean age was 34 (10) years, and median duration of disease was 7.5 (6–10) years. The mean (SD) absolute blood volume was 59 (8) ml/kg, a value −11 (7) ml/kg below the reference blood volume. Of the 12 patients, 4 had no OI and 8 had a clinical suspicion of OI. In 8 patients with OI, absolute blood volumes were significantly lower than for the 4 without OI (56 [2] vs. 66 [5]; $p < 0.05$) as were the differences between the measured and the reference blood volume (−14 [2]; vs. −4 [3]; $p < 0.02$).

Conclusions: Adults with ME/CFS had a significantly lower blood volume if they had a clinical suspicion of OI compared to those without a clinical suspicion of OI, as well as a significantly lower blood volume compared to the expected value. The data suggest that accounting for symptoms of OI could enhance the detection of the subset with reduced blood volume.

Keywords: orthostatic intolerance, chronic fatigue syndrome, myalgic encephalomyelitis, blood volume, POTS, dual isotope scan

INTRODUCTION

Myalgic encephalomyelitis/chronic fatigue syndrome (ME/CFS) is characterized by a persistent severe fatigue, diminished exercise tolerance, post exertional malaise, unrefreshing sleep, and impaired memory and concentration. A prominent feature is also dizziness and/or lightheadedness. More individuals with ME/CFS than healthy controls experience lightheadedness and syncope (1–3). Studies have shown conflicting results regarding circulating blood volume in ME/CFS patients compared to a healthy population (4–6). Lin et al. (7) identified a relation between red blood cell (RBC) volume deficiency and the presence of orthostatic intolerance (OI) in chronic OI patients and especially in those with postural orthostatic tachycardia syndrome (POTS). To explore whether this observation of OI in a non-ME/CFS subject group might also be applicable in a population with ME/CFS, the aim of the present study was to compare measured blood volume in adults with ME/CFS after sub-grouping by the presence or absence of OI symptoms.

MATERIALS AND METHODS

Individuals with ME/CFS were eligible for this study if they were being evaluated at the Stichting CardioZorg, a cardiology clinic with a special interest in ME/CFS. ME/CFS was considered present if participants met both the CFS (8) and the ME criteria (9) with no other major comorbidities.

Beginning in 2010, as part of routine care, we began measuring blood volume using the standard dual isotope erythrocyte labeling technique ($Na_2^{51}CrO_4$ and ^{125}I-human serum albumin) (10) at the department of Nuclear Medicine of the Free University Hospital Amsterdam. Blood volume was compared with the ideal weight of patients (11), using the method of Devine (12). Due to the high cost of the blood volume measurements (3500 USD) and the loss of funding for these studies, patient enrollment was limited to the first 12 individuals.

The presence or absence of a clinical suspicion of OI was based on the history taken by an experienced cardiologist (FCV) who asked how individuals felt in the following circumstances: while waiting in line, at receptions, while shopping, while sitting still for long periods, and when exposed to warm/stressful circumstances (e.g., summer weather, after hot showers, after episodes of fear or pain), (13–15). Those with increased lightheadedness and other symptoms in these settings were considered to have a clinical suspicion of OI. The use of clinical data for descriptive studies was approved by the ethics committee of the Slotervaart Hospital.

Scores were tested for normal distribution using the Shapiro Wilk test in SPSS (IBM SPSS version 21). Normally distributed data were presented as mean (SD), and data that were not normally distributed were presented as a median (IQR). Data were compared with the student' t-test for unpaired data where appropriate. A p-value < 0.05 was considered significantly different.

RESULTS

Among the 12 consecutive ME/CFS participants, the mean age was 34 (10) years, and the median duration of disease was 7.5 (6–10) years. In the total patient group the absolute blood volume was 59 (8) ml/kg. The reduction in blood volume from the reference standard based on ideal weight was −11(7) ml/kg. Based on the clinical history, 4 had no clinical suspicion of OI and 8 had a clinical suspicion of OI (two of whom had been diagnosed with POTS; in the remaining six, tilt table testing elsewhere had identified no hemodynamic abnormalities). **Table 1** shows the baseline data and blood volumes in patients without ($n = 4$) and with ($n = 8$) OI. Those with OI were significantly younger. In those who reported symptoms of OI, the absolute blood volumes were significantly lower than in those without OI, as were the differences between measured blood volume and the reference blood volume.

TABLE 1 | Demographic and volume characteristics of the study population*.

	OI absent	OI present	p-value
Female	100%	88%	ns
Height	173 (9) cm	170 (10) cm	ns
Weight	65 (9) kg	63 (13) kg	ns
Caucasian	100%	100%	ns
Age (years)	44 (4)	28 (9)	<0.01
Median duration of CFS	9 (8–11) years	7 (5.8–10) years	ns

**Unless otherwise specified, these values represent mean (SD. Diff, difference; OI, orthostatic intolerance).*

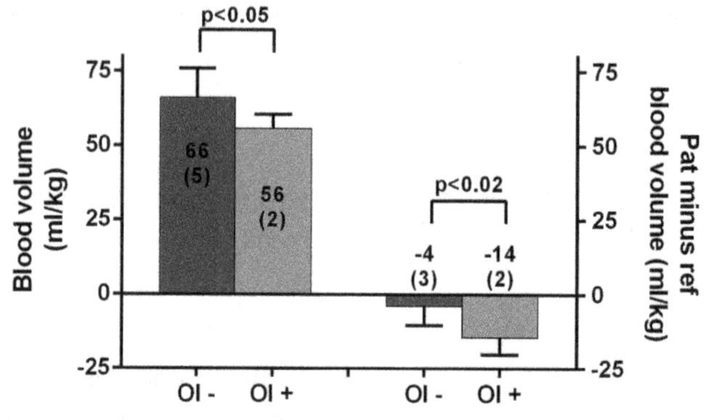

FIGURE 1 | Absolute blood volumes (ml/kg) in those without and with OI are shown on the left y-axis. The differences between the measured blood volume minus the reference value (ml/kg) are shown on the right y-axis. Values are presented as mean (SD); OI− and OI+, clinical suspicion of orthostatic intolerance absent and present; Pat, patients; ref, reference.

Figure 1 shows the differences in blood volumes for patients with and without OI: 56 (2) vs. 66 (5) ml/kg; $p < 0.05$. The difference between the measured blood volume and the reference blood volume is shown in patients with and without OI: −14 (2) vs. −4 (3); $p < 0.02$. No significant correlation was found between the disease duration and absolute blood volume or the reduction in blood volume compared to the reference blood volume.

DISCUSSION

The main finding of this study is that blood volumes were significantly lower for adults with ME/CFS whose symptoms were consistent with orthostatic intolerance compared to those with no clinical suspicion of OI. The finding was present when we compared either absolute blood volume values or the percent reduction in blood volumes from the normal reference value for each individual. Our data are similar to a study in which only OI patients were investigated (7). Lin and colleagues compared the measured red blood cell (RBC) volume with an expected RBC volume, and found RBC volumes between 78% (POTS patients) and 85% (chronic OI patients without POTS) of the reference value.

Only a limited number of studies on blood volume have been performed in those with ME/CFS. Streeten and colleagues found in 12 female CFS patients that the RBC volumes were lower than that of female control subjects, but found in contrast that plasma and whole blood volumes were not significantly different from control subjects (6). Farquhar identified no significant difference in blood volume between ME/CFS patients and simultaneously studied age-matched controls (4), although there was a non-significant trend toward lower blood volume in those with ME/CFS. Hurwitz and colleagues examined 56 with ME/CFS (30 more severely affected and 26 non-severely affected). Total blood volume, erythrocyte volume, and plasma volume were not significantly different from 21 sedentary controls (5). However, when recalculating the reduction from ideal volumes, the percent total blood, plasma, and RBC volumes were all significantly lower in those with ME/CFS than in sedentary controls and also lower in those with severe ME/CFS compared to less severely affected individuals. Of interest, the mean absolute blood volume in our patient population (59 ml/kg) was mid-way between the values for those with severe ME/CFS (57 ml/kg) and non-severe ME/CFS (61 ml/kg) reported by Hurwitz et al. Newton et al. (16) found no significant difference for whole blood volumes between 41 with CFS and 10 healthy controls, but 68% of those with ME/CFS had a RBC volume below 95% of the expected mean volume for healthy individuals. Thirty-two percent had a normalized plasma volume below the lower limit of normal of 95%, suggesting a difference in the degree of reduction between plasma and RBC volumes. None of these studies classified participants according to the presence or absence of orthostatic intolerance.

The group with was younger than the group without orthostatic intolerance. Future studies will be able to determine whether this age difference persists in a larger sample. Of the limited number of studies regarding how blood volume varies over the lifespan in healthy volunteers, the data are consistent with either stable or declining blood volume with increasing age (17, 18) If the same relationship between blood volume and age is present for those with ME/CFS, then the older age of the group without orthostatic intolerance would have reduced the likelihood of detecting the difference we observed. Similarly, an age-matched group without orthostatic intolerance would be expected to increase the difference in blood volume between groups.

LIMITATIONS

In the present study we did not include simultaneous control subjects. We acknowledge that the small sample size could have led to a type I statistical error. Thus, the data presented here should be considered preliminary and our results need to be confirmed in a larger study.

CONCLUSION

This small study identified a lower absolute measured blood volume and a greater reduction in blood volume compared to expected normal values in those with ME/CFS who reported symptoms of orthostatic intolerance. The data suggest that accounting for orthostatic symptoms has the potential to better identify the subset of individuals with ME/CFS who have a reduced blood volume, which in turn would have implications for treatment and the prevention of disabling symptoms. Because a significant reduction of blood volume is an objectively demonstrable laboratory abnormality in ME/CFS patients, larger studies are warranted.

ETHICS STATEMENT

This trial was designed, conducted, and reported in accordance with the international Conference on Harmonization (ICH) Guidelines for Good Clinical Practice (GCP), applicable local regulations (including European Directive 2001/20/EC), and following the ethical principles laid down in the Declaration of Helsinki. The protocol was approved by the METC Slotervaartziekenhuis en Raede, Amsterdam, Netherlands.

AUTHOR CONTRIBUTIONS

CvC, PR, and FV conceived the study. CvC and FV collected the data. CvC performed the primary data analysis and FV and PR performed secondary data analyses. All authors were involved in the drafting and review of the manuscript.

ACKNOWLEDGMENTS

Dr. Rowe is supported by the Sunshine Natural Wellbeing Foundation Professorship of Chronic Fatigue and Related Disorders.

REFERENCES

1. Bou-Holaigah I, Rowe PC, Kan J, Calkins H. The relationship between neurally mediated hypotension and the chronic fatigue syndrome *JAMA* (1995) 274:961–7.
2. Rowe PC, Bou-Holaigah I, Kan JS, Calkins H. Is neurally mediated hypotension an unrecognised cause of chronic fatigue? *Lancet* (1995) 345:623–4.
3. Ulas UH, Chelimsky TC, Chelimsky G, Mandawat A, McNeeley K, Alshekhlee A. Comorbid health conditions in women with syncope. *Clin Auton Res.* (2010) 20:223–7. doi: 10.1007/s10286-010-0070-x
4. Farquhar WB, Hunt BE, Taylor JA, Darling SE, Freeman R. Blood volume and its relation to peak O(2) consumption and physical activity in patients with chronic fatigue. *Am J Physiol Heart Circ Physiol.* (2002) 282:H66–71. doi: 10.1152/ajpheart.2002.282.1.H66
5. Hurwitz BE, Coryell VT, Parker M, Martin P, Laperriere A, Klimas NG, et al. Chronic fatigue syndrome: illness severity, sedentary lifestyle, blood volume and evidence of diminished cardiac function. *Clin Sci.* (2010) 118:125–35. doi: 10.1042/CS20090055

6. Streeten DH, Thomas D, Bell DS. The roles of orthostatic hypotension, orthostatic tachycardia, and subnormal erythrocyte volume in the pathogenesis of the chronic fatigue syndrome. *Am J Med Sci.* (2000) 320:1–8. doi: 10.1016/S0002-9629(15)40790-6
7. Lin CJ, Chu YK, Chern CM. RBC volume deficiency in patients with excessive orthostatic decrease in cerebral blood flow velocity. *J Chin Med Assoc.* (2014) 77:174–8. doi: 10.1016/j.jcma.2014.01.005
8. Fukuda K, Straus SE, Hickie I, Sharpe MC, Dobbins JG, Komaroff A. The chronic fatigue syndrome: a comprehensive approach to its definition and study. International Chronic Fatigue Syndrome Study Group. *Ann Intern Med.* (1994) 121:953–9.
9. Carruthers BM, van de Sande MI, De Meirleir KL, Klimas NG, Broderick G, Mitchell T, et al. Myalgic encephalomyelitis: International Consensus Criteria. *J Intern Med.* (2011) 270:327–38. doi: 10.1111/j.1365-2796.2011.02428.x
10. Fairbanks VF, Klee GG, Wiseman GA, Hoyer JD, Tefferi A, Petitt RM, et al. Measurement of blood volume and red cell mass: re-examination of 51Cr and 125I methods. *Blood Cells Mol Dis.* (1996) 22:169–86; discussion 186a–g. doi: 10.1006/bcmd.1996.0024
11. Feldschuh J, Katz S. The importance of correct norms in blood volume measurement. *Am J Med Sci.* (2007) 334:41–6. doi: 10.1097/MAJ.0b013e318063c707
12. Devine BJ. Gentamycin therapy drug. *Intell Clin Pharm.* (1974) 8:650–5.
13. Grubb BP. Clinical practice. Neurocardiogenic syncope. *N Engl J Med.* (2005) 352:1004–10. doi: 10.1056/NEJMcp042601
14. Raj SR. Postural tachycardia syndrome (POTS) *Circulation* (2013) 127:2336–42. doi: 10.1161/CIRCULATIONAHA.112.144501
15. Thieben MJ, Sandroni P, Sletten DM, Benrud-Larson LM, Fealey RD, Vernino S, et al. Postural orthostatic tachycardia syndrome: the Mayo clinic experience. *Mayo Clin Proc.* (2007) 82:308–13. doi: 10.4065/82.3.308
16. Newton JL, Finkelmeyer A, Petrides G, Frith J, Hodgson T, Maclachlan L, et al. Reduced cardiac volumes in chronic fatigue syndrome associate with plasma volume but not length of disease: a cohort study. *Open Heart* (2016) 3:e000381 doi: 10.1136/openhrt-2015-000381
17. Davy KP, Seals DR. Total blood volume in healthy young and older men. *J Appl Physiol.* (1985) (1994) 76:2059–62. doi: 10.1152/jappl.1994.76.5.2059
18. Jones PP, Davy KP, DeSouza CA, van Pelt RE, Seals DR. Absence of age-related decline in total blood volume in physically active females. *Am J Physiol.* (1997) 272:H2534–40. doi: 10.1152/ajpheart.1997.272.6.H2534

11

The Importance of Accurate Diagnosis of ME/CFS in Children and Adolescents

Keith James Geraghty and Charles Adeniji*

Division of Population Health, Health Services Research and Primary Care, Centre for Primary Care, University of Manchester, Manchester, United Kingdom

***Correspondence:**
Keith James Geraghty
keith.geraghty@manchester.ac.uk

Myalgic encephalomyelitis/chronic fatigue syndrome (ME/CFS) is a chronic illness that causes a range of debilitating symptoms. While most research has focused on adults, the illness also presents in children and adolescents. Many physicians find it difficult to diagnose the illness. In this commentary paper, we discuss a range of salient themes that have emerged from our ongoing research into the prevalence of ME/CFS in children and adolescents. We discuss reasons why pediatric prevalence estimates vary widely in the literature, from almost 0% to as high as 3%. We argue that there is considerable misdiagnosis of pediatric cases and over-inflation of estimates of pediatric ME/CFS. Many children and teenagers with general fatigue and other medical complaints may meet loose diagnostic criteria for ME/CFS. We make recommendations for improving epidemiological research and identifying pediatric ME/CFS in clinical practice.

Keywords: chronic fatigue syndrome (CFS), myalgic encephalomyelitis, diagnosis, prevalence, pediatric case

INTRODUCTION

Children and adolescents with suspected myalgic encephalomyelitis/chronic fatigue syndrome (ME/CFS) regularly present with persistent fatigue, sleep disturbance, and an array of other symptoms, such as headaches and cognitive difficulties (1). ME/CFS is noted for being a major cause of long-term school absence and has profound negative ramifications for social development, educational achievement, and future employment (2, 3). The illness is associated with co-morbid anxiety and depression (4). It is known that children with chronic health problems exhibit higher rates of distress, anxiety, and depression (5). Taking these factors together, it is vital that young patients with this illness are correctly identified, so that they might receive a speedy diagnosis and appropriate medical care and social support.

Epidemiological studies report a wide range of prevalence estimates of ME/CFS in this age group. Some estimates are as low as 0.1% (6), while others suggest rates of 2.6% (7); and rates for CFS-like illness go as high as 4.4% (8). Girls are at greater risk of developing ME/CFS, particularly post-puberty (9). This wide spread in prevalence estimates appears to result from researchers using different diagnostic criteria to classify cases and applying different methods to sample and identify cases, such as postal or telephone questionnaires, community-based surveys, and clinical interviews. Given the general lack of consistency in methodologies applied, inconsistency in prevalence estimates is not surprising. However, such inconsistency suggests a problem with the methods used to identify young ME/CFS sufferers. It is clear, with estimates as low as 0.1% and as high as 3–4%, many young patients are being misdiagnosed, either under or over. Misdiagnosis in this vulnerable group has profound implications, since a false positive diagnosis may lead to inappropriate labeling of a child with ME/CFS and improper intervention with treatment (10), while under-diagnosis might mean a child or teen not receiving the care they require. If researchers are unable to reliably identify pediatric cases of ME/CFS, how confident can we be that clinicians are able to diagnose cases at the clinic level? We know doctors often find it difficult to diagnose ME/CFS and adult sufferers commonly wait an average of 5 years for a diagnosis (11).

THE ROOT OF THE PROBLEM

The International Chronic Fatigue Syndrome Study Group Criteria (12) is one of the most cited in the literature. The Fukuda Criteria requires severe and disabling new-onset fatigue lasting at least 6 months, accompanied by four or more of eight symptoms: impaired memory or concentration, sore throat, tender cervical or axillary lymph nodes, muscle pain, multiple joint pain, headaches, unrefreshing sleep, and post-exertional malaise (PEM). However, in the UK an alternative case definition, known as the Oxford Criteria (13), is promoted, that is much broader, given it only requires a single symptom—severe and disabling fatigue of definite onset that is present for at least 6 months and affects physical and mental function. Other symptoms often found in ME/CFS patients, headaches, sleep problems, orthostatic intolerance and so on, may be present, but are not required to be diagnosed with ME/CFS using Oxford Criteria.

In 2015, a report by the US Institutes of Health found the Oxford Criteria too broad to be of value in investigations of ME/CFS (14). The report stated that use of this case definition could impair progress and cause harm by conflating fatigue as a complaint with the illness ME/CFS. The Fukuda case definition has also been criticized; while it requires the presence of other symptoms to render a diagnosis, it does not specifically mandate that patients experience post-exterional malaise (PEM), which is considered a cardinal symptom of the illness. There are newer case criteria for ME/CFS, such as the Canadian Consensus Criteria and the International Consensus Criteria or the U.S. Institute of Medicine (now known as the National Academy of Medicine) Systemic Exertional Intolerance Disease formulation, that require the presence of PEM, however there continues to be a lack of consensus on which diagnostic criteria should be used (15). Researchers studying children or teens with the illness arbitrarily select a criterion to identify cases.

Most research in ME/CFS has focused on adults with the illness. In many adult studies, broad case definitions that require little more than fatigue as the presenting complaint, have been used to recruit patients into clinical trials of treatment interventions; commonly psychological and behavioral treatments, such as cognitive behavioral therapy (CBT) and graded exercise therapy (GET). For example, the largest clinical trial of psycho-behavioral treatments in adults, the UK PACE trial, tested CBT and GET against standard medical care and a pacing therapy (16). The PACE trial reported CBT and GET to be moderately effective compared with pacing treatment or standard medical care. However, recent commentaries have questioned whether PACE recruited true-positive ME/CFS cases (17, 18)—-the Oxford Criteria was employed to select participants. Recent reanalyses of data from the PACE trial suggests treatment benefits were grossly over-stated (19).

Another major problem in this field of research is the ubiquity of "fatigue" or "chronic fatigue" as a medical complaint and its conflation with "chronic fatigue syndrome." Pediatric studies of ME/CFS that apply broad diagnostic criteria may recruit cohorts with generalized fatigue, rather than cohorts with the cardinal symptomology of myalgic encephalomyelitis (20), proposed by Ramsay (21). The Oxford Criteria requirement to only need ongoing fatigue as a presenting complaint means many young patients with general fatigue issues could be misclassified as having ME/CFS. Up to 20% of adult patients seen in community/primary care settings present to doctors complaining of fatigue and up to 33% of adolescents experience fatigue at least 4 days per week (22, 23). UK community doctors are encouraged to refer young patients with suspected ME/CFS to be treated within specialized CFS clinics that offer CBT and exercise therapy (24). However, for adult ME/CFS patients referred to these clinics, there is a diagnostic error rate of at least 40% (25, 26) and the majority of patients treated (90%+) still report having ME/CFS at long-term follow up (27). In one of these clinics, many patients were eventually diagnosed with other conditions to explain their fatigue; 47% being diagnosed with a chronic disease, 20% a primary sleep disorder, 15% a psychological/psychiatric illness (most commonly, depression, anxiety, and post-traumatic stress disorder), and 4% a cardiovascular disorder (26). Community doctors find it difficult to differentiate fatigue linked to undiagnosed medical or mental health complaints, from clear ME/CFS.

A series of epidemiological studies into ME/CFS prevalence in teenagers conducted at the University of Bristol used a birth cohort database called the Avon Longitudinal Study of Parents and Children (ALSPAC). This database includes information on 14,500 families from Bristol and the surrounding region, with health status monitored through self-reported questionnaires filled out by both parents and children. The ALSPAC database, in conjunction with follow-up questionnaires, has been used to assess pediatric chronic fatigue prevalence, with rates reported of 1.47% at age 13 years, 2.22% at age 16 years, and 2.99% at age 18 years (28). Here "chronic disabling fatigue" is used as a proxy measure of chronic fatigue syndrome. In one of these studies published in *Pediatrics*, 41% of parents (n2201) reported their teenager being tired or lacking energy in the last month. Clearly, fatigue is a common complaint among adolescents. Of 2,201 possible CFS cases identified, after exclusions (e.g., fatigue not causing loss of activity), 4.17% (n207) with fatigue > 3 months and 2.76% (n137) with fatigue > 6 months were classified as possible cases (29). After a "Life at 16 Questionnaire" was administered to this cohort to match 16-year olds with self-reported fatigue–this generated a CFS prevalence estimate of 1.9% (29). Across the ALSPAC studies, estimation of prevalence uses proxy measures of CFS (chronic disabling fatigue), parental reported fatigue, self-reported fatigue and or school absence; however, there is a lack of detailed clinical screening or the requirement for cardinal symptoms of ME/CFS to be present, such as post-exertional malaise. As such, the near 2% prevalence rate to emerge from the

ALSPAC studies, is likely to be an over-estimation of pediatric ME/CFS.

NOT ALL FATIGUE IS THE SAME

Since fatigue is a common complaint among children and adolescents and up to half of all parents perceive their children to have "a problem" with fatigue (29, 30), there is a clear need for robust clinical investigations to assess the causes of presenting fatigue in young patients–whether it is the usual fatigue many teenagers experience, or whether it is the type of fatigue that is characteristic of ME/CFS (not all fatigue is the same). Any methodological approach that conflates the symptom of fatigue with ME/CFS is likely to inflate case estimates. For example, in the 2.99% prevalence rate of chronic disabling fatigue reported at age 18 years (28), only 29% of this CDF cohort meet the US CDC/Fukuda criteria for CFS; whereas presumably most would meet UK guidelines for CFS (31). In UK pediatric prevalence studies that apply the CDC criteria, pediatric prevalence falls to 0.019–0.05% (32, 33). This is an illuminating finding.

In the Crawley et al. prevalence study of chronic disabling fatigue at age 13, only 30.7% of teens identified as possible CFS cases had presented to a doctor complaining of fatigue (34). Presumably, the other 69.3% didn't feel their fatigue was related to a medical condition like ME/CFS, that required medical attention. Even when children or teenagers (most likely with concerned parent) present to doctors complaining of fatigue, a diagnosis of ME/CFS requires a triangulation approach, using multiple strands of information to build up a clinical case profile that helps exclude other potential medical or psychological conditions (35). Where careful clinical screening is applied, with clinicians undertaking a detailed case history, laboratory tests or psychological screening, pediatric prevalence rates fall to as low as 0.1% (6) or 0.06% (36).

Depression, mental health complaints and substance abuse, are a major cause of unexplained fatigue in young ME/CFS patients (6), thus there is a clear need for pediatric patients to be carefully screened before being given a ME/CFS diagnosis (37). The difficulty for any physician will be how to differentiate co-morbid depression and anxiety from primary depression or anxiety, as the cause of presenting fatigue. Failure to robustly assess mental health as a possible cause of fatigue is likely to lead to inflated estimates of ME/CFS. In the study of CFS rates among 16 year-olds, rates of CFS fell by more than two-thirds, from 1.89 to just 0.6%, after investigators removed those with high levels of depressive symptoms from their analysis (29). This lower 0.6% figure is much closer to rates of ME/CFS reported among adults, which commonly fall between 0.1 and 0.5% (38).

IMPLICATIONS FOR TREATMENT

The problem with over-estimation of pediatric ME/CFS is an epidemiological one that is likely to impact resource allocation and health planning. However, misdiagnosis at the clinic level is even more concerning–many children and teenagers may be wrongly diagnosed with ME/CFS. These young patients will most likely trust a diagnosis given by a physician and they are likely to follow recommended care, which might include being offered psycho-behavioral therapies like CBT or graded exercise (which are recommended based on clinical trials that apply the same loose diagnostic tools that generate inflated prevalence estimates). The Bristol ALSPAC research team, that report prevalence rates as high as 2%, are active in testing CBT and GET on children and teenagers with suspected ME/CFS (39, 40). There is a concern that psychological therapies may help teenagers that perhaps have undiagnosed psychological complaints or general fatigue complaints, who are inappropriately included into clinical trials. Basically, many teenagers with general chronic fatigue issues may meet UK Oxford/NICE criteria for ME/CFS. However, data on the success of these therapies is contaminated by the inclusion of significant numbers of false-positive cases. This concern might be evidenced in data from the ALSPAC studies that show that only 11% of teens identified as possible ME/CFS cases continued to have a problem with chronic disabling fatigue over two time points: 85.25% (6 months fatigue) between the ages of 13–16 years recovered and 79.80% (6 months fatigue) between the ages of 16–18 years recovered (CMRC Conference Presentation on ALSPAC recovery rates 2014). Essentially, 8 out of every 10 teens identified as possible CFS cases recovered by age 18 (or were wrongly classified as CFS).

A current large clinical trial (FITNET) of internet-based CBT and tele-support with activity management for teenagers (age 11–17 years) with ME/CFS uses broad (Oxford/NICE) criteria to select participants (40). A major justification used by the trial team is that teenagers have a 63% chance of recovery using FITNET vs. just 8% chance using standard medical care (40). This data is taken from a pediatric CBT trial of FITNET in the Netherlands (41). The Dutch trial has been criticized for over-stating benefits via *post-hoc* selection of recovery measures and for including young patients with general fatigue issues (42). Interestingly, at long-term follow up in the Dutch FITNET study (2 years+), recovery stood at 64% for CBT-GET participants, but 52.8% for usual care participants (43). Remarkably, teenagers in the standard care group (which is often nothing more than usual general practice care) improved over time, with relatively little difference between the CBT cohort and the *de facto* no-treatment control. This same phenomenon is visible in adult CBT trials, with the gap closing between the intervention and standard care in the PACE trial (44) and FINE trial (45). What we can take from this observation is that CBT or exercise therapy perform little better than no care over the longer term. There are other reasons some trials show modest benefits over the short-term, such as selection of milder cases and strong treatment promotion effects (18, 46). Taking this into consideration, in addition to noting high rates of natural recovery in children and adolescents, the case for early intervention with psycho-behavioral therapy is rather weak. Good quality primary care support should always be available. For more severe cases, treatment in specialist secondary care should be available also. This care should include symptomatic support, advice on nutrition, sleep support, pain control, infection control, allergies, and mental health issues (35). There is no evidence to support GET for severe ME/CFS cases (clinical trials do not include severe homebound sufferers). Very little is known about patients with severe ME/CFS. They are often housebound, bedbound and are rarely studied. Overall, much more research is needed around all aspects of pediatric ME/CFS.

CONCLUSION

There is a clear need for robust prevalence estimates of childhood and adolescent ME/CFS to guide clinical practice and inform health care decision-making. The wide range of prevalence rates observed in the literature is concerning. This range reflects a lack of agreement about the diagnostic criteria used to identify pediatric cases and a lack of consistency in the methods used to collect data. Broad diagnostic criteria, such as the Oxford Criteria, result in inflated prevalence rates and fail to adequately distinguish true-positive cases from non-cases. Psychological and behavioral therapies continue to be tested on young patients with ME/CFS, but if children or teens are wrongly labeled as having ME/CFS and enrolled in trials of CBT or exercise therapy, findings from these studies are likely to be misleading and erroneous. Researchers need to agree on sampling strategies to identify true pediatric cases of ME/CFS and clinicians need to use a comprehensive triangulation approach to diagnose children and teenagers with ME/CFS, while carefully excluding young patients with health problems that mimic the illness.

AUTHOR CONTRIBUTIONS

KG conceived the paper. KG and CA contributed to the final draft. CA assisted with a systematic review of the literature discussed in this paper.

ACKNOWLEDGMENTS

We wish to thank the UK Tymes Trust for donating the open access publication fees.

REFERENCES

1. Oliver LM, Patel K. Co-morbid conditions in children with chronic fatigue syndrome/myalgic encephalomyelitis (CFS/ME)-a retrospective case note review of a large cohort. *Arch Dis Child.* (2012) 97:A105. doi: 10.1136/archdischild-2012-301885.248
2. Dowsett EG, Colby J. Long-term sickness absence due to ME/CFS in UK schools: an epidemiological study with medical and educational implications. *J Chronic Fatigue Syndr.* (1997) 3:29–42. doi: 10.1300/J092v03n02_04
3. Nijhof SL, Maijer K, Bleijenberg G, Uiterwaal CS, Kimpen JL, Van De Putte EM. Adolescent chronic fatigue syndrome: prevalence, incidence, and morbidity. *Pediatrics* (2011) 127:e1169–75. doi: 10.1542/peds.2010-1147
4. Collin SM, Nuevo R, van de Putte EM, Nijhof SL, Crawley E. Chronic fatigue syndrome (CFS) or myalgic encephalomyelitis (ME) is different in children compared to in adults: a study of UK and Dutch clinical cohorts. *BMJ Open* (2015) 5:e008830. doi: 10.1136/bmjopen-2015-008830
5. Pao M, Bosk A. Anxiety in medically ill children/adolescents. *Depress Anxiety* (2011) 28:40–9. doi: 10.1002/da.20727
6. Jones JF, Nisenbaum R, Solomon L, Reyes M, Reeves WC. Chronic fatigue syndrome and other fatiguing illnesses in adolescents: a population-based study. *J Adolesc Health* (2004) 35:34–40. doi: 10.1016/S1054-139X(03)00372-0
7. Gunn WJ, Connell DB, Randall B. Epidemiology of chronic fatigue syndrome: the centers for disease control study. *Ciba Found Symp.* (1993) 173:83–93; discussion 93–101.
8. Mears CJ, Taylor RR, Jordan KM, Binns HJ. Sociodemographic and symptom correlates of fatigue in an adolescent primary care sample. *J Adolesc Health* (2004) 35:528.e21–6. doi: 10.1016/j.jadohealth.2004.02.012
9. Haines LC, Saidi G, Cooke RW. Prevalence of severe fatigue in primary care. *Arch Dis Child.* (2005) 90:367–8. doi: 10.1136/adc.2003.039917
10. Nacul L, Lacerda EM, Kingdon CC, Curran H, Bowman EW. How have selection bias and disease misclassification undermined the validity of myalgic encephalomyelitis/chronic fatigue syndrome studies? *J Health Psychol.* (2017) 1:1359105317695803. doi: 10.1177/13591053176 95803
11. Cairns R. A systematic review describing the prognosis of chronic fatigue syndrome. *Occupat Med.* (2005) 55:20–31. doi: 10.1093/occmed/kqi013
12. Fukuda K, Straus SE, Hickie I, Sharpe MC, Dobbins JG, Komaroff A. The chronic fatigue syndrome: a comprehensive approach to its definition and study. International chronic fatigue syndrome study group. *Ann Intern Med.* (1994) 121:953–9. doi: 10.7326/0003-4819-121-12-199412150-00009
13. Sharpe MC, Archard LC, Banatvala JE, Borysiewicz LK, Clare AW, David A, et al. A report–chronic fatigue syndrome: guidelines for research. *J R Soc Med.* (1991) 84:118–21. doi: 10.1177/014107689108400224
14. Green CR, Cowan P, Elk R, O'neil KM, Rasmussen AL. National institutes of health pathways to prevention workshop: advancing the research on myalgic encephalomyelitis/chronic fatigue syndrome. *Ann Intern Med.* (2015) 162:860–5. doi: 10.7326/M15-0338
15. Nacul L, Kingdon CC, Bowman EW, Curran H, Lacerda EM. Differing case definitions point to the need for an accurate diagnosis of myalgic encephalomyelitis/chronic fatigue syndrome. *Fatigue* (2017) 5:1–4. doi: 10.1080/21641846.2017.1273863
16. White PD, Goldsmith KA, Johnson AL, Potts L, Walwyn R, Decesare JC, et al. Comparison of adaptive pacing therapy, cognitive behaviour therapy, graded exercise therapy, and specialist medical care for chronic fatigue syndrome (PACE): a randomised trial. *Lancet* (2011) 377:823–36. doi: 10.1016/S0140-6736(11)60096-2
17. Geraghty KJ. 'PACE-Gate': when clinical trial evidence meets open data access. *J Health Psychol.* (2017) 22:1106–12. doi: 10.1177/1359105316675213
18. Geraghty KJ. Further commentary on the PACE trial: biased methods and unreliable outcomes. *J Health Psychol.* (2017) 22:1209–16. doi: 10.1177/1359105317714486
19. Wilshire CE, Kindlon T, Courtney R, Matthees A, Tuller D, Geraghty K, et al. Rethinking the treatment of chronic fatigue syndrome-a reanalysis and evaluation of findings from a recent major trial of graded exercise and CBT. *BMC Psychol.* (2018) 6:6. doi: 10.1186/s40359-018-0218-3
20. Twisk F. Myalgic Encephalomyelitis (ME) or what? an operational definition. *Diagnostics* (2018) 8:64. doi: 10.3390/diagnostics8030064
21. Ramsay AM. Encephalomyelitis in north west london. *Lancet* (1957) 270:1196–200. doi: 10.1016/S0140-6736(57)90163-0
22. Rosenthal TC, Majeroni BA, Pretorius R, Malik K. Fatigue: an overview. *Am Fam Phys.* (2008) 78:1173–9.
23. Viner R, Christie D. Fatigue and somatic symptoms. *BMJ* (2005) 330:1012–5. doi: 10.1136/bmj.330.7498.1012
24. Brigden A, Loades M, Abbott A, Bond-Kendall J, Crawley E. Practical management of chronic fatigue syndrome or myalgic encephalomyelitis in childhood. *Arch Dis Child.* (2017) 102:981–6. doi: 10.1136/archdischild-2016-310622
25. Devasahayam A, Lawn T, Murphy M, White PD. Alternative diagnoses to chronic fatigue syndrome in referrals to a specialist service: service evaluation survey. *JRSM Short Rep.* (2012) 3:1–5. doi: 10.1258/shorts.2011.011127
26. Newton JL, Mabillard H, Scott A, Hoad A, Spickett G. The newcastle NHS chronic fatigue syndrome service: not all fatigue is the same. *J R Coll Physicians* (2010) 40:304–7. doi: 10.4997/JRCPE.2010.404
27. Collin SM, Crawley E. Specialist treatment of chronic fatigue syndrome/ME: a cohort study among adult patients in England. *BMC Health Serv Res.* (2017) 17:488. doi: 10.1186/s12913-017-2437-3

28. Norris T, Collin SM, Tilling K, Nuevo R, Stansfeld SA, Sterne JAC, et al. Natural course of chronic fatigue syndrome/myalgic encephalomyelitis in adolescents. *Arch Dis Child.* (2017) 19. doi: 10.1136/archdischild-2016-311198
29. Collin SM, Norris T, Nuevo R, Tilling K, Joinson C, Sterne JAC, et al. Chronic fatigue syndrome at age 16 years. *Pediatrics* (2016) 137:e20153434. doi: 10.1542/peds.2015-3434
30. Farmer A, Fowler T, Scourfield J, Thapar A. Prevalence of chronic disabling fatigue in children and adolescents. *Br J Psychiatry* (2004) 184:477–81. doi: 10.1192/bjp.184.6.477
31. Baker R, Shaw EJ. Diagnosis and management of chronic fatigue syndrome or myalgic encephalomyelitis (or encephalopathy): summary of NICE guidance. *BMJ* (2007) 335:446–8. doi: 10.1136/bmj.39302.509005.AE
32. Rimes KA, Goodman R, Hotopf M, Wessely S, Meltzer H, Chalder T. Incidence, prognosis, and risk factors for fatigue and chronic fatigue syndrome in adolescents: a prospective community study. *Pediatrics* (2007) 119:e603–9. doi: 10.1542/peds.2006-2231
33. Chalder T, Goodman R, Wessely S, Hotopf M, Meltzer H. Epidemiology of chronic fatigue syndrome and self reported myalgic encephalomyelitis in 5-15 year olds: cross sectional study. *BMJ* (2003) 327:654–5. doi: 10.1136/bmj.327.7416.654
34. Crawley E, Hughes R, Northstone K, Tilling K, Emond A, Sterne JAC. Chronic disabling fatigue at age 13 and association with family adversity. *Pediatrics* (2012) 130:e71–9. doi: 10.1542/peds.2011-2587
35. Rowe PC, Underhill RA, Friedman KJ, Gurwitt A, Medow MS, Schwartz MS, et al. Myalgic encephalomyelitis/chronic fatigue syndrome diagnosis and management in young people: a primer. *Front Pediatr.* (2017) 5:121. doi: 10.3389/fped.2017.00121
36. Jordan KM, Jason LA, Mears CJ, Katz BZ, Rademaker A, Huang CF, et al. Prevalence of pediatric chronic fatigue syndrome in a community-based sample. *J Chronic Fatigue Syndr.* (2006) 13:75–8. doi: 10.1300/J092v13n02_04
37. Jones JF, Lin J-MS, Maloney EM, Boneva RS, Nater UM, Unger ER, et al. An evaluation of exclusionary medical/psychiatric conditions in the definition of chronic fatigue syndrome. *BMC Med.* (2009) 7:57. doi: 10.1186/1741-7015-7-57
38. Nacul LC, Lacerda EM, Pheby D, Campion P, Molokhia M, Fayyaz S, et al. Prevalence of myalgic encephalomyelitis/chronic fatigue syndrome (ME/CFS) in three regions of England: a repeated cross-sectional study in primary care. *BMC Med.* (2011) 9:91. doi: 10.1186/1741-7015-9-91
39. Loades M, Brigden A, Crawley E. Current treatment approaches for paediatric CFS/ME. *Paediatr Child Health* (2017) 27:432–4. doi: 10.1016/j.paed.2017.05.007
40. Baos S, Brigden A, Anderson E, Hollingworth W, Price S, Mills N, et al. Investigating the effectiveness and cost-effectiveness of FITNET-NHS (Fatigue In Teenagers on the interNET in the NHS) compared to activity management to treat paediatric chronic fatigue syndrome (CFS)/myalgic encephalomyelitis (ME): protocol for a randomised controlled trial. *Trials* (2018) 19:136. doi: 10.1186/s13063-018-2500-3
41. Nijhof SL, Bleijenberg G, Uiterwaal CS, Kimpen JL, Van De Putte EM. Effectiveness of internet-based cognitive behavioural treatment for adolescents with chronic fatigue syndrome (FITNET): a randomised controlled trial. *Lancet* (2012) 379:1412–8. doi: 10.1016/S0140-6736(12)60025-7
42. Ghatineh S, Vink M. FITNET's internet-based cognitive behavioural therapy is ineffective and may impede natural recovery in adolescents with myalgic encephalomyelitis/chronic fatigue syndrome. A review. *Behav Sci.* (2017) 7:52. doi: 10.3390/bs7030052
43. Nijhof SL, Priesterbach LP, Uiterwaal CS, Bleijenberg G, Kimpen JL, Van De Putte EM. Internet-based therapy for adolescents with chronic fatigue syndrome: long-term follow-up. *Pediatrics* (2013) 131:e1788–95. doi: 10.1542/peds.2012-2007
44. Sharpe M, Goldsmith KA, Johnson AL, Chalder T, Walker J, White PD. Rehabilitative treatments for chronic fatigue syndrome: long-term follow-up from the PACE trial. *Lancet Psychiatry* (2015) 2:1067–74. doi: 10.1016/S2215-0366(15)00317-X
45. Wearden AJ, Dowrick C, Chew-Graham C, Bentall RP, Morriss RK, Peters S, et al. Nurse led, home based self help treatment for patients in primary care with chronic fatigue syndrome: randomised controlled trial. *BMJ* (2010) 340:c1777. doi: 10.1136/bmj.c1777
46. Geraghty KJ, Blease C. Cognitive behavioural therapy in the treatment of chronic fatigue syndrome: a narrative review on efficacy and informed consent. *J Health Psychol.* (2018) 23:127–38. doi: 10.1177/1359105316667798

12

Onset Patterns and Course of Myalgic Encephalomyelitis/Chronic Fatigue Syndrome

Lily Chu*, Ian J. Valencia, Donn W. Garvert and Jose G. Montoya

Stanford ME/CFS Initiative, Division of Infectious Diseases and Geographic Medicine, Stanford University School of Medicine, Stanford, CA, United States

***Correspondence:**
Lily Chu
lchu1@stanford.edu

Background: Epidemiologic studies of myalgic encephalomyelitis/ chronic fatigue syndrome (ME/CFS) have examined different aspects of this disease separately but few have explored them together.

Objective: Describe ME/CFS onset and course in one United States-based cohort.

Methods: One hundred and fifty subjects fitting Fukuda 1994 CFS criteria completed a detailed survey concerning the initial and subsequent stages of their illness. Descriptive statistics, graphs, and tables were used to illustrate prevalence and patterns of characteristics.

Results: The most common peri-onset events reported by subjects were infection-related episodes (64%), stressful incidents (39%), and exposure to environmental toxins (20%). For 38% of subjects, more than 6 months elapsed from experiencing any initial symptom to developing the set of symptoms comprising their ME/CFS. Over time, the 12 most common symptoms persisted but declined in prevalence, with fatigue, unrefreshing sleep, exertion-related sickness, and flu-like symptoms declining the most (by 20–25%). Conversely, cognitive symptoms changed the least in prevalence, rising in symptom ranking. Pregnancy, menopause, and menstrual cycles exacerbated many women's symptoms. Fatigue-related function was not associated with duration of illness or age; during the worst periods of their illness, 48% of subjects could not engage in any productive activity. At the time of survey, 47% were unable to work and only 4% felt their condition was improving steadily with the majority (59%) describing a fluctuating course. Ninety-seven percent suffered from at least one other illness: anxiety (48%), depression (43%), fibromyalgia (39%), irritable bowel syndrome (38%), and migraine headaches (37%) were the most diagnosed conditions. Thirteen percent came from families where at least one other first-degree relative was also afflicted, rising to 27% when chronic fatigue of unclear etiology was included.

Conclusions: This paper offers a broad epidemiologic overview of one ME/CFS cohort in the United States. While most of our findings are consistent with prior studies, we highlight underexamined aspects of this condition (e.g., the evolution of symptoms) and propose new interpretations of findings. Studying these aspects can offer insight and solutions to the diagnosis, etiology, pathophysiology, and treatment of this condition.

Keywords: chronic fatigue syndrome, myalgic encephalomyelitis, epidemiology, onset, course, systemic exertion intolerance disease, natural history

INTRODUCTION

Myalgic encephalomyelitis/ chronic fatigue syndrome is a complex, disabling, chronic illness that is estimated to affect from 0.76 to 3.28% (1) of the population worldwide and up to 2.5 million US residents (2). Although the average age of onset is in the 30 s and women are affected at two to three times the rate of men, CFS can occur at any age, also strikes children, and, contrary to its early nickname, "yuppie flu," may disproportionately affect certain ethnic minorities as well as lower socio-economic classes (2–4). Severe fatigue accompanied by musculoskeletal pain, headaches, sore throat, tender lymph nodes, concentration/ memory difficulties, unrefreshing sleep, exacerbation of these symptoms with minimal physical, or cognitive exertion (termed post-exertional malaise), and orthostatic intolerance results in patients suffering a substantial reduction in function from their pre-illness state (5, 6). Rates of unemployment can be as high as 81% (7) while ~25% of patients may be homebound or bedridden (8). Function and health-related quality of life scores have been shown to be lower than that of patients affected by multiple sclerosis, rheumatoid arthritis, congestive heart failure, and myocardial infarction (9–11). Despite these serious public health implications, after 3 decades, we still do not know what causes ME/CFS nor do we have established objective diagnostic tests or a single FDA-approved treatment (6). Since the median rate of full recovery is only 5% (12), many patients remain ill for years to decades, costing the US ~\$18–\$54 billion annually from both direct medical costs as well as lost productivity and taxes (13).

Prior studies have documented various aspects of ME/CFS including onset of illness (14, 15), symptoms (6), function (16, 17), course (18–24), co-morbidities (25–29), and family history (30–36). However, these studies have tended to focus on one or a few clinical characteristics. Alternatively, epidemiologic results from one cohort, like the US Centers for Disease Control and Prevention's Wichita ME/CFS group, are dispersed among several articles (21, 23, 37, 38). Consequently, the clinical picture of ME/CFS has had to be pieced together from studies that may have very different subjects or across multiple articles originating from one group of subjects. The few studies that have attempted to give a broad-based overview of one cohort in one article have been based in Europe, Australia, and Japan but not in the United States (39–43). Juxtaposing different aspects of ME/CFS together in one paper might allow researchers and clinicians to see connections among the aspects more easily. Secondly, commonly referenced concepts have not always been clear. For example, many studies classify subjects as having either an "acute"/ "sudden" or "gradual" onset of illness yet most do not define the time period meant by such terms. Researchers, subjects, and article readers might interpret the same term to mean different lengths of time. Third, some aspects of ME/CFS have not been examined in detail. For example, very few papers have examined how symptoms changes over more than a few years and the effect of female reproductive hormonal events on the disease.

The objective of this study was to examine the different dimensions of ME/CFS together and fill in some of these gaps, by characterizing clinical aspects of ME/CFS in detail in one cohort of subjects based in the United States. This study will also serve as a reference for other papers derived from the same cohort (44, 45) exploring relationships among immunological, genetic, microbiological, and clinical characteristics of ME/CFS. Findings from this study may inform clinical care, help generate hypotheses about etiology, pathophysiology, diagnosis, and treatment, and assist in the design and implementation of future studies.

METHODS

From March 2010 to August 2011, 200 ME/CFS subjects were recruited as part of our GESID (Genetic Expression and Immune System Dynamics) study examining the interactions among pathogen presence and load, human leukocyte antigen (HLA) types, and the immune system in ME/CFS. Some subjects originated from Stanford University's ME/CFS Clinic or the Clinic wait list while others were recruited via local support groups and electronic patient forums. All subjects were screened using a standardized telephone interview and included if they fitted Fukuda 1994 CFS criteria, lived in the San Francisco Bay area, were at least 14 years old, were non-pregnant, and had not been exposed to more than 2 weeks of antimicrobials recently. Subjects were excluded from the study if they were affected by an alternative medical or psychiatric condition that could explain their symptoms, suffered from certain immunological conditions, struggled with substance abuse issues in the last year (not including nicotine/caffeine), received an influenza vaccination within the past 4 weeks, or had limited ability communicating in English.

Fatigue severity and impact on function were assessed using the Multi-dimensional Fatigue Inventory –20 (MFI-20) (46, 47) and the Fatigue Severity Scale (FSS) (48). The MFI-20 gives a total score (ranging from 20 to 100) as well as subscores related to 5 dimensions of fatigue (general fatigue, physical fatigue, reduced motivation, reduced activity, and mental fatigue, each ranging from 4 to 20). The FSS total score ranges from 1 to 7 and is an average of the score of 9 individual items, each also rated on a 1–7 scale. For both questionnaires, a higher number indicates a greater impact of fatigue on daily life.

In 2012, to further characterize our subjects, we used the Research Electronic Data Capture (REDCap)[1] web application to design an online survey covering demographic traits, illness onset, symptoms, illness course, function, patient medical history, family medical history, social history, and medication use. Content, wording, and format of survey items were based on a review of the scientific literature, the authors' clinical/research experiences, and feedback from several patient volunteers. We included a 54-item symptom survey from the DePaul Symptom Questionnaire[2] (DSQ), which was designed to elicit the wide range of symptoms known to occur in ME/CFS and has been used in multiple other studies. This project was reviewed and approved by the Stanford University Institutional Review Board.

The aforementioned 200 subjects were re-contacted via e-mail or telephone from January 2013 to July 2013 and asked if they wished to participate in the survey. Written consent was obtained. Those expressing interest were given an individualized secured hyperlink to access the survey; if they could not finish it in one session, they were given a code so they could complete it in as many sessions as they needed. A paper version of the survey was also offered to participants who expressed technical or cognitive difficulties with the online survey. After completion, subjects submitted the survey electronically or mailed the survey back to staff.

Next, survey data were stripped of identifying information per the Health Insurance Portability and Accountability Act (HIPAA) Privacy Rule and exported to create a database. We used Microsoft Excel 2016 to generate histograms, scatterplots, and descriptive statistics (frequencies, percentages, mean, medians, standard deviation). To assess for differences between groups and for relationships among variables, we calculated chi-square statistics for categorical variables and Welch's t-test for continuous variables using the online program GraphPad[3] A two-tailed p-value of equal or <0.05 was deemed to be statistically significant.

RESULTS

A total of 150 subjects participated in the survey, equivalent to a 75% response rate. Responders were more likely to be Caucasian (95 vs. 84%, $p = 0.04$), female (80 vs. 66%, $p = 0.05$) and to be affected by sore throats or post-exertional malaise (respectively, 67 vs. 48%, $p < 0.01$; 98 vs. 92%, $p = 0.04$) than non-responders. No statistically significant differences existed otherwise in terms of age, duration of illness, fatigue severity, self-rated physical/cognitive functioning, prevalence of viral onset, or prevalence of minor Fukuda case definition symptoms (data not shown).

Eighty-four percent of the subjects ($n = 126$) completed the survey online. The number of subjects completing each survey item varied as some might not have remembered what had occurred previously or were unsure of their answers. However, for almost every item except one item concerning the onset date of their illness (see next section), more than 92% of the subjects were able to give an answer and only 5 subjects did not complete extensive, contiguous parts of the survey. For all items, statistics were performed based on the number of subjects answering that specific item.

DEMOGRAPHICS

Eighty-one percent of respondents ($n = 121$) were female while 19% were male. An overwhelming 97% of subjects were Caucasian with the remaining subjects identifying themselves as African-American (1%, $n = 1$), Hispanic-American (1%, $n = 2$), and Asian-American (2%, $n = 3$). The median age (standard deviation) of respondents was 53.7 ± 12.4 years (range, 20–75 years of age). Six subjects (4%) could not remember a time in their lives that they had not been sick and 18 subjects could not give an approximate time their illness began. Thus, duration of illness and age of onset could not be determined for these 24 (15%) subjects. Based on available data, the median age of illness onset was 36.6 ± 12.3 years and median duration of illness was 12.5 ± 10.1 years.

ILLNESS ONSET

Most subjects (90%, $n = 135$) could remember a time before they were sick and 85% ($n = 123$) noted a specific time their illness began. When asked if they believed a specific factor precipitated their illness, 88% ($n = 132$) answered affirmatively or possibly.

Although we offered 14 different factors that could be associated with onset, 61% of subjects selected only one or two factors. We chose to group subjects who responded "yes" or "not sure" (vs. a clear "no") together as illness onset has not been examined in detail and we wanted to include all possibilities. The top five factors selected were infectious illnesses (64%), stress/ major life events (39%, primarily work- or family-related), exposure to chemical/ environmental toxins (20%), recent international travel (19%), and recent domestic travel (17%) (**Table 1**).

Of the 40 individuals selecting only one factor, 58% chose an infectious event compared to 22% choosing a life event. An "other" category, selected by 17% ($n = 22$), was also included so subjects could write in responses: 36% of these were still infection-related events with the subject also checking the "infectious illness" category. Four percent of subjects cited none of the factors listed and did not write down a specific factor.

Infectious illnesses were further broken down into the type of infectious illness (**Table 2**). A little over a third of subjects (35%) reported documentation of a specific acute infection; the most common infection-related symptoms were respiratory-related

[1]https://projectredcap.org/
[2]http://condor.depaul.edu/ljason/cfs/measures.html
[3]http://www.graphpad.com/quickcalcs/

TABLE 1 | Factors reported by subjects to be associated with their ME/CFS onset.

Factor	Number of subjects[a]	Percentage of subjects[b] (%)
Infectious illness	84	64
Stress or major life event[c]	51	39
Exposure to chemical/environmental toxin[d]	26	20
Recent international travel	25	19
Recent domestic travel	23	17
Other[e]	22	17
Medical injection	13	10
Pregnancy	11	8
Surgery	10	8
Accident	10	8
Consumption of water from questionable source	10	8
Neurologic event	9	7
Cardiac event	8	6
None of the above	5	4
Raw/undercooked dairy, eggs, meat	2	2

[a]Subjects responding "yes" or possibly to factor as a precipitant. Subjects could choose more than one factor.
[b]Out of 132 subjects total who noted a precipitating event(s).
[c]Primarily family and work-related events.
[d]Subjects primarily mentioned environments which might have exposed them to higher levels of various substances. "Mold" was the most common specific answer given.
[e]8 (36%) were infection-related events with all subjects also replying "yes" to infectious illness; remainder included insect bites and other medical events.

TABLE 2 | Subject-reported infectious events related to ME/CFS-onset.

Type of infection	Number of subjects identifying infection[a]	Percentage identifying infection[b] (%)
Respiratory infection (sore throat, runny nose, cough, etc.)	33	39
Documented acute infection (herpes viruses, parvovirus B19, etc.)	29	35
Non-specific infection (fever, chills, sweats, muscle aches, etc.)	28	33
Other	15	18
Abdominal infection (diarrhea, nausea, vomiting, blood in stool, etc.)	10	12
Bladder infection (pain/burning urinating, urinating frequently, feeling of having to urinate urgently, etc.)	4	5
Prostate infection	0	0

[a]Out of 84 total respondents endorsing an infectious illness as a precipitating factor for their ME/CFS.
[b]Subjects were permitted to choose more than one type of infectious event. However, 77% chose only one event.

TABLE 3 | Elapsed time from any initial symptoms to consistent illness.

Time to onset	N	%
Within 24 h	17	12
1–6 days	5	3
7–30 days	19	13
1–6 months	32	22
7–12 months	16	11
1–2 years	11	7
More than 2 years	30	20
Do not know	17	12
No answer	3	–

(39%; sore throat, runny nose, cough, etc.) followed closely by constitutional symptoms (33%; fever, chills, etc.). Except for one case, all subjects first fell ill while in the United States.

Half of the subjects (N = 13 out of 26) selecting a toxic or chemical trigger did not cite a specific substance but described workplaces, living situations, or hobbies which might have exposed them to unusual levels of various solvents, animal droppings, metals, dust, asbestos, or volatile organic compounds. Six subjects wrote down "mold" but did elaborate further. Subjects traveled widely and no specific portion of the United States nor of the world stood out. Most did not become ill until after returning to the United States. Activities engaged in while traveling included work, visiting family, seeing tourist sites, and participating in outdoor sports. A few noted they recovered from their travel-related illness only to become sick again later (so it was unclear whether ME/CFS was related or not to their travels) while others indicated travel companions did not become sick.

Table 3 shows that the time from the first intimation of illness to becoming consistently sick varied greatly: while 28% endorsed an onset period of a month or less, 38% noted it took over 6 months. Subjects who reported an infectious precipitant were no more likely to develop ME/CFS within 1 month or within 6 months compared to those who noted no infectious precipitant (respectively, 14 vs. 21% and 51 vs. 43%, $0.05 < p$-value).

The second column of **Table 4** shows the 12 most prevalent symptoms, out of the 54 elicited by the DSQ, during the first 6 months of illness. Although fatigue/extreme tiredness, endorsed by 97% of subjects, was the most common symptom, five of the remaining symptoms were associated with physical/ cognitive exertion (range 73–85%) and 3 involved cognitive dysfunction (72–76%). Unrefreshing sleep (92%), flu-like feelings (70%), and muscle pain (76%) also figured prominently.

We also asked about the existence of several symptoms that were not included in the DSQ or the Fukuda 1994 criteria but are part of newer criteria like the Systemic Exertion Intolerance Disease/ National Academy of Medicine definition (6), Canadian Consensus Criteria (CCC) (49), and Myalgic Encephalomyelitis-International Consensus Criteria (ME-ICC) (50). Sixty-two percent of subjects reported fainting or near-fainting episodes, 66% were less able to tolerate alcohol compared to their pre-illness state, and 81% felt sick or uncomfortable waiting in lines. All three symptoms are characteristic of orthostatic intolerance. Compared to before the onset of their CFS, 32 and 52%

TABLE 4 | Prevalence and ranking of the most common 12 symptoms during the first 6 months of illness, after the first 6 months, and at the time of survey[a].

Symptom	Prevalence first 6 months (rank)[b]	Prevalence after first 6 months (rank)[c]	Prevalence at time of survey (rank)	Change from beginning of illness to time of survey[d] (%)
Fatigue/extreme tiredness	97% (1)	86% (1)	76% (1)	−23
Feeling unrefreshed after you wake up in the morning	92% (2)	81% (2)	69% (2)	−23
Physically drained or sick after mild activity	85% (3)	79% (4)	60% (11)	−25
Minimum exercise makes you physically tired	80% (4)	77% (5)	63% (7)	−17
Next day soreness or fatigue after non-strenuous exercise	76% (5)	73% (9)	64% (6)	−12
Problems remembering things	76% (6)	77% (6)	68% (4)	−8
Pain or aching in your muscles	76% (7)	71% (11)	59% (13)	−17
Mentally tired after the slightest effort	75% (8)	76% (7)	61% (9)	−14
Difficulty paying attention	74% (9)	73% (8)	64% (5)	−10
"Dead" or "heavy" feeling after starting to exercise	73% (10)	68% (16)	53% (18)	−20
Difficulty finding the right word/ expressing self	72% (11)	79% (3)	68% (3)	−4
Flu-like symptoms	70% (12)	67% (20)	46% (25)	−24

[a]*The median length of illness in our sample was 12.5 ± 10.1 years. It was explained to survey respondents that "after first 6 months" meant anytime between that time and the time of the survey. So if someone had been sick for a decade and they suffered from a symptom from years 2 through 5 of their illness, but not at the beginning of their illness or at the time of the survey, they would mark down their answer affirmatively during this period.*

[b]*Subjects were asked if a symptom was present at the specified moment in time. Fifty-four different symptoms were listed with the most common ranked as "1" and the least common as "54."*

[c]*The prevalence of these symptoms changed over time such that they would no longer be or rise to being among the 12 most common symptoms. For example, "Physically drained or sick after mild activity" was the 3rd most common symptom during the first 6 months but had fallen to the 11th most common by the time of our survey.*

[d]*Percentage change is absolute, not relative (e.g., for fatigue, 97–76% = 23%). Over time, "absentminded or forgetfulness" (19, 10, 10), "only can focus on one thing at a time" (22, 17, 8), and "sensitivity to noise" (15, 12, 12) moved up to the top 12 most common symptoms (numbers in parentheses refer to change in rank over the 3 time periods).*

of subjects, respectively, felt they were more prone to viral infections or took a longer time to recover from infections. Eighty-seven percent experienced problems with temperature regulation, especially when the weather was unusually hot or cold.

ILLNESS COURSE

For the overwhelming majority of patients (96%, $n = 141$), their illness did not improve with time although different patterns of illness were seen: 14% of subjects believed their illness was constantly worsening; 7%, relapsing-remitting (all symptoms might disappear for a time only to return); 8%, persisting with little change; 59%, fluctuating (symptoms could change in severity but were always present) and 7%, "other" pattern, although the most common response here was analogous to the "fluctuating" pattern with some symptoms worsening while others improved over time. Thirteen percent of subjects reported that they experienced remissions (i.e., no symptoms) of more than a month during their years of illness. The median duration of remission was 7 months with the range being from 1.5 to 240 months.

The symptomology of the illness generally remained unchanged with 9 of the top 12 symptoms present at the beginning of the illness continuing to stay in the top 12 after the initial 6 months and up to the time of this survey more than a decade into illness (**Table 4**). However, the prevalence of all 12 symptoms decreased over time and three symptoms ("flu-like feelings," "'dead' or "heavy' feeling after starting to exercise," "pain or aching in your muscles") dropped out of the top 12 to be replaced by "absentminded or forgetfulness," "only can focus on one thing at a time," and "sensitivity to noise." Over time, flu-like symptoms, fatigue, unrefreshing sleep, and exertion-related items decreased the most, by between 12 and 25%. For flu-like issues, 55% believed their disappearance to be spontaneously induced whereas for fatigue, exertion-related items and unrefreshing sleep, 72, 50–73, and 90%, respectively, attributed their decline to specific treatments. Cognitive symptoms present at the beginning of the illness tended to persist, declining by only 4–10%.

Like the section regarding illness onset, we presented subjects with the same 14 factors and asked which factors they believed might have affected their illness course significantly. The two most-cited factors were infectious illnesses (33%) and stress/ major life events (29%) but a quarter of our subjects cited none of the factors nor wrote in any factors (**Table 5**). Female subjects were also queried about whether and how specific hormone-related events in their lives affected their symptoms (**Figure 1**). A significant percentage of women felt that pregnancy (42% overall), menopause (38%), and monthly

TABLE 5 | Subject-reported factors which affected the course of illness.

Factor	Number of subjects	Percentage of subjects[a] (%)
Infectious illness	49	35
Stress or major life event[b]	44	31
None of the above	37	26
Exposure to chemical/environmental toxin[c]	16	11
Other[d]	16	11
Surgery	15	11
Neurologic event	15	11
Cardiac event	15	11
Accident	11	8
Recent domestic travel	8	6
Pregnancy	8	6
Recent international travel	8	5
Medical injection	3	2
Consumption of water from questionable source	1	1
Raw/ undercooked dairy, eggs, meat	1	1

[a]*Out of 141 respondents.*
[b]*Work, family, and relationship-related events.*
[c]*9 out of 16 cited mold; otherwise, a variety of occupational exposures.*
[d]*8 out of 16 may be infection-related.*

menstrual cycles (53%) negatively impacted their illness. In contrast, hormone-based contraception and replacement therapy were only cited by 11% as having a deleterious effect with about three-fourths of women citing no effect on their ME/CFS symptoms.

FUNCTION

The 1994 Fukuda CFS criteria requires that "fatigue results in substantial reduction in previous levels of occupational, educational, social, or personal activities." This level of functional impairment was reflected via the various ways we assessed the impact of ME/CFS on subject's lives. Almost all of our subjects (92%, $n = 138$) believed that the illness had reduced their function by 50% or more; only 15% were able to work more than 30 h a week whereas 47% had been designated as permanently disabled from work.

Figure 2 illustrates functional level, as assessed by ability to carry out work, school, family, and other responsibilities during various periods of an individual subject's illness. For most of their illness, 82% were unable to work or attend school full-time (functional levels 1–4). During the worst periods, nearly half (48%) were confined to their beds or could not engage in any productive activity (functional level 1). Even during their best periods, only about a third of subjects were able to engage in their work or school full-time, albeit it often still meant they had to sacrifice participating in other aspects of life.

The mean FSS score of our subjects was 5.9 ± 1.1. The mean MFI-20 scores and standard deviations were: total, 73.8 ± 13.6; general, 17.2 ± 3.0; physical, 16.6 ± 3.3; mental, 13.6 ± 4.2; reduced activity, 15.2 ± 4.1; and reduced motivation, 10 ± 4.4. Scatterplots of the total MFI-20 score and total FSS score vs. duration of illness (**Figure 3**) and age of the subject (**Figure 4**) show little correlation with R-squared values ranging from 0.0106 to 0.0234.

PERSONAL MEDICAL HISTORY

From a list of 43 different medical and psychiatric conditions, including those purported to frequently co-exist with ME/CFS, subjects indicated which conditions they had been diagnosed with by a healthcare professional. They suffered from a median of 7 ± 4.2 conditions with over 50% of the subjects citing any chronic condition as unresolved. Almost all subjects (97%) suffered from at least one other medical condition and 64% divulged at least one psychiatric condition.

The 15 most prevalent conditions are shown in **Table 6**: anxiety (48%), depression/ seasonal affective disorder/ dysthymia (43%), fibromyalgia (39%), irritable bowel syndrome (38%), and migraine (37%) comprised the 5 most common chronic diagnoses. Past history of varicella zoster infection and symptomatic infectious mononucleosis episode occurred in 82% and 37% (70% noted Epstein-Barr mononucleosis and 17% cytomegalovirus), respectively, while 27% carried a diagnosis of an autoimmune condition. Cancer afflicted 8% but was not among the top 15 conditions. Only 14% cited any history of post-traumatic stress disorder (data not shown).

FAMILY MEDICAL HISTORY: FIRST DEGREE RELATIVES

Thirteen percent recounted at least one first-degree relative (FDR, e.g., blood-related father, mother, sibling, child) who was also diagnosed with ME/CFS and 21%, at least one FDR affected by "chronic fatigue of unclear etiology." In total, 27% of subjects came from families with FDRs affected by ME/CFS or "chronic fatigue of unclear etiology." Thirty-five percent of subjects also described at least one FDR afflicted by an autoimmune disorder.

MEDICATIONS

Table 7 shows the five most common categories of medications and specific medications taken by this cohort. Medications included prescription and over-the-counter drugs as well as herbal preparations, vitamins and other supplements. Approximately or slightly over 50% of our subjects took a medication regularly or occasionally to manage symptoms related to sleep, pain (not including migraine headaches), and endocrinological issues. Mood and gastrointestinal symptoms were also noteworthy with about one-third of subjects taking medication to cope with these categories of symptoms.

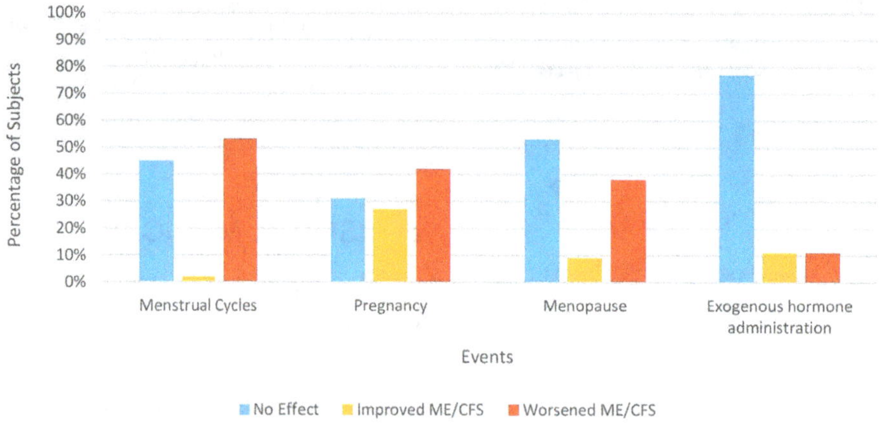

FIGURE 1 | Impact of hormonal events on ME/CFS in women. Only subjects identifying themselves as female were asked these items. 120 out of 121 women responded. The number answering for each event varies depending on both response rate and each woman's circumstances. "Exogenous hormone administration" refers to any form of reproductive hormones (e.g., pills, patch, implants, etc.) taken for contraception, relief of menopausal symptoms, or treatment of any medical condition.

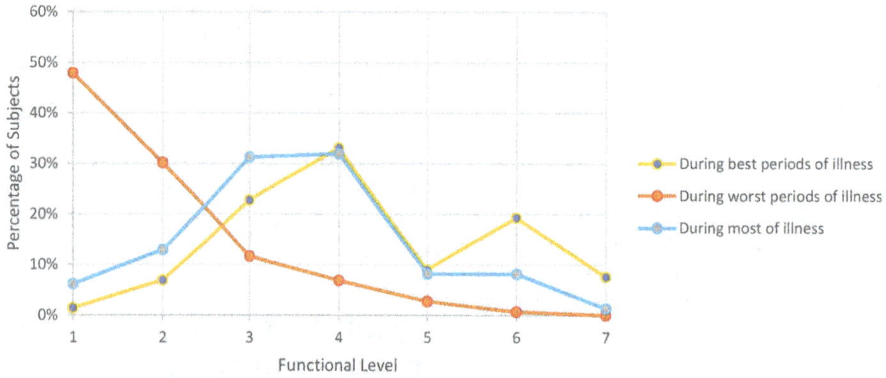

FIGURE 2 | Self-reported functional level during various periods of illness. Numbers 1–7 on x-axis correspond to the following functional levels: (1) I am not able to work, go to school, or do anything, and I am bedridden. (2) I can walk around the house, but I cannot do light housework. (3) I can do light housework, but I cannot work or go to school part-time. (4) I can only work part-time at work or school or on some family responsibilities. (5) I can work or go to school full time, but I have no energy left for anything else. (6) I can work or go to school full time and finish some family responsibilities but I have no energy left for anything else. (7) I can do all work, school, or family responsibilities without any problems with my energy.

The most prevalent specific medications matched those of the medication categories. Four of the top five medications addressed sleep (melatonin, zolpidem) or pain (ibuprofen, acetaminophen) while levothyroxine was prescribed presumably for hypothyroidism. Approximately a quarter of our subjects wrote in a medication other than those listed to treat their sleep and gut symptoms. However, no single written-in treatment was used by a significant number of subjects.

DISCUSSION

This is the first publication to give a broad epidemiologic overview of a US-based, ME/CFS cohort within one paper. While our findings concerning onset, course, function, co-morbid conditions, and personal as well as family medical history are consistent with those of prior studies, we hope to highlight under-examined aspects of this condition: (a) onset is most commonly gradual and precipitated by an infectious incident with stressful/major life events as the next most frequent precipitant; (b) problems with prolonged standing, alcohol consumption, and temperature regulation, which all may be related to circulatory impairment, are common; (c) while other symptoms may decline over time, cognitive symptoms tend to persist; (d) improvement in our cohort is rare but short, temporary remissions can occur in a minority of patients; (e) increasing age and illness duration do not necessarily portend worsening fatigue or function; (f) events associated with the female reproductive system can negatively impact ME/CFS in women; (g) patients with co-morbid medical or psychiatric conditions are the rule rather than the exception; and (h) ME/CFS, chronic fatigue of unclear etiology, and autoimmune conditions are common in family

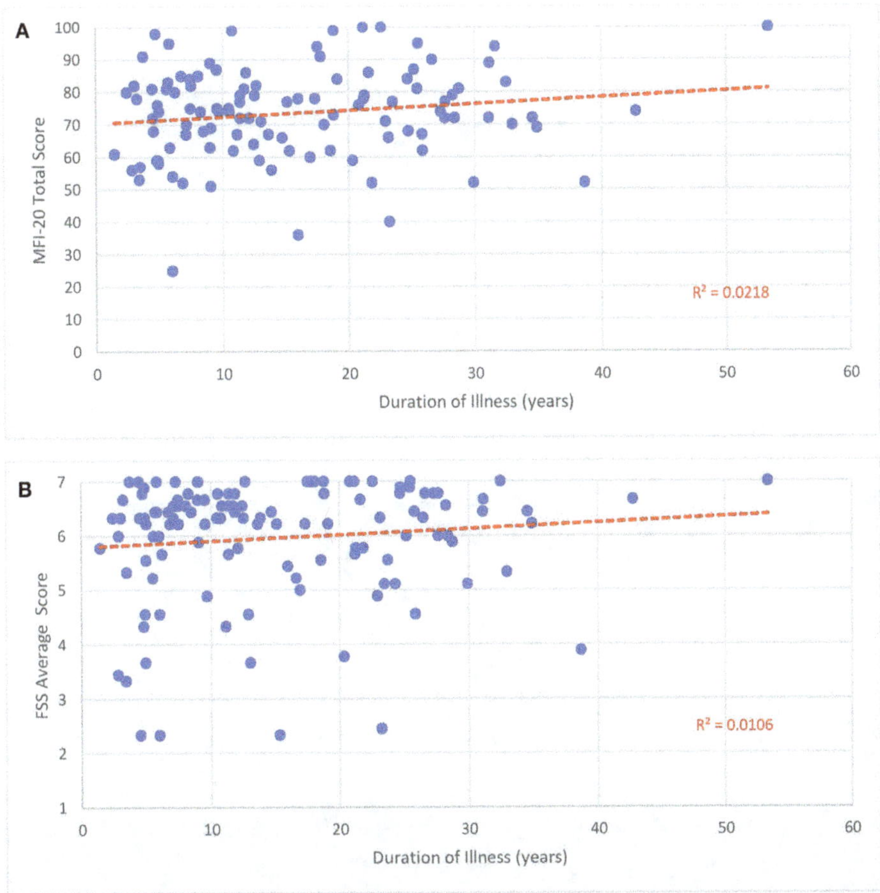

FIGURE 3 | Fatigue questionnaire scores vs. duration of illness. Each point represents one subject. **(A)** Total Multi-dimensional Fatigue Inventory-20 (MFI-20). **(B)** Average Fatigue Severity Scale (FSS) scores.

members. These findings have significant implications for the clinical care and research of patients affected by ME/CFS. We also supply information about medication usage for context.

A GRADUAL ONSET PRECEDED BY AN INFECTIOUS EVENT IS THE MOST COMMON PATTERN

The most common onset pattern was a distinct change in health heralded by an infectious event followed by a gradual progression to becoming consistently sick. Despite offering 14 possible precipitating factors and an open text box, almost two-thirds of our subjects selected only one or two factors. The top three factors were an infectious illness (64%), stress or a major life event (39%, e.g., occupational pressure, family illness, divorce), and exposure to an environmental/ chemical toxin (20%, with mold being the top answer written in) (**Table 1**). Stressful events were rarely chosen as the only precipitant though, endorsed only by 8% of our subjects, and appeared mostly in conjunction with infection or other precipitants. These results agree with prior studies: 49–93% of subjects reported an infection-like illness while 43–95% noted significant stress in the months or years preceding or surrounding the beginning of their illness (18, 41, 42, 52, 71–74). Becker (72) also found that 99% of their subjects chose only 1 or 2 factors and both he and Evans (52) showed <15% of subjects endorsed stress as the sole precipitant.

Since infectious events have been consistently found to be the foremost factor preceding ME/CFS retrospectively and prospective studies (14, 15) have confirm their progression to ME/CFS, this fact should be emphasized more in educational materials and case definitions. There are already two moves in this direction. The 2015 National Academy of Medicine criteria, also known as Systemic Exertion Intolerance Disease (SEID), incorporated failure to recover from infection as a secondary characteristic of ME/CFS (75) but perhaps this characteristic should be elevated to primary criteria. Lack of or incomplete recovery might provide a valuable clue in the diagnosis of ME/CFS for clinicians faced with a plethora of patients presenting with fatigue. Additionally, the National Institutes of Health have focused on post-infectious cases of ME/CFS in their intramural ME/CFS study (76) to try to decrease the heterogeneity of their research sample. Heterogeneity of study samples is widely acknowledged to be an obstacle for

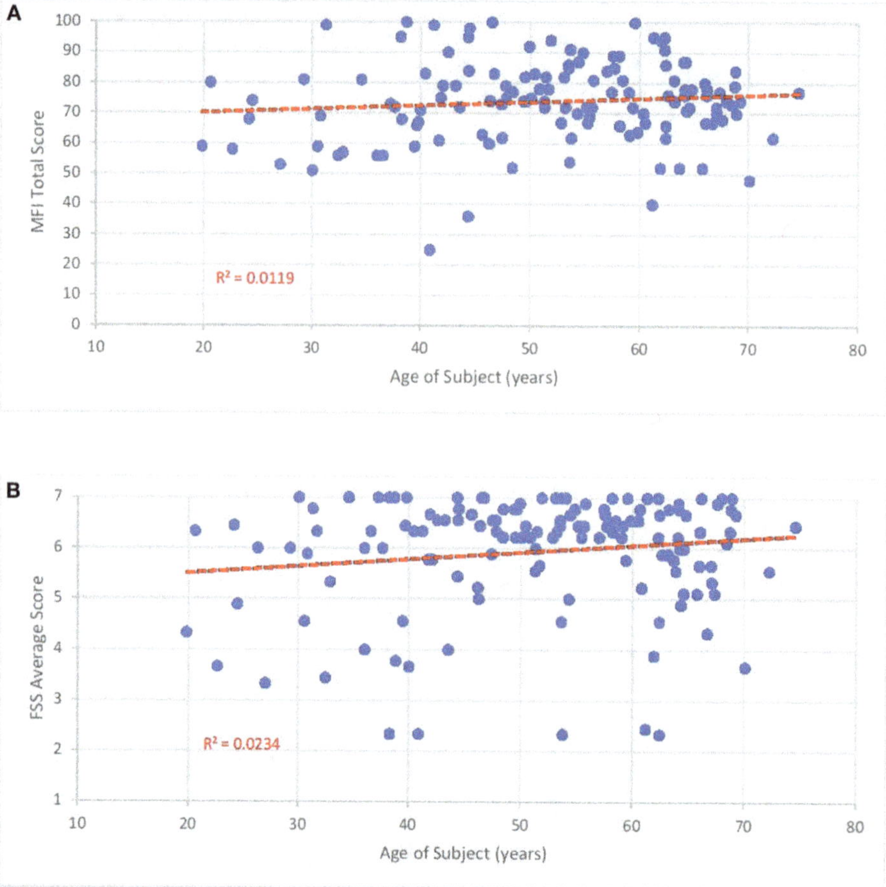

FIGURE 4 | Fatigue questionnaire scores vs. age of subject. Each point represents one subject. **(A)** Total Multi-dimensional Fatigue Inventory-20 (MFI-20). **(B)** Average Fatigue Severity Scale (FSS) scores.

ME/CFS studies (77). As shown in **Table 1**, we believe that other precipitating factors should be explored. Nevertheless, materials which do not emphasize a post-infectious onset (78) or suggest that all precipitating events are equally common or relevant (79) make it more difficult for clinicians and researchers to discern ME/CFS from other medical conditions or situations.

For a third of subjects each, their preceding infectious event manifested as respiratory symptoms (e.g. sore throat, rhinorrhea, cough, etc.) or constitutional symptoms (e.g., fever, chills, muscle aches, etc.) while 35% claimed that a specific infection was documented (**Table 2**). This is comparable to Ramsey's early accounts (80) and Becker's (72) study where upper respiratory infections (URIs) were noticed to be the chief infectious event, followed by "flu-like illness[es]," and, trailing far behind, gastrointestinal infections. In our survey, gastrointestinal (GI) infections were also rare, endorsed only by 10% of those with an infection peri-onset and 6% overall (out of 150 subjects). This might clue clinicians in to a diagnosis of ME/CFS even without a specific pinpointed microbe as certain types of infections (e.g., prostatitis, urinary tract infections, etc.) seem much less likely to progress to ME/CFS.

However, respiratory symptoms should not lead researchers to assume that the common causes of URIs (e.g., rhinoviruses, coronaviruses) are implicated in ME/CFS. In 1998, White (81) demonstrated that URIs are much less likely to cause ME/CFS than glandular fever. The pathogens which have been linked to ME/CFS are extraordinarily adept at evading the usual immune defenses through, for example, intracellular or latent states (e.g., Coxiella burnetii, herpes family viruses). Thirty-five percent of our subjects noted documentation of an acute infection, higher than the 23% Salit (71) found. Unfortunately, our survey did not ask respondents to elaborate which initial infections they were diagnosed with, a shortcoming we hope to rectify in the future. Knowledge of which pathogens contribute to the establishment of ME/CFS may stimulate new ideas about disease pathophysiology and treatment.

The frequent presence of stressful/ major life events surrounding ME/CFS onset does not automatically mean that ME/CFS is caused by or perpetuated by psychiatric or psychological factors. Some researchers have proposed or supported psychogenic or psychosomatically-infused theories of ME/CFS which have led to therapies like cognitive behavioral therapy (CBT) and graded exercise therapy (GET). These

TABLE 6 | Most common co-morbid medical and psychiatric conditions reported by our subjects with ME/CFS[a] compared to the general United States population and previously published prevalence among ME/CFS subjects.

Medical condition	Percentage (%) with medical condition ever diagnosed	Percentage (%) endorsing condition as active/unresolved	Prevalence of medical condition, ME/CFS subjects[d] in other studies (%)	Prevalence of medical condition, general US population[e] (%)
Anxiety	48	67	21–88	18
Depression, seasonal affective disorder, or dysthymia	43	63	17–47	7
Fibromyalgia	39	88	12–91	8
Irritable bowel syndrome	38	76	17–92	10–20
Symptomatic infectious mononucleosis[b]	37	1	39	30–50
Migraine headache	37	63	84	14.2
Any autoimmune condition[c]	27	66	13–27	4.5
Chronic sinusitis	33	71	66	8
Hay fever	30	86	33; 57	13–39
Hypothyroidism (non-Hashimoto's)	28	77	5–35	3.7
Peripheral neuropathy (for example, carpal tunnel syndrome)	28	86	N/A[f]	2.4
Multiple chemical sensitivity syndrome	27	87	4–72%	13%
Sleep apnea	26	65	4–46%	26%
Temporomandibular joint disorder (TMJ)	21	57	27–67%	15%
Postural orthostatic tachycardia syndrome (POTS)	20	83	13–81%	0.17%

[a] *Subjects were asked if they had ever been diagnosed by a healthcare professional with any of a list of 43 medical/ psychiatric conditions.*
[b] *Meaning presence of symptoms along with confirmatory bloodwork. Seventy percent stated their mononucleosis was due to Epstein-Barr virus while 16% noted cytomegalovirus-associated mononucleosis.*
[c] *The most common autoimmune illness was Hashimoto's thyroiditis with a prevalence of 15%. Others mentioned were vitiligo, celiac disease, psoriasis, ulcerative colitis, interstitial cystitis, Sjogren's syndrome, and multiple sclerosis.*
[d] *Prevalence figures for conditions cited are from the following references: anxiety (24, 39, 41, 51), depression (21, 24, 40, 41), fibromyalgia (19, 24, 26–28, 35, 39, 41, 51, 52), irritable bowel syndrome (19, 25–29, 52), symptomatic infectious mononucleosis (25), migraine headaches (53), autoimmune conditions (25, 40, 54), chronic sinusitis (55), hay fever (55), hypothyroidism (general) (24, 41, 55), multiple chemical sensitivities (19, 27, 35, 55), sleep apnea (41, 56), TMJ (27, 28, 51), POTS (35, 42, 52, 57, 58).*
[e] *Prevalence figures for conditions are cited from the following references: anxiety (59), depression (59), fibromyalgia (60), irritable bowel syndrome (61), symptomatic infectious mononucleosis (62), migraine headaches (63), autoimmune conditions (64), chronic sinusitis (65), hay fever (65), hypothyroidism (general) (66), peripheral neuropathy (67), multiple chemical sensitivities (68), sleep apnea (69), TMJ (70), POTS (58).*
[f] *No study found addressing this topic specifically.*

treatments are predicated on the hypothesis that patients are overly anxious or fearful about normal bodily sensations *per se* or minor discomfort related to deconditioning and thus limit their activities (82). Both treatments have been shown to not only be much less effective than initially alleged (83) but to actively cause harm to patients (84). Metabolic studies provide objective evidence that patients' bodies are unable to routinely meet energy demands (85).

Other mechanisms may be responsible for the recurring association between stressful/ major life events and ME/CFS. One theory is that stress decreases the immune system's ability to fight off and contain infections (86). Some ME/CFS patients are significantly helped by administration of antivirals (87, 88) while other studies suggest deficient control of infections (89, 90). Alternatively, peri-onset stressful events might act as the "straw that broke the camel's back," accelerating a pathological process which was already underway. A hallmark feature of ME/CFS is post-exertional malaise (PEM), a severe and often prolonged exacerbation of multiple symptoms (e.g., muscle pain, fatigue, problems thinking, sore throat) which is out-of-proportion to the physical, cognitive, emotional, or positional stressors triggering it (6, 44, 91). PEM can be triggered by activities of daily life (e.g., showering, cooking, reading, etc.) and is often deemed to be the most disabling ME/CFS symptom. Several studies provide evidence that ME/CFS patients' bodies react to these stressors abnormally. For example, compared to healthy people, the rise of serum cortisol and heart rate in response to, respectively, the stress of waking up (92) and aerobic exercise (93), are blunted in ME/CFS patients. Conversely, when the sympathetic nervous system involved in reacting to stress should be dampened, for example, during nighttime to facilitate sleep, its activity is instead elevated, possibly leading to another major ME/CFS symptoms, unrefreshing sleep (56, 94). Combining what is known about onset with these key symptoms suggests that a dysfunctional stress response system may play a major role in the pathophysiology of ME/CFS.

The stress response system in the human body depends on a complex interplay between the neurological, neuroendocrine,

TABLE 7 | Most common medication categories and specific medications[a] used by our subjects[b].

Reason for medication	Percentage using medication category/specific medication (%)
Sleep	62
Pain, inflammation, or muscle spasms (not including migraine)	52
Thyroid function, other endocrine/hormonal issues	46
Anxiety, depression, or general mental health	36
Digestive or gastrointestinal problems	35
SPECIFIC MEDICATION[c]	
Ibuprofen	25
Levothyroxine	20
Melatonin	19
Acetaminophen	17
Zolpidem	15

[a]*Subjects were initially asked if they took medications for a specific reason (e.g., sleep). Next, they were presented with a list of medications commonly used to treat that condition. A category labeled "other" accompanied by an open text box was also included. Subjects were encouraged to write in anything they took, including herbs, supplements, and over-the-counter medications.*

[b]*Out of 150 subjects total.*

[c]*27% and 24% of subjects chose the "Other" category, respectively, for sleep and gastrointestinal treatments. No one medication emerged as dominant. Examples of sleep treatments: over-the-counter pain/ cough medications containing antihistamines; herbal teas; magnesium; L-tryptophan. For gut symptoms: probiotics, prebiotics, digestive enzymes, sodium bicarbonate.*

and endocrine systems (95, 96). Components involved in the response system include the prefrontal cortex, amygdala, hypothalamus, pituitary gland, sympathetic and parasympathetic ganglia and nerves composing the autonomic nervous system, and adrenal glands. The theory behind CBT depends on defects at the beginning of this system, i.e., the cognitive appraisal and interpretation of challenges. Consequently, it is believed if patients can decrease their fear and anxiety around activity and symptoms then their ME/CFS will be largely resolved. However, problems with any downstream component of the stress response system could also lead to poor adaptation and similar consequences. Autoantibodies to both adrenergic and cholinergic muscarinic receptors (97, 98), part of the signaling pathways in the sympathetic and parasympathetic nervous systems, have been found in a subset of ME/CFS patients. They may account for some patients' bodies reacting inappropriately to stressors. Other individuals' symptoms might instead stem from other components, like the hypothalamus or adrenal glands. Different, dysfunctional components of the stress response system may potentially generate different clinical presentations while still preserving the hallmark feature of PEM.

The aforementioned concepts are not entirely new. In 1995, to explain why 95% of their ME/CFS subjects endorsed a stressful event at onset, Dobbins et al. (73) initially advanced stress as a causative factor or as a byproduct of recall bias but then also considered that "the perception of stress is [also possibly] correlated with some other variable related to the pathogenesis of CFS." These concepts are testable. By prospectively following adolescents stricken by Epstein-Barr mononucleosis, Katz et al. (99) have already demonstrated that autonomic dysfunction is predictive of ME/CFS several months later. Future studies could attempt to replicate Katz's study, especially in adults, after different types of infections known to be linked to ME/CFS, and in parallel with both subjective measures of challenges (whether physical, cognitive, emotional, or orthostatic) and objective measures of the stress response system (e.g., tilt table, serum cortisol levels, thermoregulatory sweat test, heart rate response to Valsalva maneuver).

Ideas about acuity and its link to infection should also be re-examined. Some past case definitions have included onset within a few hours or days as part of their criteria (100–102). In contrast, for the majority of our subjects, the first intimation of illness to full-blown ME/CFS often occurred over months if not years (**Table 3**). This is congruent with empirical data: while a few studies reported that around 60% and up to 91% of subjects disclose an "acute" onset (42, 52, 72), the majority of subjects (between 59 and 77%) in many studies describe a "gradual" onset. (37–39, 41, 103). Furthermore, many researchers do not define, are vague, are or inconsistent among themselves about what period of time (e.g., hours, days, weeks) is considered "acute." When interviewed in detail by Evans et al. subjects choosing a "sudden onset" described time periods ranging from a few hours to a few years and interpreted the term to mean remembering a discrete onset date, experiencing a severe onset, or having an infection around the time of ME/CFS onset (52).

We also found that there was no link between subject endorsement of an infectious precipitant and the time span of ME/CFS development. Some believe that an acute onset is necessarily infectious or an infectious onset is necessarily acute (50). Past studies examining this relationship are mixed, with some agreeing (52, 72) and others disagreeing with our result (104). Clinically, one infectious yet gradual onset sequence we have observed is a stuttering pattern whereby a subject experiences a severe infection, returns to near-normal functioning, but then experiences recurrent infections over months to years, recovering less each time, before succumbing entirely to ME/CFS. Overall, we agree with Evans that onset patterns are complicated and that simple categories do not capture this complexity. In the meantime, researchers should be careful about mandating an acute onset in order for an individual to be diagnosed with ME/CFS and should not make assumptions about the relationship between duration of onset and etiology. Future studies need to be more precise about what they are studying: if it is about time, define the time periods; if it is about infection, ask about infection. Accurate representation of onset is important as it might provide the key to the pathophysiology of ME/CFS.

FURTHER EXPLORATION OF OTHER POTENTIAL TRIGGERS IS NEEDED

Twenty percent of our subjects noted that an exposure to a chemical or environmental toxin might have a played an initiating role in their illness. Two independent Australian research groups published similar results: in Clark et al. (41), 16% endorsed "exposure to environmental toxins" while in Johnston et al. 6% reported "mold"; 11%,"toxic chemicals"; 6%, "poor[ly] recycled air"; and 4%, "heavy metals" (42). In contrast, in Friedberg's US-based study, 44% of subjects perceived "toxic exposure" to be a source of their illness (18). It is unclear why Friedberg's study yielded double the percentages we and the Australians found. None of these researchers commented further on these findings in their articles.

Since this survey was constructed as a broad overview, we did not take a comprehensive history of possible exposures. Additionally, because the published literature in this area is sparse and composed of mostly case studies [e.g., (105, 106)], it is difficult to know what specific substances to concentrate on. Written-in responses from our subjects may provide leads but were too imprecise and disparate to draw any solid conclusions. Subjects' answers might also be influenced by, for example, recall bias, misattribution, other patients' accounts, and media outlets.

Nevertheless, given how often this topic has come up, it is an area deserving of more attention. One initial approach might be to formally survey clinicians about what external, non-infectious triggers they believe to be important. Patients could be asked if anyone around them suffers from similar symptoms and if there are places where or times (of the day, week, or year) when they recurrently feel better. These traits have been suggestive of an environmental factor in other medical conditions. If patients respond affirmatively, clinicians should take a more detailed occupational, residential, and avocational history. Establishing a causal link between a particular agent and a disease is challenging. Definitive answers are often impossible to obtain although well-designed toxicological and epidemiological studies performed in parallel can reach sensible conclusions (107).

We encountered similar issues with replies to our items regarding travel. Patients have occasionally stated that they became ill during or shortly after a trip or that they have a history of widespread travel. Many wonder whether their excursions have any relationship to their illness. Responses collected in this survey were too diverse to generate concrete hypotheses. It is also plausible that the unpredictability and hassles of travel itself (i.e., stress) instead of subjects' destinations were conducive to illness onset.

ALCOHOL INTOLERANCE, THERMOREGULATION, AND DIFFICULTIES STANDING STILL ARE COMMON SYMPTOMS

Our subjects confirmed the high frequency of symptoms often considered important features of ME/CFS by clinicians but not included in the 1994 Fukuda CFS criteria. The prevalence of alcohol intolerance (66%), difficulties managing temperature extremes (87%), and issues with standing (81%) are as high or higher than some of the top 12 symptoms in our **Table 4**. Additionally, they are within the range of prevalence figures

TABLE 8 | Prevalence of self-reported alcohol intolerance, thermoregulatory issues, and difficulty standing still in this and other studies.

Symptom	Prevalence in subjects with ME/CFS (%)	Study author (references number)
Alcohol intolerance	66	This study
	45–75	Berne (108)
	60	De Becker (109)
	67	Woolley et al. (57)
	80	Bansal (110)
Problems adjusting to heat or cold	87	This study
	59	Chu et al. (16)
	75–80	Berne (108)
	54	De Becker et al. (109)
Difficulty with standing still[a]	81	This study
	81	Lapp et al. (111)
	95	Rowe et al. (112)
	90[b]	Robinson et al. (113)

[a] *Due to symptoms associated with orthostatic intolerance.*
[b] *Composite of symptoms including orthostatic intolerance.*

found previously (**Table 8**): 45–80% for alcohol intolerance (57, 108–110); 54–80% for temperature control issues (16, 108, 109); and 81–95% for problems with remaining immobile in an upright position (111–113). Bansal has suggested that since alcohol intolerance is present in 80% of his ME/CFS patients, its occurrence should increase the likelihood of an ME/CFS diagnosis if there are any doubts otherwise (110). Based on his finding that 81% of ME/CFS patients demonstrated abnormal tilt table testing results, Lapp proposed that all patients should be questioned about orthostatic intolerance (111). The symptom most predictive of an abnormal test was not fainting/ near-fainting but inability to stand in place without getting sick.

Dysfunction of the autonomic nervous system is one mechanism which may account for all three non-Fukuda symptoms. Without appropriate vasoconstriction and vasodilation of blood vessels by the autonomic nervous system, consistent blood pressure and body temperature may not be maintained, resulting in postural and thermoregulatory issues (114). Alcohol not only increases fatigue and disturbs cognition but also has been shown to exacerbate orthostatic intolerance (115), compatible with why some patients affected by ME/CFS would endorse problems with alcohol intake.

Currently, OI is already one of five symptoms highlighted by the NAM (6, 75) but intolerance to climatic shift is not. Both symptoms are included in the CCC (49) and ME-ICC (50) but buried in a long list of other symptoms and are optional. Emphasizing these symptoms would not be a new undertaking but actually a return to Dr. Melvin Ramsey's original conception of ME where "circulatory impairment" manifested as "hypersensitivity to climatic change," insufficient responses to stress, and "dysfunction of the autonomic nervous system" (80) are repeatedly mentioned. These symptoms could be especially selected for when recruiting subjects so that they may be investigated further.

DISEASE COURSE

Over time, while individual symptoms or the disease overall might fluctuate and even remit temporarily, almost all of our subjects continued to be sick and disabled. During the first 6 months of the illness (**Table 4**), the most common symptoms were fatigue-, exertion-, sleep-, pain-, cognition- and flu-related, with over 70% of subjects endorsing these symptoms. Similarly, Evans found that exhaustion (57%), cognition (43%), headaches, pain, and sleep were the top symptoms at onset (52). As months and years passed, most symptoms remained among the top 12 most common symptoms even as the percentage of subjects experiencing any symptom declined. Feeling fatigued and unrefreshed after a night's sleep retained their ranking as the most and second most common symptoms. Because the declines associated with troubles paying attention, finding the right word and remembering things were relatively small (between 4 and 10%) compared with those of flu-like symptoms, dead/heavy feelings post-exercise, and muscle pain/ aches (between 17 and 25%), these cognitive symptoms rose in their ranking while the latter three fell off the most common dozen symptoms. Similarly, because of their low declines in prevalence (between 1 and 10%), three other cognitive symptoms (absentmindedness, inability to multi-task, and sensitivity to noise) joined the top 12 symptoms by the time of the survey.

Our results agree with two published studies examining symptoms in subjects who remained sick for over a decade. Sore throat and lymph nodes tenderness tended to improve the most over a mean of 15.4 years of illness (24). On the other hand, Friedberg noted that the third, fourth, and fifth most common symptoms in subjects sick for a median of 18 years were "forgetfulness," "distractibility by noise," and "concentration difficulty" (18). Additionally, when Friedberg analyzed which symptoms were significantly more frequent in these long-term subjects vs. his short-term subjects (median length of illness = 3 years), four out of the top five symptoms were cognitive symptoms. After a median of 12.5 years of sickness, we observed remarkably similar shifts in our study sample. Inability to multi-task rose from being the 22nd most common symptom to 8th most common; forgetfulness from 19th to 10th; and nose sensitivity from 15 to 12th. In contrast, Jason (19) found little change in prevalence when comparing Fukuda-associated symptoms assessed at two time points separated by a decade. Discrepancies in findings might be traced back to the cross-sectional vs. longitudinal design of studies, how subjects were selected, whether symptoms were inquired prospectively or retrospectively, varying follow-up times and the stage of subjects' illness when they were questioned. Ideally, research investigating evolution of symptoms should be prospective, longitudinal, and endure beyond a few years.

The reasons why symptoms fluctuated differed according to the individual symptom. Patients recounted that fatigue, post-exertional malaise, and unrefreshing sleep appear to be improved by treatment whereas flu-like symptoms abated spontaneously. This latter claim is supported by Lipkin et al. (116), who found that subjects ill for <3 years demonstrated more robust pro- and anti-inflammatory activity relative to subjects who had been ill longer. We did not ask patients specifically which treatments helped the most but use of a behavioral technique called pacing along with sleep medication are often deemed to be helpful among patients (16, 117). The stubborn presence of cognitive symptoms is concerning. Clinical trials targeting the cognitive symptoms of ME/CFS or including neurocognitive outcome measures are rare: both deficiencies need to be remedied.

The dominance of infections and stressful/ major life events as significant modifiers of disease course underscores the importance of these two factors (**Table 5**). The third most common answer, "None of the above," was selected by a quarter of subjects and all other choices were selected by 11% or less of subjects. Intervening medical events (e.g., surgery, accidents, cardiac and neurologic disease) also, unsurprisingly, impacted the overall course of the disease. This result concurs with March et al. and others (24, 117, 118) who have shown that additional co-morbidities tended to worsen ME/CFS symptoms and function. The lack of long-term longitudinal studies means there is very little information about what issues or events influence disease course. Finding out more about this area may aid in understanding ME/CFS and bring up opportunities for secondary prevention (e.g., decrease functional decline). For example, Dr. Charles Lapp (119) has written previously on steps clinicians can take to prepare patients for and minimize the effects of surgery.

Surprisingly, about one-tenth of our subjects experienced complete cessation of their symptoms during their illness course even as their ME/CFS eventually recurred. Similarly, over a short follow-up period of 3 years, Nisenbaum et al. (21) found that about 10% of their subjects sustained "total" remission of at least a year's time. However, since remission was defined by operational criteria rather than direct questioning of their subjects, the authors believed that actual remission rates might be lower. In March's study (24) of long-term ME/CFS subjects, the prevalence of any remission was higher at 30% but they did not specific for how long symptoms were absent. While our median length of remission was 7 months, one subject noted normal health for a decade. This is not without precedent: online anecdotes (120, 121) support long intervening periods of good health between episodes of ME/CFS. These findings accentuate the importance of appropriate control subjects and extended follow-up times. Temporary disappearance of ME/CFS symptoms may confound the interpretation of interventional, longitudinal, and prognostic studies. With a few exceptions, most studies have lasted for <5 years when it is extremely common for study subjects to have been sick for more than a decade. Control subjects and protracted monitoring would help distinguish transient variations from long-term, lasting improvement.

Since the GEISD study was not set up to particularly assess prognosis, we cannot calculate a rate of recovery but the unrelenting illness course of our subjects is consistent with other studies. Only 4% of our subjects felt their medical condition was improving over time with 50% endorsing a fluctuating course. A

2013 survey (16) of 551 subjects found only 1.1% felt they were improving while 54.4% designated their course as "fluctuating/ remitting/ relapsing" and 27%, as "worsening." Out of 14 subjects she interviewed in-depth, Evans et al. (52) found only 1 (7%) expressing continual improvement while Underhill's rate was 5% (35). These data comport with the low median recovery rate of 5% Cairns (12) found in their 2005 systematic review of prognosis. In individual studies, higher rates of recovery, up to 66%, have been documented but Friedberg et al. (122) as well as Jason (123) have questioned the validity of such figures since recovery definitions have tended to be limited, narrow, and/or unidimensional.

EVENTS ASSOCIATED WITH THE FEMALE REPRODUCTIVE SYSTEM AFFECT ME/CFS

Considering that ~75% of people affected are women (16, 40, 41, 43, 104, 124–126) and that onset often occurs during their reproductive years, i.e., between the ages of 10–40 (16, 23, 39–42), exceptionally few studies have evaluated the impact of female reproductive events on ME/CFS. During casual conversations or in the clinic, patients will occasionally relate that their ME/CFS began during or shortly after pregnancy. In one study of stressful events surrounding onset, women who were pregnant in the previous year were found to be 31.7 times more likely (126) to become ill with ME/CFS compared to women who had not been pregnant. A small but detectable 8% of our subjects (**Table 1**) connected their illness onset to pregnancy, within the range of 3.5–10% identifying this as an initiating event in earlier studies [18. 52]. When the more ambiguous category "hormonal events" was used instead, this percentage rose slightly to 12% (18, 41).

Although women have discussed amongst themselves premenstrual aggravation of their ME/CFS symptoms for many years, only one other study besides ours has formally surveyed patients. Sixty-seven percent of Clark et al.'s (41) subjects reported worsening of ME/CFS before their periods, close to our figure of 53% (**Figure 1**). Likewise, there have been scant studies of ME/CFS symptoms during pregnancy. Schacterle (127) showed that approximately equivalent percentages of patients reported no change, deterioration, or a boost in their health status (41, 30, 29%, respectively) during pregnancy, convergent with our figures of 31, 27, and 42%. Conversely, 86% of one Australian cohort (41) reported deterioration while the impression of several US-based ME/CFS specialists (128) was that ME/CFS symptoms tended to attenuate during pregnancy, to the point of remission. One reason for these diverse conclusions might be that ME/CFS symptoms vary depending on the stage of the pregnancy (e.g., first trimester, second trimester, etc.). Without explicit questioning, some subjects might be communicating their average health status during pregnancy while others might inadvertently be focusing on one time period to the exclusion of others.

Despite the highest prevalence of ME/CFS being recorded in the 40–50 age range (124, 129), no other study has asked about the impact of menopause on symptoms. Menopausal symptoms such as increased fatigue, hot flashes, insomnia, and forgetfulness overlap with those of ME/CFS. This fact combined with the 38% of our peri- and post-menopausal subjects (**Figure 1**) who felt that menopause exacerbated their ME/CFS should prompt further research. Are amplified symptoms during this life phase due primarily to the expected changes of menopause, hormonal adjustments on ME/CFS, or a combination of the two? Should ME/CFS be a consideration when women decide whether and for how long to partake of hormone replacement therapy? In contrast, over three-quarters of women expressed no changes in symptoms while taking exogenous female hormones, whether for birth control, menopause, or other medical conditions. Only eleven percent of our subjects and 7–9% of Friedberg's (18) subjects noted worsening or onset, respectively, with hormonal medications.

Investigating these topics can shed light on the pathophysiology of the disease, answer women's questions about ME/CFS during different stages of their lives, and even result in new treatments. The oscillation of symptoms with these short-term and even repetitive events can provide a naturalistic model for understanding the relationship between biological indices and clinical characteristics. Remissions and flares of various autoimmune diseases during pregnancy have been linked, respectively, to a TH1 or TH2-dominant immunological status (130). Equipped with more knowledge, healthcare professionals can better assist women to make informed decisions about pregnancy and to prepare for menstrual cycles and menopause. New treatment options might even be introduced. For example, anecdotal evidence (131, 132) suggests that some women may be able to moderate their premenstrual intensification of ME/CFS symptoms with judicious use of birth control pills or patches. These management techniques need to be tested in formal clinical trials.

FUNCTION IS LOW BUT APPEARS STABLE OVER TIME

The high rate of unemployment we observed (47%) is in line with the 40–81% rate noted in other studies (7, 16, 21, 23, 24, 39, 41–43, 133). Commencement of ME/CFS decimated the pre-illness employment rate by at least 40% in Japan (43), Australia (41), and the United Kingdom (133). Moreover, surveys rarely asked those still employed if they were able to retain their prior hours, duties, position, salary, or even field: in the Japanese study, only 2% of respondents did not have to modify their occupation whereas both Tiersky (20) and Kingdon (133) found much reduced work hours. Functional levels echoed those of a 2013 survey of over 550 subjects (16): even during their best periods, most subjects could barely attend to school, work, or family responsibilities part-time (but not all three) and during their worst periods, over half were bedridden and unable to participate in any activities (**Figure 2**).

These low functional levels are supported by the high mean FSS and MFI-20 scores [respectively, 5.9 ± 1.1 (out of 7) and, for example, MFI General Fatigue (GF) subscale 17.2 ± 3.0 (maximum of 20)], which reflect those of prior studies (134–137), are occasionally double the score of healthy controls, and even exceed the mean values of subjects afflicted by depression, stroke, multiple sclerosis, myocardial infarct, systemic sclerosis, and human immunodeficiency virus (134, 136–140). Of the studies examined for comparison, only patients affected by fibromyalgia/ chronic widespread pain (138) or enrolled in palliative care programs for cancer (140) exhibited mean MFI-20 GF scores (respectively, 16 ± 3.2 and 17 ± 3.0) approaching those of ME/CFS subjects.

Despite how severely ME/CFS impaired our subjects, it may be reassuring to clinicians and patients that functional status does not seem to drop with the passage of time. As shown in **Figures 3, 4**, no relationship was observed between either measure of fatigue and age of subjects or duration of illness. These results agree with studies monitoring Short Form 36 physical function (SF-36 PF) subscale trends across time. In a cross-sectional survey of ~500 subjects, Chu et al. (141) found low, non-significant Pearson correlation coefficients of 0.025 and 0.019 when SF-36 PF scores were plotted against age and duration of illness. In fact, Komaroff (142) found slight improvements in SF-36 PF when following one cohort of 99 subjects over a decade and both Tiersky (20) and Kidd (125) mentioned that long-suffering subjects might develop better psychological coping techniques. One study (143) did indicate increased fatigue, autonomic symptoms and depression in older subjects relative to younger ones but it is unclear how this study's conclusion might apply to the question at hand since they emanate from a sample who did not develop ME/CFS until they were 55 years of age or older, 15–20 years beyond the mean age of ME/CFS onset. Indeed, the authors speculated that ME/CFS beginning in later stages of life might be very different from earlier-onset ME/CFS.

Our results should be interpreted with caution since a) they derive from a cross-sectional instead of longitudinal cohort and b) the FSS is subject to ceiling effects (144). Since cross-sectional designs are based on different subjects, it might not be accurate to extrapolate future function from one individual to another. Because two-thirds of our subjects displayed an average score of 6 or higher on the FSS when 7 is the maximum score, the FSS might not have the capacity to represent or distinguish between more intense levels of fatigue.

MULTIPLE CO-MORBID CONDITIONS ARE THE RULE RATHER THAN THE EXCEPTION

ME/CFS is often accompanied by other co-morbid and psychiatric conditions. Out of 43 listed conditions, almost all our subjects (97%) had been diagnosed with at least one medical condition while 64% revealed at least one psychiatric condition. The mean number of conditions affecting subjects was high, 7.0 ± 4.2. Previously, in separate studies, 80–95% of subjects have declared at least one other condition while 38–90% cited at least one psychiatric condition (19, 24, 28, 29, 39, 51, 52, 105). In Bateman et al.'s study (29), out of 17 conditions listed, women subjects suffered a mean of 2.7 ± 2.1 conditions and men, 3.6 ± 2.1 conditions.

Our 5 most common conditions (anxiety, depression, fibromyalgia, irritable bowel syndrome, and migraine, from most to least common) (**Table 6**) match 3 of the top 5 condition in Bateman's cohort (fibromyalgia, depression, anxiety, low testosterone, hypothyroidism) (29). We did not ask about low testosterone, which existed in 36.4% of their male subjects, and hypothyroidism was our ninth most common condition albeit our prevalence of 28% is close to their 35%. Their survey did not query about irritable bowel syndrome or migraine headaches.

Our prevalences for individual conditions are generally concordant with those documented in previous ME/CFS studies (**Table 6**). The exceptions in this comparison are migraine headaches (37% in our study vs. 84%) (53) and chronic sinusitis (33 vs. 66%) (55). As there is meager data on these two conditions in ME/CFS however, these comparisons should not be taken as the final word. In contrast, except for sleep apnea and symptomatic infectious mononucleosis, all 12 of the most common conditions in our study surpassed their prevalence in the general United States population [**Table 6**, (58–70)]. The similar prevalence of mononucleosis in our subjects compared to the general population [37 vs. 30–50%, (62)] suggests that mere symptomatic infection does not elevate the risk of ME/CFS but rather the severity or aftermath of the infection may be the determining factor for whether ME/CFS manifests. Intriguingly, our prevalence of cancer (8%) is approximately double that of the prevalence in the general population [4.1%, ages 50–59, 14-yr. limited prevalence, (145)], whereas Bateman's cohort had quadruple the prevalence at 16% (29). These results, along with studies showing an increased risk of lymphoma among elderly ME/CFS subjects (146) and an early mean age of death due to cancer (147), warrant further investigation.

Our data underscore the importance of the National Academy of Medicine criteria (6) moving away from ME/CFS being primarily a diagnosis of exclusion and allowing the concurrence of what some clinicians and researchers might have interpreted to be absolute exclusionary diagnoses (e.g., major depression, obstructive sleep apnea, hypothyroidism). Given the ubiquity of co-morbid conditions, many ME/CFS patients might never be diagnosed with or would have lost their ME/CFS diagnosis had the NAM criteria continued to designate exclusionary criteria. Some people (148) have expressed concerns about how the new criteria might unintentionally attract subjects to studies who are actually affected by another diagnosis or have a potentially confounding condition (e.g., major depressive disorder). However, depending on a study's purpose, researchers can always institute additional exclusionary criteria beyond the NAM criteria or alternatively, subgroup or statistically adjust for co-morbid conditions. The internal and external validity of a study must also be balanced (149): strict exclusionary criteria might permit more solid conclusions to be made but the results might not have much applicability for the average ME/CFS patient (150).

Given their unresolved/ active state, the most common co-morbid diagnoses should be actively screened for by healthcare professionals. Treatment options for ME/CFS itself are limited but many of these conditions have standardized, effective treatments. Their improvement can positively influence patients' health, function, and quality of life even as they remain ill with ME/CFS (117, 118). Finally, studying co-morbid conditions might also help provide answers to the pathophysiology of ME/CFS. For example, the high prevalence of autoimmune co-morbid conditions supports the hypothesis that ME/CFS might be an autoimmune condition for at least some subgroups or that the immune system possibly plays a major role in disease pathophysiology. On the other hand, the unexpected high prevalence of migraines reinforces the idea of ME/CFS being a condition of poor autonomic dysfunction. Some (151) have postulated that imbalance of the sympathetic and parasympathetic arms and changes in cranial blood vessel dilation are two of the many steps leading to a migraine headache.

Aside from natural variation in study samples, the wide range of prevalence for the same co-morbid condition could be due to issues like which conditions clinicians were alert to, how study subjects were asked about medical conditions, the accuracy of subject recall, and how subjects were assessed for a co-morbidity. For example, March did not ask about co-morbid conditions overall but only about conditions after onset of ME/CFS. Conditions which are less recognized by clinicians will also be less likely to be diagnosed: this might account for why only 13–40% of subjects stated they were diagnosed with POTS (**Table 6**) whereas unfiltered screening of all ME/CFS patients in Lapp's study (111) yielded an 81% prevalence of POTS.

ME/CFS, CHRONIC FATIGUE OF UNCLEAR ETIOLOGY, AND AUTOIMMUNE DISEASE ARE COMMON IN FIRST-DEGREE RELATIVES

The pervasiveness of ME/CFS, chronic fatigue of unclear etiology, and autoimmune disease in the FDRs of subjects may yield clues to the genetic basis and pathophysiology of the disease. Thirteen percent of our subjects imparted that they had at least one FDR affected by ME/CFS. Because ME/CFS is known to be widely underdiagnosed (152–154), we also asked whether any FDRs sustained chronic fatigue without a specific diagnosis. When this category was added, 21% of our subjects replied affirmatively and the percentage of subjects who did or might have a relative afflicted by ME/CFS rose to 27%. Our results are consistent with Pheby (34), who found that 12.1% of his subjects had at least one FDR affected, and the 5.3–18.3% of subjects noted in multiple studies (30, 32, 35, 36, 41, 155) to have at least one other blood-related family member, regardless of degree, affected. In two studies asking about both ME/CFS and chronic fatigue of unclear etiology in family members, 25% (31) and 46% (35) replied affirmatively.

ME/CFS has also been shown to be present in second- and third-degree relatives (33, 35) in a dose-response matter, i.e., the more genetic distance between the ME/CFS patient and a relative, the lower the risk. Since second- and third-degree relatives are less likely to share the same household or lifestyle factors as FDRs, this pattern strengthens the argument that there might be a shared genetic rather than environmental factor increasing the risk of disease. Astonishingly, hardly any studies have examined families where multiple members are sick with ME/CFS. More than 2 decades ago, Levine (156) showed a gradient of natural killer cell activity with family members affected by ME/CFS having the lowest values, followed by those unaffected but related, and finally, un-related friends of the family having the highest and normal values. By evaluating such family pedigrees, especially in conjunction with genetic or other biomarkers, we might better comprehend the risk factors behind and the mechanisms of ME/CFS.

About one-third of our subjects suffered from an autoimmune condition (**Table 6**) and a similar percentage had an FDR with an autoimmune condition. These figures are congruent with prior research: autoimmune conditions were noted in 15–27% (40, 54) of ME/CFS patients and in 18–47% (40, 54, 155) of their family members. Autoimmune thyroid disease was the most common co-morbid diagnosis while a variety of conditions, including rheumatoid arthritis, psoriasis, lupus, and Sjogren's syndrome, were observed among family members.

The commonality of autoimmune conditions within patients and among their family members is compatible with some researchers' theories (157, 158) that ME/CFS might have an autoimmune basis. It is well-known that individuals with one autoimmune disease are more likely to be affected by another autoimmune disease (159). The same but also diverse autoimmune diseases might affect families; the former phenomenon is labeled as a "familial autoimmune disease" while the latter is known as "familial autoimmunity" (160). Furthermore, many of the traits displayed by ME/CFS fit Rose and Witebsky's circumstantial criteria (161, 162) for determining when a condition qualifies as an autoimmune condition. For example, ME/CFS is more common in women, runs in families, can be triggered by infections, can be alleviated by immunosuppressants and is associated with autoantibodies [e.g., to adrenergic and cholinergic receptors (97, 98)]. Fluge et al. (163) also demonstrated *in vitro* that serum transferred from patients' bodies adversely affected the function of healthy, cultured muscle cells. This serves as a more direct piece of evidence for autoimmunity. Rose and Witebsky's criteria could operate as a guideline for future studies to prove or disprove the role of autoimmunity in ME/CFS. For example, to test maternal transfer of autoantibodies, infants of ME/CFS patients could have their blood tested for ME/CFS-specific autoantibodies and be followed serologically and clinically for ME/CFS symptoms. Four percent of our subjects and 6% of Jason's (164) admit to being sick as long as they can remember. Another project might devise animal models capable of developing ME/CFS: if exposure to patient serum or a putative antigen replicates the illness in these animals, that would corroborate the autoimmune foundations of ME/CFS.

MEDICATIONS

Unsurprisingly, the most common specific medications and categories of medications used (**Table 7**) correspond to well-known ME/CFS symptoms (sleep, muscle/ joint pain, headaches) and co-morbid conditions (mood disorders, fibromyalgia, irritable bowel syndrome, hypothyroidism). Our findings are similar to the medication survey which Reeves et al. (165) conducted in 2003. Their top six medication categories were pain relievers (88%), hormones (52%), antidepressants (41%), allergy-related drugs (32%), gastrointestinal therapies (30%), and cold medications (25%). Sixty-two percent of their subjects took supplements and vitamins.

Reeves did not ask subjects why they used specific medications and attributed allergy-related/ cold medications to the alleviation of sore throats, which are part of ME/CFS. While it also possible subjects are taking these medications for hay fever or sinusitis (see **Table 6**), subjects may also be consuming antihistamines to assist with sleep. (Reeves et al. classified antihistamines as both allergy and cold medications.) This claim is reinforced by patient comments from a survey conducted for a US Food and Drug Administration workshop in 2013 (16).

The pervasiveness of over-the-counter medications, herbal preparations, and supplements underscores the need for research directed at symptom control. For example, Gotts et al. have mentioned targeting the different phenotypes of sleep issues in ME/CFS with different medications (166). Subjects also expressed that side effects or hypersensitivity to customary doses of medications restricted what they could use. Effective management of symptoms can help patients greatly while progress is being made toward a disease-modifying treatment.

STRENGTHS AND LIMITATIONS

The major strength of this study lies in its use of a collaboratively-designed survey covering a broad range of topics relevant to clinicians, researchers, and patients. Consequently, except for a few items, the overall amount of missing data was small. Because data were collected from a single cohort, we were able to make connections between different areas (e.g., onset time and infectious onset) and confirm that, despite claims that ME/CFS is a heterogenous disease, separate aspects of epidemiological information collected from many cohorts based in different locations and at different times are in concordance with the data captured from one cohort. Our results also contribute to the paucity of data on the evolution of symptoms longitudinally and the impact of female reproductive events on ME/CFS.

Limitations of this study include the study sample recruited, reliance on subject self-report, recall bias, and relative superficiality of some survey items. Although we tried to recruit subjects from a diverse range of sources, our study population still consisted primarily of middle-aged, self-identified Caucasian women who had been sick for over a decade. Most ME/CFS studies end up with a similar sample. Therefore, the results of our study may be less applicable to younger, male, non-Caucasian, and recently afflicted patients. During the recruitment stage of this study, in 2012, the prevailing research case definition was the Fukuda 1994 criteria. In 2017, the US National Institutes of Health announced that either the CCC or NAM criteria should be used instead (167). Despite this study's use of the Fukuda 1994 criteria, we believe that our results will also apply to subjects fitting CCC or NAM criteria: at least 71 and 72% of our subjects qualified, respectively, for these criteria.

Because items answers were based on subject self-report instead of medical records or clinical examinations, some portions of the survey (e.g., peri-onset factors, comorbid conditions) might be less accurate than others. Moreover, since our subjects had been sick a median of 12.5 years, forgetfulness on the one hand or recall bias on the other might affect answers concerning onset or course. However, research on memory shows that events of great importance to a person are much more likely to be remembered accurately (52, 155, 168) than otherwise. For many patients, ME/CFS is a life-changing event so patients often pay extra attention to their condition. In fact, some patients keep extensive notes and even computerized worksheets documenting their symptoms, treatments, and other factors. The agreement between much of what our subjects describe and what other studies found also testifies to memory issues perhaps being less of a concern. Finally, since we attempted to ask about a broad range of subjects, we had to cut down on details to obtain a high survey response rate.

To overcome or reduce these limitations in the future, research should attempt to recruit subjects from various settings (e.g., from the community, primary and specialty clinics), employ the CCC and/or NAM criteria during subject recruitment, gather information prospectively rather than retrospectively, and complement subject-reported accounts with third-party reports (e.g., medical records) and/or objective measures where possible. Areas which would have benefitted from greater detail include which documented infections preceded ME/CFS, what treatments specifically helped with which symptoms, and how ME/CFS symptoms might vary depending on which stage of pregnancy, menstrual cycle, or menopause a woman is occupying.

CONCLUSION

This paper gives a broad epidemiologic overview of one ME/CFS cohort in the United States. While our findings concerning onset, course, function, co-morbid conditions, and family history support those of prior studies, by examining these topics together, we were able to interpret our findings within the complicated context of this condition and offer unique insights into how epidemiologic data can be utilized to inform both clinical care and improve future research. We also contribute new information about how ME/CFS symptoms change longitudinally and with events associated with the female reproductive system throughout a woman's life. Finally, we advance hypotheses centered around the human stress response system, autonomic nervous system, and autoimmune mechanisms to explain the similar yet heterogenous elements of ME/CFS.

In the future, we hope to investigate the relationship between clinical characteristics identified in this study and biomarkers, how epidemiological features may vary contingent on different

researchers will verify the findings in this paper and probe further into the areas and issues we have identified.
case definitions, and the influence of human leukocyte antigens on ME/CFS initiation and perpetuation. We also hope that other

ETHICS STATEMENT

This study was carried out in accordance with the recommendations of United States Federal Policy for the Protection of Human Subjects (known as the Common Rule, 45 CFR part 46) and the Belmont Report with written informed consent from all subjects. All subjects gave written informed consent in accordance with the Declaration of Helsinki. The protocol was approved by the Stanford University Institutional Review Board (Review Panel 3, Protocol 24244).

AUTHOR CONTRIBUTIONS

LC, IV, and JM conceived and designed the study, JM obtained funding and supervised the study. JM and IV recruited subjects and collected data. LC and DG analyzed the data and performed the statistical analyses. LC wrote the first draft of the manuscript. All authors contributed to manuscript revision, read, and approved the submitted version.

ACKNOWLEDGMENTS

We would like to acknowledge the precious time and energy our subjects put forth in completing our extensive survey. For some subjects, the cognitive effort might have exacerbated their ME/CFS symptoms so we are grateful for their sacrifice in helping advance understanding of this medical condition.

REFERENCES

1. Johnston S, Brenu EW, Staines D, Marshall-Gradisnik S. The prevalence of chronic fatigue syndrome/ myalgic encephalomyelitis: a meta-analysis. *Clin Epidemiol.* (2013) 5:105–10. doi: 10.2147/CLEP.S39876
2. National Academy of Medicine. *Myalgic Encephalomyelitis/Chronic Fatigue Syndrome (ME/CFS) Key Facts.* National Academy of Sciences, Engineering, Medicine (2015). Available online at: https://www.nap.edu/resource/19012/MECFS_KeyFacts.pdf (Accessed August 20, 2018).
3. Jason LA, Porter N, Brown M, Anderson V, Brown A, Hunnell J, et al. CFS: a review of epidemiology and natural history studies. *Bull IACFS ME* (2009) 17:88–106.
4. Bakken IJ, Tveito K, Gunnes N, Ghaderi S, Stoltenberg C, Trogstad L, et al. Two age peaks in the incidence of chronic fatigue syndrome/myalgic encephalomyelitis: a population-based registry study from Norway 2008-2012. *BMC Med.* (2014) 12:167. doi: 10.1186/s12916-014-0167-5
5. Fukuda K, Straus SE, Hickie I, Sharpe MC, Dobbins JG, Komaroff A. The chronic fatigue syndrome: a comprehensive approach to its definition and study. International Chronic Fatigue Syndrome Study Group. *Ann Intern Med.* (1994) 121:953–9. doi: 10.7326/0003-4819-121-12-199412150-00009
6. Institute of Medicine (U.S.), Institute of Medicine (U.S.), editors. *Beyond Myalgic Encephalomyelitis/Chronic Fatigue Syndrome: Redefining an Illness* Washington, DC: The National Academies Press (2015).
7. Klimas N, Patarca-Montero R. *Disability and Chronic Fatigue Syndrome: Clinical, Legal, and Patient Perspectives.* 1st ed. Binghamton, NY: Routledge (1998). 124 p.
8. Pendergrast T, Brown A, Sunnquist M, Jantke R, Newton JL, Strand EB, et al. Housebound versus nonhousebound patients with myalgic encephalomyelitis and chronic fatigue syndrome. *Chronic Illn.* (2016) 12:292–307. doi: 10.1177/1742395316644770
9. Komaroff AL, Fagioli LR, Doolittle TH, Gandek B, Gleit MA, Guerriero RT, et al. Health status in patients with chronic fatigue syndrome and in general population and disease comparison groups. *Am J Med.* (1996) 101:281–90. doi: 10.1016/S0002-9343(96)00174-X
10. Falk Hvidberg M, Brinth LS, Olesen AV, Petersen KD, Ehlers L. The health-related quality of life for patients with myalgic encephalomyelitis / chronic fatigue syndrome (ME/CFS). *PLoS ONE* (2015) 10:e0132421. doi: 10.1371/journal.pone.0132421
11. Núñez M, Núñez E, del Val JL, Fernández-Huerta JM, Alegre C, Bonet M, et al. Health-related quality of life in chronic fatigue syndrome versus rheumatoid arthritis as control group. *J Chronic Fatigue Syndr.* (2007) 14:31–43. doi: 10.1300/J092v14n02_04
12. Cairns R, Hotopf M. A systematic review describing the prognosis of chronic fatigue syndrome. *Occup Med.* (2005) 55:20–31. doi: 10.1093/occmed/kqi013
13. Jason LA, Benton MC, Valentine L, Johnson A, Torres-Harding S. The economic impact of ME/CFS: individual and societal costs. *Dyn Med.* (2008) 7:6. doi: 10.1186/1476-5918-7-6
14. Hickie I, Davenport T, Wakefield D, Vollmer-Conna U, Cameron B, Vernon SD, et al. Post-infective and chronic fatigue syndromes precipitated by viral and non-viral pathogens: prospective cohort study. *BMJ* (2006) 333:575. doi: 10.1136/bmj.38933.585764.AE
15. Katz BZ, Shiraishi Y, Mears CJ, Binns HJ, Taylor R. Chronic fatigue syndrome following infectious mononucleosis in adolescents: a prospective cohort study. *Pediatrics* (2009) 124:189–93. doi: 10.1542/peds.2008-1879
16. Chu L. *Patient Survey Results for FDA Drug Development Meeting for ME and CFS.* International Association for Chronic Fatigue Syndrome/ Myalgic Encephalomyelitis (2013). Available online at: http://iacfsme.org/portals/0/pdf/FDA_Survey_Results_Word_Version_July2013%20_2_.pdf (Accessed August 20, 2018).
17. Barrows DM. Functional capacity evaluations of persons with chronic fatigue immune dysfunction syndrome. *Am J Occup Ther.* (1995) 49:327–37. doi: 10.5014/ajot.49.4.327
18. Friedberg F, Dechene L, McKenzie MJ, Fontanetta R. Symptom patterns in long-duration chronic fatigue syndrome. *J Psychosom Res.* (2000) 48:59–68. doi: 10.1016/S0022-3999(99)00077-X
19. Jason LA. Natural history of chronic fatigue syndrome. *Rehabil Psychol.* (2011) 56:32–42. doi: 10.1037/a0022595
20. Tiersky LA, DeLuca J, Hill N, Dhar SK, Johnson SK, Lange G, et al. Longitudinal assessment of neuropsychological functioning, psychiatric status, functional disability and employment status in chronic fatigue syndrome. *Appl Neuropsychol.* (2001) 8:41–50. doi: 10.1207/S15324826AN0801_6
21. Nisenbaum R, Jones JF, Unger ER, Reyes M, Reeves WC. A population-based study of the clinical course of chronic fatigue syndrome. *Health Qual Life Outcomes* (2003) 1:49. doi: 10.1186/1477-7525-1-49
22. Jones DEJ, Gray J, Frith J, Newton JL. Fatigue severity remains stable over time and independently associated with orthostatic symptoms in chronic fatigue syndrome: a longitudinal study. *J Intern Med.* (2011) 269:182–8. doi: 10.1111/j.1365-2796.2010.02306.x
23. Nisenbaum R, Jones A, Jones J, Reeves W. Longitudinal analysis of symptoms reported by patients with chronic fatigue syndrome. *Ann Epidemiol.* (2000) 10:458. doi: 10.1016/S1047-2797(00)00119-8
24. March D. The natural history of chronic fatigue syndrome: evidence from a multi-site clinical epidemiology study. In: *Paper Presented at 11th Biennial International Association for Chronic Fatigue Syndrome/ Myalgic Encephalomyelitis Conference.* San Francisco, CA (2014).
25. Endicott NA. Chronic Fatigue Syndrome in Psychiatric Patients: Lifetime

and premorbid personal history of physical health. *Psychosom Med.* (1998) 60:744. doi: 10.1097/00006842-199811000-00017

26. Dansie EJ, Furberg H, Afari N, Buchwald D, Edwards K, Goldberg J, et al. Conditions comorbid with chronic fatigue in a population-based sample. *Psychosomatics* (2012) 53:44–50. doi: 10.1016/j.psym.2011.04.001
27. Aaron LA, Burke MM, Buchwald D. Overlapping conditions among patients with chronic fatigue syndrome, fibromyalgia, and temporomandibular disorder. *Arch Intern Med.* (2000) 160:221–7. doi: 10.1001/archinte.160.2.221
28. Aaron LA, Herrell R, Ashton S, Belcourt M, Schmaling K, Goldberg J, et al. Comorbid clinical conditions in chronic fatigue. *J Gen Intern Med.* (2001) 16:24–31. doi: 10.1046/j.1525-1497.2001.03419.x
29. Bateman L, Darakjy S, Klimas N, Peterson D, Levine SM, Allen A, et al. Chronic fatigue syndrome and co-morbid and consequent conditions: evidence from a multi-site clinical epidemiology study. *Fatigue* (2015) 3:1–15. doi: 10.1080/21641846.2014.978109
30. Walsh CM, Zainal NZ, Middleton SJ, Paykel ES. A family history study of chronic fatigue syndrome: *Psychiatr Genet.* (2001) 11:123–8. doi: 10.1097/00041444-200109000-00003
31. Torres-Harding SR, Jason LA, Turkoglu OD. Family medical history of persons with chronic fatigue syndrome. *J Chronic Fatigue Syndr.* (2004) 12:25–35. doi: 10.1300/J092v12n04_03
32. Njoku N, Jason L, DiPasqaule L. *Family Illnesses Among People With ME/CFS: Blood vs. Non-Blood Relatives.* Invest in ME (2009). Available online at: http://www.investinme.org/documents/journals/Journal%20of%20IiME%20Vol%202%20Issue%202.pdf (Accessed August 20, 2018).
33. Albright F, Light K, Light A, Bateman L, Cannon-Albright LA. Evidence for a heritable predisposition to chronic fatigue syndrome. *BMC Neurol.* (2011) 11:62. doi: 10.1186/1471-2377-11-62
34. Pheby D, Saffron L. Risk factors for severe ME/CFS. *Biol Med.* (2009) 1:50–74.
35. Underhill RA, O'gorman R. Prevalence of chronic fatigue syndrome and chronic fatigue within families of CFS patients. *J Chronic Fatigue Syndr.* (2006) 13:3–13. doi: 10.1300/J092v13n01_02
36. Alegre J, Castro-Marrero J, Ribases M, Alista L, Saez N, Calvo B. Family aggregation studies in CFS.In: *Paper presented at 11th Biennial International Association for Chronic Fatigue Syndrome/Myalgic Encephalomyelitis Conference.* San Francisco, CA (2014).
37. Reyes M, Nisenbaum R, Hoaglin DC, Unger ER, Emmons C, Randall B, et al. Prevalence and incidence of chronic fatigue syndrome in Wichita, Kansas. *Arch Intern Med.* (2003) 163:1530–6. doi: 10.1001/archinte.163.13.1530
38. Reeves WC, Wagner D, Nisenbaum R, Jones JF, Gurbaxani B, Solomon L, et al. Chronic Fatigue Syndrome – a clinically empirical approach to its definition and study. *BMC Med.* (2005) 3:19. doi: 10.1186/1741-7015-3-19
39. Ruiz E, Alegre J, García Quintana AM, Aliste L, Blázquez A, Fernández de et al. [Chronic fatigue syndrome: study of a consecutive series of 824 cases assessed in two specialized units]. *Rev Clin Esp.* (2011) 211:385–90. doi: 10.1016/j.rce.2010.10.007
40. Capelli E, Lorusso L, Ghitti M, Venturini L, Cusa C, Ricevuti G. Chronic fatigue syndrome: features of a population of patients from northern Italy. *Int J Immunopathol Pharmacol.* (2015) 28:53–9. doi: 10.1177/0394632015572074
41. Clark K, Del Fante P, Burnet R, Cahalan P, Briggs N, Griffith L. *Myalgic Encephalopathy/Chronic Fatigue Syndrome Longitudinal Outcomes* (2006). Available online at: http://sacfs.asn.au/download/me_cfs_pilot_study_report.pdf (Accessed September 7, 2018).
42. Johnston SC, Staines DR, Marshall-Gradisnik SM. Epidemiological characteristics of chronic fatigue syndrome/myalgic encephalomyelitis in Australian patients. *Clin Epidemiol.* (2016) 8:97–107. doi: 10.2147/CLEP.S96797
43. Japanese Ministry for Health, Welfare, and Labor. *National ME/CFS Patient Survey.* International Association for Chronic Fatigue Syndrome/ Myalgic Encephalomyelitis (2017) Available online at: http://iacfsme.org/PDFS/2017JanNewsletter/8-Japan-2014-Patient-Survey.aspx (Accessed September 7, 2018).
44. Chu L, Norris JL, Valencia IJ, Montoya JG. Patients diagnosed with Myalgic encephalomyelitis/chronic fatigue syndrome also fit systemic exertion intolerance disease criteria. *Fatigue* (2017) 5:114–28. doi: 10.1080/21641846.2017.1299079
45. Chu L, Valencia IJ, Garvert DW, Montoya JG. Deconstructing post-exertional malaise in myalgic encephalomyelitis/ chronic fatigue syndrome: a patient-centered, cross-sectional survey. *PLoS ONE.* (2018) 13:e0197811. doi: 10.1371/journal.pone.0197811
46. Smets EM, Garssen B, Bonke B, De Haes JC. The Multidimensional Fatigue Inventory (MFI) psychometric qualities of an instrument to assess fatigue. *J Psychosom Res.* (1995) 39:315–25. doi: 10.1016/0022-3999(94)00125-O
47. Lin J-MS, Brimmer DJ, Maloney EM, Nyarko E, Belue R, Reeves WC. Further validation of the Multidimensional Fatigue Inventory in a US adult population sample. *Popul Health Metr.* (2009) 7:18. doi: 10.1186/1478-7954-7-18
48. Krupp LB, LaRocca NG, Muir-Nash J, Steinberg AD. The fatigue severity scale. Application to patients with multiple sclerosis and systemic lupus erythematosus. *Arch Neurol.* (1989) 46:1121–3. doi: 10.1001/archneur.1989.00520460115022
49. Carruthers BM, Jain AK, Meirleir KLD, Peterson DL, Klimas NG, Lerner AM, et al. Myalgic cncephalomyelitis/chronic fatigue syndrome. *J Chronic Fatigue Syndr.* (2003) 11:7–115. doi: 10.1300/J092v11n01_02
50. Carruthers BM, van de Sande MI, Meirleir KLD, Klimas NG, Broderick G, Mitchell T, et al. Myalgic encephalomyelitis: International Consensus Criteria. *J Intern Med.* (2011) 270:327–38. doi: 10.1111/j.1365-2796.2011.02428.x
51. Castro-Marrero J, Faro M, Aliste L, Sáez-Francàs N, Calvo N, Martínez-Martínez A, et al. Comorbidity in chronic fatigue syndrome/myalgic encephalomyelitis: a nationwide population-based cohort study. *Psychosomatics* (2017) 58:533–43. doi: 10.1016/j.psym.2017.04.010
52. Evans MA, Jason LA. Onset patterns of chronic fatigue syndrome and myalgic encephalomyelitis. *Res Chronic Dis.* (2018) 2:1–30.
53. Ravindran MK, Zheng Y, Timbol C, Merck SJ, Baraniuk JN. Migraine headaches in chronic fatigue syndrome (CFS): comparison of two prospective cross-sectional studies. *BMC Neurol.* (2011) 11:30. doi: 10.1186/1471-2377-11-30
54. Fluge Ø, Bruland O, Risa K, Storstein A, Kristoffersen EK, Sapkota D, et al. Benefit from B-Lymphocyte depletion using the Anti-CD20 antibody rituximab in chronic fatigue syndrome. A double-blind and placebo-controlled study. *PLoS ONE* (2011) 6:e26358. doi: 10.1371/journal.pone.0026358
55. Evans M, Barry M, Im Y, Brown A, Jason LA. An investigation of symptoms predating CFS onset. *J Prev Interv Community* (2015) 43:54–61. doi: 10.1080/10852352.2014.973240
56. Jackson ML, Bruck D. Sleep abnormalities in chronic fatigue syndrome/myalgic encephalomyelitis: a review. *J Clin Sleep Med.* (2012) 8:719–28. doi: 10.5664/jcsm.2276
57. Woolley J, Allen R, Wessely S. Alcohol use in chronic fatigue syndrome. *J Psychosom Res.* (2004) 56:203–6. doi: 10.1016/S0022-3999(03)00077-1
58. Low PA, Sandroni P, Joyner M, Shen W-K. Postural tachycardia syndrome (POTS). *J Cardiovasc Electrophysiol.* (2009) 20:352–8. doi: 10.1111/j.1540-8167.2008.01407.x
59. National Alliance on Mental Illness. *Mental Health Facts in America.* National Alliance on Mental Illness. Available online at: https://www.nami.org/NAMI/media/NAMI-Media/Infographics/GeneralMHFacts.pdf (Accessed September 5, 2018).
60. National Fibromyalgia Association. *Prevalence.* National Fibromyalgia Association (NFA). Available online at: http://www.fmaware.org/about-fibromyalgia/prevalence/ (Accessed September 6, 2018).
61. Endo Y, Shoji T, Fukudo S. Epidemiology of irritable bowel syndrome. *Ann Gastroenterol.* (2015) 28:158–9.
62. Womack JP, Jimenez M. Common questions about infectious mononucleosis. *AFP* (2015) 91:372–6.
63. Burch RC, Loder S, Loder E, Smitherman TA. The prevalence and burden of migraine and severe headache in the United States: updated statistics from government health surveillance studies. *Headache* (2015) 55:21–34. doi: 10.1111/head.12482
64. Hayter SM, Cook MC. Updated assessment of the prevalence, spectrum and case definition of autoimmune disease. *Autoimmun Rev.* (2012) 11:754–65. doi: 10.1016/j.autrev.2012.02.001
65. The American Academy of Allergy, Asthma & Immunology. *Allergy Statistics.* AAAAI. The American Academy of Allergy, Asthma & Immunology. Available online at: https://www.aaaai.org/about-aaaai/newsroom/allergy-statistics (Accessed September 6, 2018).

66. Orlander PR. *Hypothyroidism: Practice Essentials, Background, Pathophysiology*. Medscape (2018). Available online at: https://emedicine.medscape.com/article/122393-overview#a5 (Accessed Sep 6, 2018).
67. Shields RW. *Peripheral Neuropathy*. Cleveland Clinic Center for Continuing Medical Education (2010). Available online at: http://www.clevelandclinicmeded.com/medicalpubs/diseasemanagement/neurology/peripheral-neuropathy/ (Accessed September 6, 2018).
68. Steinemann A. National prevalence and effects of multiple chemical sensitivities. *J Occup Environ Med.* (2018) 60:e152–6. doi: 10.1097/JOM.0000000000001272
69. American Academy of Sleep Medicine. *Rising Prevalence of Sleep Apnea in U.S. Threatens Public Health*. American Academy of Sleep Medicine – Association for Sleep Clinicians and Researchers (2014). Available online at: https://aasm.org/rising-prevalence-of-sleep-apnea-in-u-s-threatens-public-health/ (Accessed September 6, 2018 Sep 6).
70. Gauer R, Semidey MJ. Diagnosis and treatment of temporomandibular disorders. *AFP* (2015) 91:378–86.
71. Salit IE. Precipitating factors for the chronic fatigue syndrome. *J Psychiatr Res.* (1997) 31:59–65. doi: 10.1016/S0022-3956(96)00050-7
72. Becker PD, McGregor N, Meirleir KD. Possible triggers and mode of onset of chronic fatigue syndrome. *J Chronic Fatigue Syndr.* (2002) 10:3–18. doi: 10.1300/J092v10n02_02
73. Dobbins JG, Natelson B, Brassloff I, Drastal S, Sisto S-A. Physical, behavioral, and psychological risk Factors for chronic fatigue syndrome: a central role for stress? *J Chronic Fatigue Syndr.* (1995) 1:43–58. doi: 10.1300/J092v01n02_04
74. Kerr JR, Mattey DL. Preexisting psychological stress predicts acute and chronic fatigue and arthritis following symptomatic Parvovirus B19 infection. *Clin Infect Dis.* (2008) 46:e83–7. doi: 10.1086/533471
75. National Academy of Medicine. *Beyond Myalgic Encephalomyelitis/ Chronic Fatigue Syndrome: Redefining an Illness - Report Guide For Clinicians*. National Academy Press (2015) Available online at: https://www.nap.edu/resource/19012/MECFScliniciansguide.pdf (Accessed August 22, 2018).
76. National Institutes of Health. *NIH Intramural Study on Myalgic Encephalomyelitis/ Chronic Fatigue Syndrome*. National Institutes of Health (2016). Available online at: https://mecfs.ctss.nih.gov/ (cited August 23, 2018).
77. Montoya J, Chu L. *Research Update on Adult ME/CFS*. US Department of Health and Human Services (2017). Available online at: https://www.hhs.gov/sites/default/files/2017-12-cfsac-meeting-presentation-research-updates-on-adult-mecfs.pdf (Accessed September 7, 2018).
78. ME Action. What is ME? [Internet]. ME Action. [cited 23 August 2018]. Available from: https://www.meaction.net/about/what-is-me/
79. Mayo Clinic Staff. *Chronic Fatigue Syndrome - Symptoms and Causes*. Mayo Clinic (2018). Available online at: http://www.mayoclinic.org/diseases-conditions/chronic-fatigue-syndrome/symptoms-causes/syc-20360490 (Accessed August 23, 2018).
80. National Alliance for ME. *Ramsay's Definition for ME*. National Alliance for ME. Available online at: https://web.archive.org/web/20180623215524/http://www.name-us.org/DefintionsPages/DefRamsay.htm (Accessed August 23, 2018).
81. White PD, Thomas JM, Amess J, Crawford DH, Grover SA, Kangro HO, et al. Incidence, risk and prognosis of acute and chronic fatigue syndromes and psychiatric disorders after glandular fever. *Br J Psychiatry* (1998) 173:475–81. doi: 10.1192/bjp.173.6.475
82. Bavinton J, Darbishire L, White P. *PACE Manual for Therapists: Graded Exercise Therapy for CFS/ME*. Me-PediaOrg (2018). Available online at: https://me-pedia.org/images/8/89/PACE-get-therapist-manual.pdf (Accessed August 24, 2018).
83. Wilshire C, Kindlon T, Matthees A, McGrath S. Can patients with chronic fatigue syndrome really recover after graded exercise or cognitive behavioural therapy? A critical commentary and preliminary re-analysis of the PACE trial. *Fatigue* (2017) 5:43–56. doi: 10.1080/21641846.2017.1259724
84. Kindlon T. *Reporting of Harms Associated With Graded Exercise Therapy and Cognitive Behavioral Therapy in Myalgic Encephalomyelitis/ Chronic Fatigue Syndrome*. International Association for Chronic Fatigue Syndrome/Myalgic Encephalomyelitis (2011). Available online at: https://iacfsme.org/PDFS/Reporting-of-Harms-Associated-with-GET-and-CBT-in.aspx (Accessed August 24, 2018).
85. Tomas C, Newton J. Metabolic abnormalities in chronic fatigue syndrome/myalgic encephalomyelitis: a mini-review. *Biochem Soc Trans.* (2018) 46:547–53. doi: 10.1042/BST20170503
86. American Psychological Association. *Stress Weakens the Immune System*. American Psychological Association (2006). Available online at: http://www.apa.org/research/action/immune.aspx (Accessed August 24, 2018).
87. Watt T, Oberfoell S, Balise R, Lunn MR, Kar AK, Merrihew L, et al. Response to valganciclovir in chronic fatigue syndrome patients with human herpesvirus 6 and Epstein-Barr virus IgG antibody titers. *J Med Virol.* (2012) 84:1967–74. doi: 10.1002/jmv.23411
88. Montoya JG, Kogelnik AM, Bhangoo M, Lunn MR, Flamand L, Merrihew LE, et al. Randomized clinical trial to evaluate the efficacy and safety of valganciclovir in a subset of patients with chronic fatigue syndrome. *J Med Virol.* (2013) 85:2101–9. doi: 10.1002/jmv.23713
89. Loebel M, Strohschein K, Giannini C, Koelsch U, Bauer S, Doebis C, et al. Deficient EBV-specific B- and T-cell response in patients with chronic fatigue syndrome. *PLoS ONE* (2014) 9:e85387. doi: 10.1371/journal.pone.0085387
90. Lerner AM, Ariza ME, Williams M, Jason L, Beqaj S, Fitzgerald JT, et al. Antibody to Epstein-Barr virus deoxyuridine triphosphate nucleotidohydrolase and deoxyribonucleotide polymerase in a chronic fatigue syndrome subset. *PLoS ONE* (2012) 7:e47891. doi: 10.1371/journal.pone.0047891
91. VanNess JM, Stevens SR, Bateman L, Stiles TL, Snell CR. Postexertional malaise in women with chronic fatigue syndrome. *J Womens Health* (2010) 19:239–44. doi: 10.1089/jwh.2009.1507
92. Tomas C, Newton J, Watson S. A review of hypothalamic-pituitary-adrenal axis function in chronic fatigue syndrome. *ISRN Neurosci.* (2013) 2013:784520. doi: 10.1155/2013/784520
93. VanNess J, Davenport T, Stevens S, Stevens J, Snell C. Chronotropic incompetence in chronic fatigue syndrome/myalgic encephalomyelitis. *Presented at Combined Sections Meeting of the American Physical Therapy Association*. Anaheim, CA (2016).
94. Burton AR, Rahman K, Kadota Y, Lloyd A, Vollmer-Conna U. Reduced heart rate variability predicts poor sleep quality in a case-control study of chronic fatigue syndrome. *Exp Brain Res.* (2010) 204:71–8. doi: 10.1007/s00221-010-2296-1
95. Vital Lifestyle. *How Stress Works: The Anatomy & Physiology of Stress*. Vital Lifestyle. Available online at: http://www.vitallifestyle.com.au/how-stress-works/ (Accessed September 1, 2018).
96. Everly GS, Lating JM. *A Clinical Guide to the Treatment of the Human Stress Response*. 3rd ed. New York, NY: Springer (2013). 485 p. doi: 10.1007/978-1-4614-5538-7
97. Loebel M, Grabowski P, Heidecke H, Bauer S, Hanitsch LG, Wittke K, et al. Antibodies to β adrenergic and muscarinic cholinergic receptors in patients with Chronic Fatigue Syndrome. *Brain Behav Immun.* (2016) 52:32–9. doi: 10.1016/j.bbi.2015.09.013
98. Tanaka S, Kuratsune H, Hidaka Y, Hakariya Y, Tatsumi K-I, Takano T, et al. Autoantibodies against muscarinic cholinergic receptor in chronic fatigue syndrome. *Int J Mol Med.* (2003) 12:225–30. doi: 10.3892/ijmm.12.2.225
99. Jason LA, Katz BZ, Shiraishi Y, Mears CJ, Im Y, Taylor RR. Predictors of post-infectious chronic fatigue syndrome in adolescents. *Health Psychol Behav Med.* (2014) 2:41–51. doi: 10.1080/21642850.2013.869176
100. Holmes GP, Kaplan JE, Gantz NM, Komaroff AL, Schonberger LB, Straus SE, et al. Chronic fatigue syndrome: a working case definition. *Ann Intern Med.* (1988) 108:387–9. doi: 10.7326/0003-4819-108-3-387
101. ME Association (UK). *London Criteria for M.E. – For Website Discussion*. ME Association (2011). Available online at: https://www.meassociation.org.uk/2011/02/london-criteria-for-m-e/ (Accessed September 2, 2018).
102. Jason LA, Damrongvachiraphan D, Hunnell J, Bartgis L, Brown A, Evans M, et al. Myalgic encephalomyelitis case definitions. *Autom Control Physiol State Funct.* (2012) 1:1–14. doi: 10.4303/acpsf/K110601
103. Jason LA, Brown A, Evans M, Sunnquist M, Newton JL. Contrasting chronic fatigue syndrome versus myalgic encephalomyelitis/chronic fatigue syndrome. *Fatigue* (2013) 1:168–83. doi: 10.1080/21641846.2013.774556
104. Ray C, Jeffefues S, Weir W, Hayes K, Simon S, Akingbade F, et al. Making sense of chronic fatigue syndrome: patients' accounts of onset. *Psychol Health* (1998) 13:99–109.

105. Racciatti D, Vecchiet J, Ceccomancini A, Ricci F, Pizzigallo E. Chronic fatigue syndrome following a toxic exposure. *Sci Total Environ.* (2001) 270:27–31. doi: 10.1016/S0048-9697(00)00777-4
106. Behan PO. Chronic fatigue syndrome as a delayed reaction to chronic low-dose organophosphate exposure. *J Nutr Environ Med.* (1996) 6:341–50. doi: 10.3109/13590849609007262
107. Adami H-O, Berry SCL, Breckenridge CB, Smith LL, Swenberg JA, Trichopoulos D, et al. Toxicology and epidemiology: improving the science with a framework for combining toxicological and epidemiological evidence to establish causal inference. *Toxicol Sci.* (2011) 122:223–34. doi: 10.1093/toxsci/kfr113
108. Berne K. *Running on Empty: The Complete Guide to Chronic Fatigue Syndrome.* Revised ed. Alameda, CA: Hunter House (1995). 315 p.
109. De Becker P, McGregor N, De Meirleir K. A definition-based analysis of symptoms in a large cohort of patients with chronic fatigue syndrome. *J Intern Med.* (2001) 250:234–40. doi: 10.1046/j.1365-2796.2001.00890.x
110. Bansal AS. Investigating unexplained fatigue in general practice with a particular focus on CFS/ME. *BMC Fam Pract.* (2016) 17:81. doi: 10.1186/s12875-016-0493-0
111. Lapp C, Black L, Smith R. *Symptoms Predict the Outcome of Tilt Table Testing in CFS/ME/FM.* Hunter-Hopkins Center. Available online at: http://drlapp.com/wp-content/uploads/TTT_symptoms.pdf (Accessed September 1, 2018).
112. Rowe PC, Lucas KE. Orthostatic intolerance in chronic fatigue syndrome. *Am J Med.* (2007) 120:e13. doi: 10.1016/j.amjmed.2006.02.033
113. Robinson LJ, Durham J, MacLachlan LL, Newton JL. Autonomic function in chronic fatigue syndrome with and without painful temporomandibular disorder. *Fatigue* (2015) 3:205–19. doi: 10.1080/21641846.2015.1091152
114. Tansey EA, Roe SM, Johnson CD. The sympathetic release test: a test used to assess thermoregulation and autonomic control of blood flow. *Adv Physiol Educ.* (2014) 38:87–92. doi: 10.1152/advan.00095.2013
115. Narkiewicz K, Cooley RL, Somers VK. Alcohol potentiates orthostatic hypotension : implications for alcohol-related syncope. *Circulation* (2000) 101:398–402. doi: 10.1161/01.CIR.101.4.398
116. Hornig M, Montoya JG, Klimas NG, Levine S, Felsenstein D, Bateman L, et al. Distinct plasma immune signatures in ME/CFS are present early in the course of illness. *Sci Adv.* (2015) 1:e1400121. doi: 10.1126/sciadv.1400121
117. Costigan A, Elliott C, McDonald C, Newton JL. Orthostatic symptoms predict functional capacity in chronic fatigue syndrome: implications for management. *QJM* (2010) 103:589–95. doi: 10.1093/qjmed/hcq094
118. Deftereos SN, Vernon SD, Persidis A. Current therapeutic strategies for myalgic encephalomyelitis/chronic fatigue syndrome: results of an online survey. *Fatigue* (2016) 4:39–51. doi: 10.1080/21641846.2015.1126025
119. International Association for Chronic Fatigue Syndrome/ Myalgic Encephalomyelitis. *Chronic Fatigue Syndrome/ Myalgic Encephalomyelitis: Primer for Clinical Practitioners.* International Association for Chronic Fatigue Syndrome/ Myalgic Encephalomyelitis (2014). Available online at: https://iacfsme.org/portals/0/pdf/Primer_Post_2014_conference.pdf (Accessed September 3, 2018).
120. X E. *Why I Believe I Got Sick Again After Making a Full Recovery From ME/CFS.* Consciously Healthy (2016). Available online at: http://consciouslyhealthy.co.uk/thelessonslearned/ (Accessed September 3, 2018).
121. Nooram57. *Cfs Relapse After 16 Years? Anyone Else?.* Reddit/Cfs (2017). Available online at: https://www.reddit.com/r/cfs/comments/5a7hol/cfs_relapse_after_16_years_anyone_else/ (Accessed September 7, 2018).
122. Adamowicz JL, Caikauskaite I, Friedberg F. Defining recovery in chronic fatigue syndrome: a critical review. *Qual Life Res.* (2014) 23:2407–16. doi: 10.1007/s11136-014-0705-9
123. Devendorf AR, Jackson CT, Sunnquist M, Jason LA. Defining and measuring recovery from myalgic encephalomyelitis and chronic fatigue syndrome: the physician perspective. *Disabil Rehabil.* (2017) 39:1–8. doi: 10.1080/09638288.2017.1383518
124. Jason LA, Richman JA, Rademaker AW, Jordan KM, Plioplys AV, Taylor RR, et al. A community-based study of chronic fatigue syndrome. *Arch Intern Med.* (1999) 159:2129–37. doi: 10.1001/archinte.159.18.2129
125. Kidd E, Brown A, McManimen S, Jason L, Newton J, Strand E. The relationship between age and illness duration in chronic fatigue syndrome. *Diagnostics* (2016) 6:16. doi: 10.3390/diagnostics6020016
126. Gimeno Pi I, Guitard Sein-Echaluce ML, Rosselló Aubach L, Torres Puig-Gros J, Fernández Solà J. Stressful events in the onset of chronic fatigue syndrome. *Rev Esp Salud Publica.* (2016) 90:e1–7.
127. Schacterle RS, Komaroff AL. A comparison of pregnancies that occur before and after the onset of chronic fatigue syndrome. *Arch Intern Med.* (2004) 164:401–4. doi: 10.1001/archinte.164.4.401
128. Allen PR. Chronic fatigue syndrome: implications for women and their health care providers during the childbearing years. *J Midwifery Womens Health* (2008) 53:289–301. doi: 10.1016/j.jmwh.2007.12.001
129. Unger ER, Lin JMS, Brimmer DJ, Lapp CW, Komaroff AL, Nath A, et al. CDC grand rounds: chronic fatigue syndrome — advancing research and clinical education. *MMWR* (2016) 65:1434–8. doi: 10.15585/mmwr.mm655051a4
130. Tavakolpour S, Rahimzadeh G. New insights into the management of patients with autoimmune diseases or inflammatory disorders during pregnancy. *Scand J Immunol.* (2016) 84:146–9. doi: 10.1111/sji.12453
131. Rowe PC, Underhill RA, Friedman KJ, Gurwitt A, Medow MS, Schwartz MS, et al. Myalgic Encephalomyelitis/Chronic Fatigue Syndrome diagnosis and management in young people: a primer. *Front Pediatr.* (2017) 5:121. doi: 10.3389/fped.2017.00121
132. Studd J, Panay N. Chronic fatigue syndrome. *Lancet* (1996) 348:1384. doi: 10.1016/S0140-6736(05)65448-7
133. Kingdon CC, Bowman EW, Curran H, Nacul L, Lacerda EM. Functional status and well-being in people with myalgic encephalomyelitis/chronic fatigue syndrome compared with people with multiple sclerosis and healthy controls. *Pharmacoecon Open* (2018) 2:381–92. doi: 10.1007/s41669-018-0071-6
134. Pepper CM, Krupp LB, Friedberg F, Doscher C, Coyle PK. A comparison of neuropsychiatric characteristics in chronic fatigue syndrome, multiple sclerosis, and major depression. *J Neuropsychiatry Clin Neurosci.* (1993) 5:200–5. doi: 10.1176/jnp.5.2.200
135. Wise S, Jantke R, Brown A, Jason LA. Functional level of patients with chronic fatigue syndrome reporting use of alternative vs. traditional treatments. *Fatigue* (2015) 3:235–40. doi: 10.1080/21641846.2015.1097102
136. Unger ER, Lin J-MS, Tian H, Natelson BH, Lange G, Vu D, et al. Multi-Site Clinical Assessment of Myalgic encephalomyelitis/chronic fatigue syndrome (MCAM): design and implementation of a prospective/retrospective rolling cohort study. *Am J Epidemiol.* (2017) 185:617–26. doi: 10.1093/aje/kwx029
137. Thombs BD, Bassel M, McGuire L, Smith MT, Hudson M, Haythornthwaite JA. A systematic comparison of fatigue levels in systemic sclerosis with general population, cancer and rheumatic disease samples. *Rheumatology* (2008) 47:1559–63. doi: 10.1093/rheumatology/ken331
138. Hedlund L, Gyllensten AL, Hansson L. A psychometric study of the multidimensional fatigue inventory to assess fatigue in patients with schizophrenia spectrum disorders. *Community Mental Health J.* (2015) 51:377–82. doi: 10.1007/s10597-014-9746-3
139. Valko PO, Bassetti CL, Bloch KE, Held U, Baumann CR. Validation of the Fatigue Severity Scale in a Swiss cohort. *Sleep* (2008) 31:1601–7. doi: 10.1093/sleep/31.11.1601
140. Johansson S, Kottorp A, Lee KA, Gay CL, Lerdal A. Can the Fatigue Severity Scale 7-item version be used across different patient populations as a generic fatigue measure - a comparative study using a Rasch model approach. *Health Qual Life Outcomes* (2014) 12:24. doi: 10.1186/1477-7525-12-24
141. Chu L. Post-exertional malaise symptoms and abnormal cardiopulmonary exercise testing are associated with decreased physical functioning in myalgic encephalomyelitis/ chronic fatigue syndrome. In:*Poster Presented at 11th Biennial International Association for Chronic Fatigue Syndrome/ Myalgic Encephalomyelitis Conference.* San Francisco, CA (2014).
142. Matthews RM, Komaroff AL. Changes in functional status in chronic fatigue syndrome over a decade: do age and gender matter? *J Chronic Fatigue Syndr.* (2007) 14:33–42. doi: 10.1300/J092v14n01_04
143. Lewis I, Pairman J, Spickett G, Newton JL. Is Chronic fatigue syndrome in older patients a different disease? - a clinical cohort study. *Eur J Clin Investig.* (2013) 43:302–8. doi: 10.1111/eci.12046
144. Stouten B. Identification of ambiguities in the 1994 chronic fatigue syndrome research case definition and recommendations for resolution. *BMC Health Serv Res.* (2005) 5:37. doi: 10.1186/1472-6963-5-37

145. US Cancer Statistics. *United States Cancer Statistics: Data Visualizations*. Centers for Disease Control and Prevention (2015). Available online at: https://gis.cdc.gov/grasp/USCS/DataViz.html (Accessed September 6, 2018).
146. Chang CM, Warren JL, Engels EA. Chronic fatigue syndrome and subsequent risk of cancer among elderly U.S. adults. *Cancer* (2012) 118:5929–36. doi: 10.1002/cncr.27612
147. McManimen SL, Devendorf AR, Brown AA, Moore BC, Moore JH, Jason LA. Mortality in patients with myalgic encephalomyelitis and chronic fatigue syndrome. *Fatigue* (2016) 4:195–207. doi: 10.1080/21641846.2016.1236588
148. Jason LA, Sunnquist M, Kot B, Brown A. Unintended consequences of not specifying exclusionary illnesses for Systemic Exertion Intolerance Disease. *Diagnostics* (2015) 5:272–86. doi: 10.3390/diagnostics5020272
149. McKeon JMM, McKeon PO. A balancing act between control and generalizability. *Int J Athletic Ther Training* (2016) 21:1–3. doi: 10.1123/ijatt.2016-0010
150. Millar E, Dowell T, Lawrenson R, Mangin D, Sarfati D. Clinical guidelines: what happens when people have multiple conditions? *N Z Med J.* (2018) 131:73–81.
151. Burstein R, Noseda R, Borsook D. Migraine: multiple processes, complex pathophysiology. *J Neurosci.* (2015) 35:6619–29. doi: 10.1523/JNEUROSCI.0373-15.2015
152. Solomon L, Reeves WC. Factors influencing the diagnosis of chronic fatigue syndrome. *Arch Intern Med.* (2004) 164:2241. doi: 10.1001/archinte.164.20.2241
153. Jason LA, Taylor RR, Kennedy CL, Song S, Johnson D, Torres S. Chronic fatigue syndrome: occupation, medical utilization, and subtypes in a community-based sample: *J Nerv Ment Dis.* (2000) 188:568–76. doi: 10.1097/00005053-200009000-00002
154. Palacios N, Fitzgerald KC, Komaroff AL, Ascherio A. Incidence of myalgic encephalomyelitis/chronic fatigue syndrome in a large prospective cohort of U.S. nurses. *Fatigue* (2017) 5:159–66. doi: 10.1080/21641846.2017.1323576
155. Endicott NA. Chronic fatigue syndrome in private practice psychiatry: family history of physical and mental health. *J Psychosom Res.* (1999) 47:343–54. doi: 10.1016/S0022-3999(99)00013-6
156. Levine PH, Whiteside TL, Friberg D, Bryant J, Colclough G, Herberman RB. Dysfunction of natural killer activity in a family with chronic fatigue syndrome. *Clin Immunol Immunopathol.* (1998) 88:96–104. doi: 10.1006/clin.1998.4554
157. Blomberg J, Gottfries C-G, Elfaitouri A, Rizwan M, Rosén A. Infection elicited autoimmunity and myalgic encephalomyelitis/chronic fatigue syndrome: an explanatory model. *Front Immunol.* (2018) 9:299. doi: 10.3389/fimmu.2018.00229
158. Sotzny F, Blanco J, Capelli E, Castro-Marrero J, Steiner S, Murovska M, et al. Myalgic encephalomyelitis/chronic fatigue syndrome – evidence for an autoimmune disease. *Autoimmun Rev.* (2018) 17:601–9. doi: 10.1016/j.autrev.2018.01.009
159. Berkovich R. *Staying Ahead of Multiple Autoimmune Disorders*. Healio Rheumatology (2016). Available online at: https://www.healio.com/rheumatology/rheumatoid-arthritis/news/print/healio-rheumatology/%7bed6a292b-402b-402b-82ca-c2c2e9c01e3b%7d/staying-ahead-of-multiple-autoimmune-disorders (Accessed September 7, 2018).
160. Cárdenas-Roldán J, Rojas-Villarraga A, Anaya J-M. How do autoimmune diseases cluster in families? A systematic review and meta-analysis. *BMC Med.* (2013) 11:73. doi: 10.1186/1741-7015-11-73
161. Rose NR, Bona C. Defining criteria for autoimmune diseases (Witebsky's postulates revisited). *Immunol Today* (1993) 14:426–30.
162. Mackay IR, Rose NR. *The Autoimmune Diseases*. Cambridge, MA: Elsevier (2006). 1161 p.
163. Fluge Ø, Mella O, Bruland O, Risa K, Dyrstad SE, Alme K, et al. Metabolic profiling indicates impaired pyruvate dehydrogenase function in myalgic encephalopathy/chronic fatigue syndrome. *JCI Insight* (2016) 1:e89376. doi: 10.1172/jci.insight.89376
164. Sunnquist M, Jason LA, Brown A, Evans M, Berman A. Complications in operationalizing lifelong fatigue as an exclusionary criterion. *J Prev Interv Community* (2015) 43:42–53. doi: 10.1080/10852352.2014.973238
165. Jones JF, Nisenbaum R, Reeves WC. Medication use by persons with chronic fatigue syndrome: results of a randomized telephone survey in Wichita, Kansas. *Health Qual Life Outcomes* (2003) 1:74. doi: 10.1186/1477-7525-1-74
166. Gotts ZM, Deary V, Newton J, Dussen DV der, Roy PD, Ellis JG. Are there sleep-specific phenotypes in patients with chronic fatigue syndrome? A cross-sectional polysomnography analysis. *BMJ Open* (2013) 3:e002999. doi: 10.1136/bmjopen-2013-002999
167. US National Institutes of Health. *Myalgic Encephalomyelitis/Chronic Fatigue Syndrome (ME/CFS) Collaborative Research Centers (CRCs) (U54)*. US National Institutes of Health (2017). Available online at: https://grants.nih.gov/grants/guide/rfa-files/RFA-NS-17-021.html (Accessed September 10, 2018).
168. Evans M, Jason LA. Effects of time frame on the recall reliability of CFS symptoms. *Eval Health Profess.* (2015) 38:367–81. doi: 10.1177/0163278713497014

13

Healthcare Utilization in Myalgic Encephalomyelitis/Chronic Fatigue Syndrome (ME/CFS): Analysis of US Ambulatory Healthcare Data, 2000–2009

Jaeyong Bae[1,2†] *and Jin-Mann S. Lin*[1*]

[1] *Chronic Viral Diseases Branch, Division of High-Consequence Pathogens and Pathology, National Center for Emerging and Zoonotic Infectious Diseases, Centers for Disease Control and Prevention, Atlanta, GA, United States,* [2] *Department of Health Policy and Management, Rollins School of Public Health, Emory University, Atlanta, GA, United States*

Correspondence:
Jin-Mann S. Lin
dwe3@cdc.gov

Background: ME/CFS is a complex and disabling illness with substantial economic burden and functional impairment comparable to heart disease and multiple sclerosis. Many patients with ME/CFS do not receive appropriate healthcare, partially due to lack of diagnostic tests, and knowledge/attitudes/beliefs about ME/CFS. This study was to assess the utility of US ambulatory healthcare data in profiling demographics, co-morbidities, and healthcare in ME/CFS.

Methods: Data came from the National Ambulatory Medical Care Survey (NAMCS) and the National Hospital Ambulatory Medical Care Survey (NHAMCS) in the U.S. Weighted analysis was performed. We examined 9.06 billion adult visits from 2000 to 2009 NAMCS/NHAMCS data. ME/CFS-related visits were identified by ICD-9-CM code, 780.71, up to tertiary diagnosis.

Results: We estimated 2.9 million (95% CI: 1.8–3.9 million) ME/CFS-related visits during 2000–2009, with no statistical evidence (p-trend = 0.31) for a decline or increase in ME/CFS-related visits. Internists, general and family practitioners combined provided 52.12% of these visits. Patients with ME/CFS-related visits were mostly in their 40 and 50 s (47.76%), female (66.07%), white (86.95%), metropolitan/urban residents (92.05%), and insured (87.26%). About 71% of ME/CFS patients had co-morbidities, including depression (35.79%), hypertension (31.14%), diabetes (20.30%), and arthritis (14.11%). As one quality indicator, physicians spent more time on ME/CFS-related visits than non-ME/CFS visits (23.62 vs. 19.38 min, $p = 0.065$). As additional quality indicators, the top three preventive counseling services provided to patients with ME/CFS-related visits were diet/nutrition (8.33%), exercise (8.21%), and smoking cessation (7.24%). Compared to non-ME/CFS visits, fewer ME/CFS-related visits included counseling for stress management (0.75 vs. 3.14%, $p = 0.010$), weight reduction (0.88 vs. 4.02%, $p = 0.002$), injury prevention (0.04 vs. 1.64%, $p < 0.001$), and family planning/contraception (0.17 vs. 1.45%, $p = 0.037$).

Conclusions: Visits coded with ME/CFS did not increase from 2000 to 2009. Almost three quarters of ME/CFS-related visits were made by ME/CFS patients with other co-morbid conditions, further adding to complexity in ME/CFS healthcare. While physicians spent more time with ME/CFS patients, a lower proportion of ME/CFS patients received preventive counseling for weight reduction, stress management, and injury prevention than other patients despite the complexity of ME/CFS. NAMCS/NHAMCS data are useful in evaluating co-morbidities, healthcare utilization, and quality indicators for healthcare in ME/CFS.

Keywords: myalgic encephalomyelitis/chronic fatigue syndrome, National Ambulatory Medical Care Survey (NAMCS), co-morbidities, healthcare utilization, quality indicators of healthcare

BACKGROUND

Myalgic encephalomyelitis/chronic fatigue syndrome (ME/CFS) is a multi-system illness characterized by reduced functioning associated with fatigue that is not due to ongoing exertion and not significantly improved by rest. Minimal mental or physical exertion may trigger relapse (termed post-exertional malaise). Additional core or common symptoms include unrefreshing sleep, cognitive problems, increased symptoms when standing, and pain, but patients may experience numerous other symptoms (1–4). Several different etiologies have been investigated for ME/CFS but so far the etiology cannot be fully explained (4, 5). Experts have noted that the terminology "chronic fatigue syndrome" can trivialize this illness and stigmatize persons who experience its symptoms (6). A variety of other names have been used, including myalgic encephalomyelitis (ME), ME/CFS, chronic fatigue immune dysfunction, and most recently, systemic exertion intolerance disease (4). In 2010, the Chronic Fatigue Syndrome Advisory Committee recommended use of ME/CFS across federal agencies within the Department of Health and Human Services. The term ME/CFS will be used in this paper.

Previous prevalence estimates of ME/CFS have varied from 0.007 to 8.34% (7–16). In the community-based studies (with or without clinical assessment), the prevalence of ME/CFS was estimated to be 0.007–8.34%, and in the clinical-based studies in primary care setting the prevalence was estimated to be 0.006–3.00%. The large variation in the ME/CFS prevalence estimates may be due to differences in study methodology, such as study population composition, heterogeneity of source populations, data collection procedures, limitations in case ascertainment, different case definitions, and operational application of case definition criteria. Moreover, most prior studies took place at a small number of hospitals or clinics, or used a population sample from one state (9, 11, 13, 17, 18).

The economic burden and functional impairment associated with ME/CFS is substantial and comparable to heart disease and multiple sclerosis. ME/CFS accounts for $18–51 billion of economic costs including $9–14 billion in medical costs and $9–37 billion in lost productivity annually (19–21). Patients with ME/CFS suffer from worse functional impairment compared to cancer, diabetes, heart disease, lung disease, multiple sclerosis, and rheumatoid arthritis (15, 22). Additionally, many patients with ME/CFS are found to have additional overlapping pain conditions such as fibromyalgia, multiple chemical sensitivity, and irritable bowel syndrome (23–27). Adjusting to a chronic, debilitating illness sometimes leads to other problems, including depression, stress, and anxiety. Like patients with other chronic illnesses, many patients with ME/CFS develop depression during their illness course (28, 29). ME/CFS patients with other co-morbid conditions have poor health and worse functioning status than those without co-morbid conditions. Co-morbid or co-existing conditions may also increase the frequency of healthcare utilization including office visits and laboratory tests (27, 30) and further complicate the management of ME/CFS symptoms. Many ME/CFS patients do not receive appropriate healthcare, partially due to constraints US healthcare systems face in addressing chronic illnesses but also due to healthcare providers lack of knowledge and misaligned attitudes, and beliefs concerning ME/CFS (31, 32).

In this study, we sought to use US national healthcare data from ambulatory visits to evaluate trends from 2000 to 2009 in ME/CFS. Additionally, we characterized demographics, co-morbidities, and healthcare services/quality indicators related to ME/CFS visits.

METHODS

Data Sources

This analysis was based on the National Ambulatory Medical Care Survey (NAMCS) (33) and the National Hospital Ambulatory Medical Care Survey (NHAMCS) (34) from 2000 to 2009. Since 1992, both surveys have been administrated by the National Center for Health Statistics (NCHS), Centers for Disease Control and Prevention (CDC) (35–38). The NCHS Research Ethics Review Board approved the protocols for both the NAMCS and NHAMCS surveys, including a waiver of the requirement for informed consent of participating patients.

In brief, NAMCS collects healthcare data provided by non-federal office-based physicians whereas NHAMCS collects healthcare data provided by non-federal hospital outpatient departments (OPDs) and hospital emergency departments (EDs). Both surveys use multistage probability sampling procedures to allow for generating nationally representative estimates of ambulatory medical care services in the United States. The patient visit was the unit of this analysis. Between 2000 and 2009, response rates were 58.9–70.4% among physicians invited to participate in NAMCS, 68.3–91.0% among hospital OPDs, and 79.5–97.0% among EDs invited to participate in NHAMCS.

This analysis included the aggregated number of 748,464 adult visits (made by patients aged 18 years or older, 9.06 billion weighted visits) from the NAMCS and NHAMCS data during 2000–2009. This included 231,984 physician patient visits (7.49 billion weighted visits), 250,821 OPD visits (691 million weighted visits), and 265,659 ED visits (879 million weighted visits).

Measures

The US national ambulatory data includes up to three listed diagnoses (primary, secondary, and tertiary) for each visit. We classified all visits into two types: ME/CFS-related visits and non-ME/CFS-related visits. ME/CFS-related visits were identified using the International Classification of Diseases, 9th revision, Clinical Modification (ICD-9-CM) code, 780.71, up to tertiary diagnosis received in provider's diagnoses during visits. The primary outcomes of interest were: (1) co-morbidities, (2) healthcare services. We also examined the associations between types of visits and patient demographics.

Co-morbidities

In addition to the provider's diagnoses for patient visits, providers (for NAMCS and OPD only for NHAMCS) indicate the presence of 14 conditions even if the condition had been reported in the diagnosis box. The 14 conditions were arthritis, asthma, cancer, cerebrovascular disease, congestive heart failure, chronic renal failure, chronic obstructive pulmonary disease, depression, diabetes, hyperlipidemia, hypertension, ischemic heart disease, obesity, and osteoporosis. We considered these to be co-morbid conditions, and compared the percentages of ME/CFS and non-ME/CFS-related visits with these conditions.

Healthcare Services

Both NAMCS and NHAMCS surveys collected information on any service ordered or provided for patients during their visits. Our analysis included three categories of healthcare services: (1) preventive counseling/management services—asthma, diet/nutrition, exercise, family planning/contraception, growth/development, injury prevention, stress management, tobacco use/exposure, weight reduction, and other counseling, (2) diagnostic/screening services—complete blood count (CBC), glucose, glycohemoglobin (HgbA1c), lipid/cholesterol, and other blood tests, and (3) non-medication treatments—Complementary Alternative Medicine (CAM), physical therapy, psychotherapy, and other mental health counseling. We also examined the length of the patient's visit. These healthcare services have been constructed as quality indicators in other illnesses along with other illness-specific quality indicators based on the Institute of Medicine's broad criteria of clinical importance, scientific soundness, and feasibility for indicator selection (39, 40).

Other variables used in this study were: (1) patient demographics- age, sex, race/ethnicity, source of payment source including insurance type, and tobacco use (current or not), (2) vital signs—body mass index (BMI), and blood pressure (BP), and (3) physician/clinic information—geographic region (Northeast/Midwest/South/West), metropolitan statistical area (MSA or not), physician specialty (NAMCS only), clinic type (OPD only), physician practice characteristics (NAMCS only; solo practitioner physician practice characteristics employment status, ownership, office type), use of electronic medical records (EMRs), and referral status.

Statistical Analysis

Statistical analyses were performed using STATA version 12 (Stata Corporation, College Station, TX). To report national estimate, the "svy" command designed for multistage weighted probability surveys such as NAMCS and NHAMCS were utilized. The NCHS analytical guidelines establish the legitimacy of combining multiple years of data from the NAMCS and NHAMCS surveys. Comparisons of NAMCS and NHAMCS suggested limited differences in the percentage estimates of ME/CFS-related visits annually. We, therefore, combined the two surveys for subsequent analyses between ME/CFS-related and non-ME/CFS-related visits.

The Pearson correlation test was used to analyze the percentage trend of ME/CFS-related visits during 2000–2009. In addition to national estimate of ME/CFS-related visits, we examined bivariate associations of ME/CFS-related visits with the following health and healthcare outcomes: (1) co-morbidities, (2) quality of healthcare such as health education services and length of patient's visit, (3) other variables such as patient and physician/clinic information, and vital signs.

RESULTS

Demographic Characteristics of ME/CFS-Related Visits

Table 1 shows the demographics for overall visits to physician offices, hospital outpatient departments, and emergency departments. Among 784,464 visits made by patients ≥18 years of age in the 2000–2009 NAMCS and NHAMCS datasets, we identified 130 visits (unweighted counts) indicating ICD-9-CM code, 780.71 for ME/CFS. After appropriate weighting, the estimated number of visits made by patients with ME/CFS in the United States over the 10 years period was 2.9 million [95% Confidence interval (CI): 1.8–3.9 million]. ME/CFS patient visits were mostly in the fourth and fifth decade age group (48.76%), female (66.07%), white (86.95%), metropolitan/urban residents (92.04%), and insured (87.26%). There were no statistically significant difference on the distribution of age, sex, race, residential area, and insurance between ME/CFS and non-ME/CFS related visits. Of the ME/CFS-related visits to office-based physicians, 52.12% were to general/family practitioners and internists. Obstetrics and gynecology, psychiatry, and neurology combined only accounted for <10% while all other specialties accounted for 38.13% ME/CFS patient visits. Among ME/CFS-related visits to hospital outpatient departments, general medicine clinics accounted for most of the visits (72.38%). Compared to non-ME/CFS visits, a slightly higher rate of adopting electronic health

TABLE 1 | Patient and practice demographic characteristics of ambulatory adult visits in USA, 2000–2009.

Variables	All visits	ME/CFS visits	Non-ME/CFS visits	*P*-value[a]
Unweighted no. of visits	748,464	130	748,334	
Weighted no. of visits	9,061,664,246	2,911,161	9,058,753,085	
Practice setting (%)				
Office based (NAMCS)	7,491,099,961 (82.67%)	2,723,988 (93.57%)	7,488,375,973 (82.66%)	
Outpatient department (NHAMCS-OPD)	690,679,940 (7.62%)	119,850 (4.12%)	690,560,090 (7.62%)	
Emergency department (NHAMCS-ED)	879,884,345 (9.71%)	67,323 (2.31%)	879,817,022 (9.71%)	
Physician Specialty[1] (%)				0.382
General and family practice	24.97%	35.86%	24.97%	
Internal medicine	18.82%	16.26%	18.82%	
Obstetrics and gynecology	9.33%	2.06%	9.33%	
Psychiatry	3.15%	4.72%	3.15%	
Neurology	1.56%	2.96%	1.56%	
All other	42.18%	38.13%	42.18%	
Clinical Type[2] (%)				0.001
General medicine	65.75%	72.38%	65.75%	
Surgery	13.48%	16.03%	13.48%	
Pediatric	1.06%	0.00%	1.06%	
Obstetrics and Gynecology	10.45%	0.13%	10.45%	
Substance abuse	0.92%	0.00%	0.92%	
Other	8.34%	11.46%	8.34%	
	(n: 6,075,856,067)	(n: 1,673,624)	(n: 6,074,182,443)	
EHR use[3] (%)	35.91%	42.95%	35.91%	0.462
Age, mean (SD)	52.65 (18.89)	48.56 (11.60)	52.66 (18.89)	0.077
Age, median (range)	47 (18–100)	47.5(20–89)	47 (18–100)	
Age Group (%)				0.440
18 to 29	13.81%	15.22%	13.81%	
30 to 39	13.90%	11.46%	13.90%	
40 to 49	17.02%	31.44%	17.02%	
50 to 59	17.81%	17.32%	17.81%	
60 to 69	15.06%	12.01%	15.06%	
70 or older	22.40%	12.56%	22.40%	
Sex (%)				0.528
Female	61.35%	66.07%	61.35%	
Race (%)				0.800
White	83.87%	86.95%	83.87%	
Black	11.81%	9.21%	11.81%	
Other	4.32%	3.84%	4.32%	
Metropolitan status: (MSA) (%)	85.79%	92.04%	85.79%	0.140
Geographic region (%)				0.499
Northeast	20.56%	15.99%	20.56%	
Midwest	22.43%	19.88%	22.43%	
South	36.66%	32.54%	36.67%	
West	20.34%	31.59%	20.34%	
Health insurance (%)				0.077
Private	49.94%	59.62%	49.94%	
Medicare	27.04%	24.65%	27.04%	
Medicaid	8.07%	2.99%	8.08%	
Other	14.94%	12.74%	14.94%	

1. NAMCS only; 2. OPD only; 3. 03-09 NAMCS and 05-09 OPD/ED.

[a]*p-values based on adjusted Wald tests with* H_0, $Var|_{if\ ME/CFS} = Var|_{if\ NON-ME/CFS}$; *Column percentages were listed in the table.*

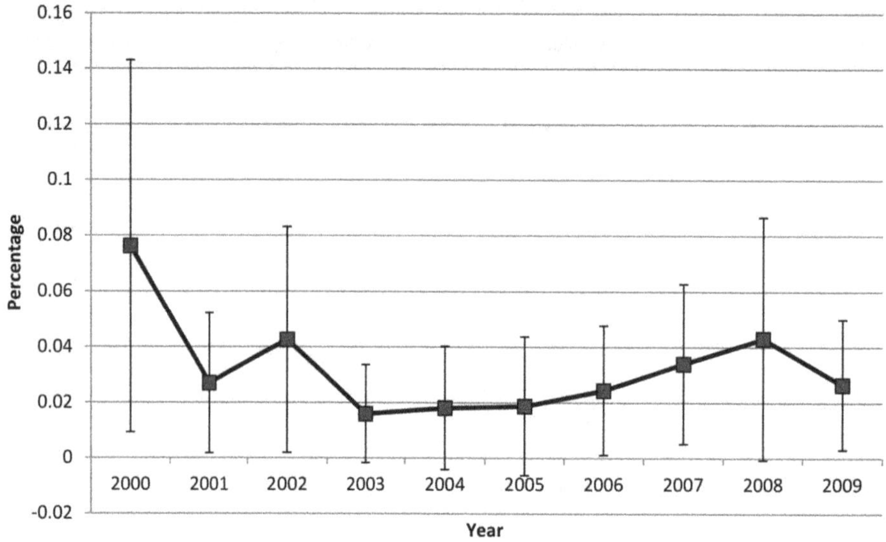

FIGURE 1 | ME/CFS patient visit trend, 2000–2009.

record (EHR) systems was observed in ME/CFS-related visits (35.91 vs. 42.95%).

ME/CFS Patient Visit Trend, 2000–2009

Overall 0.03% of ambulatory visits by patients aged 18 years or older were made by ME/CFS patients. The percentage of ME/CFS-related visits was 0.04% for physician office visits, 0.02% for OPD visits, and 0.01% for ED visits. These proportions did not change significantly over time. The percentage of ME/CFS-related visits ranged from 0.02 to 0.08% during 2000–2009, and there was no statistical evidence for a linearly increasing trend across year (p-value for the linear trend: 0.31) (**Figure 1**).

Vital Signs, Continuity of Care, Providers Seen, and Visit Disposition

Table 2 summarizes the information on vital signs, continuity of care, major reason for visits, providers seen, and visit disposition of ME/CFS and non-ME/CFS patients. The vital signs of patients visiting for ME/CFS and all others did not differ significantly. The number of visits during the past 12 months made by established ME/CFS patients was greater than that by non-CFS patients (5.60 vs. 4.35, $p = 0.202$). Of ME/CFS-related visits, the top three reasons for visits were chronic/routine problems (60.85%), new problems (14.86%), and chronic/flare up problems (11.47%). Physicians provided care for over 90% of the patient visits for both ME/CFS-related and non-ME/CFS visits. The rates of referral to other physicians did not differ significantly between ME/CFS-related and non-ME/CFS visits.

ME/CFS and Other Chronic Conditions as Co-morbidities

Table 3 shows chronic conditions recorded at ME/CFS-related and non-ME/CFS visits. The co-morbidity rate was higher in visits by patients with ME/CFS than those by patients without ME/CFS (71.30 vs. 61.18%). The most frequent chronic conditions among ME/CFS-related visits were depression (35.79%), hypertension (31.14%), diabetes (20.30%), arthritis (14.11%), and asthma (13.79%).

Healthcare Services and Quality

Table 4 compares quality of healthcare between ME/CFS-related visits and non-ME/CFS related visits. Physicians spent more time for ME/CFS-related visits than non-ME/CFS visits (23.62 vs. 19.38 min, $p = 0.065$). Fewer health counseling services were provided in ME/CFS-related visits than non-ME/CFS related visits (0.16 vs. 0.32 services per visit, $p = 0.126$). The most common counseling services provided during visits by ME/CFS patients were diet/nutrition (8.33%), exercise (8.21%), and smoking cessation (7.24%). Compared to non-ME/CFS visits, a lower proportion of ME/CFS-related visits was provided health education services on stress management (0.75 vs. 3.14%, $p = 0.010$), weight reduction (0.88 vs. 4.02%, $p = 0.002$), injury prevention (0.04 vs. 1.64%, $p < 0.001$), and family planning/contraception (0.17 vs. 1.45%, $p = 0.037$). Smoking cessation (tobacco use/expose) counseling was more prevalent in ME/CFS-related visits than non-ME/CFS visits (7.24 vs. 2.89%, $p = 0.386$). Contrary to health counseling services, more diagnostic/screening tests were provided in ME/CFS-related visits than non-ME/CFS visits (1.00 vs. 0.50 services per visit, $p = 0.132$). The most common diagnostic/screening tests provided during visits by ME/CFS patients were CBC (25.01%), glucose (19.05%), and lipids/cholesterol (12.84%), but did not reach any statistical significance level of 0.05. Non-medication treatment was more frequently provided at ME/CFS-related visits than non-ME/CFS visits (0.15 vs. 0.07 per visit, $p = 0.244$).

TABLE 2 | Vital sign and continuity of care ambulatory adult visits in USA, 2000–2009.

Variables	All visits	ME/CFS visits	Non-ME/CFS visits	*P*-value[a]
Unweighted no. of visits	748,464	130	748,334	
Weighted no. of visits	9,061,664,246	2,911,161	9,058,753,085	
Vital sign				
Body Mass Index (BMI)[1], mean (SD)	29.13 (7.18)	27.42 (4.60)	29.13 (7.18)	0.274
Body Mass Index (BMI)[1], median (range)	28.19 (8.14–98.91)	28.25 (19.66–51.58)	28.19 (8.14–98.91)	
Blood Pressure (systolic)[2], mean (SD)	128.22 (19.52)	126.38 (11.96)	128.22 (19.52)	0.607
Blood Pressure (systolic)[2], median (range)	129 (0–290)	121.5 (89–180)	129 (0–290)	
Blood Pressure (diastolic)[2], mean (SD)	76.16 (11.97)	75.72 (6.97)	76.16 (11.97)	0.803
Blood Pressure (diastolic)[2], median (range)	76 (0–190)	76 (37–109)	76 (0–190)	
Current tobacco user[3] (%)	11.51%	12.77%	11.51%	0.811
Continuity of care				
Established patient[4] (%)	87.04%	87.17%	87.04%	0.981
# of visits[5], mean (SD)	4.35 (6.29)	5.60 (3.80)	4.35 (6.29)	0.202
# of visits[5], median (range)	2 (0–99)	4 (0–21)	2(0–99)	
Prior-visit status[6]				0.144
None	8.64%	3.60%	8.64%	
1–2 visits	34.36%	29.53%	34.37%	
3–5 visits	24.43%	17.04%	24.43%	
6 or more visits	32.57%	49.83%	32.57%	
New patient[4]				0.306
Referred for this visit (%)	17.01%	10.08%	17.02%	
Not referred for this visit (%)	33.34%	44.86%	33.34%	
Unknown if referred (%)	49.65%	45.06%	49.65%	
Major reason for this visit[4]				0.007
Chronic problem, routine	35.21%	60.85%	35.21%	
New problem	32.17%	14.86%	32.18%	
Chronic problem, flare up	9.08%	11.47%	9.08%	
Preventive care	16.15%	9.55%	16.15%	
Pre-/Post-surgery	7.39%	3.26%	7.39%	
Providers at this visit				
Physician	94.21%	91.14%	94.21%	0.570
Physician assistant	3.94%	2.62%	3.94%	0.434
Nurse practitioner/Midwife	2.10%	0.00%	2.10%	0.000
RN/LPN	34.09%	29.79%	34.09%	0.537
Other	23.57%	32.09%	23.57%	0.284
Mental health provider[7]	0.55%	0.00%	0.55%	0.002
Visit disposition[3]				
Refer to other physician	8.06%	9.89%	8.06%	0.698

1. 05-09 NAMCS/OPD; 2. 03-09 NAMCS/OPD/ED; 3. 01-09 NAMCS/OPD; 4. 00-09 NAMCS/OPD; 5. 01-09 NAMCE/OPD and 07-09 ED; 6. 07-09 NAMCS/OPD/ED; 7. 07-09 NAMCS/OPD.

[a]p-values based on adjusted Wald tests with H_0, $Var|_{if\ ME/CFS} = Var|_{if\ NON-ME/CFS}$; Column percentages were listed in the table.

DISCUSSION

To our best knowledge, this is the first study that used a nationally representative healthcare sample of the U.S. to investigate the visit trend of diagnosing ME/CFS over years. This paper examined demographics, co-morbidities, and healthcare for visits by ME/CFS patients using a nationally representative sample of patient visits to physician offices, hospital outpatient departments, and emergency departments from 2000 to 2009. We found the overall estimated percentage of ME/CFS-related visits to be 0.03% with no statistical evidence (p-trend = 0.31) for a decline or increase from 2000 to 2009. Assuming no repeat visits by same patients, the percentage estimate of visits by ME/CFS patients would approximately reflect the prevalence estimates reported from previous studies in primary care settings.

Visits by ME/CFS patients report slightly more co-morbid conditions than visits by patients without ME/CFS. Over 70% of visits by ME/CFS patients report one or more co-morbid

TABLE 3 | ME/CFS and co-morbid conditions.

Variables	ME/CFS visits	Non-ME/CFS visits	*P*-value[a]
Unweighted no. of visits	130	748,334	
Weighted no. of visits[1]	1,354,662	4,307,118,192	
Chronic Conditions			
# of chronic conditions, mean (SD)	1.49 (1.05)	1.27 (1.40)	0.406
# of chronic conditions, median (range)	1 (0–6)	1 (0–13)	
# of chronic conditions (%)			0.343
No chronic condition	28.70%	37.82%	
1 chronic condition	19.19%	27.47%	
2 or more chronic conditions	52.11%	34.71%	
Depression	35.79%	10.67%	0.019
Hypertension	31.14%	30.66%	0.965
Diabetes	20.30%	13.27%	0.500
Arthritis	14.11%	15.83%	0.799
Asthma	13.79%	5.54%	0.239
Chronic obstructive pulmonary disease	12.90%	4.52%	0.372
Hyperlipidemia	11.58%	17.65%	0.443
Cancer	6.59%	6.92%	0.945
Cerebrovascular disease	1.64%	2.05%	0.808
Obesity	1.43%	8.13%	0.002
Osteoporosis	0.11%	3.18%	<0.001
Congestive heart failure	0.06%	2.20%	<0.001
Chronic renal failure	0.00%	1.84%	<0.001
Ischemic heart disease	0.00%	5.10%	<0.001

1. 05-09 NAMCS/OPD.

[a]p-values based on adjusted Wald tests with H_0, $Var|_{if\ ME/CFS} = Var|_{if\ NON-ME/CFS}$; Column percentages were listed in the table.

conditions, adding to complexity in ME/CFS healthcare. Our results on healthcare for visits by ME/CFS patients are mixed. While physicians spent more time during visits by ME/CFS patients than that by patients without ME/CFS, a lower portion of visits by ME/CFS patients was provided counseling for diet/nutrition, exercise, and weight reduction. On the other hand, a higher portion of visits by ME/CFS patients were provided diagnostic/screening tests and non-medication treatment twice as often as visits by non-ME/CFS patients.

Conclusion

In conclusion, we found that there is no increasing or decreasing trend in the percentage of ME/CFS-related visits during 2000–2009. Compared to visits by non-ME/CFS patients, visits by ME/CFS patients are provided more direct care time by physicians, more diagnostic/screening tests, and more non-medication treatments but less health counseling services. Future research should consider developing basic guidelines or recommendations for appropriate healthcare in ME/CFS-diagnosed visits such as providing weight reduction or nutrient/diet counseling for ME/CFS patients with greater BMI. When providing exercise counseling, one should be cautious of the impact of exercise. An individualized exercise

TABLE 4 | Quality indicators of healthcare between ME/CFS-related and non-ME/CFS related visits.

Variables	ME/CFS visits	Non-ME/CFS visits	*P*-value[a]
Unweighted no. of visits	130	748,334	
Weighted no. of visits	1,354,662	4,307,118,192	
Time Spent with Physician[1], mean (SD)	23.62 (14.86)	19.38 (13.83)	0.065
Time Spent with Physician[1], median (range)	20 (0–90)	15 (0–240)	
Health Education Services[2]			
# of services ordered, mean (SD)	0.16 (0.57)	0.32 (0.74)	0.126
# of services ordered, median (range)	0 (0–3)	0 (0–5)	
None (%)	92.00%	80.30%	
One (%)	0.21%	11.05%	
2 or more (%)	7.79%	8.65%	
Type of Health Education Services			
Diet/Nutrition[3]	8.33%	12.48%	0.306
Exercise[3]	8.21%	9.79%	0.677
Weight reduction[4]	0.88%	4.02%	0.002
Stress management[5]	0.75%	3.14%	0.010
Tobacco use/exposure[5]	7.24%	2.89%	0.386
Growth/Development[3]	2.97%	0.54%	0.412
Asthma education[4]	2.38%	0.91%	0.531
Injury prevention[7]	0.04%	1.64%	<0.001
Other health education[5]	23.74%	19.86%	0.702
Family planning/Contraception[8]	0.17%	1.45%	0.037
Diagnostic/Screening Services[9]			
# of services ordered, mean (SD)	1.00 (1.51)	0.50 (1.06)	0.132
# of services ordered, median (range)	0 (0–5)	0 (0–5)	
None (%)	57.73%	76.74%	
One (%)	20.32%	8.77%	
2 or more (%)	21.95%	14.49%	
Blood tests ordered: (%)			
CBC[10]	25.01%	15.03%	0.191
Glucose[11]	19.05%	8.63%	0.248
HgbA1c[12]	3.24%	3.53%	0.916
Lipids/Cholesterol[13]	12.84%	8.11%	0.330
Other blood test[14]	33.94%	15.12%	0.065
Non-Medication Treatment[5]			
# of treatments ordered, mean (SD)	0.15 (0.36)	0.07 (0.27)	0.244
# of treatments ordered, median (range)	0 (0–2)	0 (0–3)	
None (%)	84.78%	93.72%	
One (%)	15.17%	5.80%	
2 or more (%)	0.06%	0.48%	
CAM[7]	8.55%	1.09%	0.125
Physical therapy[5]	2.70%	2.65%	0.984
Psychotherapy[3]	0.61%	2.24%	0.003
Other mental health counseling[5]	0.06%	1.47%	<0.001

1. 00-09 NAMCS and 00 OPD; 2. 05-09 NAMCS/OPD; 3. 00-09 NAMCS/OPD; 4. 01-09 NAMCS/OPD; 5. 05-09 NAMCS/OPD; 6. 05-09 NAMCS/OPD; 7. 00, 05-09 NAMCS/OPD; 8. 00 & 09 NAMCS/OPD; 9. 05-09 NAMCS/OPD and 03-04 ED; 10. 01-09 NAMCS/OPD and 00-09 ED; 11. 03-09 NAMCS/OPD and 01-09 ED; 12. 03-09 NAMCS/OPD and 01-04 ED; 13. 00-09 NAMCS/OPD and 01-04 ED; 14. 00, 05-09 NAMCS/OPD and 00, 03-09 ED.

[a]p-values based on adjusted Wald tests with H_0, $Var|_{ifCFS} = Var|_{ifNON-CFS}$; Column percentages were listed in the table.

or activity management plan should be emphasized to balance rest and activity to avoid post-exertional malaise flare-ups. Before starting any individualized exercise or activity management program, one should be carefully assessed and monitored periodically on their muscle strength and functional status for any physical activity.

It will also allow for identifying the potential interrupted time series that might be resulted from future ICD coding transition/change and the impact of the 2015 IOM recommendation on ME/CFS. Future investigation on this topic is warranted.

Study Limitation

Several limitations of this study should be mentioned. First, NAMCS, and NHAMCS do not include identifiers for individual patients; therefore, some patients who made visits more than once may have had their visits counted independently, which would yield inaccurate estimates of the variance. The surveys used a randomly selected sampling unit (a physician or facility) with a reporting period of the randomly assigned 1-week for NAMCS and 4-week for NHAMCS. Although our results showed that on average ME/CFS patients made about 5.6 visits per year and that translated into one visit every 2 months, it's less likely that the same patient would visit to the same selected physician or facility during the randomly assigned 1-week reporting period. Therefore, we believe that this limitation might affect our conclusion only to a small degree. Second, the NAMCS and NHAMCS included at most only three diagnosis codes and chief complaints. A greater number of listed diagnosis codes was associated with a higher likelihood of identifying ME/CFS. Thus, we may not have been able to identify some ME/CFS patients who were diagnosed as ME/CFS in 4th or later diagnosis. There is an ICD-9-CM code 780.79 for "Other malaise and fatigue" which converts approximately to ICD-10-CM G93.3 for Postviral fatigue syndrome ([Benign] myalgic encephalomyelitis) but 780.79 was not commonly documented in this data source. Therefore, in our analysis we focused on visits with ICD-9-CM code, 780.71 for chronic fatigue syndrome. One should also be aware that the ME/CFS related visits might be under-reported due to the possibility of a substantial level of omissions by healthcare providers. Finally, due to the small number of cases identified one should be cautious of generalizing the results beyond the general healthcare setting.

ETHICS STATEMENT

This is a secondary analysis using publicly available data. This analysis was based on the National Ambulatory Medical Care Survey (NAMCS) (33) and the National Hospital Ambulatory Medical Care Survey (NHAMCS) (34) from 2000 to 2009. Since 1992, both surveys have been administrated by the National Center for Health Statistics (NCHS), Centers for Disease Control and Prevention (CDC) (35–38). The NCHS Research Ethics Review Board approved the protocols for both the NAMCS and NHAMCS surveys, including a waiver of the requirement for informed consent of participating patients.

AUTHOR CONTRIBUTIONS

JML had the original idea for the study. JML developed the analysis plan and JB performed all statistical analyses with guidance and support from JML. JB and JML drafted the paper and contributed to the interpretation and the final manuscript.

ACKNOWLEDGMENTS

This work was conducted primarily while JB was supported in part by an appointment to the Research Participation Program at the Centers for Disease Control and Prevention administered by the Oak Ridge Institute for Science and Education through an inter-agency agreement between the U.S. Department of Energy and the Centers for Disease Control and Prevention.

REFERENCES

1. Fukuda K, Straus SE, Hickie I, Sharpe MC, Dobbins JG, Komaroff A. The chronic fatigue syndrome: a comprehensive approach to its definition and study. *Ann Intern Med.* (1994) 121:953–9. doi: 10.7326/0003-4819-121-12-199412150-00009
2. Whiting P, Bagnall AM, Sowden AJ, Cornell JE, Mulrow CD, Ramírez G. Interventions for the treatment and management of chronic fatigue syndrome. *JAMA.* (2001) 286:1360–8. doi: 10.1001/jama.286.11.1360
3. Afari N, Buchwald D. Chronic fatigue syndrome: a review. *Am J Psychiatry.* (2003) 160:221–36. doi: 10.1176/appi.ajp.160.2.221
4. Institute of Medicine. *Beyond Myalgic Encephalomyelitis/Chronic Fatigue Syndrome: Redefining an Illness.* Washington, DC: The National Academies Press (2015). Available online at: http://www.nationalacademies.org/hmd/reports/2015/me-cfs.aspx
5. Rowe PC, Underhill RA, Friedman KJ, Gurwitt A, Medow MS, Schwartz MS, et al. Myalgic encephalomyelitis/chronic fatigue syndrome diagnosis and management in young people: a primer. *Front Pediatr.* (2017) 5:121. doi: 10.3389/fped.2017.00121
6. Komaroff AL. Myalgic encephalomyelitis/chronic fatigue syndrome: a real illness. *Ann Intern Med.* (2015) 162:871–2. doi: 10.7326/M15-0647
7. Price RK, North CS, Wessely S, Fraser VJ. Estimating the prevalence of chronic fatigue syndrome and associated symptoms in the community. *Public Health Rep.* (1992) 107:514–22.
8. Lawrie SM, Pelosi AJ. Chronic fatigue syndrome in the community. Prevalence and associations. *Br J Psychiatry.* (1995) 166:793–7. doi: 10.1192/bjp.166.6.793
9. Jason LA, Jordan KM, Richman JA, Rademaker AW, Huang CF, Mccready W, et al. A community-based study of prolonged fatigue and chronic fatigue. *J Health Psychol.* (1999) 4:9–26. doi: 10.1177/135910539900400103
10. Bates DW, Schmitt W, Buchwald D, Ware NC, Lee J, Thoyer E, et al. Prevalence of fatigue and chronic fatigue syndrome in a primary care practice. *Arch Intern Med.* (1993) 153:2759–65. doi: 10.1001/archinte.153.24.2759
11. Wessely S, Chalder T, Hirsch S, Wallace P, Wright D. The prevalence and morbidity of chronic fatigue and chronic fatigue syndrome: a prospective primary care study. *Am J Public Health.* (1997) 87:1449–55. doi: 10.2105/AJPH.87.9.1449
12. Ranjith G. Epidemiology of chronic fatigue syndrome. *Occup Med.* (2005) 55:13–9. doi: 10.1093/occmed/kqi012
13. Reeves W, Jones JF, Maloney E, Heim C, Hoaglin DC, Boneva RS, et al. Prevalence of chronic fatigue syndrome in metropolitan, urban, and rural Georgia. *Popul Health Metr.* (2007) 5:5 doi: 10.1186/1478-7954-5-5

14. Dinos S, Khoshaba B, Ashby D, White PD, Nazroo J, Wessely S, et al. A systematic review of chronic fatigue, its syndromes and ethnicity: prevalence, severity, co-morbidity and coping. *Int J Epidemiol.* (2009) 38:1554–70. doi: 10.1093/ije/dyp147
15. Nacul LC, Lacerda EM, Campion P, Pheby D, Drachler MDL, Leite JC, et al. The functional status and well being of people with myalgic encephalomyelitis/chronic fatigue syndrome and their carers. *BMC Public Health.* (2011) 11:402. doi: 10.1186/1471-2458-11-402
16. Johnston S, Brenu EW, Staines D, Marshall-Gradisnik S, Johnston S, Brenu EW, et al. The prevalence of chronic fatigue syndrome/myalgic encephalomyelitis: a meta-analysis. *Clin Epidemiol.* (2013) 5:105–10. doi: 10.2147/CLEP.S39876
17. Steele L, Dobbins J, Fukuda K, Reyes M, Randall B, Koppelman M, et al. The epidemiology of chronic fatigue in San Francisco. *Am J Med.* (1998) 105:83S—90S. doi: 10.1016/S0002-9343(98)00158-2
18. Vincent A, Brimmer DJ, Whipple MO, Jones JF, Boneva R, Lahr BD, et al. Prevalence, incidence, and classification of chronic fatigue syndrome in olmsted county, minnesota, as estimated using the rochester epidemiology project. *Mayo Clin Proc.* (2012) 87:1145–52. doi: 10.1016/j.mayocp.2012.08.015
19. Reynolds KJ, Vernon SD, Bouchery E, Reeves WC. The economic impact of chronic fatigue syndrome. *Cost Effect Resource Allocation.* (2004) 2:4. doi: 10.1186/1478-7547-2-4
20. Jason LA, Benton MC, Valentine L, Johnson A, Torres-Harding S. The economic impact of ME/CFS: individual and societal costs. *Dynamic Med.* (2008) 7:6. doi: 10.1186/1476-5918-7-6
21. Lin JMS, Resch SC, Brimmer DJ, Johnson A, Kennedy S, Burstein N, et al. The economic impact of chronic fatigue syndrome in Georgia: direct and indirect costs. *Cost Effect Resource Allocation.* (2011) 9:1. doi: 10.1186/1478-7547-9-1
22. Komaroff AL, Fagioli LR, Geiger AM, Doolittle TH, Lee J, Kornish RJ, et al. An examination of the working case definition of chronic fatigue syndrome. *Am J Med.* (1996) 100:56–4. doi: 10.1016/S0002-9343(96)90012-1
23. Goldenberg DL, Simms RW, Geiger A, Komaroff AL. High frequency of fibromyalgia in patients with chronic fatigue seen in a primary care practice. *Arthritis Rheum.* (1990) 33:381–7. doi: 10.1002/art.1780330311
24. Buchwald D, Garrity D. Comparison of patients with chronic fatigue syndrome, fibromyalgia, and multiple chemical sensitivities. *Arch Intern Med.* (1994) 154:2049–53. doi: 10.1001/archinte.1994.00420180053007
25. Jason LA, Taylor RR, Kennedy CL. Chronic fatigue syndrome, fibromyalgia, and multiple chemical sensitivities in a community-based sample of persons with chronic fatigue syndrome-like symptoms. *Psychosom Med.* (2000) 62:655–63. doi: 10.1097/00006842-200009000-00009
26. Warren JW, Langenberg P, Clauw DJ. The number of existing functional somatic syndromes (FSSs) is an important risk factor for new, different FSSs. *J Psychosom Res.* (2013) 74:12–7. doi: 10.1016/j.jpsychores.2012.09.002
27. Rusu C, Gee ME, Lagacé C, Parlor M. Chronic fatigue syndrome and fibromyalgia in Canada: prevalence and associations with six health status indicators. *Health Promot Chronic Dis Prev Can.* (2015) 35:3–11. doi: 10.24095/hpcdp.35.1.02
28. DeJean D, Giacomini M, Vanstone M, Brundisini F. Patient experiences of depression and anxiety with chronic disease: a systematic review and qualitative meta-synthesis. *Ont Health Technol Assess Ser.* (2013) 13:1–33.
29. Nater UM, Lin JM, Maloney EM, Jones JF, Tian H, Boneva RS, et al. Psychiatric comorbidity in persons with chronic fatigue syndrome identified from the Georgia population. *Psychosom Med.* (2009) 71:557–65. doi: 10.1097/PSY.0b013e31819ea179
30. Aaron LA, Herrell R, Ashton S, Belcourt M, Schmaling K, Goldberg J, et al. Comorbid clinical conditions in chronic fatigue: a co-twin control study. *J Gen Intern Med.* (2001) 16:24–31. doi: 10.1046/j.1525-1497.2001.03419.x
31. Lin JMS, Brimmer DJ, Boneva RS, Jones JF, Reeves WC. Barriers to healthcare utilization in fatiguing illness: a population-based study in Georgia. *BMC Health Serv Res.* (2009) 9:13. doi: 10.1186/1472-6963-9-13
32. Brimmer DJ, Fridinger F, Lin JMS, Reeves WC. US healthcare providers' knowledge, attitudes, beliefs, and perceptions concerning Chronic Fatigue Syndrome. *BMC Family Pract.* (2010) 11:28. doi: 10.1186/1471-2296-11-28
33. National Center for Health Statistics: The National Ambulatory Medical Care Survey. *Centers for Disease Control and Prevention, U.S. Department of Health and Human Services.* Available online at: http://www.cdc.gov/nchs/ahcd/about_ahcd.htm
34. National Center for Health Statistics: The National Hospital Ambulatory Medical Care Survey. *Centers for Disease Control and Prevention, U.S. Department of Health and Human Services.* Available online at: http://www.cdc.gov/nchs/ahcd/about_ahcd.htm
35. Schappert SM, Rechtsteiner EA. Ambulatory medical care utilization estimates for 2007. *Vital and Health Stat.* (2011) 169:1–38.
36. Hing E, Hall MJ, Ashman JJ, XU J. National hospital ambulatory medical care survey: 2007 outpatient department summary. *National Health Stat Rep.* (2010) 28:1–32.
37. Hsiao CJ, Cherry DK, Beatty PC, Rechtsteiner EA. National ambulatory medical care survey: 2007 summary. *National Health Stat Rep.* (2010) 27:1–32.
38. Niska R, Bhuiya F, Xu J. National hospital ambulatory medical care survey: 2007 emergency department summary. *Natl Health Stat Rep.* (2010) 386:1–31. doi: 10.1037/e587172010-001
39. Ma J, Stafford RS. Quality of US outpatient care: temporal changes and racial/ethnic disparities. *Arch Intern Med.* (2005) 165:1354–61. doi: 10.1001/archinte.165.12.1354
40. Edwards ST, Mafi JN, Landon BE. Trends and quality of care in outpatient visits to generalist and specialist physicians delivering primary care in the United States, 1997-2010. *J Gen Intern Med.* (2014) 29:947–55. doi: 10.1007/s11606-014-2808-y

Disclaimer: The findings and conclusions in this report are those of the authors and do not necessarily represent the official position of the Centers for Disease Control and Prevention.

14

Low Sensitivity of Abbreviated Tilt Table Testing for Diagnosing Postural Tachycardia Syndrome in Adults with ME/CFS

C. (Linda) M. C. van Campen[1]*, Peter C. Rowe*[2*] *and Frans C. Visser*[1]

[1] *Stichting CardioZorg, Hoofddorp, Netherlands,* [2] *Department of Pediatrics, Johns Hopkins University School of Medicine, Baltimore, MD, United States*

***Correspondence:**
Peter C. Rowe
prowe@jhmi.edu

Introduction: Orthostatic intolerance is common among individuals with myalgic encephalomyelitis/chronic fatigue syndrome (ME/CFS). In some ME/CFS case definitions, orthostatic intolerance is considered a core feature of the disorder. Some studies have employed tilt table tests lasting 2–5 min to diagnose one common form of orthostatic intolerance, postural tachycardia syndrome (POTS). We examined the diagnostic yield of abbreviated durations of tilt testing in adults meeting criteria for ME/CFS, and identified the proportion with POTS misdiagnosed using testing of <10 min.

Methods: Eligible participants were consecutive individuals satisfying study criteria for ME/CFS and POTS evaluated at the Stichting CardioZorg (SCZ, Hoofddorp, NL) between November 2012 and August 2018. Individuals being treated with medications commonly used to manage orthostatic intolerance were excluded. Head-up tilt table testing involved 15 min of supine posture then 20 min at 70 degrees upright. Only the data from the first 10-min upright were used. POTS was defined as an increase in HR during a maximum of 10 min of upright tilt of at least 30 beats per minute (bpm), in the absence of either classical or delayed orthostatic hypotension. We measured the time until HR criteria for POTS were reached using survival curves, and compared survival curves between subgroups divided by age, sex, disease duration, and degree of hypocapnia during the test.

Results: Of 627 individuals with ME/CFS evaluated during the study period, 155 met criteria for POTS. The median time to reaching HR criteria for POTS was 3 min. A two-minute tilt table test would miss 55% (95% CI, 48–63%) of those meeting POTS criteria over the course of 10 min upright. The median time to reaching HR criteria for POTS did not differ by sex, age, duration of ME/CFS, or hypocapnia during tilt.

Conclusions: Abbreviated tilt table testing misses a substantial proportion of those ultimately diagnosed with POTS during a 10-min tilt table test, and should be abandoned for the clinical diagnosis and in epidemiologic studies designed to estimate the prevalence of POTS among those with ME/CFS.

Keywords: postural tachycardia syndrome, orthostatic intolerance, tilt table test, myalgic encephalomyelitis, chronic fatigue syndrome

INTRODUCTION

Orthostatic tachycardia has been associated with clinical syndromes that resemble myalgic encephalomyelitis/chronic fatigue syndrome (ME/CFS) since at least 1940, when McLean and Allen described a group of patients who experienced excessive heart rate acceleration and hypotension after shifting from a recumbent to an upright posture (1, 2). Studies in the 1990s brought further attention to the association between ME/CFS and various forms of orthostatic hypotension or postural tachycardia syndrome (POTS) (3–8). Although neglected in the Fukuda criteria for CFS (9), and underemphasized in the ME criteria (9, 10), orthostatic intolerance is now considered a core feature in the Institute of Medicine ME/CFS criteria (11).

The various consensus criteria for POTS all require a heart rate (HR) increase of at least 30 beats per minute over the course of 10 min upright for adults (or at least 40 bpm for those 12–19 years) compared to measurements in the supine position (12–14). These HR changes can be assessed using either passive or active standing maneuvers, or head-up tilt testing (15–21). The diagnosis of POTS also requires the absence of orthostatic hypotension (OH), although the 2011 consensus criteria are somewhat unclear as to whether this refers just to OH during the first 3 min or also to delayed OH after the 3-min point. While all of the criteria mention that POTS is usually associated with chronic orthostatic symptoms, not all criteria specifically require this.

When POTS is diagnosed using the 2011 consensus criteria, the duration upright would need to be 10 min. Questions have been raised about whether a shorter period of study would be sufficient, or could identify a more impaired patient population. For example, the seminal early study by Schondorf and colleagues used a 5-min period of head-up tilt (22). Braune and colleagues have suggested that a 2-min duration of upright posture is sufficient for the diagnosis in most instances (20). A 2-min period of standing was adopted by Hoad and colleagues in defining a 27% prevalence of POTS among those with ME/CFS (23). Stewart and colleagues suggested a 5-min tilt test might suffice for diagnosing POTS in the pediatric population (14).

Roma and colleagues have recently reported that an abbreviated 2-min test would miss 53% of those who ultimately satisfy heart rate criteria for POTS over 10 min of passive standing (24). In that study of young people (median age 17 years) the median time to POTS was 3 min. Those diagnosed in the first 5 min upright had higher peak heart rates than those diagnosed in the final 5 min, and were more likely to reach a peak HR > 120 bpm. Symptom provocation during the standing test, however, was similar for the sub-groups meeting POTS criteria early vs. late in the 10 min upright.

We sought to re-examine the diagnostic yield of abbreviated orthostatic testing in a sample of patients from an adult as opposed to a primarily adolescent population with ME/CFS, using tilt testing as the form of orthostatic stress rather than passive standing.

MATERIALS AND METHODS

Eligible Participants

Consecutive individuals satisfying study criteria for ME/CFS and POTS were included in this study if they had been evaluated at the SCZ (Stichting CardioZorg) between November 2012 and August 2018. The SCZ is a specialty clinic in Hoofddorp, The Netherlands. All participants had been referred by their general practitioners for either ME/CFS or orthostatic intolerance. No participants were self-referred. The use of clinical data for descriptive studies was approved by the ethics committee of the Slotervaart Hospital.

ME/CFS was considered present if participants met both the 1994 International Chronic Fatigue Syndrome Study Group criteria for CFS (25) and the 2011 international consensus definition of ME (10). Participants with ME/CFS entered the study with the expectation that they would be followed and treated clinically.

All participants were evaluated by the same experienced clinician (FV), who conducted a history and physical examination to confirm or establish the diagnosis of ME/CFS, and also conducted a tilt table test. For the tilt testing component, individuals being treated with medications that could lower heart rate or blood pressure (for example, beta-adrenergic antagonists, anti-hypertensive medications, or ivabradine) were excluded, as were those being treated with midodrine, fludrocortisone, desmopressin, pyridostigmine bromide, or stimulant medications. Individuals being treated with selective serotonin reuptake inhibitors or serotonin norepinephrine reuptake inhibitors continued to take these medications.

Tilt Test Methods

Participants were studied in a climate-controlled room where the temperatures range from 22 to 24 degrees C. No intravenous or intra-arterial cannulation was employed. Nasal prongs were placed to measure expired carbon dioxide ($CO2$) concentrations. Individuals were positioned supine for 15 min before a motorized table brought them to a 70-degree upright position over approximately 30 s. Participants remained in the head-up tilt position for up to 20 min. The test was prematurely stopped at the request of the patient, or if the individual developed syncope or presyncope. For this study, only the data from the first 10-min upright were used. Testing was conducted at least 3 h after a light meal. Participants were encouraged to ingest an ample amount of fluid on the day of the procedure, but did not drink fluids in the 2 h before the test. Heart rate (HR), systolic, diastolic, and mean blood pressures (SBP, DBP, and MAP) were continuously recorded by finger plethysmography using the Nexfin device (BMeye, Amsterdam, NL). HR and BP data were extracted from the Nexfin device and imported into an Excel spreadsheet, and a curve-fitting procedure was used to define heart rate and BP data for the pre-test supine HR and at each discrete 1-min interval during the test (GraphPad Prism, version 6.05, GraphPad Software, La Jolla, California, USA, www.graphpad.com).

Definition of POTS

We used the 2011 consensus definition for POTS, which requires a sustained increase in HR during a maximum of 10 min of upright tilt of at least 30 beats per minute (bpm) in those >19 years (12). The peak HR was compared to the calculated HR value at the end of the 15-min supine period. POTS was diagnosed only if there was no orthostatic hypotension (a decrease in systolic blood pressure of 20 mmHg or a decrease in diastolic blood pressure of 10 mmHg) within the first 3 min of tilt (classical OH), and additionally if there was no delayed OH during the 10 min upright.

We considered the HR criteria for POTS to have been reached when the HR during tilt first reached a 30 bpm increase from the HR at the end of the 15 min supine. We analyzed the survival curves of the time until HR criteria for POTS were reached using Graph Pad Prism. We compared survival curves between subgroups divided by age, sex, disease duration, end-tidal CO2, and serotonin reuptake inhibitor status with the Mantel-Haenszel hazard ratio, using the Mantel-Cox log rank test to determine whether differences between curves were significant. We used 95% confidence intervals (CI) for the estimates of the proportion of patients with POTS who would be missed if the test were stopped at each 1-min interval.

RESULTS

A total of 627 individuals with ME/CFS were evaluated at the Stichting CardioZorg during the study period. We excluded those with classical OH ($N = 16$), delayed OH ($N = 91$), vaso-vagal syncope ($N = 6$), and a normal BP and HR response to tilt ($N = 351$). We also excluded subjects whose diagnosis of POTS was based on having a HR over 120 bpm standing ($N = 4$) but who did not reach a 30 bpm HR increase. Four others were excluded because insufficient data were available ($N = 4$). No participants had a co-morbid diagnosis of diabetes mellitus, SLE, rheumatoid arthritis, or Sjogren syndrome. We did not ascertain whether participants had antibodies to adrenergic receptors or an auto-immune form of POTS. This left 155 participants who met study criteria for both ME/CFS and POTS. **Table 1** shows the demographic characteristics of the study population as well as baseline pre-tilt circulatory values and highest HR and BP or lowest CO2 values during tilt. Eighteen of the 155 participants (12%) were being treated with serotonin reuptake inhibitor medications at the time of tilt testing.

Figure 1 illustrates the cumulative incidence of reaching HR criteria for POTS during the 10 min of upright tilt testing. The median time to reaching HR criteria for POTS was 3 min. In all participants, the HR remained elevated for the duration of the testing. **Table 2** shows the proportion of participants in whom the diagnosis of POTS would have been missed if shorter durations of orthostatic stress were employed.

Figures 2A–D shows the survival curve differences by sex, age, duration of disease, and end tidal CO2 values, respectively. The median time to reaching HR criteria for POTS was 3 min for females and 4 min for males (Mantel-Haenszel ratio, 1.3; 95% CI, 0.69–2.41; $P = 0.42$). Using a cut-point for age at the median age of our study population, there was no difference in the time to reaching HR criteria for POTS by those under 33 vs. 33 or older (Mantel-Haenszel ratio, 1.1; 95% CI, 0.72–1.58; $P = 0.74$). Using a cut-point for disease duration at the median for participants in the study, there was no difference in the time to reaching HR criteria for POTS among subjects with a disease duration of <7 years vs. more than 7 years (Mantel-Haenszel ratio, 1.12; 95% CI, 0.76–1.66; $P = 0.56$). There was no difference in the time to reaching HR criteria for POTS among subjects with an end-tidal CO2 level at the end of 10 min of <30 vs. 30 mm Hg or more (Mantel-Haenszel ratio, 1.22; 95% CI 0.89–1.85; $P = 0.28$). There was no difference in the time to reaching HR criteria for POTS for those being treated with serotonin reuptake inhibitors compared

TABLE 1 | Demographic and circulatory characteristics of the study population*.

DEMOGRAPHIC	
Female	91%
Height	173 (8) cm
Weight	69 (15) kg
Caucasian	100%
Age (years)	33 (10)
Median duration of ME/CFS	7 years
CIRCULATORY	
Supine systolic BP	131 (15)
Supine diastolic BP	79 (8)
Supine end-tidal CO2‡	36 (4)
Supine HR	79 (14)
Peak HR during tilt	118 (20)
Peak systolic BP	125 (18)
Peak diastolic BP	85 (11)
10 min upright end-tidal CO2‡	26 (6)

Unless otherwise specified, these values represent mean (SD). Blood pressure and end-tidal CO2 units are mm Hg.
‡End-tidal CO2 measures were available for 147/155 participants.

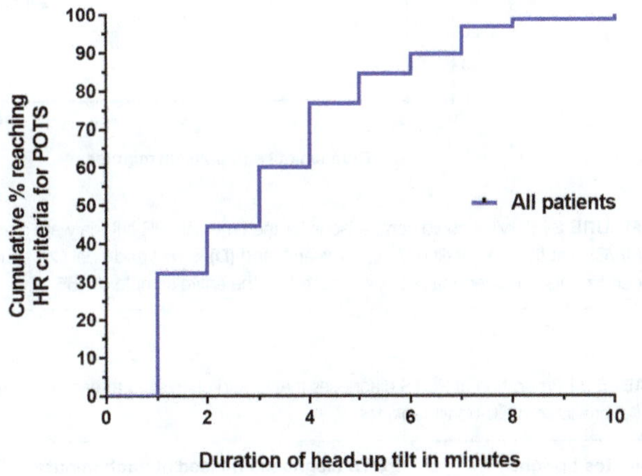

FIGURE 1 | Survival curve of the time until HR criteria for POTS were reached for all 155 participants with ME/CFS.

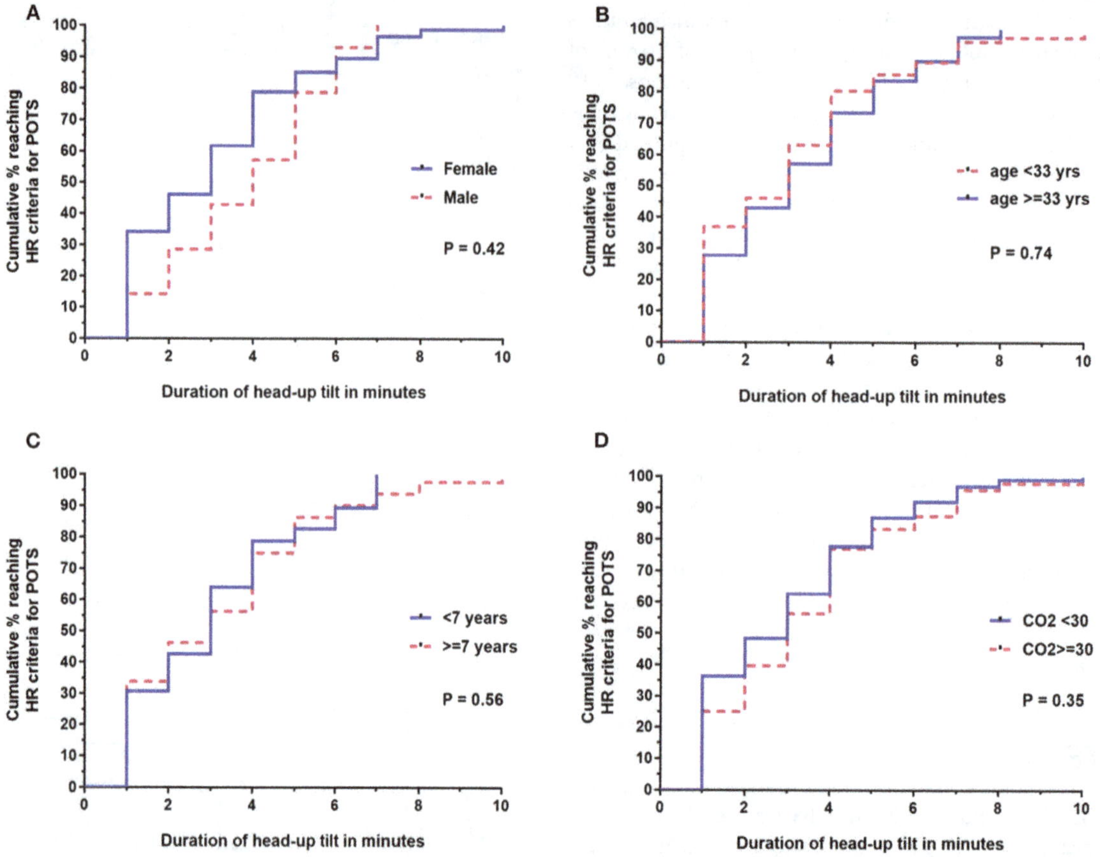

FIGURE 2 | Survival curve comparisons for the time until HR criteria were reached for ME/CFS subsets based on **(A)** sex, **(B)** age (<33 vs. ≥33 years), **(C)** duration of ME/CFS at the time of tilt (<7 vs. ≥7 years), and **(D)** lowest end-tidal CO2 during tilt (<30 vs. ≥30 mm Hg). End-tidal CO2 data were available for 147/155 participants; all other analyses were based on the entire sample of 155.

TABLE 2 | Proportion of POTS diagnoses that would be missed at each minute of an abbreviated head-up tilt table test.

Minutes upright	POTS diagnoses missed at each minute	
	%	(95% CI)
1	68	(60–75)
2	55	(48–63)
3	40	(33–48)
4	23	(17–30)
5	15	(11–22)
6	10	(6–16)
7	3	(1–7)
8	2	(0–4)
9	2	(0–4)
10	0	

to those not being treated (Mantel-Haenszel ratio, 0.89; 95% CI, 0.0.50–1.59; $P = 0.69$).

One hundred thirty-one (85%) met HR criteria for POTS during the first 5 min upright vs. 24 (15%) in the last 5 min upright. The proportion with a peak HR of ≥ 120 was 47% in the early group and 21% in the late group ($P = 0.02$, Fisher's exact test).

DISCUSSION

The main finding of this study is that for adults with ME/CFS, abbreviated tilt table testing has the potential to miss a substantial proportion of those ultimately diagnosed with POTS during a 10-min tilt table test. A two-minute test would miss 55% (95% CI, 48–63%), emphasizing the limitations of POTS prevalence estimates based on abbreviated orthostatic testing. The median time to reaching HR criteria for POTS during tilt testing was 3 min, identical to the findings of Roma and colleagues in younger individuals who were studied using a passive standing test (24). We found no differences in the time to reaching the HR criteria for POTS based on age, sex, duration of ME/CFS, or the end-tidal CO2 levels at the end of the 10 min upright.

Other studies have examined the optimal time to tilt testing for the diagnosis of POTS (26). In 28 patients selected for tilt testing based on a suspicion of POTS, but in whom the ME/CFS status was not reported, Carew and colleagues reported that all 28 meeting HR criteria for POTS had done so by 7 min of 70-degree tilt, whereas none of 28 age-matched controls had developed a sustained tachycardia (26). While our study identified an additional 3% with POTS after the 7-min point, this minor variability in outcomes is likely related to the larger sample size in our study. Carew and colleagues concluded that the full 10 min of tilt was required to diagnose POTS.

The time to reaching HR criteria for POTS in our study among adults was the same as that for a primarily adolescent and young adult population. However, the proportion with a peak HR of 120 bpm or higher in the first 5 min of tilt was 47%, which compares to just 26% in the Roma study (24 Plash and colleagues reported a mean HR increase for those with POTS that was five beats higher after 5 min of upright tilt than after the same period of active standing, although this difference did not reach statistical significance until participants with POTS and healthy controls were combined (17). In their combined study population, a higher HR during passive tilt vs. active standing was present for all 5-min intervals of the 30 min of upright posture. A potential contributor to this difference, among other physiologic changes, is that active standing involves greater use of the leg muscles, more postural sway than tilt, and greater engagement of the abdominal muscles, all of which can combine to increase venous return to the heart (17). The "passive" element of a passive standing test involves leaning back against a wall, which reduces postural sway, but the leg and abdominal muscles are nonetheless expected to be more actively engaged while standing than during upright tilt. As a result, we believe the more robust HR changes in the first 5 min of tilt testing in this study compared to that of Roma and colleagues could be related in part to differences between the forms of orthostatic testing in the two studies. Other important differences such as age and disease duration could also play a role.

Among the strengths of this study are its relatively large sample size, the lack of variability in the application of diagnostic criteria due to a single examiner, a consistent tilt testing protocol, and the fact that participants satisfied the definitions for both ME and CFS. One limitation is that the study may not be applicable to all individuals with POTS, as the study enrolled only those with POTS and ME/CFS. Adults meeting case definitions for both ME/CFS and POTS report a significantly greater prevalence of severe fatigue, unrefreshing sleep, muscle pain, post exertional fatigue, and headaches than those with POTS alone (27). Similar observations of increased symptom burden for those with CFS and POTS vs. POTS alone results have been found in pediatric patients (8). Without data on time to reaching HR criteria for those with POTS in the absence of ME/CFS, we are unsure what effect the differences in general symptom burden would have on our results, and we do not have data to suggest that our findings can be extrapolated with confidence to those with POTS alone.

All individuals in this study had chronic orthostatic symptoms. The proportion of individuals with ME/CFS who have exaggerated postural tachycardia during tilt in the absence of chronic orthostatic intolerance symptoms is difficult to determine. All those with ME/CFS have chronic symptoms of fatigue and exercise intolerance, which are viewed in the autonomic literature to be features consistent with orthostatic intolerance. A high proportion with ME/CFS have lightheadedness, 96% in some studies (5), and 61% report intolerance of being on their feet (28). Across several studies, over 90% with ME/CFS report cognitive dysfunction, but in most ME/CFS studies, little effort is made to distinguish whether these symptoms are a consequence of orthostatic stress or due to some other contributor to ME/CFS pathophysiology. Some of the variability in the reporting of orthostatic symptoms in the ME/CFS literature is due to differences in the comprehensiveness with which orthostatic intolerance symptoms are ascertained (11). We are not aware of data reporting an exaggerated tachycardia among those with ME/CFS in the absence of chronic orthostatic symptoms.

We did not perform more extensive autonomic testing using quantitative sudomotor axon reflex testing, Valsalva, or heart rate variability measures to identify specific pathophysiologic subgroups of those with POTS, nor did we evaluate for small fiber neuropathy. Our focus was to determine whether abbreviated testing would miss a high proportion of those meeting the current definitions for POTS. Future studies will be able to examine whether specific POTS subgroups have different heart rate responses to upright tilt, and whether healthy controls have a parallel HR elevation at different points of the tilt test. Future studies with healthy controls will also be able to ascertain whether the interaction between time and HR elevation is similar in healthy individuals.

Participants in this study were not being treated with medications typically used to directly modulate heart rate and blood pressure, and only 18 individuals (12%) were being treated with SSRI or SNRI medications at the time of tilt testing. The survival curves of the time to reaching HR criteria for POTS, however, did not differ between those on SSRI/SNRI medications and those not being treated, suggesting that medication status did not affect the results. We acknowledge that serotonin has the potential to affect vascular tone (both vasoconstriction and vasodilation) (29), and the SNRI medications in the clinical setting can raise BP, but our data suggest a limited or absent impact on the detection of POTS among those with ME/CFS. The impact of these medications on other forms of orthostatic intolerance remains to be determined.

We conclude that abbreviated orthostatic testing should be abandoned in epidemiologic and clinical studies designed to estimate the prevalence of POTS among those with ME/CFS, in whom a full 10-min of tilt testing improves the sensitivity of the test for identifying POTS.

AUTHOR CONTRIBUTIONS

CvC, PR, and FV conceived the study, CvC and FV collected the data, CvC performed the primary data analysis and FV and PR performed secondary data analyses. All authors were involved in the drafting and review of the manuscript.

ACKNOWLEDGMENTS

We thank the ME/CFS patients whose participation made this study possible and Colleen L. Marden for help with the Figures. PR is supported by the Sunshine Natural Wellbeing Foundation Professorship of Chronic Fatigue and Related Disorders.

REFERENCES

1. MacLean AR, Allen EV. Orthostatic hypotension and orthostatic tachycardia: treatment with the "head-up" bed. *JAMA* (1940) 115:2162–7.
2. MacLean AR, Allen EV, Magath TB. Orthostatic hypotension and orthostatic tachycardia: defects in the return of venous blood to the heart. *Am Heart J* (1944) 27:145–63. doi: 10.1016/S0002-8703(44)90720-9
3. Streeten DHP, Anderson GH. Delayed orthostatic intolerance. *Arch Int Med.* (1992) 152:1066–72. doi: 10.1001/archinte.1992.00400170138025
4. Rowe PC, Bou-Holaigah I, Kan JS, Calkins H. Is neurally mediated hypotension an unrecognised cause of chronic fatigue? *Lancet* (1995) 345:623–4.
5. Bou-Holaigah I, Rowe PC, Kan J, Calkins H. Relationship between neurally mediated hypotension and the chronic fatigue syndrome. *JAMA* (1995) 274:961–7. doi: 10.1001/jama.1995.03530120053041
6. Freeman R, Komaroff AL. Does the chronic fatigue syndrome involve the autonomic nervous system? *Am J Med.* (1997) 102:357–64. doi: 10.1016/S0002-9343(97)00087-9
7. De Lorenzo F, Hargreaves J, Kakkar VV. Pathogenesis and management of delayed orthostatic hypotension in patients with chronic fatigue syndrome. *Clin Autonom Res.* (1997) 7:185–90. doi: 10.1007/BF02267980
8. Stewart JM, Gewitz MH, Weldon A, Arlievsky N, Li K, Munoz J. Orthostatic intolerance in adolescent chronic fatigue syndrome. *Pediatrics* (1999) 103:116–21. doi: 10.1542/peds.103.1.116
9. Carruthers BM, Jain AK, De Meirleir KL, Peterson DL, Klimas NG, Lerner AM, et al. Myalgic encephalomyelitis/chronic fatigue syndrome: clinical working case definition. *J Chronic Fatigue Synd.* (2003) 11:7–115. doi: 10.1300/J092v11n01_02
10. Carruthers BM, Van de Sande MI, De Meirleir KL, Klimas NG, Broderick G, Mitchell T, et al. Myalgic encephalomyelitis: International consensus criteria. *J Int. Med.* (2011) 270:327–38. doi: 10.1111/j.1365-2796.2011.02428.x
11. Institute of Medicine. *Committee on the Diagnostic Criteria for Myalgic Encephalomyelitis/Chronic Fatigue Syndrome. Beyond Myalgic Encephalomyelitis/Chronic Fatigue Syndrome: Redefining an Illness* Washington, DC: The National Academies Press (2015).
12. Freeman R, Wieling W, Axelrod FB, Benditt DG, Benarroch E, Biaggioni I, et al. Consensus statement on the definition of orthostatic hypotension, neurally mediated syncope and the postural tachycardia syndrome. *Clin Auton Res.* (2011) 21:69–72. doi: 10.1007/s10286-011-0119-5
13. Sheldon RS, Grubb BP, Olshansky B, Shen W-K, Calkins H, Brignole M, et al. Society expert consensus statement on the diagnosis and treatment of postural tachycardia syndrome, inappropriate sinus tachycardia, and vasovagal syncope. *Heart Rhythm.* (2015) 12:e41–63. doi: 10.1016/j.hrthm.2015.03.029
14. Stewart JM, Boris JR, Chelimsky G, Fischer PR, Fortunato JE, Grubb BP, et al. Pediatric disorders of orthostatic intolerance. *Pediatrics* (2018) 141:e20171673. doi: 10.1542/peds.2017-1673
15. Hyatt KH, Jacobson LB, Schneider VS. Comparison of 70° tilt, LBNP, and passive standing as measures of orthostatic tolerance. *Aviat Space Environ Med.* (1975) 46:801–8.
16. Streeten DHP, Thomas D, Bell DS. The roles of orthostatic hypotension, orthostatic tachycardia, and subnormal erythrocyte volume in the pathogenesis of chronic fatigue syndrome. *Am J Med Sci.* (2000) 320:1–8. doi: 10.1016/S0002-9629(15)40790-6
17. Plash WB, Diedrich A, Biaggioni I, Garland EM, Paranjape SY, Black BK, et al. Diagnosing postural tachycardia syndrome: Comparison of tilt testing compared with standing haemodynamics. *Clin Science.* (2012) 124:109–14. doi: 10.1042/CS20120276
18. Kirbis M, Grad A, Meglic B, Bajrovic F. Comparison of active standing test, head-up tilt test and 24-hour ambulatory heart rate and blood pressure monitoring in diagnosing postural tachycardia syndrome. *Funct Neurol.* (2013) 28:39–46.
19. Winker R, Prager W, Haider A, Salameh B, Rudiger HW. Schellong test in orthostatic dysregulation: a comparison with tilt-table testing. *Wien Klin Wochenschr* (2005) 117:36–41. doi: 10.1007/s00508-004-0288-5
20. Braune S, Wrocklage C, Schutle-Monting J, Schnitzer R, Lucking CH. Diagnosis of tachycardia syndromes associated with orthostatic symptoms. *Clin Autonom Res.* (1999) 9:97–101. doi: 10.1007/BF02311766
21. Arnold AC, Ng J, Raj SR. Postural tachycardia syndrome—diagnosis, physiology, and prognosis. *Auton Neurosci.* (2018). doi: 10.1016/j.autneu.2018.02.005. [Epub ahead of print].
22. Schondorf R, Low PA. Idiopathic postural orthostatic tachycardia syndrome: an attenuated form of acute pandysautonomia? *Neurology* (1993) 43:132–7. doi: 10.1212/WNL.43.1_Part_1.132
23. Hoad A, Spickett G, Elliott J, Newton J. Postural orthostatic tachycardia is an under-recognized condition in chronic fatigue syndrome. *Q J Med.* (2008) 101:961–5. doi: 10.1093/qjmed/hcn123
24. Roma M, Marden CL, Rowe PC. Passive standing tests for the office diagnosis of postural tachycardia syndrome: new methodological considerations. *Fatigue* (2018) 6:179–92. doi: 10.1080/21641846.2018.1512836
25. Fukuda K, Straus SE, Hickie I, Sharpe M, Dobbins JG, Komaroff A, et al. Chronic fatigue syndrome: a comprehensive approach to its definition and study. *Ann Int Med.* (1994) 121:953–9. doi: 10.7326/0003-4819-121-12-199412150-00009
26. Carew S, Cooke J, O'Connor M, Donnelly T, Costelloe A, Sheehy C, et al. What is the optimal duration of tilt testing for the assessment of patients with suspected postural tachycardia syndrome? *Europace* (2009) 11:635–7. doi: 10.1093/europace/eup044
27. Okamoto LE, Raj SR, Peltier A, Gamboa A, Shibao C, Diedrich A, et al. Neurohumoral and haemodynamic profile in postural tachycardia and chronic fatigue syndromes. *Clin Sci.* (2012) 122:183–92. doi: 10.1042/CS20110200
28. Nacul LC, Lacerda EM, Pheby D, Campion P, Molokhia M, Fayyaz S, et al. Prevalence of myalgic encephalomyelitis/chronic fatigue syndrome (ME/CFS) in three regions of England: a repeated cross-sectional study in primary care. *BMC Med.* (2011) 9:91. doi: 10.1186/1741-7015-9-91
29. Watts SW, Morrison SF, Davis RP, Barman SM. Serotonin and blood pressure regulation. *Pharm. Rev.* (2012) 64:359–88. doi: 10.1124/pr.111.0 04697

15

Genetic Predisposition for Immune System, Hormone and Metabolic Dysfunction in Myalgic Encephalomyelitis/Chronic Fatigue Syndrome

Melanie Perez[1], *Rajeev Jaundoo*[2,3], *Kelly Hilton*[1], *Ana Del Alamo*[1,3], *Kristina Gemayel*[1], *Nancy G. Klimas*[1,3,4], *Travis J. A. Craddock*[1,2,3,5]* *and Lubov Nathanson*[1,3]*

[1] *Dr. Kiran C. Patel College of Osteopathic Medicine, Nova Southeastern University, Fort Lauderdale, FL, United States,* [2] *Department of Psychology and Neuroscience, Nova Southeastern University, Fort Lauderdale, FL, United States,* [3] *Institute for Neuro Immune Medicine, Nova Southeastern University, Fort Lauderdale, FL, United States,* [4] *Veterans Affairs Medical Center, Miami, FL, United States,* [5] *Department of Computer Science, Nova Southeastern University, Fort Lauderdale, FL, United States*

Correspondence:
Travis J. A. Craddock
tcraddock@nova.edu
Lubov Nathanson
lnathanson@nova.edu

Introduction: Myalgic Encephalomyelitis/ Chronic Fatigue Syndrome (ME/CFS) is a multifactorial illness of unknown etiology with considerable social and economic impact. To investigate a putative genetic predisposition to ME/CFS we conducted genome-wide single-nucleotide polymorphism (SNP) analysis to identify possible variants.

Methods: 383 ME/CFS participants underwent DNA testing using the commercial company 23andMe. The deidentified genetic data was then filtered to include only non-synonymous and nonsense SNPs from exons and microRNAs, and SNPs close to splice sites. The frequencies of each SNP were calculated within our cohort and compared to frequencies from the Kaviar reference database. Functional annotation of pathway sets containing SNP genes with high frequency in ME/CFS was performed using over-representation analysis via ConsensusPathDB. Furthermore, these SNPs were also scored using the Combined Annotation Dependent Depletion (CADD) algorithm to gauge their deleteriousness.

Results: 5693 SNPs were found to have at least 10% frequency in at least one cohort (ME/CFS or reference) and at least two-fold absolute difference for ME/CFS. Functional analysis identified the majority of SNPs as related to immune system, hormone, metabolic, and extracellular matrix organization. CADD scoring identified 517 SNPs in these pathways that are among the 10% most deleteriousness substitutions to the human genome.

Keywords: myalgic encephalomyelitis/chronic fatigue syndrome, genome-wide, single-nucleotide polymorphism, immune system, hormone, metabolic

INTRODUCTION

Myalgic Encephalomyelitis/Chronic Fatigue Syndrome (ME/CFS) is a complex illness characterized by disabling fatigue, disturbed sleep patterns, pain, and flu-like symptoms. Patients report a high degree of physical disability, and a decreased quality of life with 24% being homebound (1), causing a US economic loss ranging from of $9.1 to $51 billion (2). Currently, there are three main sources of diagnosis criteria, the Center for Disease Control (CDC) Empiric (3), Fukuda (4), and Canadian Consensus (5), showing 2.54, 1.0, and 0.10% of the population affected, respectively. This variation highlights the lack of a concrete illness definition. Although research studies have identified various aspects such as immune abnormalities and exposure to toxins relevant to the pathogenesis of ME/CFS (6), ME/CFS is still not yet fully understood. The genetic and environmental pathogenesis of ME/CFS remains unclear. Currently, treatment of ME/CFS is dependent on management of symptomology and improvement on quality of life (6). An improved understanding of the molecular mechanisms affected and dysfunction in the regulatory systems will translate into better diagnostic methods and more targeted approaches to treatment. There are numerous studies suggesting that genes and single nucleotide polymorphisms (SNPs) within those genes might play a role in the development and progression of ME/CFS (7–9). Results of these studies are very interesting and useful, however, one of these studies was focused on mitochondrial DNA (7), and the other two were limited by 80 study subjects (8, 9). The aim of the current study is to increase the size of the ME/CFS cohort and identify the most harmful variants associated with ME/CFS.

MATERIALS AND METHODS

Patient Population

Individuals with ME/CFS were selected through an online English pre-screening questionnaire via the RedCap platform. The study was restricted to adults (18–70 years of age) that endorsed a clinically diagnoses of chronic fatigue syndrome (CFS), post-infection fatigue (IF), or myalgic encephalomyelitis (ME) and endorsed criteria meeting the 1994 CDC definition of CFS (4): four or more of the following symptoms over a minimum of 6 consecutive months and not predating fatigue: sore throat, tender cervical or axillary lymph nodes, muscle pain, multiple joint pain without swelling or redness, headaches of new type, pattern or severity, unrefreshing sleep, post-exertional malaise, and impaired memory or concentration. Furthermore, study subjects were excluded if they had HIV infection, or dementia precluding full participation/consent. Qualified prescreened participants then completed an online consent form describing the study in detail, asking them to accept or decline the opportunity to continue with the study, via the RedCap online platform. Consenting participants then securely uploaded their genotyping data received from 23andMe into a secure database using the RedCap online platform.

Ethics Approval and Consent to Participate

All study subjects signed an informed consent approved by the Institutional Review Board (IRB) of Nova Southeastern University (NSU). Ethics review and approval for data analysis was also obtained by the IRB of NSU.

23andME Genotyping

23andME processes saliva containing DNA that was sent by the study subjects collected with the 23andMe kits according to the supplied instructions. The 23andMe CLIA-certified lab extracted DNA and processed the DNA on a genotyping chip that reads hundreds of thousands of variants in the human genome. Samples were collected starting in July 2016 until August 2018 and processed with 23andMe chip versions 4 (~570 k SNPs; prior to August 2017) and version 5 (~640 k SNPs; after August 2017). Genotyping calls were performed by 23andMe. Personalized reports based on well-established scientific and medical research were returned to study subjects and subsequently uploaded to the NSU RedCap online platform.

SNP Filtering and Analysis

All variants received from study participants were annotated using SeattleSeq 138 (10) for Genes, Distance-To-Nearest Splice Site, and microRNAs. Based on the annotation we focused our analysis on only non-synonymous and non-sense SNPs located in the gene's coding regions, near the splice sites and in microRNAs. The frequency of each of these SNPs was calculated in ME/CFS cohort (study participants). We compared these frequencies with the frequencies of the corresponding SNPs from the reference database Kaviar [hg19 (GRCh37)] (11). Kaviar contains over 162 million SNPs from 35 projects, including dbSNP, 1000Genomes and other and does not include the data from cancer genomes.

For functional analysis we selected SNPs that satisfied following criteria: the frequency at least 10% in either reference or ME/CFS cohort and the ratio in frequencies between the ME/CFS cohort and the reference cohort is more than two in either direction (**Supplementary Table 1**).

All variants that prevail in ME/CFS cohort were also scored using the Combined Annotation Dependent Depletion algorithm (CADD) (12) (**Supplementary Table 2**).

Functional Annotation

Functional annotation of SNPs was performed using the ConsensusPathDB (13–15) to provide biological pathway information. Over-representation analysis (13) incorporating the Kyoto Encyclopedia of Genes and Genomes (KEGG) (73.0) (16), Netpath (1.1.2015) (17), the Integrating Network Objects with Hierarchies (INOH) (1.1.2015) (18), Biocarta (2009_05_12) (19), Humancyc (18.5) (20), Signalink (8.1.2015) (21), Edinburgh human metabolic network (Ehmn) (1.1.2015) (22), Reactome (51) (23), Wikipathways (9.1.2015) (24) and the Pathway Interaction Database (PID) (2014_02_14) (25) pathway sets was used to interpret the functions the identified SNPs may play. Here the significance of the observed overlap between the gene module and the members of known pathways, compared to random expectations, was calculated based on a hypergeometric distribution. A minimum overlap of two genes between the gene module and the pathway set at a p-value cutoff of 0.01 was required. Specifically, the p-value was calculated as the probability of randomly finding k or more successes from the population in N total draws. Thus, small p-values indicate a greater over-representation than expected by chance. As many of the identified pathways share SNP genes the relation between functions was mapped as a network between identified pathway nodes where edges indicate a number of shared genes. These networks were visualized with Cytoscape version 3.3.0 (26). Pathways sharing at least 30% of SNPs were clustered and organized via circular layout, while the remainder were organized via a perfuse force-directed layout based on the number of shared genes.

RESULTS AND DISCUSSION

Functional analysis of SNPs identified three main clusters of pathways as sharing at least 30% SNP related genes (**Figure 1**). The first is dominated in size via the pathway Cytokine Signaling in Immune System and includes other immune-related pathways such as interferon signaling, autoimmune responses, and T-cell receptor signaling. This cluster highlights a module of immune-related SNPs.

The second cluster is dominated in size via the Nuclear-Receptors Meta-Pathway and includes hormone related pathways such as steroid hormone, estrogen, and androgen biosynthesis, glucuronidation, and the pregnane x receptor pathway. This cluster highlights modules of hormone-related SNPs.

The final cluster is dominated in size by Pathways in Cancer, however, closer inspection shows many metabolic processes such as enzyme reactions (protein kinase A, calcium and calmodulin signaling), and G proteins signaling which regulate metabolic enzymes, which are all involved in the regulation of glycogen, sugar and lipid metabolism. This cluster highlights a module of metabolism-related SNPs.

While there is an overlap between the metabolic and immune modules, the hormone module remains isolated with main connections only formed via Ovarian Steroidogenesis and the Wnt signaling pathway. Finally, there is a group of loosely connected pathways involved in an extracellular matrix organization.

While this organization highlights the interplay between immune, hormone and metabolic activity underlying ME/CFS, overlay of the location of CADD scores illustrates where the most deleterious effects occur (**Figure 1**; lower panel).

Of the 11,485 SNPs that passed prefiltering according to the annotations (see Methods), 8,593 SNPs had frequency more than 10% in either reference or ME/CFS cohort. Out of them, 5,693 SNPs had a two-fold difference between ME/CFS and the reference cohorts in either direction (**Supplementary Table 1**).

SNPs that prevailed in ME/CFS cohort were scored using the CADD algorithm (12). According to the CADD algorithm, C-scores above 10 indicate that these SNPs are predicted to be among the 10% most harmful, and C-scores above 20 indicate the 1% most deleterious substitutions (12). **Table 1** shows 50 SNPs that are the most frequent in the ME/CFS cohort and have C-scores above 10.

Of the 50 most frequent deleterious SNPs found in our ME/CFS cohort compared to the reference database (**Table 1**), 10 were found to have a frequency of 70% or more in the ME/CFS group. This includes *CYP2D6*, *PRRT4*, and *PRSS56* at a frequency over 90%, *C14orf37*, *ANKDD1B*, at over 80%, and *GPBAR1*, *LHB*, *ADAMTS19*, *VARS2*, and *CPLX2* at over 70%.

CYP2D6 (Cytochrome P450 2D6) is primarily expressed in the liver, but also highly expressed in areas of the central nervous system, including the substantia nigra, and is one of the most important enzymes involved in the metabolism of xenobiotics in the body. A significantly higher frequency of polymorphisms *CYP2D6* was found in ME/CFS study subjects with Fibromyalgia than in controls and could differentiate these study subjects s from study subjects with multiple chemical sensitivity (27). *CYP2D6* was found in the xenobiotics metabolism, androgen and estrogen biosynthesis and metabolism, tyrosine metabolism, codeine and morphine metabolism, oxidation by cytochrome P450, metapathway biotransformation phase I and II, and cytochrome P450—arranged by substrate type pathways all of which belong to the hormone related cluster.

PRSS56 (putative serine protease 56) is a serine protease that has been implicated in human eye development (28) and in the regulation of cerebellum activity of mice in exercise (29). It was not found to be a member of any of the annotated pathways.

GPBAR1 (G Protein-Coupled Bile Acid Receptor) functions as a cell surface receptor for bile acids and participates in the production of intracellular cAMP and activation of a MAP kinase signaling pathway. This receptor plays a big role in the suppression of macrophage functions and regulation of energy homeostasis by bile acids (30). Finding of the deleterious SNP in GPBAR1 (**Table 1**) is in agreement with the results of the recent study that showed disturbances in bile acid metabolism in ME/CFS study subjects (31). *GPBAR1* was not among any of the pathways annotated.

LHB (luteinizing hormone beta polypeptide) is expressed in the pituitary gland and is essential for spermatogenesis and ovulation by stimulating the testes and ovaries to synthesize steroids (32, 33). *LHB* was found among the GnRH signaling pathway and ovarian steroidogenesis pathway.

ADAMTS19 is a member of the large *ADAMTS* (a desintegrin-like and metalloprotease with thrombospondin type 1 motif) family of metalloproteases (metal binding enzymes). ADAM proteins are responsible for the proteolytic cleavage of many transmembrane proteins and the release of their extracellular domain. *ADAMTS19* is considered as a possible candidate for premature ovarian failure (34). Only the O-linked glycosylation pathway was found to contain ADAMTS19.

VARS2 (valyl-tRNA synthetase 2, mitochondrial) is important for the mitochondrial protein synthesis. Mutations in this gene are associated with cardiomyopathy (35), microcephaly and epilepsy (36), deficiency of the mitochondrial respiratory chain complex I and oxidative phosphorylation deficiency (37). *VARS2* was not found among any of the annotated pathways.

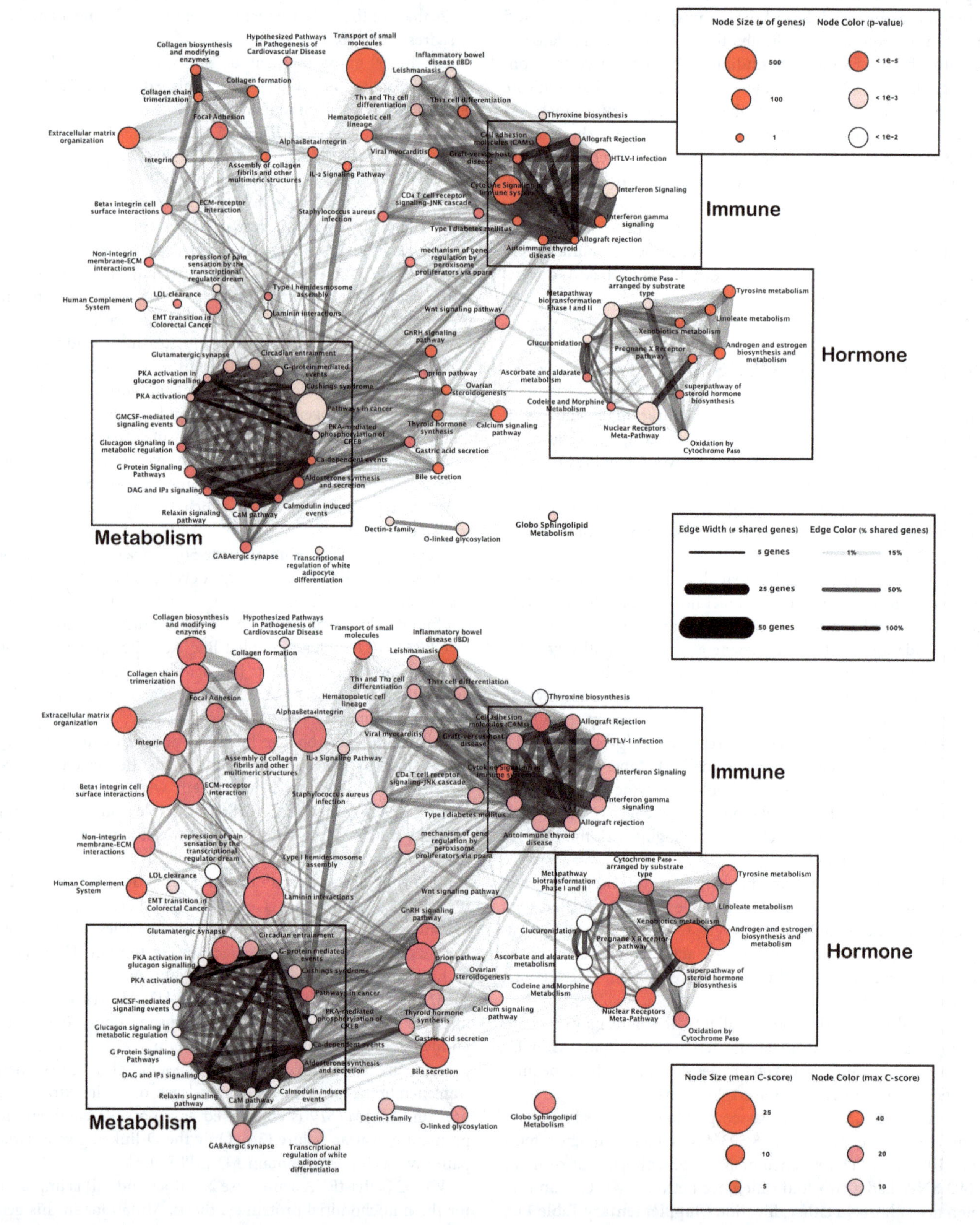

FIGURE 1 | Pathway overlap networks. Pathways identified via over-representation analysis (nodes) connected by shared genes with SNPs (edges). Upper panel gives total number of SNPs per pathway and likelihood of annotation (*p*-value). Lower panel shows pathways most affected by deleterious SNPs.

TABLE 1 | 50 most frequent deleterious SNPs in ME/CFS cohort compared to reference cohort.

Gene	ID	ME/CFS frequency	Kaviar frequency	Frequency ratio	C-score
GPBAR1	rs199986029	7.73E-01	6.00E-06	1.29E+05	36.00
HLA-C	rs41560916	6.27E-01	1.30E-05	4.82E+04	15.55
BCAM	rs3810141	1.02E-01	6.00E-06	1.70E+04	33.00
AAAS	rs150511103	1.93E-01	1.30E-05	1.49E+04	33.00
FGA	rs146387238	1.93E-01	1.30E-05	1.49E+04	33.00
SLC25A13	rs80338723	1.93E-01	1.30E-05	1.49E+04	32.00
MYBPC3	rs112738974	1.93E-01	1.90E-05	1.02E+04	34.00
PEX6	rs112298166	1.93E-01	1.90E-05	1.02E+04	26.80
CYP2D6	rs1135830	4.54E-01	9.70E-05	4.68E+03	24.30
HLA-DRB1	rs112796209	4.15E-01	1.09E-04	3.81E+03	26.10
PLA2G4D	rs147516345	1.59E-01	1.03E-04	1.55E+03	25.60
CYP2A6	rs5031017	3.86E-01	2.64E-04	1.46E+03	24.20
CYP2D6	rs199535154	9.43E-01	2.31E-03	4.08E+02	22.10
DDX51	rs201101053	1.59E-01	7.08E-04	2.25E+02	49.00
LHB	rs34349826	7.42E-01	6.44E-03	1.15E+02	13.18
HLA-A	rs1137110	1.38E-01	2.49E-03	5.57E+01	16.35
HLA-DRB1	rs1136756	4.39E-01	1.00E-02	4.38E+01	14.71
HLA-DRB1	rs9269744	4.05E-01	1.30E-02	3.12E+01	23.80
TPTE	rs1810540	3.45E-01	1.16E-02	2.97E+01	35.00
HLA-DQA1	rs1061172	1.57E-01	1.33E-02	1.18E+01	15.33
C6orf183	rs399561	6.32E-01	6.46E-02	9.78E+00	15.17
C14orf37	rs3829765	8.15E-01	9.75E-02	8.36E+00	15.58
EFCAB4B	rs11062745	2.79E-01	3.39E-02	8.25E+00	21.60
PLD5	rs2810008	5.54E-01	6.71E-02	8.25E+00	16.00
MUC19	rs11564109	2.40E-01	2.95E-02	8.15E+00	24.70
ARHGAP42	rs17647207	1.44E-01	1.82E-02	7.91E+00	23.30
ADAMTS19	rs30645	7.65E-01	9.75E-02	7.85E+00	18.74
LINC01171	rs11605546	2.30E-01	2.97E-02	7.73E+00	15.31
ANKDD1B	rs34358	8.33E-01	1.09E-01	7.65E+00	45.00
ZBED5	rs2232919	1.20E-01	1.61E-02	7.45E+00	24.20
CTC-441N14.4	rs9112	6.03E-01	8.44E-02	7.15E+00	21.70
SLC35B2	rs3187	1.31E-01	1.85E-02	7.07E+00	11.89
PRSS41	rs61747737	1.15E-01	1.63E-02	7.06E+00	13.70
OTOG	rs12422210	2.64E-01	3.76E-02	7.01E+00	15.38
MTCH2	rs1064608	4.57E-01	6.58E-02	6.95E+00	25.00
SULF1	rs6990375	5.12E-01	7.49E-02	6.83E+00	14.77
OTOG	rs11024333	2.95E-01	4.34E-02	6.80E+00	10.26
ART3	rs14773	4.33E-01	6.41E-02	6.76E+00	14.51
PPHLN1	rs12658	3.63E-01	5.45E-02	6.66E+00	15.95
PRICKLE1	rs12658	3.63E-01	5.45E-02	6.66E+00	15.95
VARS2	rs2249464	7.47E-01	1.14E-01	6.56E+00	16.14
MORN2	rs3099950	2.19E-01	3.37E-02	6.50E+00	25.50
AC007956.1	rs2270424	3.68E-01	5.99E-02	6.15E+00	33.00
AREL1	rs2270424	3.68E-01	5.99E-02	6.15E+00	33.00
PRRT4	rs359642	9.50E-01	1.55E-01	6.12E+00	10.83
HUS1	rs2307252	1.67E-01	2.76E-02	6.05E+00	12.72
PRSS56	rs1550094	9.22E-01	1.62E-01	5.68E+00	16.32
C5orf52	rs10051838	2.40E-01	4.35E-02	5.52E+00	17.68
ZNHIT1	rs17319250	4.05E-01	7.41E-02	5.46E+00	10.74
CPLX2	rs3822674	7.05E-01	1.29E-01	5.46E+00	10.05

CPLX2 gene encodes the complexin 2 protein that participates in neurotransmitter release by directly interacting with the neuronal SNARE complex (38). *CPLX2* is known to be overexpressed in aging and downregulated by sleep deprivation (39), and this shows a connection of *CPLX2* expression to fatigue. *CPLX2* was also not found among any of the annotated pathways.

The remaining genes *PRRT4*, *C14orf37*, and *ANKDD1B* are obscure without much literature to support their function and not found among any of the annotated pathways. It was determined that *PRRT4* (proline-rich transmembrane protein 4) showed biased expression in adult ovary, lung, adrenals, CNS and whole brain, while *C14orf37* showed bias in brain, kidney, and ovary (ncbi.nlm.nih.gov). Little information was found for *ANKDD1B* (ankyrin repeat and death domain containing 1B).

Although SNPs in *MYBPC3* and *HLA* genes have lower frequencies in ME/CFS cohort (0.19 for *MYBPC3* and 0.13-0.44 for various *HLA* isoforms, respectively), these SNPs could be used for subgrouping of ME/CFS study subjects in larger studies because of their possible association with ME/CFS and fatigue. Multiple deleterious SNPs in *HLA* genes are in agreement with known impairment of the immune system in ME/CFS (40). Increased frequency of *HLA-DQA1* alleles and decreased expression of *HLA-DRB1* was found to be associated with ME/CFS (41). *MYBPC3* (myosin binding protein C, cardiac) dysfunction is also associated with hypertrophic cardiomyopathy and corresponding fatigue (42).

These results contrast with previous SNP studies in ME/CFS (9, 43–45) which have found statistically significant associations in multiple loci including in neuroendocrine effector and receptor genes (43), TRP ion channels and AChRs (44, 45), and genes regulating the HPA axis (9, 46). This difference is most likely due to a combination of factors such as, (i) differences in array types used between studies, (ii) difference in the methods of analysis, (iii) differences between cohorts and the general heterogeneity of ME/CFS, and (iv) small-effect variants due to the relatively small sample sizes in each of these previous studies, compared to our relatively large cohort.

To date, this is the largest study known using SNP data and its affected pathways in combination with study subjects' self-reported symptoms. The results generated from our study will enhance the current understanding of ME/CFS and will generate new studies, all of which will lead to a better method for diagnosis and targeted genetic therapy. Replicative larger studies are warranted to improve the reliability of the results.

While these results are novel there are some limitations to the current analysis that are worth noting. First, there is no control over the chip version used by 23andMe for genotyping. This can result in loss of precision in the determination of study subject genotyping signature. Second, this initial pilot analysis was only conducted on SNPs in protein coding regions, miRNA regions, and regions close to splice junctions. SNPs in non-coding regions may be important in the cause of the illness. Finally, this analysis does not include rare variants. Moving forward, future studies based on this on-going collection of study subject information will address these limitations, will increase sample size, and provide more detailed statistical analyses. Building on this dataset we also aim to correlate these findings with our ongoing research on gene expression (47), miRNA expression and DNA methylation (48).

ETHICS STATEMENT

All subjects signed an informed consent approved by the Institutional Review Board of Nova Southeastern University. Ethics review and approval for data analysis was also obtained by the IRB of Nova Southeastern University.

AUTHOR CONTRIBUTIONS

NK, LN, and TC conceived the study. MP, RJ, TC, and LN analyzed data. NK consulted on ME/CFS symptoms. AD, KH, KG, and MP led the recruitment of study participants.

ACKNOWLEDGMENTS

We acknowledge the student of Dr. Kiran C. Patel College of Osteopathic Medicine of Nova Southeastern University Christopher Larrimore for his help in managing RedCap database. We would like to thank students of Halmos College of Natural Sciences and Oceanography of Nova Southeastern University Valentina Ramirez, Maria Cash and Pallavi Samudrala for their help with the analysis of data. This study was partially supported by the Health Professions Division grant from Nova Southeastern University awarded to KH.

REFERENCES

1. Pendergrast T, Brown A, Sunnquist M, Jantke R, Newton JL, Strand EB, et al. Housebound versus nonhousebound patients with myalgic encephalomyelitis and chronic fatigue syndrome. *Chronic Illn.* (2016) 12:292–307. doi: 10.1177/1742395316644770
2. Lin J-MS, Resch SC, Brimmer DJ, Johnson A, Kennedy S, Burstein N, et al. The economic impact of chronic fatigue syndrome in Georgia: direct and indirect costs. *Cost Eff Resour Alloc.* (2011) 9:1. doi: 10.1186/1478-7547-9-1
3. Brurberg KG, Fønhus MS, Larun L, Flottorp S, Malterud K. Case definitions for chronic fatigue syndrome/myalgic encephalomyelitis (CFS/ME): a systematic review. *BMJ Open.* (2014) 4:e003973. doi: 10.1136/bmjopen-2013-003973
4. Fukuda K, Straus SE, Hickie I, Sharpe MC, Dobbins JG, Komaroff A. The chronic fatigue syndrome: a comprehensive approach to its definition and study. *Ann Intern Med.* (1994) 121:953–9. doi: 10.7326/0003-4819-121-12-199412150-00009
5. Reeves WC, Jones JF, Maloney E, Heim C, Hoaglin DC, Boneva RS, et al. Prevalence of chronic fatigue syndrome in metropolitan, urban, and rural Georgia. *Popul Health Metr.* (2007) 5:5. doi: 10.1186/1478-7954-5-5
6. Bested AC, Marshall LM. Review of myalgic encephalomyelitis/chronic fatigue syndrome: an evidence-based approach to diagnosis and management by clinicians. *Rev Environ Health.* (2015) 30:223–49. doi: 10.1515/reveh-2015-0026
7. Billing-Ross P, Germain A, Ye K, Keinan A, Gu Z, Hanson MR. Mitochondrial DNA variants correlate with symptoms in myalgic encephalomyelitis/chronic fatigue syndrome. *J Transl Med.* (2016) 14:19. doi: 10.1186/s12967-016-0771-6
8. Smith AK, Fang H, Whistler T, Unger ER, Rajeevan MS. Convergent genomic studies identify association of GRIK2 and NPAS2 with chronic fatigue syndrome. *Neuropsychobiology.* (2011) 64:183–94. doi: 10.1159/000326692
9. Schlauch KA, Khaiboullina SF, De Meirleir KL, Rawat S, Petereit J, Rizvanov AA, et al. Genome-wide association analysis identifies genetic variations in subjects with myalgic encephalomyelitis/chronic fatigue syndrome. *Transl Psychiatry.* (2016) 6:e730. doi: 10.1038/tp.2015.208
10. Ng SB, Turner EH, Robertson PD, Flygare SD, Bigham AW, Lee C, et al. Targeted capture and massively parallel sequencing of 12 human exomes. *Nature.* (2009) 461:272–6. doi: 10.1038/nature08250
11. Glusman G, Caballero J, Mauldin DE, Hood L, Roach JC. Kaviar: an accessible system for testing SNV novelty. *Bioinformatics.* (2011) 27:3216–7. doi: 10.1093/bioinformatics/btr540
12. Kircher M, Witten DM, Jain P, O'Roak BJ, Cooper GM, Shendure J. A general framework for estimating the relative pathogenicity of human genetic variants. *Nat Genet.* (2014) 46:310–5. doi: 10.1038/ng.2892
13. Kamburov A, Wierling C, Lehrach H, Herwig R. ConsensusPathDB—a database for integrating human functional interaction networks. *Nucleic Acids Res.* (2009) 37:D623–8. doi: 10.1093/nar/gkn698
14. Kamburov A, Pentchev K, Galicka H, Wierling C, Lehrach H, Herwig R. ConsensusPathDB: toward a more complete picture of cell biology. *Nucleic Acids Res.* (2011) 39:D712–7. doi: 10.1093/nar/gkq1156
15. Kamburov A, Stelzl U, Lehrach H, Herwig R. The ConsensusPathDB interaction database: 2013 update. *Nucleic Acids Res.* (2013) 41:D793–800. doi: 10.1093/nar/gks1055
16. Kanehisa M, Goto S, Sato Y, Furumichi M, Tanabe M. KEGG for integration and interpretation of large-scale molecular data sets. *Nucleic Acids Res.* (2011) 40:A109–14. doi: 10.1093/nar/gkr988
17. Kandasamy K, Mohan SS, Raju R, Keerthikumar S, Kumar GSS, Venugopal AK, et al. NetPath: a public resource of curated signal transduction pathways. *Genome Biol.* (2010) 11:R3. doi: 10.1186/gb-2010-11-1-r3
18. Yamamoto S, Sakai N, Nakamura H, Fukagawa H, Fukuda K, Takagi T. INOH: ontology-based highly structured database of signal transduction pathways. *Database.* (2011) 2011:bar052. doi: 10.1093/database/bar052
19. Nishimura D. BioCarta. *Biotech Softw Internet Rep.* (2001) 2:117–20. doi: 10.1089/152791601750294344
20. Romero P, Wagg J, Green ML, Kaiser D, Krummenacker M, Karp PD. Computational prediction of human metabolic pathways from the complete human genome. *Genome Biol.* (2004) 6:R2. doi: 10.1186/gb-2004-6-1-r2
21. Fazekas D, Koltai M, Türei D, Módos D, Pálfy M, Dúl Z, et al. SignaLink 2–a signaling pathway resource with multi-layered regulatory networks. *BMC Syst Biol.* (2013) 7:7. doi: 10.1186/1752-0509-7-7
22. Hao T, Ma H-W, Zhao X-M, Goryanin I. Compartmentalization of the Edinburgh human metabolic network. *BMC Bioinformatics.* (2010) 11:393. doi: 10.1186/1471-2105-11-393
23. Croft D, Mundo AF, Haw R, Milacic M, Weiser J, Wu G, et al. The reactome pathway knowledgebase. *Nucleic Acids Res.* (2014) 42:D472–7. doi: 10.1093/nar/gkt1102
24. Kelder T, van Iersel MP, Hanspers K, Kutmon M, Conklin BR, Evelo CT, et al. WikiPathways: building research communities on biological pathways. *Nucleic Acids Res.* (2012) 40:D1301–7. doi: 10.1093/nar/gkr1074
25. Schaefer CF, Anthony K, Krupa S, Buchoff J, Day M, Hannay T, et al. PID: the pathway interaction database. *Nucleic Acids Res.* (2009) 37:D674–9. doi: 10.1093/nar/gkn653
26. Shannon P, Markiel A, Ozier O, Baliga NS, Wang JT, Ramage D, et al. Cytoscape: a software environment for integrated models of biomolecular interaction networks. *Genome Res.* (2003) 13:2498–504. doi: 10.1101/gr.1239303
27. Caccamo D, Cesareo E, Mariani S, Raskovic D, Ientile R, Curro M, et al. Xenobiotic sensor- and metabolism-related gene variants in environmental sensitivity-related illnesses: a survey on the Italian population. *Oxid Med Cell Longev.* (2013) 2013:831969. doi: 10.1155/2013/831969
28. Nowilaty SR, Khan AO, Aldahmesh MA, Tabbara KF, Al-Amri A, Alkuraya FS. Biometric and molecular characterization of clinically diagnosed

posterior microphthalmos. *Am J Ophthalmol.* (2013) 155:361–72 e7. doi: 10.1016/j.ajo.2012.08.016

29. Caetano-Anolles K, Rhodes JS, Garland T Jr, Perez SD, Hernandez AG, Southey BR, et al. Cerebellum transcriptome of mice bred for high voluntary activity offers insights into locomotor control and reward-dependent behaviors. *PLoS ONE.* (2016) 11:e0167095. doi: 10.1371/journal.pone.0167095
30. Jiang Y, Luo L, Gustafson EL, Yadav D, Laverty M, Murgolo N, et al. Identification and characterization of a novel RF-amide peptide ligand for orphan G-protein-coupled receptor SP9155. *J Biol Chem.* (2003) 278:27652–7. doi: 10.1074/jbc.M302945200
31. Germain A, Ruppert D, Levine SM, Hanson MR. Metabolic profiling of a myalgic encephalomyelitis/chronic fatigue syndrome discovery cohort reveals disturbances in fatty acid and lipid metabolism. *Mol Biosyst.* (2017) 13:371–9. doi: 10.1039/C6MB00600K
32. Potorac I, Rivero-Muller A, Trehan A, Kielbus M, Jozwiak K, Pralong F, et al. A vital region for human glycoprotein hormone trafficking revealed by an LHB mutation. *J Endocrinol.* (2016) 231:197–207. doi: 10.1530/JOE-16-0384
33. Katsikis I, Karkanaki A, Misichronis G, Delkos D, Kandaraki EA, Panidis D. Phenotypic expression, body mass index and insulin resistance in relation to LH levels in women with polycystic ovary syndrome. *Eur J Obstet Gynecol Reprod Biol.* (2011) 156:181–5. doi: 10.1016/j.ejogrb.2011.01.023
34. Knauff EA, Franke L, van Es MA, van den Berg LH, van der Schouw YT, Laven JS, et al. Genome-wide association study in premature ovarian failure patients suggests ADAMTS19 as a possible candidate gene. *Hum Reprod.* (2009) 24:2372–8. doi: 10.1093/humrep/dep197
35. Bruni F, Di Meo I, Bellacchio E, Webb BD, McFarland R, Chrzanowska-Lightowlers ZMA, et al. Clinical, biochemical, and genetic features associated with VARS2-related mitochondrial disease. *Hum Mutat.* (2018) 39:563–78. doi: 10.1002/humu.23398
36. Diodato D, Melchionda L, Haack TB, Dallabona C, Baruffini E, Donnini C, et al. VARS2 and TARS2 mutations in patients with mitochondrial encephalomyopathies. *Hum Mutat.* (2014) 35:983–9. doi: 10.1002/humu.22590
37. Taylor RW, Pyle A, Griffin H, Blakely EL, Duff J, He L, et al. Use of whole-exome sequencing to determine the genetic basis of multiple mitochondrial respiratory chain complex deficiencies. *JAMA.* (2014) 312:68–77. doi: 10.1001/jama.2014.7184
38. Pabst S, Hazzard JW, Antonin W, Sudhof TC, Jahn R, Rizo J, et al. Selective interaction of complexin with the neuronal SNARE complex. Determination of the binding regions. *J Biol Chem.* (2000) 275:19808–18. doi: 10.1074/jbc.M002571200
39. Porter NM, Bohannon JH, Curran-Rauhut M, Buechel HM, Dowling AL, Brewer LD, et al. Hippocampal CA1 transcriptional profile of sleep deprivation: relation to aging and stress. *PLoS ONE.* (2012) 7:e40128. doi: 10.1371/journal.pone.0040128
40. Klimas NG, Salvato FR, Morgan R, Fletcher MA. Immunologic abnormalities in chronic fatigue syndrome. *J Clin Microbiol.* (1990) 28:1403–10.
41. Smith J, Fritz EL, Kerr JR, Cleare AJ, Wessely S, Mattey DL. Association of chronic fatigue syndrome with human leucocyte antigen class II alleles. *J Clin Pathol.* (2005) 58:860–3. doi: 10.1136/jcp.2004.022681
42. Viswanathan SK, Sanders HK, McNamara JW, Jagadeesan A, Jahangir A, Tajik AJ, et al. Hypertrophic cardiomyopathy clinical phenotype is independent of gene mutation and mutation dosage. *PLoS ONE.* (2017) 12:e0187948. doi: 10.1371/journal.pone.0187948
43. Goertzel BN, Pennachin C, de Souza Coelho L, Gurbaxani B, Maloney EM, Jones JF. Combinations of single nucleotide polymorphisms in neuroendocrine effector and receptor genes predict chronic fatigue syndrome. *Pharmacogenomics.* (2006) 7:475–83. doi: 10.2217/14622416.7.3.475
44. Marshall-Gradisnik S, Huth T, Chacko A, Johnston S, Smith P, Staines D. Natural killer cells and single nucleotide polymorphisms of specific ion channels and receptor genes in myalgic encephalomyelitis/chronic fatigue syndrome. *Appl Clin Genet.* (2016) 9:39–47. doi: 10.2147/TACG.S99405
45. Marshall-Gradisnik S, Johnston S, Chacko A, Nguyen T, Smith P, Staines D. Single nucleotide polymorphisms and genotypes of transient receptor potential ion channel and acetylcholine receptor genes from isolated B lymphocytes in myalgic encephalomyelitis/chronic fatigue syndrome patients. *J Int Med Res.* (2016) 44:1381–94. doi: 10.1177/0300060516671622
46. Smith AS, Tabbaa M, Lei K, Eastham P, Butler MJ, Linton L, et al. Local oxytocin tempers anxiety by activating GABAA receptors in the hypothalamic paraventricular nucleus. *Psychoneuroendocrinology.* (2016) 63:50–8. doi: 10.1016/j.psyneuen.2015.09.017
47. Jeffrey MG, Nathanson L, Aenlle K, Barnes ZM, Baig M, Broderick G, et al. Treatment avenues in myalgic encephalomyelitis/chronic fatigue syndrome: a split-gender pharmacogenomic study of gene-expression modules. *Clin Ther.* (2019). doi: 10.1016/j.clinthera.2019.01.011. [Epub ahead of print].
48. Trivedi MS, Oltra E, Sarria L, Rose N, Beljanski V, Fletcher MA, et al. Identification of myalgic encephalomyelitis/chronic fatigue syndrome-associated DNA methylation patterns. *PLoS ONE.* (2018) 13:e0201066. doi: 10.1371/journal.pone.0201066

16

School Functioning in Adolescents with Chronic Fatigue Syndrome

Sarah Jenette Knight[1,2,3*], *Jennifer Politis*[1,4], *Christine Garnham*[1,4], *Adam Scheinberg*[1,2,3,5] *and Michelle Anne Tollit*[1,2,4,6]

[1] Murdoch Children's Research Institute, Melbourne, VIC, Australia, [2] The Royal Children's Hospital, Melbourne, VIC, Australia, [3] Department of Pediatrics, The University of Melbourne, Melbourne, VIC, Australia, [4] Melbourne Graduate School of Education, The University of Melbourne, Melbourne, VIC, Australia, [5] Department of Pediatrics, Monash University, Melbourne, VIC, Australia, [6] The Royal Children's Hospital Education Institute, Parkville VIC Australia, Melbourne, VIC, Australia

***Correspondence:**
Sarah Jenette Knight
Sarah.knight@mcri.edu.au

Background: It is well known that adolescents with chronic fatigue syndrome (CFS) experience greater school absenteeism compared to healthy adolescents. Less is known about other important aspects of school functioning including school participation, school connectedness, and academic performance in students with CFS. The aim of this study was to compare school functioning as a multifaceted construct in adolescents with CFS to healthy adolescent peers. We also explored whether illness factors were associated with school functioning in adolescents with CFS.

Methods: Thirty-nine participants with CFS and 28 healthy controls (aged 13–17 years) completed a range of subjective and objective measures of school functioning, as well as measures of fatigue and emotional symptoms.

Results: Adolescents with CFS demonstrated significantly higher rates of school absence, as well as poorer school-related quality of life, reduced school participation, poorer connectedness with school, and reduced academic performance. Fatigue severity and emotional symptoms were significantly associated with most aspects of school function.

Conclusions: Adolescents with CFS are at increased risk for poor school functioning across a range of indicators which extend beyond school absenteeism.

Keywords: adolescents, chronic fatigue syndrome, school absence, academic performance, school, chronic health condition

Adolescent chronic fatigue syndrome (CFS) is a complex condition that is characterized by intense, medically unexplained fatigue together with a range of sleep, pain, cognitive, neuroendocrine, and immune symptoms (1). The estimated incidence of CFS in children and adolescents varies widely (from 0.003 and 2.0%); however, it is consistently found to be more common in females (2, 3). CFS is associated with significant functional disability and this has a considerable impact on emotional, physical, and social functioning (4–9).

Due to the significant functional disability associated with CFS, several studies have associated CFS with high rates of school absence (4, 9–14). The average amount of time away from school for students with CFS has been estimated to be 1 year across their school life (15).

Most studies evaluating school functioning in the context of CFS have been limited by the use of relatively narrow definitions of school functioning, such as defining school functioning solely in terms of school attendance/absence (16). Adolescents with CFS have described difficulties with completing subject requirements and keeping up with academic work (17) and have also reported that their condition impacted on their education or career plans (18). Beyond school attendance, domains of functioning including academic performance, school participation, and school connectedness, have seldom been formally investigated in students with CFS despite their demonstrated links to school success and positive adjustment (16, 19). Taking a broader, more holistic approach to assessing school functioning is crucial in order to more comprehensively understand the impact of CFS and to help inform targeted strategies to optimizing educational outcomes in this vulnerable group (16). There is also limited research directly comparing school functioning in adolescents with CFS with their healthy peers (16). The lack of available normative rates of school absence and other indicators of school functioning makes it difficult to interpret findings and understand the extent and implications of school difficulties for students with CFS. This is in contrast to the larger body of research that has enhanced our understanding of the impact on school functioning in other chronic health conditions, such as childhood cancer, asthma, attention-deficit hyperactivity disorder, gastrointestinal diseases, and chronic pain (20–22).

The relationships between illness factors (e.g., fatigue severity), emotional symptoms, and school functioning in CFS have seldom been a focus of research. In a large sample of patients with CFS, Crawley and Sterne (13) found that children with better physical functioning were more likely to attend school. However, there was no evidence that gender, age, illness duration, anxiety, depression, or pain were associated with school attendance.

To summarize, there is substantial evidence that adolescents with CFS miss large amounts of school; however, our understanding of the impact of CFS on specific aspects of school functioning is limited and requires further exploration. A more thorough understanding of school functioning is an important step toward identifying risk and protective factors associated with school outcomes in the context of CFS. The aim of the current study was to compare adolescents with CFS to healthy peers across multiple aspects of school functioning, including school absence, quality of life in the school setting, school participation, school connectedness, and academic achievement. We also sought to determine whether fatigue severity and emotional symptoms were associated with aspects of school functioning in adolescents with CFS.

MATERIALS AND METHODS

Participants

Patients aged between 13 and 17 years with a diagnosis of CFS were recruited from a pediatric tertiary hospital, The Royal Children's Hospital, Melbourne, Australia. To be included in the CFS group, participants required a formal diagnosis of CFS made by a pediatrician specializing in CFS at the tertiary institution. Diagnoses were made via diagnostic interview, laboratory examinations and a medical examination using the Canadian criterion reference (1).

Control participants aged between 13 and 17 years were recruited via convenience sampling (i.e., researchers approached family members, friends, and work colleagues with children in the study age range).

Eligibility of both groups required the ability to speak or read sufficient English to complete the self-report questionnaire and assessments, and at least one parent with sufficient English to complete questionnaires. Exclusion criteria for the CFS group included severe cognitive impairment, learning disability, and/or permanent school absence or home schooling. Participants in the control group were excluded if there was a severe cognitive impairment, neurological disorder, learning disability, chronic health condition, psychiatric diagnosis, and/or permanent school absence or home schooling.

Measures

Demographics and Medical Information

Basic demographic information (age, gender, ethnicity, and parental education status) were collected via an online questionnaire completed by parents. Parents were asked when their child first started displaying signs of fatigue. Estimated illness duration was calculated in months, from date of initial signs of illness to date of assessment.

Estimated Intelligence

Level of general intellectual function was estimated using the Wechsler Abbreviated Scale of Intelligence—Second Edition (WASI-II) (23). The WASI-II is a brief standardized measure that provides an estimate of general intellectual ability in 6–89 year olds (Full Scale IQ-2 score or FSIQ-2) across two subtests, including Vocabulary and Matrix Reasoning. The Vocabulary subtest provides a measure of verbal crystallized knowledge. The Matrix Reasoning subtest measures nonverbal fluid abilities. Reliability coefficients for the FSIQ-2 for adolescents range from 0.92 to 0.95, with an average of 0.93 (23).

Fatigue Symptoms Severity

Symptoms of fatigue were measured in the CFS group and control group using The Pediatric Quality of Life Inventory-Multidimensional Fatigue Scale, self-report version (12–18 years; PedsQL MFS) (24, 25). The PedsQL MFS is comprised of 18 items and three dimensions, including; General, Sleep/Rest and Cognitive fatigue, as well as a Total Fatigue score. The 18 items are rated on a five-point scale: "Never," "Almost Never," "Sometimes," "Often," and "Almost Always." Respondents were asked how much of a problem each item had been during the past 1 month. For example, "I feel too tired to spend time with my friends"; "I sleep a lot"; "It's hard for me to think quickly." Items are reverse scored and linearly transformed to a 0–100 scale (0 = 100, 1 = 75, 2 = 50, 3 = 25, 4 = 0), higher scores indicate fewer problems with symptoms of fatigue, lower scores indicate greater problems with symptoms of fatigue. The scale scores of this measure have demonstrated good to excellent patient self-report reliability and validity across a number of pediatric chronic health conditions, including chronic fatigue syndrome (25, 26).

Emotional Symptoms

Emotional symptoms were measured using the self-report version of the Strengths and Difficulties Questionnaire (SDQ) (27). The SDQ is a 25 item questionnaire that explores common child and adolescent behavioral and emotional problems using a three-point Likert scale (0 = "Not true," 1 = "Somewhat True," and 2 = "Certainly True"). A high score on the Emotional Symptoms sub-scale indicates greater problems. The SDQ is one of the most widely used measures in child mental health research and has demonstrated acceptable reliability and content validity (28).

Measures of School Functioning

Extra Educational Supports

Parents of adolescents in both the CFS group and control group were asked the following question in order to obtain data on external educational support: "Does your child receive any extra educational support or modifications to their schooling?" The following categories were provided; "Modified curriculum," "Reduced work load," "Visiting teacher service," "Private tutoring," "Individual school tutoring or regular individual student/teacher contact," "Access to distance education," "Access to distance education as a dual enrolment with their regular school," "Access to the Program for Students with Disabilities funding (DEECD)," "Other."

School Absence

School absence was measured by asking parents of adolescents in the CFS group and control group: "How much school on average has your child missed due to illness or being sick or unwell in the last term?" The degree of absence was indicated using the following response set: None (My child didn't miss any school), About 10% (e.g., one half day per week), About 20% (e.g., 1 day per week), About 30% (e.g., one and a half days per week), About 40% (e.g., 2 days per week), About 50% (e.g., two and a half days per week), About 60% (e.g., 3 days per week), About 70% (e.g., three and a half days per week), About 80% (e.g., 4 days per week), About 90% (e.g., four and a half days per week), 100% (My child did not attend school), Not applicable (N/A).

Quality of Life in the School Setting

Quality of life in the school setting was measured using the 5-item School Functioning subscale of the Pediatric Quality of Life Inventory—self report (PedsQL, V 4.0) (29). The School Functioning scale is comprised of five items, which are rated on a five-point scale in terms of the degree to which the respondent reports having problems with school functioning: "Never," "Almost Never," "Sometimes," "Often," and "Almost Always." The PedsQL 4.0 School Functioning scale score has good reliability ($\alpha = 0.72$) and validity in a range of health conditions, including CFS (25, 29). Items are reverse scored and linearly transformed to a 0–100 scale (0 = 100, 1 = 75, 2 = 50, 3 = 25, 4 = 0). The School Functioning score was calculated by averaging the five school functioning items. Higher scores indicate better overall school functioning. Items on the subscale assess problems regarding "keeping up with school work," "paying attention in class," and "forgetting things" in the context of school.

School Participation

To assess the extent to which participants take part in school activities all participants completed The Child and Adolescent Scale of Participation (CASP) (30), school participation sub-test. The CASP is a reliable and valid measure with high internal consistency ($\alpha = 0.96$) (30). This measure consists of 20 ordinal-scaled items and four subsections: (1) Home Participation, (2) Community Participation, (3) School Participation, and (4) Home and Community Living Activities. The 20 items are rated on a four-point scale: "Age Expected (Full participation)," "Somewhat Restricted," "Very Restricted," and "Unable." A total school participation score was obtained by averaging the sum of all five school participation items. Higher scores indicate better school participation.

School Connectedness

To obtain a measure of school connectedness The Psychological Sense of School Membership (PSSM) (31) scale was completed by all participants. This scale measured student's perceptions of belonging, connectedness and psychological engagement in school. The PSSM is a reliable and valid measure with good internal consistency ($\alpha = 0.88$) (31). The PSSM includes 18 items rated on a five-point Likert scale, ranging from 1 = "Not at all True" to 5= "Completely true." Reverse scoring is necessary for five of the items; the scores are then summed into a total score. Higher scores on the PSSM indicate better connectedness and psychological engagement with school.

Academic Performance

Participants were administered the Wechsler Individual Academic Achievement Test—Australian Abbreviated—Second Edition (WIAT-II-A) (32), to assess their current academic ability. The WIAT-II-A is a reliable and valid, age-standardized measure that assesses the academic achievement of individuals across three subtests: Word Reading, Numeral Operations, and Spelling. Scores from subscales are added to provide an overall academic composite. Standard scores have a mean of 100 and standard deviation of 15. Higher scores indicate better academic functioning.

Procedure

Ethics approval was obtained from The Royal Children's Hospital's Human Research Ethics Committee (HREC#34060) and written, informed consent was obtained from all participants and their parents. Participants were recruited for this study over a 15 month period (April 2014–July 2015). Families interested in participating in the study were screened over the phone to confirm that they met study criteria. Families were emailed a link to complete the secure online questionnaire. Study data was collected and managed using REDCap electronic data capture tool (33). REDCap is a secure, web-based application designed to support data capture for research studies. Formal assessments using the WASI-II and WIAT-II-A were completed in a quiet room dedicated to such assessments at the hospital.

Data Analysis

All data were analyzed using Stata 14 (34). Preliminary analyses included chi-square, Mann-Whitney U, and independent samples t-tests to assess group differences on demographic and illness characteristics. Group differences in reported school supports was also evaluated using chi-square statistics. Effect sizes were also reported. Cohen's d was used for continuous data and Cramer's V for categorical data.

For the first aim, due to group differences in age and estimated intelligence, separate linear regression analyses were conducted to evaluate group differences in school functioning, where each individual school functioning variable was the outcome and "group" (i.e., CFS/control group) was the predictor, adjusting for age and estimated FSIQ. Mean differences (i.e., unstandardized regression coefficients [*b*]) with *p* values were reported. Given the multiple comparisons made in this study, standardized regression coefficients (β) were also evaluated. The standardized regression coefficients were used as measures of the effect size (cutoff points: 0.1 = weak prediction, 0.3 = moderate prediction, 0.5 = strong prediction).

For the second aim, separate linear regression analyses were conducted for the CFS group only to investigate the association between the school functioning variables and illness duration, fatigue, physical health, and emotional symptoms. The *b* values, significance level, coefficient of determination (R2 as a percentage) and β values of each model were reported. Significance for all analyses was determined at an alpha level of 0.05.

RESULTS

Sample Characteristics

Out of the 78 CFS patients who were invited to participate in the study, 39 consented and participated, constituting a recruitment rate of 50%. Of the families who did not consent ($n = 39$), reasons for non-participation included health reasons, distance from hospital, time, disinterest in study, unable to be contacted, and unable to schedule academic assessment during study period.

The overall sample in this study comprised 67 adolescents (39 CFS, 28 healthy controls). Of the 39 patients in the CFS group, 4 participants did not compete the CASP. There was no missing data in the control group.

On key demographic variables, there were no significant group differences with the exception of small, but statistically significant differences in age ($p = 0.003$) and estimated intelligence ($p = 0.011$) (**Table 1**). Correspondingly, these variables were used as covariates in further between group analyses. Both groups had a higher preponderance of females. Parental educational status was similar in both groups with the majority of mothers (primary caregiver) reporting a minimum of tertiary education. In the CFS group, the majority reported an infectious illness as a trigger for their child's illness and illness duration varied greatly (11–75 months). As shown in **Table 2**, compared to the healthy control group, the CFS group were significantly more likely to have a modified curriculum ($p = 0.001$), reduced work load ($p < 0.001$) and access to the visiting teacher service ($p < 0.001$), but not private tutoring, individual school tuition or access to distance education.

Group Differences in School Functioning

The first aim was to investigate group differences in aspects of school functioning between participants with CFS and the healthy control group. As shown in **Table 3**, the CFS group reported significantly greater school absence, poorer quality of life in the school setting, and reduced participation (all $p < 0.0001$, $\beta > 0.5$) compared to the control group. Significantly reduced school connectedness and academic performance were also observed in the CFS group, but with smaller effect ($p < 0.05$, $\beta < 0.3$). As expected, participants with CFS reported significantly higher levels of fatigue ($p < 0.0001$, $\beta = 0.80$) and emotional symptoms ($p = 0.015$, $\beta = 0.33$), compared to healthy controls (**Table 3**).

Influence of Fatigue and Emotional Symptoms on School Functioning in CFS Group

The second aim was to investigate the relationship between fatigue and emotional symptoms, and school functioning within the CFS group. Regression results are shown in **Table 4**. Fatigue levels were strongly associated with all aspects of school functioning (all $p < 0.001$, $\beta = 0.53$–0.69) with the exception of academic performance. Fatigue levels were able to explain a substantial amount of the variance in school absence, quality of life in the school setting, school participation and school connectedness ($R^2 = 28$–48%). Emotional symptoms were significantly associated with quality of life in the school setting ($p < 0.001$, $\beta = 0.51$), school participation ($p = 0.01$, $\beta = 0.18$), and school connectedness $p < 0.0001$, $\beta = 0.55$), but not school absence or academic performance. Overall, the amount of variance explained by emotional symptoms appeared slightly lower compared to fatigue levels ($R^2 = 18$–31%). All findings for the second aim held when re-run with age and estimated FSIQ as covariates.

DISCUSSION

The aim of this study was to extend our knowledge about school functioning in adolescents with CFS. Overall, compared to healthy adolescents, school functioning was compromised for adolescents with CFS across several specific domains (including school absence, quality of life in the school setting, school participation, school connectedness, and academic performance). Further, greater severity of fatigue in adolescents with CFS was associated with lower levels of school attendance, quality of life in the school setting, participation and connectedness, but not academic performance. Emotional symptoms were significantly associated with quality of life in the school setting, participation and connectedness, but not school absence or academic performance.

Group Differences in School Functioning

Current study findings suggest that adolescents with CFS receive significantly more external education support or modifications to the curriculum compared to healthy controls. Further, the CFS group reported poorer school functioning across all areas compared to the control group. As expected and consistent with previous studies reporting high rates of school absence (12–15, 18, 35–37), school absence rates due to illness for the CFS group were substantially higher than in the control group. On average, the control group missed less than one half a day per week

TABLE 1 | Sample characteristics.

	CFS group (n = 39)	Control group (n = 28)	p-value, effect size
Age, M (SD, range)	16.34 (1.15, 13.59–17.93)	15.41 (1.38, 13.0–17.38)	0.003, 0.74
Female sex, % (n)	76.74 (33)	62.07 (18)	0.18, 0.16
Ethnicity, % (n)			0.53, 0.18
Caucasian or European	95.12 (39)	92.86 (26)	
Asian	2.44 (1)	3.57 (1)	
Aboriginal or Torres Strait Islander	2.44 (1)	–	
Other	–	3.57 (1)	
Highest level of education (Mother), % (n)			0.53, 0.21
Did not complete high school	12.2 (5)	3.57 (1)	
Completed high school	4.88 (2)	10.71 (3)	
Some university, TAFE or certification course	21.95 (9)	14.29 (4)	
University degree	39.02 (16)	50.00(14)	
Postgraduate degree	21.95 (9)	21.43 (6)	
Estimated intelligence, M (SD, range)	108.26 (9.69, 88–129)	114.11 (8.38, 89–128)	0.011, 0.64
Illness trigger, % (n)			
Infectious illness	60.4 (17)	–	
Trip or vacation	4.7 (2)	–	
Surgery	2.3 (1)	–	
Stress	20.9 (9)	–	
Other	16.3 (7)	–	
No identifiable trigger	11.6 (5)		
Estimated illness duration (months), M(SD, range)	37.96 (17.71, 11–75)	–	

TABLE 2 | Extra educational support.

Extra educational support, % (n)	CFS group (n = 39)	Control group (n = 28)	p-value, effect size
Modified curriculum	37.2 (16)	3.5 (1)	0.001, 0.39
Reduced workload	41.9 (18)	3.5 (1)	<0.001, 0.56
Visiting teacher service	11.6 (5)	0	<0.001, 0.56
Private tutoring	14.0 (6)	3.5 (1)	0.14, 0.17
Individual school tuition	14.0 (6)	3.5 (1)	0.14, 0.17
Access to distance education	11.6 (5)	0	0.06, 0.22
Other educational supports	14.0 (6)	6.9 (2)	0.35, 0.11
No educational supports	4.7 (2)	69.0 (20)	<0.001, 0.68

over the last term due to illness, as opposed to the CFS group who were absent for, on average, 40% of the school term due to illness. These findings suggest that students with CFS are missing substantial amounts of school and report restrictions to school participation. Not only do these limitations have implications for the development of core academic skills, but such functional impairment also has potential to impact on social competencies which are integral for healthy adolescent development. Schools need to work toward supporting these students to ensure they remain connected and engaged with school when their medical condition impacts on their ability to physically attend school on a full-time basis.

When controlling for age and intelligence, the adolescents with CFS showed significantly reduced academic functioning compared to the healthy control sample, overall. Of note, both groups displayed high SES (based on educational status of primary caregiver) as well as above average intelligence. While the mean score for academic functioning for the CFS group fell within the average range in the context of normative population expectations, given the relatively high SES of the group and the overall above average level of intellectual functioning, these results suggest that compared to healthy controls, these adolescents may not be performing to their full potential academically (38). These are valuable findings as to the author's knowledge this is the first analysis of academic performance in adolescents with CFS using a standardized achievement test. Other studies exploring school performance in CFS using patient self-reports (17, 39) have also reported concerns regarding academic achievement.

Relationships Between Fatigue and Emotional Symptoms, and School Functioning in the CFS Group

As expected, greater fatigue severity was associated with higher school absence rates due to illness, as well as poorer school-related quality of life, lower school participation and connectedness. This is commensurate with findings from previous research whereby severity of physical health, were associated with school attendance (18, 40). Further, while greater

TABLE 3 | Mean differences between CFS group and controls on school functioning, fatigue and emotional symptoms.

	CFS group (n = 39)	Control group (n = 28)	Mean difference* (95% CI)	p-value, β
M (SD, range)				
School absence, %	42.10 (29.75, 0–100)	5 (8.39, 0–30)	−36.7 (−49.74, −23.65)	<0.0001, 0.62
Quality of life in the school setting	37.25 (16.60, 0–70)	77.59 (14.05, 50–100)	38.30 (29.82, 46.78)	<0.0001, 0.76
School participation†	81.70 (13.74, 40–100)	98.36 (4.64, 80–100)	15.87 (9.63, 22.12)	<0.0001, 0.58
School connectedness	67.0 (13.10, 38–87)	73.59 (11.03, 44–90)	6.98 (.10, 13.86)	0.047, 0.27
Academic performance	101.11 (12.38, 70–125)	111.81 (11.58, 82–129)	5.98 (0.78, 11.17)	0.025, 0.23
Fatigue	36.01 (15.0, 11.11–77.78)	73.23 (12.20, 41.67–95.83)	37.99 (30.13, 45.84)	<0.0001, 0.80
Emotional symptoms	4.29 (2.84, 0–9)	2.34 (1.80, 0–7)	−1.70 (−3.05, −0.35)	0.015, 0.33

All variables are adjusted for age and estimated FSIQ; CFS, chronic fatigue syndrome.
† $N_{CFS} = 35$, $N_{Control} = 28$.

TABLE 4 | Association of fatigue and emotional symptoms with school functioning in CFS group.

	Fatigue		Emotional symptoms	
	b, R^2 (95% CI)	p-value, β	b, R^2 (95% CI)	p-value, β
School absence, %	−0.10, 0.28 (−0.16, −0.49)	<0.001, 0.53	0.29, 0.08 (−0.04, 0.63)	0.09, 0.29
Quality of life in the school setting	0.76, 0.48 (0.50, 1.03)	<0.0001, 0.69	−2.99, 0.26 (−4.70, −1.29)	<0.001, 0.51
School participation†	0.58, 0.45 (0.35–0.81)	<0.0001, 0.67	−2.08, 0.18 (−3.66, −0.50)	0.01, 0.18
School connectedness	0.51, 0.35 (0.28, 0.75)	<0.0001, 0.59	−2.53, 0.31 (−3.81, −1.24)	<0.0001, 0.55
Academic performance	0.04, 0.00 (−0.24, 0.32)	0.76, 0.05	−0.30, 0.00 (−1.88, 1.27)	0.70, 0.07

CFS, chronic fatigue syndrome.
† $N_{CFS} = 35$.

emotional symptoms did not appear to relate to school absence, they were associated with poorer school-related quality of life, lower school participation and connectedness, suggesting that while school attendance may not be additionally affected for adolescents with CFS with more significant emotional symptoms, other less obvious aspects of school functioning may be further affected.

No significant associations were observed between fatigue and emotional symptoms, and academic functioning. The explanation for this discrepancy is unclear; although it is possible that more complex academic skills not assessed in the current study (e.g., comprehension, written expression) could be affected by these factors and further research into this area is warranted.

Strengths and Limitations

To the author's knowledge, this is the first study to comprehensively compare multiple aspects of school functioning in adolescents with a formal diagnosis of CFS with a control group of healthy adolescents. This study has several strengths including the use of a control group, as an indication of how this clinic group is functioning at school compared to their healthy peers.

There are limitations to the study that should be considered when interpreting results. Foremost is the employment of a small sample size in both groups. It is acknowledged that this has implications in terms of statistical power; however, given the uniqueness of such a study in the CFS literature the findings of the current study are of importance. These results should be replicated in future studies that employ a larger sample to confirm current study findings.

This study investigated school functioning from the perspective of the adolescent. Future research could incorporate reports from other informants about school functioning (e.g., parents and teachers) to obtain a more thorough understanding of school functioning. Discussion is also warranted around the representativeness of the CFS sample. Importantly, this study employed a strict diagnostic criterion, the Pediatric Canadian Criterion reference guidelines (1). While the sample characteristics (e.g., age, gender, and SES) are similar to what has been found in epidemiological studies of adolescents with CFS (3, 4, 12, 41, 42), it should be acknowledged that the adolescents participating in this study were recruited from a tertiary hospital and were required to attend the hospital in person for the academic assessment. Therefore, they may not be representative of all adolescents with CFS in the community (e.g., adolescents less severely affected may be managed in primary care and adolescents more severely affected by the illness may not have been well enough to attend the hospital for assessment).

Lastly, the cross-sectional nature of analysis employed in the study prevents exploration of the trajectory of school functioning over time as well as factors or mediators that might influence change in school functioning over time. To expound these questions, future studies could incorporate longitudinal methods to follow the course of CFS and school functioning over time.

Despite the present study containing a number of limitations requiring consideration, given the novelty of this research, the study provides a large contribution to our preliminary understanding of school functioning in adolescents with CFS and highlights directions for future research. Future studies should consider investigating academic performance beyond basic reading, spelling and mathematics, as well as the relative contributions of factors such as absenteeism, fatigue, cognitive difficulties, and emotional symptoms, to academic performance.

CONCLUSIONS

The findings from this study indicate that school functioning in adolescents with CFS is significantly poorer than that of healthy adolescents. This study highlights that expanding the indicators of school functioning beyond school absenteeism in adolescents with CFS provides a more comprehensive picture of school functioning that is likely useful in both research and school contexts. School absence due to illness does not accurately capture compromised school functioning in adolescents with CFS, and instead, more sensitive and specific domains such as those employed in the current study should be considered. This study demonstrated that in addition to increased school absence, CFS is also associated with poorer school-related quality of life, school participation, connectedness with school, and academic achievement when compared to healthy adolescent peers. School is the principle location for the development of not only academic skills, but also cognitive, social, and community-related skills during childhood and adolescence. Therefore, the impact that CFS has on school functioning may place these adolescents at a heightened risk of long-term maladjustment across a range of key developmental areas.

Implications for School Health

The findings from the current study have implications for the school health of adolescents with CFS. From a school health perspective, the findings support the early monitoring and careful analyses of specific aspects of school functioning in adolescents diagnosed with CFS, which may in turn help inform targeted intervention programs, designed to minimize the long term impact of poor school functioning. Aspects of school functioning should be screened by professionals working with students with CFS in schools, and frequent liaison between health professionals and school staff is likely to be beneficial. Given the significant impact on school functioning for adolescents with CFS noted by the current study, school staff should be provided with professional development aimed at increasing their understanding of CFS and how it can impact on the school functioning of students. Given the unique needs of each adolescent, as well as vast differences across school settings, tailored and individualized school planning that addresses not only school attendance, but also strategies to minimize the impact of the illness on school-related quality of life, school participation, school connectedness, and academic outcomes, will be crucial.

AUTHOR CONTRIBUTIONS

SK and MT lead the study design, data analysis and completed the first draft of the manuscript. They also supervised data collection. CG and JP completed data collection and contributed to data analysis and writing of the manuscript draft. AS contributed to study design and reviewed and contributed to manuscript drafts. All authors approved final version of the manuscript prior to submission.

ACKNOWLEDGMENTS

We would like to acknowledge the Mason Foundation and Victorian Government's Infrastructure Grant who provided funding to support this study. We would also like to acknowledge Diana Zannino and Elisha Josev who provided guidance for the statistical analyses.

REFERENCES

1. Jason LA, Bell DS, Rowe K, Van Hoof ELS, Jordan K, Lapp C, et al. A pediatric case definition for myalgic encephalomyalitis and chronic fatigue syndrome. *J Chron Fat Synd.* (2006) 13:1–44. doi: 10.1300/J092v13n02_01
2. Nijhof SL, Maijer K, Bleijenberg G, Uiterwaal C, Kimpen J, van de Putte EM. Adolescent chronic fatigue syndrome: prevalence, incidence, and morbidity. *Pediatrics* (2011) 127:e1169–75. doi: 10.1542/peds.2010-1147
3. Rimes KA, Goodman R, Hotopf M, Wessely S, Meltzer H, Chalder T. Incidence, prognosis, and risk factors for fatigue and chronic fatigue syndrome in adolescents: a prospective community study. *Pediatrics* (2007) 119:e603–9. doi: 10.1542/peds.2006-2231
4. Crawley E, Hughes R, Northstone K, Tilling K, Emond A, Sterne JAC. Chronic disabling fatigue at age 13 and association with family adversity. *Pediatrics* (2012) 130:e71–9. doi: 10.1542/peds.2011-2587
5. Crawley E, Hunt L, Stallard P. Anxiety in children with CFS/ME. *Eur Child Adolesc Psychiatry* (2009) 18:683–9. doi: 10.1007/s00787-009-0029-4
6. Davies S, Crawley E. Chronic fatigue syndrome in children aged 11 years old and younger. *Arch Dis Childhood* (2008) 93:419–21. doi: 10.1136/adc.2007.126649
7. Garralda ME, Rangel L. Impairment and coping in children and adolescents with chronic fatigue syndrome: a comparative study with other paediatric disorders. *J Child Psychol Psychiatry Allied Discipli.* (2004) 45:543–52. doi: 10.1111/j.1469-7610.2004.00244.x
8. Dickson A, Toft A, O'Carroll RE. Neuropsychological functioning, illness perception, mood and quality of life in chronic fatigue syndrome, autoimmune thyroid disease and healthy participants. *Psychol Med.* (2009) 39:1567–76. doi: 10.1017/S0033291708004960
9. Kennedy G, Underwood C, Belch JJ. Physical and functional impact of chronic fatigue syndrome/myalgic encephalomyelitis in childhood. *Pediatrics* (2010) 125:e1324–30. doi: 10.1542/peds.2009-2644
10. Bell DS, Jordan K, Robinson M. Thirteen-year follow-up of children and adolescents with chronic fatigue syndrome. *Pediatrics* (2001) 107:994–8. doi: 10.1542/peds.107.5.994
11. Bould H, Collin SM, Lewis G, Rimes K, Crawley E. Depression in paediatric chronic fatigue syndrome. *Arch Dis Child.* (2013) 98:425–8. doi: 10.1136/archdischild-2012-303396
12. Crawley E, Emond A, Sterne J. Unidentified chronic fatigue syndrome/myalgic encephalomyelitis (CFS/ME) is a major cause of school absence: surveillance outcomes from school-based clinics. *BMJ Open.* (2011) 1:e000252. doi: 10.1136/bmjopen-2011-000252

13. Crawley E, Sterne JA. Association between school absence and physical function in paediatric chronic fatigue syndrome/myalgic encephalopathy. *Arch Dis Child.* (2009) 94:752–6. doi: 10.1136/adc.2008.143537
14. Knight SJ, Harvey A, Lubitz L, Rowe K, Reveley C, Veit F, et al. Paediatric chronic fatigue syndrome: Complex presentations and protracted time to diagnosis. *J Paediatr Child Health* (2013) 49:919–24. doi: 10.1111/jpc.12425
15. Rangel L, Garralda ME, Levin M, Roberts H. The course of severe chronic fatigue syndrome in childhood. *J R Soc Med.* (2000) 93:129–34. doi: 10.1177/014107680009300306
16. Tollit M, Politis J, Knight S. Measuring school functioning in students with chronic fatigue syndrome: a systematic review. *J School Health* (2018) 88:74–89. doi: 10.1111/josh.12580
17. Van Hoof E, De Becker P, Lapp CW, De Meirleir K. How do adolescents with chronic fatigue syndrome perceive their social environment? a quantitative study. *Bull IACFS/ME* (2009) 17:16–31. Available online at: http://www.iacfsme.org/Portals/0/pdf/Van%20Hoof%20vol17%20n1.pdf
18. Sankey A, Hill CM, Brown J, Quinn L, Fletcher A. A follow-up study of chronic fatigue syndrome in children and adolescents: symptom persistence and school absenteeism. *Clin Child Psychol Psychiatr.* (2006) 11:126–38. doi: 10.1177/1359104506059133
19. Cole DA, Maxwell SE, Martin JM, Peeke LG, Seroczynski AD, Tram JM, et al. The development of multiple domains of child and adolescent self-concept: a cohort sequential longitudinal design. *Child Dev.* (2001) 72:1723–46. doi: 10.1111/1467-8624.00375
20. DuPaul GJ, Morgan PL, Farkas G, Hillemeier MM, Maczuga S. Eight-Year latent class trajectories of academic and social functioning in children with attention-deficit/hyperactivity disorder. *J Abnormal Child Psychol.* (2018) 46:979–92. doi: 10.1007/s10802-017-0344-z
21. Lum A, Wakefield CE, Donnan B, Burns MA, Fardell JE, Marshall GM. Understanding the school experiences of children and adolescents with serious chronic illness: a systematic meta-review. *Child* (2017) 43:645–62. doi: 10.1111/cch.12475
22. Gorodzinsky AY, Hainsworth KR, Weisman SJ. School functioning and chronic pain: a review of methods and measures. *J Pediatr Psychol.* (2011) 36:991–1002. doi: 10.1093/jpepsy/jsr038
23. Wechsler D. *Wechsler Abbreviated Scale of Intelligence (WASI-II). 2nd Edn.* San Antonio, TX: The Psychological Corporation (2011).
24. Varni JW, Burwinkle TM, Szer IS. The PedsQL Multidimensional Fatigue Scale in pediatric rheumatology: reliability and validity. *J Rheumatol.* (2004) 3112:2494–500.
25. Knight SJ, Harvey A, Hennel S, Lubitz L, Rowe K, Reveley C, et al. Measuring quality of life and fatigue in adolescents with chronic fatigue syndrome: estimates of feasibility, internal consistency and parent–adolescent agreement of the PedsQLTM. *Fatigue* (2015) 3:220–34. doi: 10.1080/21641846.2015.1090816
26. Crichton A, Knight SJ, Oakley E, Babl F, Anderson V. Fatigue in child chronic health conditions: a systematic review of assessment instruments. *Pediatrics* (2015) 135: e1015–31. doi: 10.1542/peds.2014-2440
27. Goodman R. The strengths and difficulties questionnaire: a research note. *J Child Psychol Psychiatry* (1997) 38:581–6. doi: 10.1111/j.1469-7610.1997.tb01545.x
28. Vostanis P. Strengths and difficulties questionnaire: research and clinical applications. *Curr Opin Psychiatry* (2006) 19:367–72. doi: 10.1097/01.yco.0000228755.72366.05
29. Varni JW, Seid M, Kurtin PS. PedsQL^{TM} 4.0: reliability and validity of the pediatric quality of life inventory^{TM} version 4.0 generic core scales in healthy and patient populations. *Med Care* (2001) 39:800–12. doi: 10.1097/00005650-200108000-00006
30. Bedell G. Further validation of the child and adolescent scale of participation (CASP). *Dev Neurorehabil.* (2009) 12:342–51. doi: 10.3109/17518420903087277
31. Goodenow C. The psychological sense of school membership among adolescents: scale development and educational correlates. *Psychol Schools* (1993) 30:79–90.
32. Wechsler D. *Wechsler Individual Achievement Test-Australian Abbreviated (WIAT-II Abbreviated). 2nd Ed.* Sydney: Pearson Clinical (2007).
33. Harris PA, Taylor R, Thielke R, Payne J, Gonzalez N, Conde JG. Research electronic data capture (REDCap) - a metadata-driven methodology and workflow process for providing translational research informatics support. *J Biomed Inform.* (2009) 42:377–81. doi: 10.1016/j.jbi.2008.08.010
34. StataCorp. *Stata Statistical Software: Release 14.* College Station, TX: StataCorp LP (2015).
35. Crawley E, Collin SM, White PD, Rimes K, Sterne JA, May MT. Treatment outcome in adults with chronic fatigue syndrome: a prospective study in England based on the CFS/ME National outcomes database. *QJM* (2013) 106:567. doi: 10.1093/qjmed/hct122
36. Lim A, Lubitz L. Chronic fatigue syndrome: successful outcome of an intensive inpatient programme. *J Paediatr Child Health* (2002) 38:295–9. doi: 10.1046/j.1440-1754.2002.00786.x
37. van Geelen SM, Bakker RJ, Kuis W, van de Putte EM. Adolescent chronic fatigue syndrome: a follow-up study. *Arch Pediatr Adolesc Med.* (2010) 164:810–4. doi: 10.1001/archpediatrics.2010.145
38. Sirin SR, Rogers-Sirin L. Components of school engagement among African American adolescents. *Appl Dev Sci.* (2005) 9:5–13. doi: 10.1207/s1532480xads0901_2
39. Carter BD, Edwards JF, Kronenberger WG, Michalczyk L, Marshall GS. Case control study of chronic fatigue in pediatric patients. *Pediatrics* (1995) 95:179–86.
40. Nagane M. Relationship of subjective chronic fatigue to academic performance. *Psychol Rep.* (2004) 95:48–52. doi: 10.2466/pr0.95.1.48-52
41. Farmer A, Fowler T, Scourfield J, Thapar A. Prevalence of chronic disabling fatigue in children and adolescents. *Br J Psychiatry* (2004) 184:477–81. doi: 10.1192/bjp.184.6.477
42. Lloyd AR, Hickie I, Boughton CR, Spencer O, Wakefield D. Prevalence of chronic fatigue syndrome in an Australian population. *Med J Australia* (1990) 153:522–8.

17

The UK ME/CFS Biobank: A Disease-Specific Biobank for Advancing Clinical Research into Myalgic Encephalomyelitis/Chronic Fatigue Syndrome

Eliana M. Lacerda, Kathleen Mudie, Caroline C. Kingdon, Jack D. Butterworth, Shennae O'Boyle and Luis Nacul*

Department of Clinical Research, Faculty of Infectious and Tropical Diseases, London School of Hygiene and Tropical Medicine, London, United Kingdom

***Correspondence:**
Eliana M. Lacerda
eliana.lacerda@lshtm.ac.uk

Myalgic encephalomyelitis/chronic fatigue syndrome (ME/CFS) is a disabling disease characterized by unexplained incapacitating fatigue, accompanied by variable multi-systemic symptoms. ME/CFS causes a significant personal and public health burden, and urgently requires the coordination of research efforts to investigate its etiology and pathophysiology and to develop and validate sensitive and specific biomarkers to confirm diagnosis. This narrative paper describes how people with ME/CFS, together with a multidisciplinary team of researchers, have established the UK ME/CFS Biobank (UKMEB), a unique research infrastructure specifically designed to expedite biomedical research into ME/CFS. We describe the journey that led to its conceptualization and operation, and how the resource has served as a model disease-specific biobank, aggregating human biospecimens alongside comprehensive health information on participants. The UKMEB currently has data and samples from 600 donors including people with ME/CFS and a comparison group with multiple sclerosis and healthy controls. A longitudinal sub-cohort has been established of participants having follow-up assessments at multiple time-points. As an open resource for quality and ethical research into ME/CFS, biological samples and data have not only been analyzed within our research team but have also been shared with researchers across Europe, America and the Middle East. We continue to encourage researchers from academic and commercial sectors to access the UKMEB. Major steps have been taken and challenges remain; these include sustainability and expansion, and harmonization of processes to facilitate integration with other bioresources and databanks internationally.

Keywords: ME/CFS, research infrastructure, biobank, partnership, patient engagement PE

INTRODUCTION

This paper describes a journey, beginning with extensive conversations between medical researchers, people with myalgic encephalomyelitis/chronic fatigue syndrome (ME/CFS), their carers, ME charities, and a multidisciplinary team of professional experts, and continuing with the establishment and operation of the UK ME/CFS Biobank (UKMEB) (1).

The UKMEB is, to our knowledge, the only biorepository in the United Kingdom, and one of few worldwide, dedicated to the study of ME/CFS. Such disease-specific biobanks hold high quality anonymised samples enriched by comprehensive datasets with information about the donors, all appropriately and securely stored until required for use in research. We delineate the progress our team have achieved and the remaining challenges that need to be addressed in order for the UKMEB to be able to realize its full potential.

Using a combination of qualitative methods (1, 2), we carried out extensive consultations with people with ME/CFS (PWME), a multidisciplinary group of experts in tissue banking, ethics and law, and clinicians and researchers with expertise in ME/CFS. The resultant unanimous view was that a disease-specific biobank would be a highly desirable way to enhance biomedical research in ME/CFS. In the safety of the participatory environment, PWME were able to express their justifiable concern that, in the absence of biomarkers, their illness is frequently dismissed as trivial or psychosocial (3–5), even though many are more debilitated by their disease than people with other chronic and severe diseases such as cancer and rheumatoid arthritis (6, 7). PWME told us that they would be willing to donate tissues, including blood, oral fluid and urine for research, as part of a process centered on the needs and priorities of those with ME/CFS (1). They believed that an ME/CFS Biobank would be feasible and cost-effective, and that its implementation would strengthen and further ME/CFS research.

FEATURES OF THE UKMEB PROTOCOL

The input from both PWME and the multidisciplinary group led to the development of a robust protocol, incorporating recommendations, which included:

- Comprehensive patient phenotyping and depth of any information provided by biobank donors;
- The use of rigorous standards for data and sample collection, processing, and storage;
- The inclusion of patients who are *"severely affected, including those that are bed-ridden"* (quote from a person with ME/CFS during focus-groups discussions); and
- The inclusion of control or comparison group(s).

Participants of the UKMEB were recruited through the National Health Services (NHS) general practices (GPs) and specialist services with support from the clinical and research networks of the National Institute of Health Research (NIHR). Those with ME/CFS required a previous medical diagnosis of ME/CFS and those with MS a previous diagnosis given by a NHS consultant. Healthy controls were also recruited through GP practices, other participants' contacts and higher education institutes.

The UKMEB received ethical approval from the London School of Hygiene & Tropical Medicine (LSHTM) Ethics Committee (ref. 6123), the National Research Ethics Service (NRES) London-Bloomsbury Research Ethics Committee (REC; ref. 11/LO/1760, IRAS ID: 77765), and the NHS Research Governance and Developments Offices (R&D), which oversee the recruitment of research participants from government health services. LSHTM and UCL-RFH Biobank hold Human Tissue Act licenses—HTA-12066 and HTA-11016, respectively.

Possible barriers to participation in a potential biobank resource were also discussed, and were mostly related to concerns with the misuse of the resource:

> *"if you're trying to get as much people as you can, they are afraid of what you're going to do, whether the government would get a hold of it, whether the insurance companies could use it, or whether benefit agencies would use it"* (quote from a person with ME/CFS during focus-groups discussions).

It was agreed that such misuse could be avoided by the implementation of robust ethical standards, which is reflected in the UKMEB mission statement that reads—"*The UKMEB is to conduct high quality, ethical investigations into ME/CFS and to create an open resource to enable translational research for the clinical and biomedical understanding of the illness while fostering cooperation and collaboration between researchers and thereby enhancing the opportunity for breakthrough discoveries.*"

Other key aspects of the final protocol informed by PWME together with experts include:

Control Groups

In addition to ME/CFS cases of different severities, we have recruited donors who serve as healthy controls; these individuals are grouped matched by age and sex and have no history of fatigue or fatigue-causing diseases, including cancer, hepatitis B or C, major depression or psychiatric illness, obesity, and diabetes. We also recruited people with Multiple Sclerosis (MS)—who often experience chronic fatigue as a major symptom—for a disease comparison group.

Clinical Phenotyping

Detailed questioning of potential participants with ME/CFS enables their disease to be classified according to different case definitions. To be accepted as a participant with ME/CFS, potential donors must meet either the Canadian Consensus Criteria (8) or CDC-1994 criteria (9); many fulfill both. The assessment process for compliance with study criteria includes baseline questionnaires about symptoms, a clinical assessment performed by a clinical member of the research team, and urinalysis screening and baseline blood tests, which are used to exclude alternative diagnoses.

In some association studies bias can be minimized by using samples from participants who meet at least both sets of criteria (10).

Extensive data collection together with the results of molecular analyses facilitates disease stratification, which aims to identify subgroups of patients with distinct mechanisms of disease (or other features), which may require quite different treatment approaches. Initial sub-grouping can be based on readily available variables obtained from patient questionnaires, examples of which include age, sex, type of disease onset (e.g., sudden or gradual; post-infection or not), co-morbidities, clinical severity, and disease phase and duration. The "Participant Phenotyping Questionnaire" completed by all UKMEB participants has been used to characterize individuals according to the presence and severity of seven groups of symptoms (or symptom clusters), which are largely based on the Canadian Consensus Criteria (8). **Table 1** compares study groups according to some of these variables, including general indicators of disease severity and the severity of symptoms related to each of the clusters described. For the latter, the scores are obtained from the severity of individual symptoms, each expressed as a value from 0 to 3; scores from each symptom within the cluster are added together, resulting in the cluster score, which is adjusted on a scale from 0 to 100, where "0" represents no symptoms and "100" symptoms experienced with maximum severity. For example, the severity of post-exertion malaise symptoms is highest in the severely affected cases of ME/CFS (median = 80), also high in those with mild/moderate disease (median = 67), and modest in people with MS (median = 27).

Inclusion of the Severely Affected

The systematic inclusion of participants with very severe ME/CFS for research purposes is, we believe, unique to the UK ME/CFS Biobank. This patient group usually has poor access to services and has often been excluded from research studies, not only because they are home- or bed-bound, but also because PWME often disengage from statutory medical services when they encounter skepticism or when the treatment offered is of limited value. Reaching them involves complex logistic and economic considerations.

> *"Arranging to see these extremely ill participants presents its own challenges, including the timing of appointments and the length of time that it may take to clinically assess participants, whose every move can take an enormous effort and for whom the process can require days of preparation and weeks of recovery time. Any external stimuli including touch, light and sound can exacerbate symptoms, so strategies must be undertaken to reduce the impact on participants. Certain clinical assessment procedures may not be feasible and blood samples are sometimes taken with the light from a torch in a darkened room. Nonetheless, the materials generated by these severely affected participants could provide crucial insight into the pathology of the disease, as they may present with exaggerated biochemical and/or immunological changes."* (Quote from CK (co-author) on the task of the Research Nurse)

Longitudinal Data and Samples

Through the systematic longitudinal collection of clinical data and blood samples, it is possible to investigate associations between clinical characteristics and changes in disease severity over time, as well as in a range of molecular markers, e.g., immune and genetic expression phenotypes.

We employ several validated measures of disease severity (11), while acknowledging the need for further development of ME/CFS-specific outcome measures. For example, patient-based assessments of disease impact or severity, such as the SF-36v2^{TM}, have been used in a variety of clinical settings and are monitored in clinical research to add to our understanding of disease severity, treatment outcomes, and therapeutic response (12). Changes between baseline and follow-up assessment-points can be compared with differences in biomarkers to help characterize clinical phenotypes. By using the suggested minimally important difference (MID) in SF-36v2^{TM} normalized scores, e.g., of ± 4.7 points for the Physical Component Summary (PCS) and ± 5.8 points for the Mental Component Summary (MCS), it is possible to ascertain improvement or worsening of scores with 95% confidence (12).

Figure 1 shows that <50% of the PWME demonstrated significant changes in these indicators from baseline to subsequent assessment. If there are persistent trends toward improvement or deterioration in repeated assessments, these may reflect disease progress or pathophysiological changes that may differ from those related to a fluctuation of symptoms.

UKMEB POTENTIAL: CURRENT STATUS AND ENHANCING RESEARCH

Resource Sharing

Between 2013 and 2017, biological samples alongside questionnaire and clinical data were collected from 600 participants (including 350 PWME), forming an extensive dataset. A second round of data collection took place 6–12 months after recruitment, with 140 PWME and 130 controls followed-up after baseline. From 2018 to 2020, a further 650 participants are planned to be seen at least once and a subset of 110 PWME to be seen on at least four occasions (and up to six), creating robust data that enables powerful longitudinal analyses.

The UKMEB currently holds over 35,000 aliquots of blood derivatives. Blood taken from each participant is processed to produce seven different types appropriate to the expected end use of the samples and suitable for a wide range of assays. After fractioning, an average of 46 aliquots is stored following each participant-contact as follows: serum ($n = 10$), plasma (processed from sodium heparin vacutainers $n = 7$, and from EDTA vacutainers $n = 3$), peripheral blood mononuclear cells (PBMCs) (processed from sodium heparin vacutainers $n = 17$, and from EDTA vacutainers $n = 3$), whole blood ($n = 4$), and RNA ($n = 1$–2). Additionally, for each participant contact, the UKMEB stores red blood cells/granulocyte pellet ($n = 1$), and PAXGENE tubes ($n = 1$–2).

Some of these are available to researchers at the LSHTM, the home of the UKMEB team, contributing to their ongoing projects in immunology, genomics, transcriptomics, virology, and clinical research. The rest of the samples are stored for the use of researchers from the academic and commercial sectors in biomedical research, following an established protocol for the release of samples, subject to ethical review and an approved, peer-reviewed application https://cureme.lshtm.ac.uk/researchers/accessing-the-biobank/.

Biobanks facilitate the sharing of biological samples and data in a cost- and time-effective way over many years (13). The cost savings to researchers vary depending on multiple factors, such as the type and size of the study, but have

TABLE 1 | Characteristics of cases (both mild/moderately affected and severely affected) and controls (healthy controls and MS diseased controls) within UKMEB, with cases of ME/CFS defined using a combination of three diagnostic criteria: CDC-1994, CCC, and IOM.

	Characteristic		Cases			Controls	
			CDC94+CCC+IOM $N = 232(38)$	Mild/ moderately affected[†] $N = 177(76)$	Severely Affected‡ N=55(24)	HC $N = 153(25)$	MS $N = 90$ (15)
	Age, in years	Median(IQR)	48 (38,56)	48 (40,57)	50 (37,55)	47 (35,56)	55 (48,60)
	Sex, female	N(%)	155 (76)	114 (76)	41 (76)	84 (62)	59 (78)
	Disease duration (years)	Median(IQR)	12 (6, 18)	10 (5, 17)	16 (9, 22)	-	12 (8, 20)
Disease Severity*	Fatigue severity scale	Median(IQR)	6.7 (6.3,7.0)	6.7 (6.2,7.0)	6.7 (6.3,6.9)	2.0 (1.6,2.8)	5.7 (4.1,6.4)
	Fatigue analog scale	Median(IQR)	7.3 (6.2,8.2)	6.9 (6.1,7.8)	7.6 (6.6,8.3)	1.1 (0.2,2.1)	6.2 (3.6,7.2)
	Pain analog scale	Median(IQR)	5.8 (3.2,7.2)	5.8 (3.1,7.1)	5.9 (3.2,7.4)	0.5 (0.0,1.2)	2.8 (0.7,6.2)
	PCS	Median(IQR)	26 (20,33)	28 (24,36)	20 (16, 22)	58 (56,60)	38 (29,48)
	MCS	Median(IQR)	41 (33,49)	40 (32,46)	46 (38,51)	55 (49,58)	48 (39,55)
Severity score for clusters of symptoms**	Post-exertional Malaise	Median(IQR)	67 (53,67)	67 (53,67)	80 (73,80)	0.0 (0.0,0.0)	27 (13,53)
	Pain	Median(IQR)	47 (27,67)	53 (27,67)	47 (27,80)	3.5 (0.0,10)	20 (7,40)
	Neurological/cognitive symptoms	Median(IQR)	50 (33,67)	43 (31,60)	62 (50,83)	0.0 (0.0,5.0)	36 (21,52)
	Autonomic	Median(IQR)	40 (23,57)	37 (22,50)	52 (40,77)	0.0 (0.0,3.0)	19 (10,32)
	Neuroendocrine	Median(IQR)	47 (33,67)	47 (27,60)	60 (47,80)	0.0 (0.0,0.0)	33 (20,53)
	Sleep dysfunction	Median(IQR)	83 (67,100)	67 (67,100)	100 (67,100)	0.0 (0.0,33)	50 (25,67)
	Immune	Median(IQR)	33 (22,50)	33 (22,50)	33 (22,56)	0.0 (0.0,6.0)	6.0 (0.0,11)
Disease onset	Suddenly	N(%)	91 (46)	60 (42)	31 (58)	-	30 (39)
	Over time	N(%)	80 (41)	63 (44)	17 (32)	-	31 (41)
	Not sure	N(%)	25 (13)	20 (14)	5 (9)	-	15 (20)

*CDC94: Centres for Disease Control-1994; CCC: Canadian Consensus Criteria; IOM: Institute of Medicine; HC: healthy controls; MS: Multiple Sclerosis; PCS: Summary Physical Component Score from SF-36; MCS: Summary Mental Component Score from SF-36v2[TM]. *For Fatigue Severity and Analog Scales and Pain Analog Scales; values vary from 0 to 10, where 10 indicates maximum severity. Normalized Physical and Mental Component summaries are presented; higher values represent better health status/quality of life.**Severity of symptoms within the cluster; values range from 0 (no symptom) to 100 (most severe symptoms). [†]Mild/moderately affected defined as participants who are ambulatory. ‡Severely affected defined as participants who are house- or bed-bound.*

been estimated to provide a 90% saving (14). These are in addition to significant time savings in selection, recruitment, and data and sample acquisition. This centralization of data and samples creates economies of scale, enabling and accelerating research.

In May 2016, the UKMEB opened to external researchers, who are able to apply for access to samples and data. Academic, non-commercial, and commercial researchers have since been eligible to apply to use the Biobank, when the proposed study has a sound scientific rationale and all ethical permissions are in place. Priority of research applications is given to studies testing or generating new hypotheses on the pathophysiology of ME/CFS, improving diagnosis and phenotyping, or in basic science (e.g., pharmacological *in vitro* studies potentially leading to clinical trials on therapeutic approaches).

The procedures for this access to data and samples, approved by the UKMEB Biobank Steering Committee, a multidisciplinary body comprising PWME, carers, researchers, and clinicians, include: (i) a review of outline proposals by Steering Committee members, (ii) a peer review of full proposals, (iii) ethical approval by the UCL-RFH ethics committee (BERC), and (iv) Data and/or Material Transfer Agreements (DTA and/or MTA). All proposals must also receive ethical approval from their local ethics committee.

Since the UK ME/CFS Biobank opened its doors, it has received applications from institutions in the UK and other European countries, North and South America, and the Middle East - encompassing diverse research topics including immunology, metabolomics, genetics, transcriptomics, and microbiology.

Sustainability

The UKMEB has relied on support from charities and has benefited from research grants, which have helped with recruitment, sample acquisition, data entry, and storage. This funding has supported core infrastructure, but only for the time period in which projects were taking place. To survive and thrive in the long term, plans were made for the continuing storage of samples and data, and particularly for the release of samples to external researchers. This necessitated the creation of a UKMEB Business Plan, which evolved with input from the Steering Committee.

A fee structure was calculated and agreed upon - fees are requested from biobank users on a cost-reimbursement basis, so

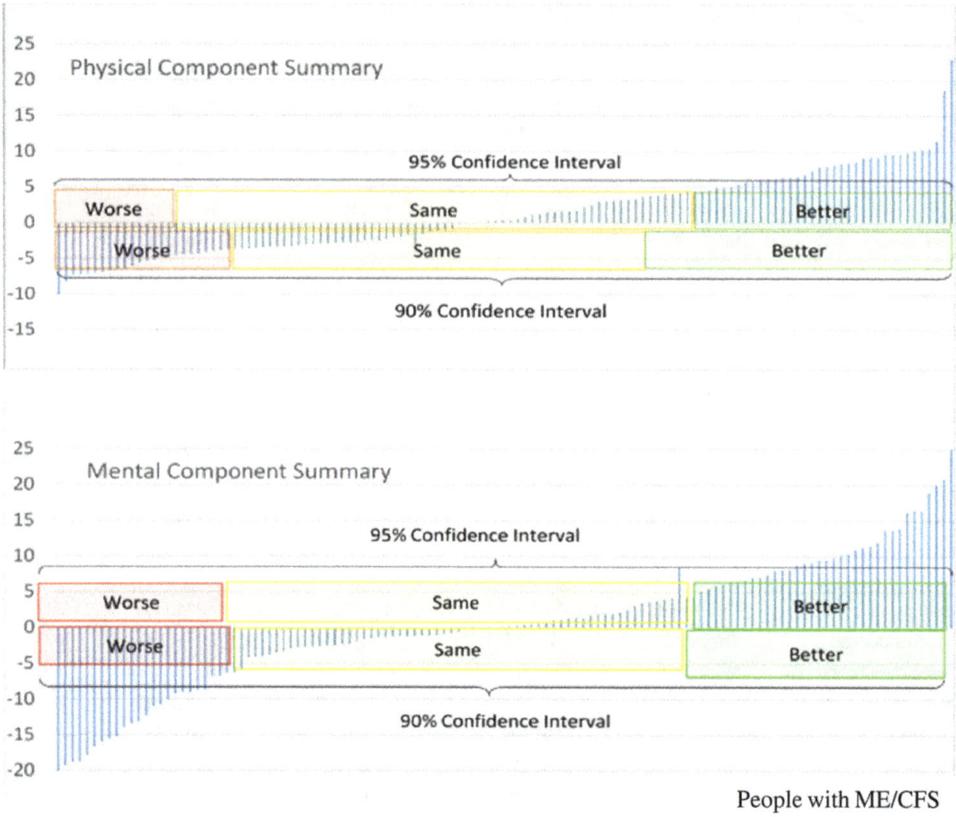

FIGURE 1 | Longitudinal changes in SF-36v2™ Component Summary scores, in people with ME/CFS who participate in the UK ME/CFS Biobank, between baseline and first follow-up*. *First follow up occurred between 6 and 12 months from baseline, Y-axis represents difference in scores between first follow-up assessment and baseline assessment; positive values indicate scores are higher at follow-up assessment, and therefore represent improvement. PCS, Normalized Physical Component Summary scores from SF-36v2™; MCS, Normalized Mental Component Summary score from SF-36v2™.

that sample stores can be replenished in the future and, where possible, additional recruitment or follow-up can be facilitated.

The long-term sustainability of the UKMEB relies upon multiple income streams, minimizing the risk of being exposed overly to any one source of funding. In financial year August 2015—July 2016, charity funding formed around 90% of gross revenue, but in financial year August 2017–July 2018, that had reduced to around 60%, with donations and cost recovery charged forming the remaining of 40% of total gross. The key elements of future UKMEB income are (i) fees for using the samples and data, (ii) philanthropic donations, (iii) crowdfunding and regular giving, and (iv) research grant support, which have to coexist to ensure long-term sustainability (14, 15). The opening of other income streams in the past financial year has shown that it is possible to move to a multi-source revenue system in biobanking, once appropriate start-up capital has been invested to enable fundraising and awareness-raising efforts.

Engagement With the Community

Social media, websites and web fora play a fundamental role in the lives of many with ME/CFS, facilitating social connection with others in the community as well as with researchers and charities, particularly when the physical demands of face-to-face interaction are not feasible. For PWME, online platforms can be one of the few places where their voices are heard and can be an invaluable resource in encouraging ongoing partnership between the ME/CFS community and researchers.

Engagement with these communities remains a key pillar of the UKMEB's strategy. We endeavor to remain transparent in our research objectives and stay engaged with PWME online, so that the communities we serve are actively involved in how we progress. In addition, we strive to be accountable to our donors by sharing whatever news and findings we can via social media and via our website.

This renewed focus on public engagement (since August 2017) has coincided with an increase in our donation income, as well as an increase in applications received from researchers wanting to use our resource. While any concrete causal relationship is difficult to prove, we feel that an active and open public engagement strategy supports several of the income streams delineated above, and helps contribute to the UKMEB's sustainability efforts, while also building trust between the research team and the community.

FINAL REMARKS—WHERE THIS JOURNEY IS HEADING?

Biobanks are recognized as key to biomedical research; and their numbers have been increasing globally, as human bio-specimens, combined with health information on their donors, provide a critical resource for biomedical research (16). Disease-specific biobanks, in particular, are useful for addressing conditions such as ME/CFS, where there remain important unanswered questions around causes, diagnosis, pathophysiology and treatment (17, 18). We believe that the UKMEB can be used as a model for others contemplating developing bio-resources in the field of ME/CFS; or indeed for other specific diseases, one that incorporates participatory approaches, partnership, time and cost-effectiveness, and sustainability into the design and implementation.

The integration of the UKMEB with other ME/CFS-specific biobanks could involve the sharing of protocols or at least an agreement to collect some common data and samples, and will be essential for accelerating much-needed ME/CFS research. Such research will likely include the investigation of potential biomarkers, transcriptomics, metabolomics, genomic and genetic studies; biobanks may also be accessed by those seeking to improve diagnosis and treatment, and undertake validation studies.

The poor recognition of and stigma that surrounds the disease are still present, and the wider needs of PWME in relation to healthcare, social, occupational and education support remain largely unmet (3). We have previously described the perceived needs of PWME, and some aspects of the care they receive (19). In this article, we focused on how the UKMEB evolved as we sought, in partnership, to help address some of these needs and to advance research into the disease. We described a journey that evolved from conversations with people with ME to an established resource facilitating biomedical research into ME/CFS locally and internationally. The journey has only just begun.

The enthusiasm from the ME/CFS community and from participants, including those with MS and healthy controls, has contributed to the success of a project developed while keeping the needs of patients and the research community in mind. With follow-up rates presently over 90% and an increasing number of external researchers using data and samples, the UKMEB is successfully delivering. However, the real benefits will only be felt when the results of research are effectively translated into better health for PWME.

There is no doubt that ME/CFS research can further be accelerated through the integration of bio-resources and the facilitation of consistent data collection globally. We are actively discussing and engaging with other bio-resources globally. The Common Data Elements project developed by the National Institute of Neurological Disorders and Stroke (20), is one example of an initiative aimed at data harmonization and integration in ME/CFS research. Another is the European Network on ME/CFS (EUROMENE), which combines resources, technologies, and expertise from over 20 European countries in a multidisciplinary approach to optimize knowledge production in the field. The harmonization of ME/CFS related data and bio-resources across the continent is one of the objectives of the network (21).

Improved research is only one of many challenges that needs addressing in the field, and we hope that our experiences presented here represent some contribution to this effort. It is only with substantial increases in research and research-infrastructure funding, and significant improvement in services for those with ME/CFS, that the individual journeys of PWME will be improved.

AUTHOR CONTRIBUTIONS

EL, LN, KM, and CK conceptualized the article, KM, LN, and EL conducted the clinical and epidemiological analyses. All authors contributed to drafting and to revising the manuscript critically for important intellectual content. All authors approved the final version of the manuscript to be published.

ACKNOWLEDGMENTS

We thank the University College London/Royal Free Hospital Biobank staff and the Norfolk UK Primary Care Network and National Institutes of Health Research and our collaborators at Royal Free Hospital Immunology and Clinical Pathology Departments, Norwich and Norfolk University Hospital, Imperial College Healthcare NHS Trust staff at the Charing Cross Hospital Neurology Department, Royal London Hospital for Integrated Medicine, ME/CFS Clinic (University College Hospitals, London) and all participating General Practices. We are especially grateful to the many people who have generously contributed to the biobank by donating their time, resources, and (often low) energy to participate in the study.

REFERENCES

1. Lacerda EM, Caroline CK, Erinna WB, Luis N. Using a participatory approach to develop and implement the UK ME/CFS biobank. *Fatigue* (2018) 6:1–4. doi: 10.1080/21641846.2018.1396021
2. Leung MW, Yen IH, Minkler M. Community-based participatory research: a promising approach for increasing epidemiology's relevance in the 21st century. *Int J Epidemiol.* (2004) 33:499–506. doi: 10.1093/ije/dyh010
3. De Drachler ML, Leite JC, Hooper L, Hong CS, Pheby D, Nacul L, et al. The expressed needs of people with chronic fatigue syndrome/myalgic encephalomyelitis: a systematic review. *BMC Public Health* (2009) 9:1–15. doi: 10.1186/1471-2458-9-458
4. Jason LA. Small wins matter in advocacy movements: giving voice to patients. *Am J Communtiy Psychol* (2010) 49:307–16. doi: 10.1007/s10464-011-9457-7
5. Jason LA, Taylor RR, Stepanek Z, Plioplys S. Attitudes regarding chronic fatigue syndrome: the importance of a name. *J. Health Psychol.* (2001) 6:61–71. doi: 10.1177/135910530100600105
6. Kingdon CC, Bowman EW, Curran H, Nacul L, Lacerda EM. Functional status and well-being in people with myalgic encephalomyelitis/chronic fatigue

syndrome compared with people with multiple sclerosis and healthy controls. *PharmacoEconomics* (2018) 2:381–92. doi: 10.1007/s41669-018-0071-6

7. Nacul LC, Eliana ML, Peter C, Derek P, De Maria LD, José CL, et al. The functional status and well being of people with myalgic encephalomyelitis/chronic fatigue syndrome and their carers. *BMC Public Health* (2011) 11:402. doi: 10.1186/1471-2458-11-402
8. Carruthers BM, Jain AK, DeMeirleir KL, Nancy G, Peterson D, Klimas MIL, et al. Myalgic encephalomyelitis / chronic fatigue syndrome : clinical working case definition, diagnostic and treatment protocols. *J Chron Fat Synd.* (2003) 11:7–36. doi: 10.1300/J092v11n01
9. Fukuda K, Straus SE, Hickie I, Sharpe MC, Dobbins JG, Komaroff A. The chronic fatigue syndrome: a comprehensive approach to its definition and study. *Int Chron Fat Synd Study Group Ann Int Med.* (1994) 121:953–9. doi: 10.7326/0003-4819-121-12-199412150-00009
10. Nacul L, Kingdon CC, Bowman EW, Curran H, Lacerda EM. Differing case definitions point to the need for an accurate diagnosis of myalgic encephalomyelitis/chronic fatigue syndrome. *Fatigue* (2017) 5:1–4. doi: 10.1080/21641846.2017.1273863
11. Lopes LV, Fernando M, Helga F, Antonio T, Salvador P, Clara C, et al. Stage at presentation of breast cancer in Luanda, angola - a retrospective study. *BMC Health Serv Res.* (2015) 15:471. doi: 10.1186/s12913-015-1092-9
12. Ware J, Snoww KK, Kosinski MA, Gandek BG, Gandek B, Ware JEJr, et al. *SF36 Health Survey: Manual and Interpretation Guide.* Lincoln, RI: Quality Metric, Inc (1993).
13. Watson PH, Nussbeck SY, Carter C, O'Donoghue S, Cheah S, Matzke LA, et al. A framework for biobank sustainability. *Biopreserv Biobank.* (2014) 12:60–8. doi: 10.1089/bio.2013.0064
14. Bromley RL. Financial stability in biobanking: unique challenges for disease-focused foundations and patient advocacy organizations. *Biopreserv Biobank.* (2014) 12:294–9. doi: 10.1089/bio.2014.0053
15. Vaught J, Joyce R, Todd C, Carolyn C. Biobankonomics: developing a sustainable business model approach for the formation of a human tissue biobank. *J Natl Cancer Inst.* (2011) 42:24–31. doi: 10.1093/jncimonographs/lgr009
16. Olson JE, Bielinski SJ, Ryu E, Winkler EM, Takahashi PY, Pathak J, et al. Biobanks and personalized. *Medicine* (2016) 86:50–5. doi: 10.1111/cge.12370.Biobanks
17. Gurwitz D, Fortier I, Lunshof JE, Knoppers BM. Children and population biobanks. *Res Ethics* (2009) 325:818–9. doi: 10.1126/science.1173284
18. Budimir D, Polasek O, Marusić A, Kolcić I, Zemunik T, Boraska V, et al. Ethical aspects of human biobanks: a systematic review. *Croatian Med J.* (2011) 52:262–79. doi: 10.3325/cmj.2011.52.262
19. Horton SM, Poland F, Kale S, de Drachler ML, de Carvalho Leite JC, McArthur MA, et al. Chronic fatigue syndrome/myalgic encephalomyelitis (CFS/ME) in adults: a qualitative study of perspectives from professional practice. *BMC Fam Pract.* (2010) 11:89. doi: 10.1186/1471-2296-11-89
20. Sheehan J, Hirschfield S, Foster E, Ghitza U, Goetz K, Karpinski J, et al. Improving the value of clinical research through the use of common data elements (CDEs). *Clin Trials* (2016) 13:6. doi: 10.1177/1740774516653238.Improving
21. COST. *European Network on Myalgic Encephalomyelitis/Chronic Fatigue Syndrome (EUROMENE).* (2015). Available online at: http://www.cost.eu/COST_Actions/ca/CA15111
22. Serepkaite J, Zivile V, Eugenijus G. 'Mirroring' the ethics of biobanking: what should we learn from the analysis of consent documents[Corrected]? *Sci. Eng. Ethics* (2014) 20:1079–93. doi: 10.1007/s11948-013-9481-0

18

Medically Documenting Disability in Myalgic Encephalomyelitis/Chronic Fatigue Syndrome (ME/CFS) Cases

Barbara B. Comerford [1*] ***and Richard Podell*** [2]

Law Offices of Barbara Comerford, Paramus, NJ, United States, [2] *Robert Wood Johnson Medical School, Rutgers, The State University of New Jersey, New Brunswick, NJ, United States*

***Correspondence:**
Barbara B. Comerford
bcomerford@barbaracomerfordlaw.com

Patients with severe myalgic encephalomyelitis/Chronic fatigue syndrome (ME/CFS) experience debilitating physical and cognitive symptoms, which often result in the need to file disability claims. A significant number of ME/CFS patients are children or adolescents. ME/CFS patients often turn to physicians who are not trained to recognize and diagnose ME/CFS, and who might or might not understand that ME/CFS is a multi-system primarily physical illness. Such misperceptions can adversely affect the doctor-patient relationship, the clinical outcomes, as well as the results of disability claims. According to the National Academies of Science, Engineering and Medicine, "Between 836,000 and 2.5 million Americans suffer from myalgic encephalomyelitis/chronic fatigue syndrome... This disease is characterized by profound fatigue, cognitive dysfunction, sleep abnormalities, autonomic manifestations, pain, and other symptoms that are made worse by exertion of any sort. ME/CFS can severely impair patients' ability to conduct their normal lives.[1]" The prevalence of MECFS among children and adolescents has been estimated variously as between 0.11 and 4% (1). A large percentage of children and adolescents with ME/CFS suffer from orthostatic intolerance due to one or both of these syndromes: Neurally Mediated Hypotension (NMH) and Postural Orthostatic Tachycardia Syndrome (POTS). These elements of ME/CFS often respond well to proper treatment (2, 3).

Keywords: CFS, physician education, chronic fatigue sydrome, myalgic encephalomyelitis, ME

MEDICALLY DOCUMENTING A SOCIAL SECURITY DISABILITY CLAIM

Under the Social Security Regulations, a person is disabled if he is unable to engage in substantial gainful activity by reason of a medically determinable impairment which can be expected to last for a continuous period of not < 12 months or result in death[2]. In April 2014, SSA issued updated guidelines for evaluating disability claims involving ME/CFS[3]. Social Security Ruling (SSR) 14-1p provides guidance on how to develop evidence and to establish that a person has a medically determinable impairment (MDI) of ME/CFS and explains how SSA evaluates those disability claims. Under 14-1p determination of an MDI includes a diagnosis of ME/CFS

[1] http://www.nationalacademies.org/hmd/Reports/2015/ME-CFS.aspx
[2] See SSR 14-1p.
[3] SSR 14-1p "CFS is a systemic disorder consisting of a complex of symptoms that may vary in frequency, duration, and severity..."
[4] SSR 14-1p and https://www.ssa.gov/disability/professionals/documents/64-063.pdf

by a licensed physician using the CDC case definition for CFS, and to a lesser extent, the Canadian Consensus Criteria and the International Consensus Criteria supported by specific medical evidence consisting of signs, symptoms and lab findings. Physicians must therefore know what medical evidence is necessary for patients to qualify for Social Security Disability benefits. Under 14-1p licensed physicians must provide medical reports which include a "thorough medical history including onset, duration, diagnosis of CFS/ME, and the prognosis. Any co-morbid conditions should also be included. Treatment prescribed, the patient response and all clinical findings such as the results of physical and mental status exams, lab findings or any other clinically accepted form of objective testing should also be included. Medical signs observed by the physician including orthostatic intolerance, palpably swollen or tender axillary or cervical lymph nodes, persistent, reproducible muscle tenderness on exam, abnormal immune function, non-exudative pharyngitis" are a few examples[5].

It is especially important to ask patients, including children and adolescents about orthostatic symptoms. At a minimum blood pressure and pulse should be documented lying down, sitting, immediately after standing, and then after remaining upright without moving for 2 to 5 min. Patients with orthostatic symptoms and/or substantial declines in blood pressure and/or tachycardia should be considered for specialty referral.

Physicians should also note symptoms or other effects of ME/CFS including: "persistent or relapsing fatigue resulting in reduction or impairment in the ability to carry out daily or work-related activities; post exertional malaise (worsening of symptoms after physical, cognitive or emotional effort); waking unrefreshed; disturbed sleep patterns; cognitive impairments (e.g., difficulty with information processing, short-term memory, reduced concentration and attention); persistent muscle pain, tenderness, stiffness, or weakness, multi-joint pain without swelling or redness; headaches of a new type, pattern or severity; frequent or re-occurring sore throats; cardiovascular abnormalities such as palpitations; gastrointestinal discomfort such as nausea, bloating, or abdominal pain; respiratory difficulties such as labored breathing or sudden breathlessness; urinary or bladder problems such as urinary frequency, nocturia, dysuria or pain in the bladder region or visual difficulties such as difficulty with focus, impaired depth perception or severe photosensitivity[6]."

Physicians should also provide an opinion about the patient's ability to perform daily activities at home, at school or at work. For example, getting dressed in the morning, organizing the day's activities, concentrating at school or at work, the ability to sustain prolonged periods of walking, sitting, typing etc, and whether these activities often cause a prolonged flare up of symptoms and decline of function (Post Exertional Malaise/ PEM).

[5]Id.

[6]Id.

Most disability claims made on behalf of children and adolescents with ME/CFS are supplemental security income claims (SSI) claims. SSI claims are filed on behalf of disabled children whose parents' income fall below federal poverty levels[7]. And in many states children on SSI can qualify for Medicaid[8].

Unlike adults, children with ME/CFS (and any other disabling conditions) must provide documentation of the existence of a medically determinable physical or mental impairment or impairments which result in *marked and severe functional limitations*; and that the impairment(s) lasted or can be expected to last for a continuous period of at least 12 months or be expected to result in death.

[7]https://www.ssa.gov/ssi/text-child-ussi.htm. WHO IS A "CHILD" FOR SSI?
A person who is neither married (as determined by Social Security) nor head of a household and: under age 18; or under age 22 and is a student regularly attending school (as determined by Social Security).
To be eligible for SSI benefits, a child must be either blind or disabled.
A child may be eligible for SSI disability benefits beginning as early as the date of birth; there is no minimum age requirement.
A child may be eligible for SSI disability benefits until attainment of age 18 (see definition of disability for children).
When the child attains age 18, we evaluate impairments based on the definition of disability for adults (see definition of disability for adults).
The child has a medically determinable physical or mental impairment or impairments ***which result in marked and severe functional limitations; and***
The impairment(s) has lasted or can be expected to last for a continuous period of at least 12 months or be expected to result in death; or

[8]If a child is under age 18, not married, and lives at home with parent(s) who do not receive SSI benefits, we may consider a portion of the parents' income and resources as if they were available to the child. We may also count a portion of a stepparent's income and resources if the child lives with both a parent and a stepparent (or an adoptive parent and a stepparent). We also do this when a child is temporarily away at school, returns home during weekends, holidays or during the summer and remains subject to parental control. We call this process "deeming".
We make deductions from deemed income for parents and for other children living in the home. After we subtract these deductions, we use the remaining amount to decide if the child meets the SSI income and resource requirements for a monthly benefit.
Deeming from the parent stops when a child attains age 18, marries, or no longer lives with a parent. Deeming does not apply, and we may pay up to $30 plus the applicable State supplement when: a disabled child receives a reduced SSI benefit while in a medical treatment facility; and the child is eligible for Medicaid under a State home care plan; and deeming would otherwise cause ineligibility for SSI benefits.
Also, we do not consider the income of a parent for deeming purposes if the parent receives a Public Income Maintenance payment (PIM) such as Temporary Assistance for Needy Families (TANF) and his or her other income was used to compute the PIM payment.
If either child or parent is temporarily absent from the household (less than 60 days), the rules about deemed income still apply.
In most States, a child who gets SSI benefits can get Medicaid to help pay medical bills.
In some cases, a child may be eligible for Medicaid while in an institution, but not be eligible when living at home either because of the parents' income and resources or because of other income.
At the State's option, children under age 18 who need institutional–level care and live at home may keep Medicaid eligibility while getting home care, if that care is less costly to the government.
Even if the child is not eligible for SSI benefits, the child still may be eligible for Medicaid under other State rules. Always check on Medicaid eligibility with the State.
For more information about Medicaid, you can look on the internet on the Centers for Medicare & Medicaid Services website at http://www.medicaid.gov/index.html or call toll–free, 1–800–633–4227.
In addition, other State services may also be available.

In determining whether a child experiences marked and severe functional limitations in the context of a child SSI case, SSA will consider proof[9] regarding all the child's impairments, including their interactive and cumulative effects, and all the relevant information in (the child's) case record that helps determine functioning, including signs, symptoms, and laboratory findings, and the descriptions about functioning from the child's parents, teachers, and other people who know, and other relevant factors.

"The medical evidence may include formal testing that provides information about the child's development or functioning in terms of percentiles, percentages of delay, or age or grade equivalents. Standard scores (e.g., percentiles) can be converted to standard deviations. When such scores (are produced), (SSA) will consider them together with the information (SSA has) about (the child's) functioning to determine whether the child has a "marked" or "extreme" limitation in a domain[10].

Children and adolescents can be diagnosed with ME/CFS if they suffer from the following symptoms:

- severe disabling fatigue that lasts for at least 3 months
- headaches
- sleep problems
- cognitive problems
- sore throat
- muscle aches and pains
- nausea, and dizziness
- Post-exertional malaise is a core symptom and the most useful when making a diagnosis[11].

Children experience an increase in fatigue, malaise and symptoms after an increase in exertion. For many, this means they attend 1 or 2 days of school, before becoming too unwell to attend school at all. Some children are severely affected and post-exertional malaise presents as an increase in symptoms after, for example, taking a shower or walking down the stairs. Other symptoms that are almost universal in children and adults are cognitive dysfunction and disturbed/unrefreshing sleep[12]."

Since there is no impairment listing for ME/CFS for either adults or children within the Code of Federal Regulations[13] governing SS cases, both adult and children cases require documentation of severe functional limitations. For an impairment to equal the listings in an SSI child case through the domains of functioning, the ME/CFS must cause severe (marked) limitations that affect at least two of the six domains of functioning or an extreme limitation that affects at least one domain[14].

SSA reviews a child/adolescent SSI case by examining whether there are marked and extreme functional deficits in one or more of six domains[15]. The Domains of Functioning evaluates a different area of functioning important in everyday life:

---

[9]https://secure.ssa.gov/poms.nsf/lnx/0425225020

[10]https://secure.ssa.gov/poms.nsf/lnx/0425225020

"We will find that you have a "marked" limitation in a domain when your impairment(s) interferes seriously with your ability to independently initiate, sustain, or complete activities. Your day-to-day functioning may be seriously limited when your impairment(s) limits only one activity or when the interactive and cumulative effects of your impairment(s) limit several activities. "Marked" limitation also means a limitation that is "more than moderate" but "less than extreme." It is the equivalent of the functioning we would expect to find on standardized testing with scores that are at least two, but less than three, standard deviations below the mean.

If you have not attained age 3, we will generally find that you have a "marked" limitation if you are functioning at a level that is more than one-half but not more than two-thirds of your chronological age when there are no standard scores from standardized tests in your case record.

If you are a child of any age (birth to the attainment of age 18), we will find that you have a "marked" limitation when you have a valid score that is two standard deviations or more below the mean, but less than three standard deviations, on a comprehensive standardized test designed to measure ability or functioning in that domain, and your day-to-day functioning in domain-related activities is consistent with that score. (See DI 25225.020D).

For the sixth domain of functioning, "Health and physical well-being," we may also consider you to have a "marked" limitation if you are frequently ill because of your impairment(s) or have frequent exacerbations of your impairment(s) that result in significant, documented symptoms or signs. For purposes of this domain, "frequent" means that you have episodes of illness or exacerbations that occur on an average of 3 times a year, or once every 4 months, each lasting 2 weeks or more. We may also find that you have a "marked" limitation if you have episodes that occur more often than 3 times in a year or once every 4 months but do not last for 2 weeks, or occur less often than an average of 3 times a year or once every 4 months but last longer than 2 weeks, if the overall effect (based on the length of the episode(s) or its frequency) is equivalent in severity.

C. Policy – Extreme Limitation

We will find that you have an "extreme" limitation in a domain when your impairment(s) interferes very seriously with your ability to independently initiate, sustain, or complete activities. Your day-to-day functioning may be very seriously limited when your impairment(s) limits only one activity or when the interactive and cumulative effects of your impairment(s) limit several activities. "Extreme" limitation also means a limitation that is "more than marked." "Extreme" limitation is the rating we give to the worst limitations. However, "extreme limitation" does not necessarily mean a total lack or loss of ability to function. It is the equivalent of the functioning we would expect to find on standardized testing with scores that are at least three standard deviations below the mean.

If you have not attained age 3, we will generally find that you have an "extreme" limitation if you are functioning at a level that is one-half of your chronological age or less when there are no standard scores from standardized tests in your case record.

If you are a child of any age (birth to the attainment of age 18), we will find that you have an "extreme" limitation when you have a valid score that is three standard deviations or more below the mean on a comprehensive standardized test designed to measure ability or functioning in that domain, and your day-to-day functioning in domain-related activities is consistent with that score. (See DI 25225.020D).

For the sixth domain of functioning, "Health and physical well-being," we may also consider you to have an "extreme" limitation if you are frequently ill because of your impairment(s) or have frequent exacerbations of your impairment(s) that result in significant, documented symptoms or signs substantially in excess of the requirements for showing a "marked" limitation in DI 25225.020B.4. However, if you have episodes of illness or exacerbations of your impairment(s) that we would rate as "extreme" under this definition, your impairment(s) should meet or medically equal the requirements of a listing in most cases. See DI 25220.010.

[11]https://www.ncbi.nlm.nih.gov/pmc/articles/PMC5919160/

[12]https://www.ncbi.nlm.nih.gov/pmc/articles/PMC5919160/

[13]CFR Part 404, Subpart P Appendix 1.

[14]https://www.disabilitycarecenter.org/medical-qualifications/domains-of-functioning/

[15]https://www.disabilitycarecenter.org/medical-qualifications/domains-of-functioning/

1) "Acquiring and using information[16]
2) Attending and completing tasks[17]
3) Interacting and relating with others[18]
4) Moving about and manipulating objects[19]
5) Caring for yourself[20]
6) Health and Physical well-being[21]."

Under the SSA sixth domain of functioning, "Health and physical well-being," to determine whether a child suffers from a "marked limitation," it will consider whether a child is frequently ill because of her impairment(s) or has frequent exacerbations of his impairment(s) that result in significant, documented symptoms or signs. For purposes of this domain, "frequent" means that the child has episodes of illness or exacerbations that occur on an average of 3 times a year, or once every 4 months, each lasting 2 weeks or more. A Marked Limitation—is a limitation that severely interferes with a child's ability to engage in activities related to a domain of functioning. A marked limitation is more severe than a moderate limitation and is less severe than an extreme limitation[22,23].

SSA may also find that the child has a "marked" limitation if he has episodes that occur more often than 3 times in a year or once

[16]Acquiring and Using Information
This domain considers how well a child can learn and acquire information as well as their ability to utilize the information. From birth, children start learning and acquiring information through exploring the world and receiving formal education by attending school. As they grow up, children should adapt and acquire skills in communication, arithmetic, reading, writing, and reasoning through their experiences. These skills should progress with complexity as they age and eventually can be utilized in a workplace or community environment.
A child may have a marked or extreme limitation in this domain if he or she:
He or she cannot show understanding of works related to size, space, or time
He or she is unable to rhyme words
He or she has difficulty remembering important concepts learned the day beforehand
He or she has difficulty solving math or arithmetic problems
He or she talks in simple, short sentence and has trouble explaining what they mean
[17]https://www.disabilitycarecenter.org/medical-qualifications/domains-of-functioning/
Attending and Completing Tasks
This domain evaluates a child's ability to focus and maintain attention as well as their ability to begin, continue, and complete activities at a normal pace for their age. Typically a child should be able to regulate alertness, filter out distractions, and maintain focus on a task or activity. While attending school, these abilities are critical for a child to effectively follow instructions, keep organized, and complete assignments.
A child may have a marked or extreme limitation if he or she:
Is easily startled, distracted or overreacts to touch, sounds, or movements
Is slow to focus on, or unable to finish activities of interest
Frequently becomes sidetracked from activities or repeatedly interrupts other
Becomes frustrated easily and gives up on tasks
Requires additional supervision to maintain engagement in an activity
[18]https://www.disabilitycarecenter.org/medical-qualifications/domains-of-functioning/
Interacting and Relating to Others
This domain focuses on a child's ability to connect and cooperate with others, abide by rules or restrictions, respond to authority or criticism, respect the possessions of others, and develop a sense of community. A child should develop close personal relationships with family and friends, and work cooperatively with other children in school or the community. A child should also understand and respect social rules in various environments such as what is behavior is acceptable at home compared to being in public at a grocery store.
A child may have a marked or extreme limitation if he or she:
Does not reach out to be picked up by his or her guardians
Has no close friends of the same age
Avoids contact with others including people they know
Has problems with adequate fluency when speaking
Has difficulty engaging in activities with rules (such as board games or sports)
Has difficulty with communication; He or she struggles with expressing emotions, continuing a conversation, or asking for help
[19]https://www.disabilitycarecenter.org/medical-qualifications/domains-of-functioning/
Moving About and Manipulating Objects
This domain involves how well a child can move his or her body from one location to another and how he or she moves and manipulates objects. These movements are known as "gross" and "fine" motor skills and are described below.
Gross and Fine Motor Skills
Gross motor skills involve movement and coordination of the limbs (arms and legs) and other large body parts while fine motor skills refer to the movement and coordination of smaller body parts such as the hands, fingers, wrists, feet, ankles and toes. Gross motor skills include movements such as running, kneeling, bending, and crawling. Fine motor skills include movements such as grasping, gripping, and writing.
The physical capabilities of a child depend on his or her age. A 6 year old is not expected to have the same complex motor skills as a 16 year old. As children age, they should develop more complex motor skills appropriate for their age. Below are some examples of limitations for this domain.
A child may have a marked or extreme limitation if he or she:
Experiences sensory loss, muscle weakness, or joint stiffness
Has difficulty keeping balance, climbing stairs, or maintaining organized locomotion
Has trouble with coordinating gross motor movement
Has trouble with fine motor movement
Has difficulty with complex finger or hand movements
Has poor hand-eye coordination while using scissors or a pencil
[20]https://www.disabilitycarecenter.org/medical-qualifications/domains-of-functioning/
Caring for Self
This domain evaluates how well a child is able to take care of him or herself. This includes a child's ability to meet his or her emotional and physical wants and needs as well as how the child deals with changes in his or her environment. As children grow, they should learn to understand how to regulate themselves independently and take care of their own personal needs, possessions, health, and safety (appropriate for their age).
A child may have a marked or extreme limitation if he or she:
Repeatedly places inedible objects in his or her month
Consistently engages in self-soothing activities exhibiting developmental regression
Is unable to dress or bathe properly for his or her age
Often engages in self-harming behavior or disregards safety rules
Does not seek out activities of interest
Has disturbed sleeping and eating patterns
[21]Id.
[22]https://www.disabilitycarecenter.org/medical-qualifications/domains-of-functioning/
Health and Physical Well-Being
This domain considers the cumulative physical effects of the child's impairment(s) and its associated medications or treatments that are not considered in the "Caring for Self" domain. Physical and mental disabilities can have physical effects that vary in severity and can inhibit a child's ability to perform activities effectively or independently. The medication a child takes for his or her disability may potentially create physical side effects that interfere with daily activities.
A child may have a marked or extreme limitation if he or she:
Needs intensive medical care to maintain health and well-being
Physical limitations manifested from treatments, medication, or surgeries
Has generalized symptoms caused by his or her condition such as dizziness, lethargy, weakness, agitation, or psychomotor retardation.
[23]https://www.disabilitycarecenter.org/medical-qualifications/domains-of-functioning/

every 4 months but do not last for 2 weeks, or occur less often than an average of 3 times a year or once every 4 months but last longer than 2 weeks, if the overall effect (based on the length of the episode(s) or its frequency) is equivalent in severity.

The functional limitations a child or adolescent who suffers from ME/CFS might experience "marked" limitation if the child is frequently ill because of the following symptoms: severe fatigue, lightheadedness, headaches, muscle aches and pains, sore throats, nausea, dizziness, sleep and cognitive deficits. If the child attends school but cannot sit the length of time other children can, and must lay down, that is a marked functional limitation most likely because of orthostatic intolerance. If the child is like that for weeks at a time, it is clearly a marked limitation. If the child is always like that, it may fall into the extreme category. And remember that under the functional child limitations, you need to document marked limitations in two domains or one extreme limitation in one domain. If the child cannot stay vertical for long because of orthostatic symptoms, that will impact the child's ability to engage in sports, or other school related activities. If the child has cognitive deficits, it is unlikely he will be able to participate in class as other children do. They may also require special testing with additional time due to slow processing speed. If they do participate in any of these activities, they may require extended rest, or miss days of school as a result of "crashes" also known as post exertional malaise.

Any diagnostics that can confirm these deficits are acceptable sources of medical evidence under SSR 14-1p.

To establish a disability, a child with ME/CFS (or any other disability) must also establish that she also suffers from a severe limitation. "Severe" in this context requires proof that the impairments very seriously interfere with a child's ability to engage in activities related to a domain of functioning. An extreme limitation is rather rare and is only given to the worst limitations.

A child or adolescent with ME/CFS can establish disability by demonstrating two marked limitations or one extreme limitation within these domains[24].

Adult ME/CFS patients experience good days and bad days and post exertional malaise following exertion which impairs sustained, predictable function which significantly impacts the ability to perform any activities on a regular and sustained basis. Therefore, the physician should discuss good day/bad day and post exertional malaise presentation of symptoms. Cognitive deficits such as difficulties processing information, remembering, concentrating, and focusing should be addressed in the report. These same limitations exist in children.

Adult ME/CFS patients may also seek benefits under a disability insurance policy provided by an employer, or through purchase of a disability insurance policy from an insurance broker. Children and adolescents do not participate in the work force such that they are entitled to private long term disability insurance so the following discussion only pertains to adults.

[24]https://www.ssa.gov/disability/professionals/bluebook/evidentiary.htm

MEDICALLY DOCUMENTING A LONG TERM DISABILITY INSURANCE CLAIM (LTD)

Some private employers offer short and long-term disability insurance coverage to eligible employees as part of an ERISA (Employee Retirement Income Security Act) welfare benefit plan. The LTD Plan provides a percentage of pre-disability income in the event the worker becomes disabled.

Individuals can also privately purchase disability income (DI) insurance directly through an insurance broker for a specific monthly benefit amount. The latter are not governed by ERISA, but rather state insurance laws.

Just as a physician must provide medical documentation for an ME/CFS SSD claim, she must also medically document the LTD claim. A patient must accurately report the ME/CFS symptoms/limitations to the physician to assist in devising a treatment plan and to clinically document the medical chart for both SSD and LTD claims.

MEDICAL DOCUMENTATION FOR ALL DISABILITY CLAIMS

ME/CFS Patients or Their Parents Should Keep a Daily Journal With Complaints and Limitations to Provide for the Physician at Each Office Visit

ME/CFS patients often complain of brain fog or other cognitive issues which may adversely impact reporting symptoms/limitations to the physician. The physician should request the patient keep a daily journal of complaints and limitations to ensure the medical chart documents the actual state of the patient's health, and the functional limitations which result. The symptom/limitation journal can therefore provide a more accurate picture of the patient's symptoms and limitations and, when given to the physician during a visit, becomes part of the chart for a physician to review for treatment purposes, and to answer questions posed by the disability insurance company or the Social Security Administration.

Good Day/Bad Day Constellation of Symptoms

ME/CFS patients often experience "good days" and "bad days" and a patient's chronicling activities on those days is important. For example, if taking a shower on a good day requires the ME/CFS patient to rest after for a period because he is exhausted, the journal can document that.

ME/CFS patients often define a "good day" as a day when she can perform one or two activities with rest intervals, hardly a good day to most people.

On bad days, the level of function can plummet to little more than eating, drinking and going to the bathroom. A contemporaneous description of such days is critical in this context, especially when LTD insurance companies frequently employ surveillance to undermine ME/CFS claims.

The U.S. General Accounting Office also conducts surveillance in Social Security Disability (SSD) claims. As a result, the patient journal entries may not simply put that surveillance in context, it can support disability.

For example, if an investigator records an ME/CFS claimant's outside the house performing a chore or two, the investigator might extrapolate from this brief period of normal activity that the person has the ability to sustain normal function throughout a full school or work day for 5 days each week. But if the claimant's journal entry on that day, records a post exertional flare up of physical pain, fatigue, or mental exhaustion, that documented evidence can undermine the insurer's attempt to pain the claimant's functional abilities in a false light. And often, good day activity is followed by physical and/or cognitive crashes which adversely impact the patient's function the next day. Therefore, the journal's description should continue for at least 24 h or more.

A common tactic of private LTD insurers is to schedule a medical exam by one of its medical vendors and then employ surveillance before and after to document the claimant's conduct. In ME/CFS cases, claimants often experience a worsening of symptoms following the insurance medical exam. A patient's journal entry can document what surveillance does not– including the worsening of symptoms during the hours or days following the exam.

The patient journal will also likely document the unpredictability of the symptoms and limitations from 1 day to the next, and often from 1 h to the next and the frequency of post exertional malaise when activities are performed.

An ME/CFS Claimant Should not Participate in a Standard Functional Capacity Evaluation Scheduled by the LTD Insurer

Private LTD insurance companies often try to schedule standard functional capacity evaluations (FCE) (as opposed to a cardio pulmonary exercise test (CPET) performed in ME/CFS cases) to determine whether an ME/CFS claimant has the physical capacity to work. Use of the FCE for that purpose has been discredited for a variety of reasons [25].

On February 20, 2019, Richard Podell, M.D. conducted a search of the National Library of Medicine database searching keywords: Functional Capacity Evaluation, Chronic Fatigue Syndrome and located 11 citations and found there were zero studies published that claim to demonstrate any validity for the FCE as standardly used to predict or certify whether a person with chronic fatigue syndrome is well enough to be able to work. Dr. Podell has written extensively on the topic and has useful information on his website regarding documenting disability in ME/CFS cases[26].

If an LTD carrier demands the ME/CFS claimant attend a standard FCE, a treating physician should prepare a letter explaining any deleterious effect that test will have on the patient's health. The most common effect of a prolonged standard FCE is post exertional malaise, and exacerbation of other physical and cognitive ME/CFS symptoms[27].

It is a basic tenet of insurance law, that an insured is disabled when the activity in question would aggravate a serious condition affecting the insured's health. *Lasser v. Reliance Standard Life Ins. Co.*, 344 F.3d 381 (3rd Cir. 2003). The treatise definition of disability holds that "[t]he insured is considered to be permanently and totally disabled when it is impossible to work without hazarding his or her health. . . ," *31 John Alan Appleman, Appleman on Insurance § 187.05[A]*, at 214 (2d ed.2007). *Lasser v. Reliance Standard Life Ins. Co., 146 F.Supp.2d 619, 628 (D.N.J. 2001) [Citing Herring v. Canada Life Assur. Co., 207 F.3d 1026 (8th Cir. 2000)].*

Whenever Possible, Objectively Document the Symptoms and Functional Limitations

The clinical longitudinal medical record is the first place the long-term disability insurer and SSA will look to determine the length of the illness, the signs and symptoms documented in the record, and what, if any, objective documentation of signs, symptoms and functional limitations exist. This is another reason why incorporating the patient journal entries into the medical record is critical in this context.

The primary concern of most treating physicians is to document and address patient signs and symptoms, not necessarily to record functional limitations. A hallmark of ME/CFS is debilitating fatigue and post exertional malaise (PEM)[28]. The LTD insurer will examine the medical record to determine whether the physician has recorded fatigue and PEM complaints during each visit, if medications were prescribed to address those complaints, the response, positive or negative the patient had to the medications, and any objective testing done to document it. The insurance reviewer will also often ask the treating physician to answer questions about the claimant's functional abilities.

Once again, the patient's journal record of complaints and functional limitations within the chart will give the physician the ability to reply to those questions.

In disability claims, medical documentation of physical exam findings during each visit, as well as, signs and symptoms, treatment plans, and objective test results often control the outcome of the claim. The patient chart charts the course of the claim[29].

Cardio pulmonary exercise testing (CPET) is a diagnostic test ordered by some ME/CFS specialists to determine the extent of the functional limitations associated with fatigue and PEM. CPET testing is administered over 2 days when the patient pedals on a stationary bike while resistance is added incrementally. It monitors cardiovascular, respiration and recovery responses, workload, effort and metabolic response/oxygen consumption. Very often the MECFS patient performs significantly worse

[25]https://www.aafp.org/afp/2007/0715/p247.html and https://www.prohealth.com/library/functional-capacity-evaluation-fce-and-your-disability-insurance-benefits-33900

[26]http://www.fmnetnews.com/coping-resources/disability-issues, https://www.drpodell.org/

[27]Id.

[28]https://www.ncbi.nlm.nih.gov/pmc/articles/PMC5983853/

[29]https://law.justia.com/cases/federal/district-courts/new-jersey/njdce/2:2015cv06197/323449/44/

on day two, which objectively documents the existence of functionally limiting post-exertional malaise[30].

While CPET is considered the "gold standard" to objectively document PEM in CFS/ME patients, it must be performed by a provider who understands ME/CFS to avoid misinterpreting the results.

ME/CFS patients often complain of many cognitive deficits including impaired information processing speed, decline in verbal fluency, memory and concentration issues[31]. The ME/CFS patient should be tested by a neuropsychologist familiar with ME/CFS to ensure the test results are accurately interpreted.

The more objective documentation of the ME/CFS patient complaints, the stronger the case. (with, for example the above tests and tilt table testing[32], EEGs[33], QEEGs[34], SPECT scans[35], PET scans[36] MRIs[37] etc.,)[38] BEAM results indicated that the energy values of δ, θ, and α_1 waves significantly increased in the observation group, compared with the control group ($P < 0.05$, $P < 0.01$, respectively), which suggests that the brain electrical activities in CFS patients were significantly reduced and stayed in an inhibitory state; 2) the increase of δ, θ, and α_1 energy values in the right frontal and left occipital regions was more significant than other encephalic regions in CFS patients, indicating the region-specific encephalic distribution; 3) the correlation dimension in the observation group was significantly lower than the control group, suggesting decreased EEG complexity in CFS patients.

In ERISA LTD cases, the contents of the administrative record often determine whether the case is later won or lost not merely during the administrative appeal stage, but in litigation. Courts in ERISA LTD cases are often limited to determining whether the insurance claim reviewer abused its discretion in denying the claim. In such cases, the Court may not substitute its opinion for that of the insurance company unless an abuse of that discretion is found. As a result, if the LTD insurer ignores the substantial evidence of record, cherry picks only unfavorable evidence from the record to deny a claim, or otherwise fails to conduct a full and fair review of the claim, it may be found to have abused its discretion. For these reasons, the medical evidence of record in support of disability, and the ME/CFS claimant documentation of complaints and functional limitations incorporated into the medical chart are crucial. A similar review occurs in SSD cases.

Provide a "Before and After" Record of Occupational and Everyday Functional Abilities

Disability insurers and SSA require all claimants to describe their work history, especially the occupational demands prior to disability onset. When a patient requests a physician respond to a disability inquiry or provide a report on their behalf, the physician should inquire about the patient's job demands to assess whether the patient's ME/CFS symptoms, limitations and restrictions reasonably prevent the patient from performing his own occupational demands or the demands of any occupation. If an ME/CFS claimant was physically active and engaged prior to disability, but has abandoned all or many of those activities, that should also be documented in the medical record.

CONCLUSION

The ME/CFS claimant must document the total adverse effect the constellation of symptoms has on his/her functional abilities and should provide that documentation in journal form to his treating physician during each visit. No claim can succeed without medical support and documentation of symptoms and functional limitations (physical and cognitive) by informed ME/CFS medical providers. The ME/CFS claimant medical record of functional limitations, and objective documentation of those limitations provided by the treating physician is crucial to support the ME/CFS disability claim.

If keeping a daily journal is not practical, we recommend that the patient or parent at each doctor visit submit 3 or 4 recent real life examples of episodes when the patient did "too much," how the symptoms then flared and functional abilities declined, and how many hours or days were needed before symptoms and functional abilities regained their pre-exertional baselines.

AUTHOR'S NOTE

BC, Esq has been practicing disability insurance law, and Social Security Disability law since 1985 (www.tristatedisabilitylaw.com). She has lectured extensively and presented papers on these topics to lawyers, judges and disability organizations around the nation. Recently, she and her senior associate, Sara Kaplan-Khodorovsky, successfully represented a Washington Post reporter disabled with ME/CFS in an ERISA LTD lawsuit

---

[30] https://www.ncbi.nlm.nih.gov/pmc/articles/PMC4482824/ and http://neuroimmune.cornell.edu/research/physiology/; https://www.ncbi.nlm.nih.gov/pmc/articles/PMC4734796/

[31] https://www.ncbi.nlm.nih.gov/pmc/articles/PMC3655280/ and http://www.ncf-net.org/library/sp.htm

[32] http://iacfsme.org/ME-CFS-Primer-Education/Bulletins/2010/Results-of-Head-Upright-Tilt-Table-Test-Full-Artic.aspx

[33] https://www.ncbi.nlm.nih.gov/pmc/articles/PMC4734796/

[34] https://books.google.com/books?id=g_xcAgAAQBAJ&pg=PA54&lpg=PA54&dq=CFS$+$patients$+$tested$+$with$+$QEEGs&source=bl&ots=bBcUSL7DJy&sig=SSGbTXul6il-Zmhi1FFZAkvCQYY&hl=en&sa=X&ved=2ahUKEwir_Z7Z-tPdAhWDNd8KHaDkD3gQ6AEwBHoECAYQAQ#v=onepage&q=CFS%20patients%20tested%20with%20QEEGs&f=false

[35] http://www.spl.harvard.edu/publications/item/view/1351

[36] https://www.ncbi.nlm.nih.gov/pmc/articles/PMC5111735/

[37] https://www.ncbi.nlm.nih.gov/pmc/articles/PMC5633338/

[38] http://www.ncf-net.org/library/sp.htm

Patients with chronic fatigue syndrome and depression had similar numbers of defects per patient (6.53 and 6.43, respectively). In all groups, defects were located predominantly in the frontal and temporal lobes. The midcerebral uptake index was found to be significantly lower ($p < 0.002$) in the patients with chronic fatigue syndrome (0.667) and patients with AIDS dementia complex (0.650) than in patients with major depression (0.731) or healthy control subjects (0.716). Also, a significant negative correlation was found between the number of defects and midcerebral uptake index in patients with chronic fatigue syndrome and AIDS dementia complex, but not in depressed patients or control subjects.

against Prudential Insurance Company. See Vastag v. Prudential Ins. Co. of Am., 2018 WL 2455921 (D.N.J. May 31, 2018). RP, M.D., MPH serves as clinical professor in the Department of Family Medicine at Rutgers-Robert Wood Johnson Medical School and as a Visiting Investigator at Rockefeller University.

AUTHOR CONTRIBUTIONS

All authors listed have made a substantial, direct and intellectual contribution to the work, and approved it for publication.

REFERENCES

1. Crawley C. Pediatric chronic fatigue syndrome: current perspectives. *Pediatric Health Med Ther.* (2017) 9:27–33 doi: 10.2147/PHMT.S126253
2. Kizilbash S, Ahrens S, Bruce B, Chelimsky G, Driscoll S, Harbeck-Weber C, et al. Adolescent fatigue, POTS and recovery: a guide for clinicians. *Curr Probl Adolesc Health Care.* (2014) 44:108–33. doi: 10.1016/j.cppeds.2013.12.014
3. Rowe P, Underhill, R Friedman K, Gurwitt A, Medow M, Schwartz M, et al. Myalgica encephalomyelitis/chronic fatigue syndrome diagnosis and management in young people: a primer. *Front Pediatar.* (2017) 5:121. doi: 10.3389/fped.2017.00121

19

The Development of the DePaul Symptom Questionnaire: Original, Expanded, Brief and Pediatric Versions

Leonard A. Jason* and Madison Sunnquist

Center for Community Research, DePaul University, Chicago, IL, United States

***Correspondence:**
Leonard A. Jason
ljason@depaul.edu

One of the key requirements of a reliable case definition is the use of standardized procedures for assessing symptoms. This article chronicles the development of the DePaul Symptom Questionnaire (DSQ) to assess symptoms of the major chronic fatigue syndrome (CFS) and myalgic encephalomyelitis (ME) case definitions. The original questionnaire has been modified and expanded over time to more fully capture symptoms from various adult case definitions, and a brief as well as pediatric version have also been developed. The DSQ has demonstrated very good psychometric properties in terms of test-retest reliability and sensitivity/specificity, as well as construct, predictive, and discriminant validity. The DSQ allows for a clear characterization of a patient's illness and allows scientists and clinicians to improve diagnostic reliability and validity when employing case definitions of ME and CFS.

Keywords: myalgic encephalomyelitis, chronic fatigue syndrome, case definition, DePaul Symptom Questionnaire, instrument development

Since 1994, many researchers have used the Fukuda et al. (1) chronic fatigue syndrome (CFS) case definition to select cases, but problems emerged in part due to this case definition not requiring core symptoms of CFS (2). In contrast, myalgic encephalomyelitis (ME) and CFS specialists have developed several adult case definitions that require essential symptoms of ME and CFS: the Canadian Consensus Criteria [CCC; (3)], ME (4), ME-International Consensus Criteria [ME-ICC; (5)], and Systemic Exertion Intolerance Disease [SEID; (6)]. These case definitions are a set of rules that allows investigators and clinicians to determine who has and who does not have an illness. In other words, the goals involve sensitivity (selecting those with the illness) and specificity (not selecting those without the illness).

Criterion variance represents the largest source of diagnostic unreliability for case definitions, and it involves specifying symptoms to classify patients' symptoms into diagnostic categories (7). Criterion variance can occur when there are multiple case definitions without a consensus on which symptoms need to be manifested to arrive at a diagnosis. In addition, case definition unreliability occurs when there is no consensus on scoring rules that specify how to determine whether a particular symptom is severe enough to qualify as satisfying criteria for the case definition, or when symptoms are not assessed by standardized instruments (8). These issues can result in investigators selecting samples of patients who are different on fundamental aspects of this illness. The consequences of these types of unreliability include difficulties replicating findings at different laboratories, estimating prevalence rates, identifying biomarkers, and determining effective treatments (9).

ME and CFS case definitions (1, 3–6, 10) have some overlapping and some different diagnostic criteria. In spite of the fact that there are currently alternative case definitions, it is still important to develop standardized ways to measure the symptoms just as this has occurred with other illnesses (11). The National Institutes of Health/Centers for Disease Control and Prevention (NIH/CDC) Common Data Elements (CDE) working group has recently recommended a set of instruments to be used by researchers, and for baseline symptoms the working group recommended using either the DePaul Symptom Questionnaire [DSQ; (12)] or a combined instrument using both the CDC's Symptom Inventory [SI; (13)] as well as items from the DSQ (even though the SI and DSQ differ on a number of dimensions, including the time period in which symptoms are measured and anchor points for the assessment of symptoms). Because of the recommendation for the use of the DSQ, this article reviews the genesis and psychometric properties of the different versions of the DSQ.

EARLY EFFORTS TO ASSESS SYMPTOMS

The DePaul research team's first attempt to measure CFS symptoms based on the Fukuda et al. (1) case definition involved the development of the CFS Screening Questionnaire. The instrument assessed 22 symptoms and was administered to four groups including those with CFS, lupus, multiple sclerosis (MS), and healthy controls (14). While the screening scale had excellent test-retest and interrater reliability, and patients with CFS could be differentiated from healthy controls, those with CFS could not be differentiated from the other illnesses. Subsequently, Hawk et al. (15) developed the CFS Questionnaire, which assessed whether each of a patient's symptoms had been present for 6 months or longer, how often the symptoms were experienced (never, seldom, often/usually, always), and the intensity of each symptom on a 100 point scale (0 = no problem and 100 = the worst problem possible). We decided to measure both symptom frequency and severity, as a severe symptom that occurs infrequently, or a very mild symptom that occurs frequently might not negatively affect patients. The items had adequate reliability, and Hawk et al. (16) later found that just six variables (i.e., percentage of time fatigue reported, postexertional malaise severity, unrefreshing sleep severity, confusion–disorientation severity, shortness of breath severity, and self-reproach) could differentiate with 100% accuracy patients with CFS from those with major depressive disorder (MDD).

In the next DePaul investigation, Jason et al. (17) administered a 22-item ME/CFS Fatigue Types Questionnaire to patients with ME and CFS, and controls. Factor analyses revealed a five-factor structure for participants with ME and CFS (with one factor being PEM, whose items were later used in the original DSQ), but the controls evidenced only a one-factor solution. This questionnaire focused on different aspects of fatigue, and our next effort attempted to assemble a more comprehensive questionnaire of symptoms.

DSQ-1

The original version of the DSQ (termed "DSQ-1") is a self-report measure of ME and CFS symptoms, demographic characteristics, and medical, occupational, and social history (12). The DSQ-1 includes 99 items, 54 of which assess the frequency and severity of ME and CFS symptoms required by several case definitions (See **Data Sheet 1**). A particular focus is placed on symptoms that fall within domains specified in the CCC (3), including fatigue, PEM, neurocognitive, sleep, pain, autonomic, neuroendocrine, and immune. Participants rate each symptom's frequency over the past 6 months on a 5-point Likert-type scale (e.g., 0=none of the time, 2=about half the time, 4=all of the time). Likewise, participants rate each symptom's severity over the past 6 months on a 5-point Likert-type scale (e.g., 0=symptom not present, 2=moderate, 4=very severe). While frequency and severity scores are considered separately in order to determine whether participants fulfill case definitions (see **Data Sheet 1**), researchers can also examine each symptom's intensity by multiplying frequency and severity scores by 25 to create 100-point scales (for ease of interpretation), then averaging each symptom's frequency and severity score to create a symptom composite score.

Considerable developmental work and testing have occurred over time with this instrument. For example, Jason et al. (8) found that that a symptom of moderate or greater severity occurring at least half of the time accurately distinguishes patients from controls. A study by Evans and Jason (18) suggested that the DSQ-1's 6-month timeframe (compared to 1-week or 1-month timeframes) led to the most reliable reports of ME and CFS symptoms. Jason et al. (19) found that the DSQ exhibited good to excellent test–retest reliability, with Pearson's or kappa correlation coefficients that were 0.70 or higher for the majority of items. An early factor analysis of the DSQ-1 symptoms (n = 189) resulted in a three-factor solution (which included one named PEM), and these factors evidenced good internal consistency (20). A later factor analysis with a larger sample (n = 969) found four factors: PEM, cognitive dysfunction, sleep difficulties, and a factor consisting of neuroendocrine, autonomic, and immune symptoms (21). Using the DSQ-1, Huber et al. (22) were able to extract six potential illness subtypes after performing a latent class analysis of symptoms that loaded onto the combined factor, including those who were likely to endorse all non-core symptoms; none of the non-core symptoms; primarily gastrointestinal symptoms; primarily circulatory symptoms; gastrointestinal and circulatory symptoms; and finally those with circulatory symptoms and orthostatic intolerance.

Other research has also confirmed different psychometric properties of the DSQ-1.When Murdock et al. (23) evaluated the performance of three self-report symptom measures (the DSQ-1, Multidimensional Fatigue Inventory, and RAND SF-36) in a sample of ME and CFS patients and controls, Cronbach's alpha statistics of the 40 DSQ-1 items that loaded onto four previously-identified factors (8) were indicative of excellent internal consistency reliability (α = 0.89–0.96). This study also found that the DSQ-1 PEM items were able to differentiate between patients and controls. Furthermore, the DSQ-1 did not have problems of ceiling effects that occurred with two other patient-reported symptom measures. In another study, Jason et al. (24) found that the five PEM items from the DSQ-1 captured the widest group of patients (97%), which was higher than any other item or series of items from different scales designed to measure PEM. Strand et al. (25) compared the agreement between a physician's diagnosis [using the Canadian ME/CFS criteria; (3)] and the DSQ-1's, and found a sensitivity of 98% (n = 55/56); while this study initially reported a specificity of 38% (n = 3/8), a correction was made after subsequent analyses revealed that the five DSQ-1 "false positive" participants had documented exclusionary conditions in their DSQ-1 responses and therefore should have been classified as true negatives. In addition, our group has recently developed a subscale to measure PEM (called the DSQ-PEM scale) that includes 10 items from the DSQ-1, and findings indicate it has good sensitivity (82%) and specificity (83%) (26).

The DSQ-1 has been used for a variety of purposes, including documenting specific ME and CFS vision-related abnormalities (27). In addition, using QEEG recordings, Zinn et al. (28) estimated cortical sources and perform a functional connectivity analysis on 84 Brodmann areas representing the entire cortex. Neurocognitive impairment, as measured by the DSQ-1's cognitive composite score, was negatively associated with small-worldness index for the delta band under observation. Finally, Kemp et al. (29) found seven DSQ-1 self-reported symptoms of autonomic dysfunction [seven autonomic symptoms: bladder problems, irritable bowel problems, nausea, feeling unsteady on feet (like you might fall), shortness of breath or trouble catching your breath, dizziness or fainting, and irregular heartbeats] were found to have a significant association with low frequency heart rate variability, a measure of increased sympathetic activity.

The DSQ-1 has been translated in multiple languages, including Norwegian, Spanish, Japanese, and Persian, and used in countries around the world including Canada, England, Iran, Norway, Spain, Mexico, France, and Japan. It has been employed in data collection efforts with the Solve ME/CFS Initiative's Biobank, the CDC multi-site study, and the Chronic Fatigue Initiative.

Consistent with its primary purpose, the DSQ-1 has been successfully utilized to operationalize various ME and CFS case definitions in order to compare the symptom profiles and functional status associated with different criteria (30–33). Scoring rules enable investigators to determine which of a variety of case definitions are met (see **Data Sheet 1** for the syntax of the scoring rules as well as the questionnaire). The DSQ-1 is freely available at REDCap's (34) shared library: https://redcap.is.depaul.edu/surveys/?s=H443P9TPFX. Participants are able to save their responses and return to the questionnaire as many times as needed, as severely ill individuals many not be able to complete the full questionnaire at once. This feature is available for all of the DSQ instruments that are described in this article.

DSQ-2

After several years of using the DSQ-1, feedback from patients and researchers as well as new developments in the field prompted our group to revise the DSQ-1. The revised questionnaire is called the "DSQ-2" (see **Data Sheet 2**), and we added several symptoms described in the ME-ICC case definition and primer for medical practitioners (5, 35) (See **Table 1**). Given that the DSQ-1's development coincided with the publication of the ME-ICC (5), we were only able to use approximations for several symptoms included in this criteria. As an example, rather than ratings of frequency and severity, we only asked whether patients had experienced intolerance to extremes of temperature or viral infections with prolonged recovery periods. The DSQ-2 now collects frequency and severity data on these two ME-ICC items. We also added other items due to findings related to orthostatic intolerance and mold sensitivity, and the DSQ-2 included new PEM items based on Ramsay's (36) writings. Furthermore, two items were added based upon feedback from patients who had completed the DSQ-1. Additionally, past participants reported difficulty answering questions related to exercise and activity that referenced the past 6 months, as they had purposefully limited activity in concordance with the Energy Envelope Theory (37). To address this limitation, we added an item to address this issue. In addition, we realized that two of our items on the DSQ-1 were double-barreled, meaning they measured more than one domain. With the DSQ-2, both of these items were split into two separate symptoms. Finally, we learned that the issue of alcohol intolerance was not well-phrased in the DSQ-1, as many patients did not have this symptom over the past 6 months due to not drinking during this period of time. We thus made this a hypothetical question asking what would occur if the respondent were to drink alcohol.

Using this expanded list of 78 symptoms from the DSQ-2, our team was able to extract an eight-factor structure (i.e., PEM, cognitive impairment, fever and flu, pain, sleep disruption, orthostatic intolerance, genitourinary problems, and temperature intolerance) that better tapped domains of a number of case definitions (38). In addition, using machine learning with the DSQ-2, we were able to differentiate those with ME and CFS from those with MS utilizing five symptoms, including one of our PEM items ("Next-day soreness after non-strenuous activities") (39). Current work with the DSQ-2 has also found that patients with ME have more severe symptoms than those with MS (40) and post-polio syndrome (41).

As the DSQ-2 includes almost all of the items found in the DSQ-1, it can also be used to operationalize various ME and CFS case definitions. The DSQ-2 is freely available at REDCap's (34) shared library: https://redcap.is.depaul.edu/surveys/?s=4NJ9CKW7JD.

TABLE 1 | New Items added to the DSQ-2.

Items from the ME-ICC case definition and primer
Feeling disoriented
Slowed speech
Difficulty reading (dyslexia) after mild physical or mental activity
Aching of the eyes or behind the eyes
Sensitivity to pain
Pressure on parts of your body causes pain in other parts of your body
Daytime drowsiness
Sensitivity to vibration
Poor coordination
Sinus infections
Urinary urgency
Waking up at night because you need to urinate
Inability to tolerate an upright position
Fluctuations in temperature throughout the day
Items revised that better approximated the ME-ICC case definition
Intolerance to extremes of temperature
Viral infections with prolonged recovery periods
Items added due to findings related to orthostatic intolerance and mold sensitivity
Heart beats quickly after standing
Blurred or tunnel vision after standing
Graying or blacking out after standing,
Sensitivity to mold
Items based on Ramsay (36)
Muscle fatigue after mild physical activity
Worsening of symptoms after mild physical activity
Worsening of symptoms after mild mental activity
Items added based upon patient feedback
Since the onset of your fatigue/energy related illness
Have you stopped getting sick with colds or flus
Item added in concordance with the Energy Envelope Theory
If you were to engage in exercise or vigorous activity, would you feel physically drained or sick?
Revised double-barreled questions
Unable to focus vision
Unablle to focus attention
Losing weight without trying
Gaining weight without trying
Issue of alcohol intolerance
What would occur if you were to drink alcohol

DSQ-SF (SHORT FORM)

In response to the expressed need of researchers and clinicians for a shorter symptom screen, our team has developed a short form of the DSQ (termed "DSQ-SF") (see **Data Sheet 3**). In validating our DSQ-SF, we used two distinct samples: a multisite sample [comprised of individuals with ME and CFS (n = 928) and controls (n = 46)] and a chronic illness sample [comprised of individuals with ME and CFS (n = 294), and a control group of individuals with MS (n = 111)]. We aimed to select a small number of symptoms from each of the domains identified in the CCC [i.e., fatigue, PEM, neurocognitive, sleep, pain, autonomic, neuroendocrine, and immune; (3)], as the DSQ-1 was originally developed to measure these criteria.

Based upon the prevalence rate of symptoms and outcomes from decision trees, the following 14 items were selected for inclusion in the DSQ-SF: fatigue (fatigue domain), next-day soreness after non-strenuous activities (PEM domain), minimum exercise makes you physically tired (PEM domain), unrefreshing sleep (sleep domain), muscle pain (pain domain), bloating (pain domain), problems remembering things (neurocognitive domain), difficulty paying attention for a long period of time (neurocognitive domain), irritable bowel problems (autonomic domain), feeling unsteady on your feet, like you might fall (autonomic domain), cold limbs (neuroendocrine domain), feeling hot or cold for no reason (neuroendocrine domain), flu-like symptoms (immune domain), and some smells, foods, medications, or chemicals make you feel sick (immune domain). Sunnquist et al. (42) found, for example, in the multisite sample that relatively similar numbers of patients were identified by the DSQ-1 and the DSQ-SF (69.7% met the CCC case definition as measured by the DSQ-1, and 65.8% met the CCC as measured by the DSQ-SF algorithm).

Our findings suggest that the DSQ-SF may serve as an effective, brief symptom screen for use in time-limited research studies and clinical practice. The DSQ-SF is freely available at REDCap's (34) shared library: https://redcap.is.depaul.edu/surveys/?s=HCT7J8EWPC

DSQ-PED (PEDIATRIC)

Prior to the development of the DSQ-1, our research group had been using a pediatric symptom inventory (43) based on the CCC case definition (3). This symptom inventory was used to assess symptoms found in the Pediatric ME/CFS case definition developed by Jason et al. (43), which had been endorsed by the International Association of Chronic Fatigue Syndrome. We called this instrument the DePaul Pediatric Health Questionnaire, but we will now refer to it as the "DSQ-Ped." This instrument consists of a parent form (**Data Sheet 4**) and a child form (**Data Sheet 5**). Researchers are encouraged to collect data from both children and their parents (i.e., use both forms) to obtain a thorough understanding of the child's illness. Children under the age of 12, or those with reading or comprehension difficulties, complete this questionnaire with the assistance of a parent or guardian. The symptom categories that were assessed in order to meet diagnostic criteria included fatigue, PEM, unrefreshing sleep or disturbance of sleep quantity, pain (myofascial, joint, abdominal, and/or head pain), two or more neurocognitive manifestations, and at least one symptom from two of the following categories: autonomic, neuroendocrine, or immune manifestations. There are a list of symptoms within these categories, and as with the other DSQ instruments, if the respondent indicates that a symptom meets the required frequency and severity rating, then it is counted as fulfilling that domain criterion. Rather than inquiring about symptoms within the past 6 months [as seen in the adult (1) case definition], we used a 3-month time frame. This decision was supported by the work of Fowler et al. (44), as no significant differences emerged between 8 and 17 years old with 3 vs. 6 months of chronic fatigue.

Jason et al. (45) used the DSQ-Ped in a study that compared 33 physician-referred young people with ME and CFS to 21 controls. Findings indicated that the Fukuda et al. (1) criteria in comparison to the Pediatric ME/CFS criteria were less accurate (43) in identifying cases of the illness (24% of patients would be misdiagnosed using the Fukuda criteria vs. only 3% with the Pediatric ME/CFS criteria). Jason et al. (46) also found that the DSQ-Ped was effective in distinguishing between those with severe vs. moderate pediatric ME and CFS. The severe vs. moderate categories were defined by how many symptoms the pediatric samples met, with more symptoms required for the severe category.

We are currently using an updated version of the DSQ-Ped in a community-based epidemiologic study of pediatric ME and CFS (47). This updated version, which is completed by both children and their parents/guardians in the present study, has some small differences from the original instrument, including the elimination of items that may be difficult for children to understand (e.g., next day soreness, muscle twitches, or bloating) as well as the inclusion of child-friendly phasing (e.g., using "no appetite," "some smells, foods, or chemicals make your child feel sick," and "upset stomach" in lieu of "nausea"). While psychometric studies of this updated questionnaire are ongoing, the symptoms assessed in this questionnaire were explicitly derived from pediatric case definitions, and the structure of the instrument mirrors that of other well-validated DSQ instruments. Furthermore, to our knowledge, the DSQ-Ped is the only pediatric-specific instrument that assesses all ME and CFS symptoms identified in case definitions. In one recent study, Schultz and Jason (48) found the orthostatic domain of the DSQ-Ped (dizziness, chest pain, shortness of breath, feeling unsteady when standing, and irregular heartbeat) significantly correlated ($r = 0.58$) with the Autonomic Symptom Checklist, which is a valid questionnaire for assessing various autonomic symptoms.

The DSQ-Ped is freely available at REDCap's (34) shared library:

DSQ-Ped (Parent Report Form): https://redcap.is.depaul.edu/surveys/?s=3FPRX49778

DSQ-Ped (Child Report Form): https://redcap.is.depaul.edu/surveys/?s=7N399W47JF

DSQ-PSQ (PEDIATRIC SCREENER)

We developed a pediatric screening questionnaire (termed "DSQ-PSQ," see **Data Sheet 6**) for use in large-scale epidemiological studies to screen potential participants for symptoms of ME and CFS, as full medical evaluations of all participants would not be feasible. Through this questionnaire, parents or guardians are asked to report upon the health status of each of their children. There are three parts of this questionnaire; the first part focuses on whether any children in the household are experiencing prolonged fatigue or exhaustion; the second part has questions pertaining to whether any of the children are experiencing cognitive difficulties or a disruption in their school activities, as some children may be more likely to report school or cognitive challenges to their parents instead of describing the fatigue (a more complex construct to verbalize) that is causing these challenges (49). The third part of the questionnaire evaluates the (1) presence, (2) frequency, and (3) severity of 13 additional ME and CFS-related symptoms, including: frequent headaches, sore throat, joint pain, muscle pain, abdominal pain, lymph node pain, rashes, fever/chills/shivers, eye pain/light sensitivity, problems sleeping, impaired memory or concentration, feeling worse, sick, or being exhausted after exercise, and dizziness.

The DSQ-PSQ "screen positive" criteria are purposefully broad in order to avoid overlooking children with non-traditional presentations, as children who screen positive should subsequently participate in thorough medical and psychiatric exams prior to diagnosis. To screen positive, a parent must endorse that their child reports either fatigue (of at least moderate severity and present at least half of the time) or one of the school or cognitive difficulties listed in the second part of the questionnaire (at any frequency or severity level). Finally, consistent with guidelines from the Fukuda et al. (1) criteria [one of the least restrictive research criteria (30)], screen positive youth must experience at least four symptoms from the third part of the questionnaire (at any frequency or severity). Preliminary psychometric analyses show that parent ratings of their child's symptoms according to these 18 items among screen-positive children and controls, internal reliability is good ($\alpha = 0.83$).

The DSQ-PSQ is also freely available at REDCap's (34) shared library: https://redcap.is.depaul.edu/surveys/?s=MFF8TXRPC8.

DISCUSSION

In 1994, our team began the initial development of a ME and CFS symptom scale (14). After multiple rounds of testing and refinement, we believed that we have arrived at an instrument, the DSQ-1, that is capable of effectively capturing many of the critical symptoms of ME and CFS. The evidence reviewed in this article suggests that the DSQ-1 has very good psychometric properties including test-retest reliability, sensitivity/specificity, construct, predictive, and discriminant validity. Over the past decade, ongoing efforts have broadened the instrument to include new symptoms (DSQ-2), a briefer version (DSQ-SF), a pediatric version (DSQ-Ped), and a pediatric screener (DSQ-PSQ). Developing questionnaires to ensure that key information is elicited from an interview is one of the critical tasks in operationalizing any case definition.

There are other instruments with excellent psychometric properties that have been developed to measure symptoms such as fatigue and pain (11). However, these instruments have not captured some of the core symptoms of patients with ME and CFS, such as PEM. For example, individuals with other chronic illnesses do experience some version of PEM, but their exertion-induced symptoms are primarily within the fatigue domain, whereas those with ME and CFS have post-exertion symptoms that involve multiple domains, including immune functioning such as flu-like symptoms or swollen lymph nodes (24). In addition, the onset (sometimes delayed) and duration (frequently over 24 h) of their symptoms can vary, which is also not typical of other chronic illnesses. Finally, sometimes symptoms can be reduced significantly by reducing dramatically the amount of activity engaged in. But the individuals would still experience that symptom if they exerted themselves by exceeding their energy boundaries (37). Certainly, the unique characteristics of these atypical symptoms need to be considered when assessing patients with ME and CFS.

While reliability of a case definition is enhanced with the development of questionnaires to standardize the collection of symptom data, it is also essential that a consensus be reached within the scientific community on the symptoms that must be present to satisfy a particular case definition. It is instructive to follow developments in another research area regarding issues involving the reliability of criteria for case definitions. In the 1950s and 1960s, the American Psychiatric Diagnostic and Statistical Manual (DSM)I and -II were comprised of unreliable clinical descriptions of psychiatric illnesses (7). Low interrater reliability in determining a psychiatric diagnosis was due to the inability of two interviewers to agree on the symptoms needed to be present before making a diagnosis. Low interrater reliability was due to criterion variance, deciding what symptoms or criteria were to be used to classify patients' into diagnostic categories.

In 1972, the psychiatric diagnostic Feighner criteria were developed for 16 diagnostic categories of the DSM II. This effort to be explicit about what symptoms were included within each of the 16 categories led to improvements in clinician to clinician diagnostic reliability (50). But it was not enough to have explicit, objective criteria because clinicians also needed to ensure that the diagnostic information could be elicited from an interview. Next, structured interview schedules were developed such as the Structured Clinical Interview for DSM-IV (51), and now diagnostic criteria are elicited by standardized the questions. In other words, these questionnaires reduce differences in the way clinical information is elicited. There are several lessons learned from the DSM; it is essential to develop explicit, objective criteria for a case definition, and standardized interviews can significantly improve the reliability of clinical diagnosis.

In addition to symptoms used in case definitions being clearly identified and assessed through standardized procedures, there is also a need to develop rules regarding whether a symptom is severe enough to count as a symptom for a particular case definition. As an example, the DSQ defines symptom presence as symptoms of at least moderate severity that occur at least half of the time, and there is empirical support for this cut-off. Jason et al. (32) employed a data analytic system whereby the threshold was dynamically adjusted for each DSQ-1 symptom based on observed frequency and severity scores. The results were similar to the cut-off involving at least moderate severity and occurring at least half the time, thus confirming the usefulness of this simpler-to-use criterion. Yet other cut-offs have been recommended, such as Baraniuk et al. (52), who considered complaints of *mild* or *more severe* sufficient for CFS attribution. In addition, even case definitions have at times been unclear about these cut-off points. For example, the ME-ICC case definition initially published (5) indicated a severity level of "*mild*" was equated to a 50% reduction in activity levels but later (35) a "*moderate*" severity level was equated to a 50% reduction. The above suggests there is still not a consensus on whether to use mild vs. moderate severity as cut-off thresholds, and consequently, this will influence the number of individuals identified as having ME or CFS symptoms.

As another example of this variation, Reeves et al. (53) Symptom Inventory requires symptoms to occur within the past month rather than the past 6 months (as required by the DSQ). The 1-month requirement may inflate the number individuals classified as having ME and CFS and capture, for example, those who experienced severe sore throats in the past month due to influenza. It is not just the rules governing cut-off thresholds and length of time that varies among investigators, but also how symptoms are summed to determine whether a person meets ME or CFS criteria. For example, the case definition proposed by Reeves et al. (53) would be met if an individual rated only two symptoms as occurring all the time, and one was of moderate and the other of severe severity. Therefore, the overall level of symptoms might be low for some patients with this summary method.

The reliability of a case definition also depends upon the operationalization of other frequently included criteria. For example, this includes a "substantial reduction in functioning" (54–56), "lifelong fatigue" (57), "fatigue not substantially alleviated by rest," and "fatigue that is the result of excessive exertion" (56). Attempts to concretely define these criteria have been met with considerable controversy [e.g., (58)]. For example, Reeves et al. (53) operationalized the way a patient's substantial reduction in functioning was measured using what was called the "empiric criteria." These researchers selected an instrument [i.e., the 36-Item Short Form Health Survey; SF-36, (59)], and if a patient met criteria for one of several specified subscales within the SF-36, the patient would meet the substantial reduction criteria for having CFS. However, one of these domains was "role emotional" functioning, and every person with a diagnosis of MDD would meet the criteria for "role emotional" functioning (60). This example demonstrates the necessity of specifying not only the instruments to be used, but also which of the instrument's subscales are appropriate and what the cut-off points are for meeting the threshold for disability. If mistakes occur on these critical choice points, it is possible that individuals with other illnesses will be misdiagnosed. To illustrate this point, using the Reeves et al. (53) "empiric criteria", with its decision to use "role emotional" functioning as a measure of substantial reduction, over one-third of individuals with MDD might have been inappropriately classified as having CFS (60). These types of decisions on how to assess substantial reductions in functioning as well as other decisions such as counting a symptom as needing to occur for only 1 rather than 6 months could be responsible for the estimated 10-fold increase in CDC prevalence estimates of CFS that occurred from 2003 to 2007 (9).

As mentioned in the introduction, the CDC/NIH CDE tasks were to recommend instruments that could be used by investigators to study ME and CFS, but they did not specify what subscales to use or scoring rules regarding thresholds that needed to be met. Criterion variance can occur when specifications of subscales, scoring rules or case definition are not specified. Without such specification, the same symptoms may not be described in different case definitions (1, 3, 5, 6, 61). As stated by Janson et al. (9), in addition to recommending measures, reducing criterion variance will only occur when there is a consensus on what subscales, scoring rules, and research case definition is to be employed in different settings (7).

A report from the IOM (6) recommended a "continuing surveillance of the evidence and revisiting of the criteria in no more than 5 years" (p. 188). Two years later, an NIH request for funding of ME/CFS centers recommended "that the investigators utilize the Canadian Consensus Criteria for ME/CFS as proposed by Carruther[s] and colleagues in 2003 and revised by Jason and colleagues in 2010, and the recent case definition from the Institute of Medicine Report on ME/CFS" (62). This NIH funding request suggests that the federal government has preferences for grant applications that use these two sets of criteria. Yet these case definitions were developed as clinical rather than research case definitions. Some prefer a broader perspective and others a more narrow one in the diagnosis and case definition, and both positions have some merit, and we might eventually call one more clinical criteria and the more research oriented. As an example, Jason et al. (63) suggested the following classification system, those with just chronic fatigue of 6 or more months would be the broadest category (similar to the Oxford criteria), those who meet a ME/CFS clinical criteria would be represented by the IOM (6) criteria (with few exclusionary illnesses), and a purer ME criteria could be based either on the Canadian Consensus Criteria (3) or work of Ramsay (36). Sophisticated and methodologically sound research methods could also be used to select and operationalize criteria for a research case definition (22, 31, 32, 64).

Our article highlights the development of DSQ in various forms. This type of interview schedule ensures that necessary symptom information is elicited reliably from an interview. This instrument is one of a variety of measures being recommended by the CDC NIH/CDE to assess ME and CFS domains, but there is now a need to also recommend a research case definition, as well as reach a consensus on other critical case definition criteria, such determining which subscales to use, what thresholds determine symptoms counting as a problem, and how to operationalize substantial reduction in functioning, lifelong fatigue, fatigue not substantially alleviated by rest, and fatigue that is the result of excessive exertion. Using large data sets and sophisticated research methods, we can work toward coming to a consensus on these issues.

An international, transparent, and inclusive effort, involving scientists, patient organizations, and government groups, could be assembled to resolve these fundamental reliability and diagnostic issues.

AUTHOR CONTRIBUTIONS

LJ wrote the first draft of this article and was engaged in the research efforts on various versions of the DSQ over the past few decades. He also helped with the development of the Supplemental Materials. MS helped write the article and was primarily responsible for writing the Supplemental Materials that involved scoring rules and syntax for the case definitions.

ACKNOWLEDGMENTS

The authors appreciate the valuable suggestions as well as organizational and editorial help from the following people: Kayla Huber, Helen Bedree, Bernardo Loiacono, Carly Holtzman, Lauren Klebek, Katie Ramian, Joseph Cotler, Damani McClellan, Catherine Dudun, Julia Terman, Mark Zinn, Marcie Zinn, and Shaun Bhatia.

REFERENCES

1. Fukuda K, Straus SE, Hickie I, Sharpe MC, Dobbins JG, Komaroff A. The chronic fatigue syndrome: a comprehensive approach to its definition and study. International Chronic Fatigue Syndrome Study Group. *Ann Intern Med.* (1994) 121:953–9.
2. McManimen SL, Jason LA, Williams YJ. Variability in symptoms complicates utility of case definitions. *Fatigue* (2015) 3:164–72. doi: 10.1080/21641846.2015.1041336
3. Carruthers BM, Jain AK, De Meirleir KL, Peterson DL, Klimas NG, Lerner AM, et al. Myalgic encephalomyelitis/chronic fatigue syndrome: Clinical working case definition, diagnostic and treatment protocols. *J Chronic Fatigue Syndr.* (2003) 11:7–115. doi: 10.1300/J092v11n01_02
4. Goudsmit E, Shepherd C, Dancey CP, Howes S. ME: Chronic Fatigue Syndrome or a distinct clinical entity? *Health Psychol Update* (2009) 18:26–31.
5. Carruthers BM, van de Sande MI, De Meirleir KL, Klimas NG, Broderick G, Mitchell T,., et al. Myalgic encephalomyelitis: International consensus criteria. *J Intern Med.* (2011) 270:327–38. doi: 10.1111/j.1365-2796.2011.02428.x
6. IOM. Beyond myalgic encephalomyelitis/chronic fatigue syndrome: an IOM report on redefining an illness. *JAMA* (2015) 313:1101–2. doi: 10.1001/jama.2015.1346
7. Jason LA, Choi M. Dimensions and assessment of fatigue. In: Yatanabe Y, Evengard B, Natelson BH, Jason LA, Kuratsune H, editors. *Fatigue Science for Human Health.* Tokyo: Springer (2008). p. 1–16.
8. Jason LA, Sunnquist M, Brown A, Evans M, Vernon SD, Furst J, et al. Examining case definition criteria for chronic fatigue syndrome and Myalgic Encephalomyelitis. *Fatigue* (2014) 2:40–56. doi: 10.1080/21641846.2013.862993
9. Jason LA, Fox PA, Gleason KD. The importance of a research case definition. *Fatigue* (2018) 6:52–8. doi: 10.1080/21641846.2018.1389336
10. National Task Force. *ME/PVFS - The UK Patient Organisations (1993) "London Criteria." In Report from the National Task Force on Chronic Fatigue Syndrome (CFS), Post Viral Fatigue Syndrome (PVFS), and Myalgic Encephalomyelitis.* Bristol: Westcare (1994). p. 96–8.
11. PROMIS. *Patient Reported Outcomes Measurement Information System* (2018). Available online at: https://commonfund.nih.gov/promis/tools

12. Jason LA, Evans M, Porter N, Brown M, Brown AA, Hunnell J, et al. The development of a revised Canadian myalgic encephalomyelitis chronic fatigue syndrome case definition. *A J Biochem Biotechnol.* (2010) 6:120–35.
13. Wagner D, Nisenbaum R, Heim C, Jones JF, Unger ER, Reeves WC. Psychometric properties of the CDC Symptom Inventory for assessment of chronic fatigue syndrome. *Pop. Health Met.* (2005) 3:8. doi: 10.1186/1478-7954-3-8
14. Jason LA, Ropacki MT, Santoro NB, Richman JA, Heatherly W, Taylor RR, et al. A screening instrument for Chronic Fatigue Syndrome: Reliability and validity. *J Chronic Fatigue Syndr.* (1997) 3:39–59. doi: 10.1300/J092v03n01_04
15. Hawk C, Jason LA, Torres-Harding S. Reliability of a chronic fatigue syndrome questionnaire. *J Chronic Fatigue Syndr.* (2006) 13:41–66. doi: 10.1300/J092v13n04_05
16. Hawk C, Jason LA, Torres-Harding S. Differential diagnosis of chronic fatigue syndrome and major depressive disorder. *Int J Behav Med.* (2006) 13:244–51. doi: 10.1207/s15327558ijbm1303_8
17. Jason LA, Jessen T, Porter N, Boulton A, Njoku MG, Friedberg F. Examining types of fatigue among individuals with ME/CFS. *Disabil Stud Quart.* (2009) 29. doi: 10.18061/dsq.v29i3.938
18. Evans M, Jason LA. The impact of symptom stability on timeframe and recall reliability in CFS. *Cogent Psychol.* (2015) 2:1079945. doi: 10.1080/23311908.2015.1079945
19. Jason LA, So S, Brown AA, Sunnquist M, Evans M. Test-retest reliability of the DePaul Symptom Questionnaire. *Fatigue* (2015) 3:16–32. doi: 10.1080/21641846.2014.978110
20. Brown AA, Jason LA. Validating a measure of myalgic encephalomyelitis/chronic fatigue syndrome symptomatology. *Fatigue* (2014) 2:132–52. doi: 10.1080/21641846.2014.928014
21. Jason LA, Sunnquist M, Brown A, Furst J, Cid M, Farietta J, et al. Factor analysis of the DePaul Symptom Questionnaire: Identifying core domains. *J Neurol Neurobiol.* (2015) 1. doi doi: 10.16966/2379-7150.114
22. Huber K, Sunnquist M, Jason LA. Latent class analysis of a heterogeneous international sample of patients with myalgic encephalomyelitis/chronic fatigue syndrome. *Fatigue* (2018) 6:163–78. doi: 10.1080/21641846.2018.1494530
23. Murdock KW, Wang XS, Shi Q, Cleeland CS, Fagundes CP, Vernon SD. The utility of patient-reported outcome measures among patients with myalgic encephalomyelitis/chronic fatigue syndrome. *Qual Life Res.* (2016) 26:913–21. doi: 10.1007/s11136-016-1406-3
24. Jason LA, McManimen S, Sunnquist M, Holtzman C. Patient perceptions of post exertional malaise. *Fatigue* (2018) 6:92–105. doi: 10.1080/21641846.2018.1453265
25. Strand EB, Lillestøl K, Jason LA, Tveito K, Diep LM, Valla SS, et al. Comparing the DePaul Symptom Questionnaire with physician assessments: a preliminary study. *Fatigue* (2016) 4:52–62. doi: 10.1080/21641846.2015.1126026
26. Cotler J, Holtzman C, Dudun C, Jason LA. A brief questionnaire to assess post-exertional malaise. *Diagnostics* (2018) 8:66. doi: 10.3390/diagnostics8030066
27. Hutchinson CV, Maltby J, Badham SP, Jason LA. Vision-related symptoms as a clinical feature of Chronic Fatigue Syndrome/Myalgic Encephalomyelitis? Evidence from the DePaul Symptom Questionnaire. *Br J Ophthalmol.* (2014) 98:144–5. doi: 10.1136/bjophthalmol-2013-304439
28. Zinn MA, Zinn ML, Jason LA. Small-world network analysis of cortical connectivity in Chronic Fatigue Syndrome using quantitative EEG. *Neuroregulation* (2017) 4:125–37. doi: 10.15540/nr.4.3-4.125
29. Kemp J, Sunnquist M, Jason LA, Newton JL. Autonomic dysfunction in Myalgic Encephalomyelitis and Chronic Fatigue Syndrome: Comparing self-report and objective measures (2018). [Epub ahead of print].
30. Jason LA, Brown A, Evans M, Sunnquist M, Newton JL. Contrasting chronic fatigue syndrome versus myalgic encephalomyelitis/chronic fatigue syndrome. *Fatigue* (2013) 1:168–83. doi: 10.1080/21641846.2013.774556
31. Jason LA, Kot B, Sunnquist M, Brown A, Evans M, Jantke R, et al. Chronic fatigue Syndrome and myalgic encephalomyelitis: toward an empirical case definition. *Health Psychol Behav Med.* (2015) 3:82–93. doi: 10.1080/21642850.2015.1014489
32. Jason LA, Kot B, Sunnquist M, Brown A, Reed J, Furst J, et al. Comparing and contrasting consensus versus empirical domains. *Fatigue* (2015) 3:63–74. doi: 10.1080/21641846.2015.1017344
33. Jason LA, Sunnquist M, Brown A, Newton JL, Strand EB, Vernon SD. Chronic fatigue syndrome versus systemic exertion intolerance disease. *Fatigue* (2015) 3:127–41. doi: 10.1080/21641846.2015.1051291
34. Harris PA, Taylor R, Thielke R, Payne J, Gonzalez N, Conde JG. Research electronic data capture (REDCap)—a metadata-driven methodology and workflow process for providing translational research informatics support. *J Biol Inform.* (2009) 42:377–81. doi: 10.1016/j.jbi.2008.08.010
35. Carruthers BM, van de Sande MI, De Meirleir KL, Klimas NG, Broderick G, Mitchell T, et al. *Myalgic Encephalomyelitis—Adult & Paediatric: International Consensus Primer for Medical Practitioners.* Vancouver, BC: Carruthers & van de Sande (2012).
36. Ramsay AM. *Myalgic Encephalomyelitis and Post Viral Fatigue States: The Saga of Royal Free Disease.* 2nd ed. London: Gower Publishing Co (1988).
37. Jason LA, Brown M, Brown A, Evans M, Flores S, Grant-Holler E, et al. Energy Conservation/Envelope Theory interventions to help patients with chronic fatigue syndrome. *Fatigue* (2013) 1:27–42. doi: 10.1080/21641846.2012.733602
38. Bedree H, Sunnquist M, Jason LA. A factor analysis of the revised DePaul Symptom Questionnaire (2018). [Epub ahead of print].
39. Ohanian D, Brown A, Sunnquist M, Furst J, Nicholson N, Klebek L, et al. Identifying key symptoms differentiating Myalgic Encephalomyelitis and Chronic Fatigue Syndrome from Multiple Sclerosis. *Neurology* (2016) 4:41–5.
40. Jason LA, Ohanian D, Brown A, Sunnquist M, McManimen S, Klebek L, et al. Differentiating multiple sclerosis from myalgic encephalomyelitis and chronic fatigue syndrome. *Insights Biomed.* (2017) 2:11. doi: 10.21767/2572-5610.10027
41. Klebek L, Sunnquist M, Jason LA. Differentiating post-polio from ME and CFS (2018). [Epub ahead of print].
42. Sunnquist M, Lazarus S, Jason LA. The development of a short form of the DePaul Symptom Questionnaire (2018). [Epub ahead of print].
43. Jason LA, Bell DS, Rowe K, Van Hoof ELS, Jordan KR, Lapp, C,et al. A pediatric case definition for myalgic encephalomyelitis and chronic fatigue syndrome. *J Chronic Fatigue Syndr* (2006) 13:1–44. doi: 10.1300/J092v13n02_01
44. Fowler T, Duthie P, Thapar A, Farmer A. The definition of disabling fatigue in children and adolescents. *BMC Fam. Pract.* (2005) 6:33. doi: 10.1186/1471-2296-6-33
45. Jason L, Porter N, Shelleby E, Lindsay T, Bell D, Lapp C, et al. Examining criteria to diagnose ME/CFS in pediatric samples. *J Behav Health Med.* (2010) 1:186–95. doi: 10.1037/h0100551
46. Jason L, Porter N, Shelleby E, Lindsay T, David B, Lapp C, et al. and De Meirleir K. (2009). Severe versus moderate criteria for the new pediatric case definition for ME/CFS. *Child Psychol Hum. Dev.* (2009). 40:609–20. doi: 10.1007/s10578-009-0147-8
47. Jason LA, Katz BZ, Mears C, Jantke R, Brown A, Sunnquist M, et al. Issues in estimating rates of pediatric chronic fatigue syndrome and myalgic encephalomyelitis in a community-based sample. *Avicen J Neurol Psychol Physiol.* (2015) 2:37281. doi: 10.17795/ajnpp-37281
48. Schultz K, Jason LA. Relationships between autonomic and Orthostatic self-report and physician ratings (2018). [Epub ahead of print].
49. Jordan KM, Kolak AM, Jason LA. Research with children and adolescents with chronic fatigue syndrome: Methodologies, designs, and special considerations. *J. Chronic Fatigue Syndr.* (1997) 3:3–13. doi: 10.1300/J092v03n02_02
50. Helzer J, Robins L, Taibleson M, Woodruff R, Reich T, Wish E. Reliability of psychiatric diagnosis. *Arch Gen Psychol.* (1977) 34:129–33. doi: 10.1001/archpsyc.1977.01770140019001
51. First MB, Spitzer RL, Gibbon M, Williams JBW. *Structured Clinical Interview for DSM-IV Axis Disorders – Patient Edition.* New York, NY: Biometrics Research Department, New York State Psychiatric Institute (1995).
52. Baraniuk JN, Adewuyi O, Merck SJ, Ali M, Ravindran MK, Timbol CR, et al. A Chronic Fatigue Syndrome (CFS) severity score based on case designation criteria. *Am J Transl Res.* (2013) 5:53–68.
53. Reeves WC, Wagner D, Nisenbaum R, Jones JF, Gurbaxani B, Solomon L, et al. Chronic fatigue syndrome – a clinically empirical approach to its definition and study. *BMC Med.* (2005) 3:19. doi: 10.1186/1741-7015-3-19<underline
54. Gleason KD, Stoothoff J, McClellan D, McManimen S, Thorpe T, Katz BZ, et al. (2018). Operationalizing substantial reduction in functioning among young

60. Jason LA, Najar N, Porter N, Reh C. Evaluating the Centers for Disease Control's empirical chronic fatigue syndrome case definition. *J Disabil Pol Stud.* (2009) 20:93–100. doi: 10.1177/1044207308325995
61. Sunnquist M, Jason LA, Nehrke P, and Goudsmit EM. (2017). A comparison of case definitions for Myalgic Encephalomyelitis and Chronic Fatigue Syndrome. *J Chronic Dis Manage.* **2**:1013.
62. *Department of Health and Human Services [internet]*. Washington, DC: Myalgic encephalomyelitis/chronic fatigue syndrome (ME/CFS) collaborative research centers (CRC). FOA: RFA-NS-17-021 (2017).
63. Jason LA, McManimen S, Sunnquist M, Brown A, Furst J, Newton JL, et al. Case definitions integrating empiric and consensus perspectives. *Fatigue* (2016) 4:1–23. doi: 10.1080/21641846.2015.1124520
64. Jason LA, McManimen SL, Sunnquist ML, Newton JL, Strand EB. Clinical criteria versus a possible research case definition in chronic fatigue syndrome/myalgic encephalomyelitis. *Fatigue* (2017) 5:89–102. doi: 10.1080/21641846.2017.1299077
65. Rowe PC, Underhill RA, Friedman KJ, Gurwitt A, Medow MS, Schwartz MS, et al. Myalgic encephalomyelitis/chronic fatigue syndrome diagnosis and management in young people: a primer *Front Pediatr.* (2017) 5:121. doi: 10.3389/fped.2017.00121

adults with chronic fatigue syndrome. *Int J Behav Med.* (2018) 25:448–55. doi: 10.1007/s12529-018-9732-1

55. Jason LA, Brown M, Evans M, Anderson V, Lerch A, Brown A, et al. Measuring substantial reduction in functioning in patients with chronic fatiguesyndrome. *Disabil Rehab.* (2011) 33:589–98. doi: 10.3109/09638288.2010.503256
56. Schafer C, Evans M, Jason LA, So S, Brown A. Measuring substantial reductions in activity. *J Prev Interv Community* (2015) 43:5–19. doi: 10.1080/10852352.2014.973242
57. Sunnquist M, Jason LA, Brown A, Evans M, Berman A. Complications in operationalizing lifelong fatigue as an exclusionary criterion. *J Prev Interv Community* (2015) 43:42–53. doi: 10.1080/10852352.2014.973238
58. Jason LA, Porter N, Brown M, Brown A, Evans M. A constructive debate with the CDC on the CFS empirical case definition. *J Disabil Pol Stud.* (2010) 20:251–6. doi: 10.1177/1044207309359515
59. Ware JE, and Sherbourne CD. The MOS 36-item short-form health survey (SF-36). I. Conceptual framework and item selection. *Med Care* (1992) 30:473–83.

20

Cardiopulmonary Exercise Test Methodology for Assessing Exertion Intolerance in Myalgic Encephalomyelitis/Chronic Fatigue Syndrome

*Staci Stevens[1], Chris Snell[1], Jared Stevens[1], Betsy Keller[2] and J. Mark VanNess[1,3]**

Workwell Foundation, Ripon, CA, United States, [2] Department of Exercise and Sport Sciences, Ithaca College, Ithaca, NY, United States, [3] Health and Exercise Science, University of the Pacific, Stockton, CA, United States

Correspondence:
J. Mark VanNess
mvanness@pacific.edu

Background: Concise methodological directions for administration of serial cardiopulmonary exercise testing (CPET) are needed for testing of patients with Myalgic Encephalomyelitis/Chronic Fatigue Syndrome (ME/CFS). Maximal CPET is used to evaluate the coordinated metabolic, muscular, respiratory and cardiac contributions to energy production in patients with ME/CFS. In this patient population, CPET also elicits a robust post-exertional symptom flare (termed, post-exertional malaise); a cardinal symptom of the disease. CPET measures are highly reliable and reproducible in both healthy and diseased populations. However, evidence to date indicates that ME/CFS patients are uniquely unable to reproduce CPET measures during a second test, despite giving maximal effort during both tests, due to the effects of PEM on energy production.

Methodology: To document and assess functional impairment due to the effects of post-exertional malaise in ME/CFS, a 2-day CPET procedure (2-day CPET) has been used to first measure baseline functional capacity (CPET1) and provoke post-exertional malaise, then assess changes in CPET variables 24 h later with a second CPET to assess the effects of post-exertional malaise on functional capacity. The second CPET measures changes in energy production and physiological function, objectively documenting the effects of post-exertional malaise. Use of CPET as a standardized stressor to induce post-exertional malaise and quantify impairment associated with post-exertional malaise has been employed to examine ME/CFS pathology in several studies. This article discusses the results of those studies, as well as the standardized techniques and procedures for use of the 2-day CPET in ME/CFS patients, and potentially other fatiguing illnesses.

Conclusions: Basic concepts of CPET are summarized, and special considerations for performing CPET on ME/CFS patients are detailed to ensure a valid outcome. The 2-day CPET methodology is outlined, and the utility of the procedure is discussed for assessment of functional capacity and exertion intolerance in ME/CFS.

Keywords: functional capacity, stress test, oxygen consumption, post exertional malaise, functional impairment

BACKGROUND

A 2-day cardiopulmonary exercise test methodology (2-day CPET) was cited by the *Institute of Medicine* (IOM) (1) as a potentially useful tool to aid in the diagnosis and assessment of functional capacity in patients with Myalgic Encephalomyelitis/Chronic Fatigue Syndrome (ME/CFS). The IOM report concluded that ME/CFS is a neuroimmune pathology that affects multiple systems and contributes to exertion intolerance or an inability to recover normally following physical, cognitive or emotional exertion (1, 2). The IOM determined that "ME/CFS patients often have a level of fatigue that is more profound, more devastating, and longer lasting than that observed in patients with other fatiguing disorders" (1). The fatigue in ME/CFS differs from that experienced by controls and is unlike the fatigue associated with deconditioning. It is often described as "flu-like" and frequently includes "brain fog" or cognitive difficulties and other symptoms. This abnormal response to exertion is a hallmark symptom of ME/CFS referred to as post-exertional malaise (PEM). PEM is among the primary debilitating symptoms of ME/CFS, as well as fatigue-related impairment lasting more than 6 months, unrefreshing sleep, and usually cognitive impairment (brain fog) and/or dysautonomia. Muscle and/or joint pain often accompany these other symptoms, any of which could force a person with ME/CFS to stop work, avoid physical activity and, consequently, further reduce functional ability.

The lack of definitive biomarkers and no known cause or cure for ME/CFS contribute to patients suffering through medical misinterpretation, misunderstanding, and an overt bias toward characterizing the illness as a psychosomatic disorder. However, studies of exercise capacity reveal that a 2-day CPET procedure can provide evidence of the pathophysiology underlying the PEM that characterizes patients with ME/CFS (3–6). CPET methodology is standardized as a well-accepted procedure to assess physiological responses to exertion in many illness conditions (7). Adaptation of this valid, standardized and reliable procedure to assess abnormalities associated with PEM is particularly useful for identifying impairment in patients with fatigue-related illnesses. The purpose of this paper is to provide guidelines and helpful practices to applying CPET techniques in patients with ME/CFS.

Cardiopulmonary Exercise Testing

Analysis of expired gases during an exercise test generates values that are useful in the assessment of functional capacity, illness severity, and illness characterization in ME/CFS. For instance, peak oxygen consumption (VO_2peak) is a well-recognized objective indicator of functional capacity (8–11), and may be used to assess disease severity and predict coronary heart disease and all-cause mortality (12–14). Additionally, VO_2peak provides a foundation to evaluate metabolic functional impairment. A CPET allows for the comprehensive and integrated analyses of cardiovascular, respiratory, metabolic and work indices to help discern the etiology of exertion intolerance in a growing population of patients with multiple chronic comorbidities (15). It can be applied similarly to better understand disease pathology in ME/CFS.

Classically, a single CPET provides physiological measures at rest and throughout incremental exercise to determine energy producing capacity at metabolically relevant time points including anaerobic threshold and peak effort. However, for ME/CFS patients, serial exercise tests are particularly useful to explore the unique post-exertional pathology associated with the illness. With a 2-day CPET, baseline functional capacity is determined with the first test, which also serves as a standardized stressor to elicit a post-exertional symptom flare. The second exercise test 24 h later provides a metric of change in physiological function due to the post-exertional response, and can indicate magnitude of impairment associated with a patient's compromised recovery. Doing the second exercise test 24 h following the first test allows comparison of performance capability without confounding influences of delayed onset muscle soreness. This serial CPET methodology is not unique to ME/CFS, and was reported previously to assess hormonal responses following an exercise stressor in overtrained athletes (16). Use of the 2-day CPET methodology in ME/CFS is of increasing interest for the same purpose; to assess a patient's ability to recover normally following exertion.

CPET Measures Are Reliable and Reproducible

The 2-day CPET methodology is useful for assessing impaired recovery because CPET measures are readily reproduced in both healthy and diseased populations. Therefore, a failure to reproduce CPET measures on a subsequent test, despite peak effort on both tests, indicates a derangement of homeostasis.

Peak Oxygen Consumption

VO_2peak is a highly reliable and objective measure of functional capacity (11, 17, 18). The reproducibility, or variability of this measure from one day to the next is also low. This is true across a broad population of healthy adults (11, 13, 17), children (19), and in those with pathologies such as heart failure (20–22), pulmonary hypertension (23), end-stage renal disease (24), cystic fibrosis (25), mild-moderate COPD (26), and stroke (27). Thus, VO_2peak provides an objective measure of baseline functional capacity or maximal ability to produce energy for work. Failure to reproduce VO_2peak during a second serial CPET, despite peak effort on both tests, implicates impairment of recovery mechanisms. This impaired recovery is consistent with PEM and suggests an underlying pathophysiology that contributes to an abnormal post-exertional state. Further, the magnitude of a test-retest decrement in VO_2peak can be used to quantify the degree of impairment associated with PEM.

Abbreviations: BP, Blood pressure; CPET, Cardiopulmonary exercise test; ECG, Electrocardiogram; HR, Heart rate; ME/CFS, Myalgic Encephalomyelitis/Chronic Fatigue Syndrome; O_2pulse, oxygen pulse; PEM, Post-exertional malaise; RPE, Rating of perceived exertion; SEID, Systemic Exertion Intolerance Disease; VAT, Ventilatory anaerobic threshold; V_{CO2}, Ventilatory removal of carbon dioxide; V_E, Minute ventilation; VO_2peak, Maximal oxygen consumption; VO_2@VAT, oxygen consumption at ventilatory anaerobic threshold; VT, Ventilatory threshold.

Anaerobic Threshold

While VO_2 at peak effort is an objective measure of maximum energy producing capacity; perhaps one of the most metabolically and functionally relevant transition points during an incremental exercise test is VO_2 at anaerobic threshold. The VO_2 and work intensity at anaerobic threshold are important indices of capacity to do continuous work, as activity above the anaerobic threshold is rapidly fatiguing and cannot be sustained. Anaerobic threshold is the exercise intensity at which the anaerobic contribution to energy generation is significant enough to cause non-linear increases in muscle and blood pH, lactate and carbon dioxide concentration. This transition is typically identified using serial measures of blood lactate obtained throughout an incremental exercise test to ascertain at which VO_2 a non-linear increase in blood lactate occurs. The ventilatory stimulus of carbon dioxide causes a similar response in expired ventilation to that of blood lactate. This makes the ventilatory threshold a good non-invasive metric for the anaerobic threshold, which is referred to as the ventilatory anaerobic threshold (VAT).

Test-retest measures of oxygen consumption and work that correspond with VAT are stable over time with the same test modality, and vary within about 7–12% in both healthy individuals (5, 6, 18, 28) and a number of other pathological conditions (21, 22). Because VO_2@VAT is a reliable and reproducible measure, a reduction in VO_2@VAT over serial exercise tests indicates an underlying limitation in the capacity to meet daily energy demands via aerobic energy production.

Functional Capacity of ME/CFS Patients

Peak oxygen consumption of ME/CFS patients obtained during a single CPET has been used to characterize functional status in adults with ME/CFS (5, 29–35) as well as adolescents (36, 37). However, patients and/or physicians typically seek this type of assessment after an individual has been physically inactive or low active for at least 6 months. Because of this it is often argued that low VO_2peak in a patient with ME/CFS is due simply to physical deconditioning.

Compared to healthy controls, VO_2peak of adults with ME/CFS varies from about 30-91% of predicted values for age and sex (5, 30–35, 38). This compares to values for adolescents with ME/CFS between 86 and 90% of predicted VO_2peak for healthy controls of similar age and sex (36, 37). While low, values for some ME/CFS patients may be consistent with physical deconditioning, and may not be considered clinically remarkable. Consequently, VO_2peak measured during a single CPET does not necessarily provide objective evidence of impaired recovery or PEM, whereas PEM is a cardinal symptom of ME/CFS, and management of PEM is a primary goal of treatment. Therefore, provocation of PEM may be accomplished using a standardized stressor of a single CPET. However, quantifying functional decrement due to PEM following the first CPET requires a second CPET administered 24 h later to determine if the patient can reproduce CPET measures within normal test-retest variability. Assessing the severity of PEM is useful for treatment for ME/CFS, and also provides objective evidence of impairment for purposes of disability review. The balance of this paper will detail the effects of PEM on recovery in ME/CFS and special considerations for testing those with ME/CFS for a valid and objective assessment of functional capacity and exertion intolerance.

RESULTS

Studies of 2-Day CPET in ME/CFS

Studies of exertion intolerance in ME/CFS using a 2-day CPET methodology indicate an impaired ability of patients to reproduce CPET results. Several studies have shown that ME/CFS patients are unable to reproduce values for VO_2peak on serial CPETs (5, 6), VO_2 at ventilatory threshold (6), and/or peak workload, or workload at ventilatory threshold (4). Additionally, abnormal responses to exercise such as hemodynamic or ventilatory responses may be observed in ME/CFS patients. Abnormalities in hemodynamic and ventilatory responses may or may not appear in some patients during the first exercise test, whereas others only display abnormalities during CPET2 following the onset of PEM.

Values for VO_2, work rate and heart rate obtained at the VAT can also be examined for reproducibility. For example, test-retest VO_2@VAT values are reliable and reproducible in both normal subjects and in various pathological conditions (22). But ME/CFS subjects often fail to reproduce values measured at VAT (3, 4). Compared to VO_2peak, VO_2@VAT is more indicative of the capacity to perform activities of daily living. Sustained activity at intensities that exceed VO_2@VAT will eventually result in fatigue (15). Measures that coincide with VAT are important indicators of metabolic impairment and delayed recovery in ME/CFS patients. The failure to reproduce measures that correspond to VAT may be useful for identifying metabolic anomalies of energy production, and describing the magnitude of impairment due to PEM.

DISCUSSION

CPET1 to CPET2 Decrement Indicates Post-exertional Malaise

The post-exertional effect on energy production are signaled by changes in values measured across two CPETs. Diminished responses, or abnormal changes in metabolic, cardiac or hemodynamic measures during incremental exercise indicate impaired recovery due to muscular, cardiovascular, pulmonary or autonomic dysfunction. Changes in these values from CPET1 to CPET2 should be compared to normal ranges for test-retest reproducibility. Abnormal variability between tests is evidence of impaired recovery where both symptoms and changes in CPET values represent abnormal perturbation. An assessment of 2-day CPET data should include comparisons with normal age/sex values, and between CPETs for peak and VAT measures of VO_2, work output, heart rate, blood pressure, minute ventilation, oxygen saturation, as well as transitional (rest to peak) changes in all measures. Additionally, the V_E/VCO_2 slope or lowest value during a CPET should be scrutinized for ventilatory decompensation. The magnitude of change from CPET1 to CPET2 is considered abnormal if in excess of normal test-retest variability. CPET measures and normal test values appear in **Table 1**. Additionally, patient reports of symptom flares with

TABLE 1 | Typical CPET values of intrest for ME/CFS patients.

CPET variables	Description/ significance	Normal values/response	References
Peak VO_2	-Highest VO_2 obtained during exercise -indicates biological functional capacity	Wide range by age, sex, fitness level % predicted value should be 85-100%	(11)
VO_2@VAT	-Submaximal VO_2 -occurs at point of dislinear increase in V_E -generally associated with anaerobic threshold -represents upper limit of workload that can be sustained for prolonged period	45–65% peak VO_2	(39)
Peak RER	-ratio of VCO_2/VO_2 -best non-invasive indicator of exercise effort	>1.1-maximal effort 1.0–1.1-good effort <1.0-poor effort	(40)
Ve/VCO_2 slope@VAT; Ve/VCO_2 slope@RCP*; Lowest Ve/VCO_2	-Indicates ventilatory efficiency and matching of ventilation to pulmonary perfusion	Generally <30, however normal values are age and sex dependent	(41)
$PetCO_2$	-also represents matching of ventilation and perfusion and cardiac function	Rest: 36-42 mmHg From rest to VAT, increases 3–8 mmHg Decreases following VAT intensity	(42)
O_2pulse	-ratio VO_2/HR -indirect indicator of cardiac work	Continual linear rise thru exercise with possible plateau approaching peak effort	(43)
Peak heart rate	-highest HR during CPET -in patients not prescribed beta blockers provides insight into chronotropic competence and cardiac response to exercise -peak HR should not be used as primary indicator of subject effort given its wide variability	Chronotropic incompetence is ≤ 85% age-predicted heart rate reserve	(44)
HR recovery@1 min post peak effort	-Difference between peak HR and HR@1 min into recovery -provides insight into parasympathetic reactivation	Should have >12–18 bpm recovery in 1st min following peak exertion	(15)
Exercise BP	Provides insight into CV response to exercise and left ventricular afterload	During exercise SBP should increase 10 mmHg/3.5 $ml \cdot kg^{-1} \cdot min^{-1}$ VO_2; DBP should not change >±10 mmHg from rest	(45)
SpO_2	-non-invasive indicator of arterial hemoglobin saturation	>95% at rest and throughout exercise	(46)
ECG	-rate, rhythmicity and perfusion of the heart	Minimal waveform changes, no significant deviation from normal sinus rhythm	(47)
Subjective symptoms	-to determine subject perception of symptoms limiting exercise -Rating of Perceived Exertion (RPE) -dyspnea scale -pain scale	Limiting factor is muscular fatigue with no significant difference in dyspnea, pain	(48, 49)

PEM following a CPET further support the pathological recovery response to exertion evidenced by the 2-day CPET results.

Other CPET Measures

In addition to VO_2, other measures should also be assessed both within and between CPETs to confirm normal responses to incremental exercise including hemodynamic, ventilatory variables, and work rate measures. Abnormal responses to incremental exercise for heart rate, blood pressure, minute ventilation (V_E), workload (e.g., VO_2/work) and temperature implicate specific aspects of energy production and physiological systems affected by ME/CFS which may contribute to PEM. Immediate post-test recovery measures (e.g., HR, BP, ECG, O_2sat, recovery time) should be closely monitored as well to determine normal post-CPET recovery responses. Post-test recovery dynamics should also be compared between CPET1 and CPET2. Disrupted post-test recovery dynamics, particularly following CPET2, are not unusual in this population. Signs and symptoms should be documented before during and after exercise, including pain and dyspnea.

VAT Is Highly Relevant for an ME/CFS Patient

The majority of daily energy demand is met via aerobic metabolic processes, which typically provides energy for daily activities such as normal speed walking, seated tasks, and other activities of daily living. A reduction in VAT following exertion in persons with ME/CFS may force reliance on anaerobiosis to support lower intensity work and subsequently lead to premature fatigue. From a practical standpoint, a reduction in the workload at which VAT occurs is believed to be consistent with the post-exertional decrease in function that coincides with PEM in ME/CFS patients. For example, with PEM induced by CPET1, it is not uncommon for patients to present with anaerobic predominance (early anaerobiosis), even during seated rest at the start of CPET2. Functionally, such patients rely on energy produced via anaerobic metabolism simply to perform resting and/or low level activities. It is not surprising when fatigue occurs under these circumstances.

To determine the point at which VAT occurs during a CPET, there may be several algorithms in the software of a metabolic measurement system to identify the VAT breakpoint. Perhaps most notable, the V-slope method, originally described by Beaver, Wasserman and Whipp (50), makes use of the relationship between minute ventilation (V_E) and ventilatory removal of carbon dioxide (V_{CO2}) during incremental exercise to determine the VAT. For consistency, the same algorithm should be used to identify VAT for both tests within the 2-day CPET method. An additional concern when testing ME/CFS patients is how a potentially abnormal ventilatory response may impact the determination of VAT. For this reason, VAT identified by an algorithm should always be scrutinized by a person(s) familiar with the determination of VAT to ascertain agreement with the algorithm-derived VAT.

METHODOLOGY

Exercise Testing Considerations for ME/CFS Patients

The objectives of the 2-day CPET method are to; (1) assess VO_2peak and VO_2 at VAT during the first CPET, in addition to other test variable kinetics, and (2) compare measures from CPET1 and CPET2 to assess test reproducibility and normality of recovery response following CPET1. To ascertain the magnitude of change in CPET2 due to CPET1, it is critical that the ME/CFS patient begin the test in a baseline state representative of the patient's well-rested capacity. Characteristics unique to ME/CFS patients require special pre-test preparations that should be addressed beginning as early as 2–3 weeks prior to a scheduled 2-day CPET. The objective is to minimize pre-fatigue and PEM in a patient who is preparing to travel in order to complete the 2-day CPET.

Pre-test Considerations

Factors such as travel to the test site, immediate pre-test (day of or even day before) paperwork that taxes cognitive function, and prolonged time in a common waiting area, even if seated, can all contribute to pre-test fatigue. Fatigue and PEM are exacerbated by physical, cognitive and emotional stressors (1), so every effort should be made to reduce such stressors where possible. Likewise, many ME/CFS patients experience hypersensitivity to light, noise, temperature, odors, and/or chemicals, so it is helpful to minimize environmental stimuli and maintain a generally low level of activity in the waiting area and testing environment.

Pretest directions/instructions should be in writing and given to the patient at least 1–2 weeks prior to arrival at a clinic. Included in these materials should be a clearly written pre-test checklist to assure that the patient adheres to pre-test preparation instructions (e.g., alcohol, caffeine, exercise and food restrictions prior to CPET, appropriate attire, etc.). Directions to the facility should include availability of disabled parking close to the building, and clear directions to the elevator or other lift assist as needed. Stairs (up and down) and long walks to the clinic should be avoided if possible as this will pre-fatigue the patient. It is reasonable to ask the patient prior to arrival if wheelchair assistance is indicated. Likewise, it is essential that the patient understands the importance of not becoming fatigued prior to the test, and plans travel to the test site with that in mind. When the test site is more than 1 h away, if feasible the patient should be encouraged to arrive the day before the scheduled test and spend the night locally. For some patients, 2 days of rest following air travel to a clinic may be necessary. It is essential that patients understand they should not drive a motor vehicle away from the clinic following either CPET, and plan accordingly. These recommendations may limit patient accessibility to testing, but should be considered to optimize quality of CPET data and patient safety.

Pre-test Forms/Questionnaires

Forms and questionnaires should be sent to the patient at least 2–3 weeks prior to a scheduled test. Completion of forms can be cognitively taxing for a person with ME/CFS and contribute to PEM, so sufficient time should be allowed for completion and return of forms to the clinic. In a clinic environment where a physician is present only part-time, prior arrangements are necessary to provide medical supervision during the 2-day CPET when testing a patient that meets criteria for high risk (7, 45). Similarly, sufficient time is necessary for the patient's physician to complete and return the referral form prior to testing the ME/CFS patient. Information provided to the patient should include explicit pretest instructions. Patients who experience cognitive impairment may be unable to process and respond quickly to copious or complex information, so providing simple, easily understood documentation helps improve adherence to pretest instructions. Paperwork that should be sent to the patient 2–3 weeks prior to a scheduled test may include the following:

- General information about test, payment options, clinic contact information
- Directions to clinic/parking, elevator, etc.
- Area lodging information, indicating hotels that provide shuttle service to your clinic
- Physician consent form
- Medical/health history form
- Informed consent document
- Fatigue status questionnaire; e.g., Bell Fatigue Scale (51), Short Form 36 Health Survey (SF-36.org), Multidimensional Fatigue Inventory (52), Fatigue Impact Scale (53)
- List of medications/non-prescription medications/ supplements
- Day of test instructions (what not to eat/drink, appropriate clothing, etc.)
- Release of information form
- Recovery strategies/aids

Medications/Supplements

The use of medications prior to testing must be clarified with the patient. If the purpose of testing is for clinical evidence of impairment or assessment of PEM, medications, including OTC medications, and supplements should be taken as prescribed, and at the same time of day prior to each CPET. However, for both research purposes and clinical diagnosis, limiting medications would be determined after consultation with the referring physician.

Test-Day Considerations

-Seek to minimize time in the waiting area prior to preparations for a CPET. A place to recline or semi-recline is helpful for a waiting patient, or when reviewing or clarifying pretest paperwork and procedures with the patient.

-Provide water throughout testing, and following CPET2, electrolyte replacement beverages can be helpful. Many ME/CFS patients have orthostatic intolerance so maintaining hydration with fluid and electrolytes (e.g., coconut water, sport drink) following CPET2 is helpful for expediting recovery. There are a number of anecdotal reports of plasma volume or salt loading reducing recovery time. Patients may consider arranging with their physician for a prescription of 1 L of IV normal saline infusion following completion of the 2-day CPET. However, if possible, there should be no intervention between the two CPETs.

Pretest Procedures

-CPET1 session should begin by explaining the entire test day procedure in detail. Prior to obtaining informed consent, respond to all patient questions.

-Review the completed pretest forms, and seek clarification of information if necessary. Additional questionnaires or procedures (e.g., title table test, cognitive tests, lung function measures, etc.) should be limited to minimize pre-fatiguing the patient. Body weight should be measured (not self-reported) prior to each CPET, and height should be measured before CPET1. After 5 min of supine rest, obtain resting heart rate, blood pressure, O_2 saturation, temperature, and monitor ECG. Monitoring the ECG throughout exercise testing is important for determining rate, rhythm and potential ischemia of cardiac tissue. Since many patients experience orthostatic symptoms, it is important to take measures after 5 min of supine rest and also during seated rest on the cycle ergometer prior to exercise.

-Explain use of the facemask or two-way valve to collect expired gases while the patient is supine. At this time, introduce and explain the Rating of Perceived Exertion (RPE)/Borg scale (48). Specify anchor intensities of 6 and 20 (or 0 and 10 for the modified scale) as the lowest and highest ratings of perceived exertion.

-Pain and dyspnea scales should be explained at this time as well. The seat height of the cycle ergometer should be adjusted to fit the subject and recorded, and the subject allowed to pedal at 0 Watts for a short period (<1 min). This will help the subject feel comfortable on the ergometer and reduce anxiety. To ensure safety during and after the CPET the patient should be monitored closely for adverse effects with continuous measures of blood pressure, oxygen saturation, ECG, and other indicators of stress.

Test Modality

A cycle ergometer is preferred to a treadmill for CPET testing of ME/CFS patients. While walking is a familiar activity for most and involves larger muscle groups, a cycle ergometer allows for easy quantification of work output and metabolic cost of exercise. There is less noise artifact for cardiac monitoring and measurement of blood pressure on a cycle ergometer, and fluctuation in work output from holding treadmill handrails, and biomechanical efficiency is less of a concern. Additionally, problems with balance and instability in some patients, particularly when close to maximum effort, are minimized when using a cycle ergometer. Patients generally feel more secure and comfortable on a cycle vs. a treadmill. Although VO_2peak may be 10–15% lower in healthy individuals when measured using a cycle ergometer compared to a treadmill, the benefits of safety and security on the cycle ergometer for the ME/CFS patient outweigh the risks associated with treadmill exercise for this population (54). Lastly, for accurate interpretation of test-retest findings it is critical to precisely reproduce the CPET1 workload protocol during CPET2, which can be accomplished more readily with the cycle ergometer. Ideally, an electronically-braked cycle ergometer affords the most accurate workload measures, and also provides smooth workload transitions for the patient. Cycle seat height should be the same for both CPETs.

Test Protocol

Selection of the test protocol should be matched closely with the anticipated ability of the patient. The goal of the test protocol is to incrementally challenge energy production such that the patient is able to complete at least 8 min but no more than 12 min of cycling (45). For *moderately ill* ME/CFS patients who complete this protocol, workload increments of 10–15 W/min, beginning at 0 watts, is appropriate to achieve an 8–12 min test to maximum effort duration. However, for a patient with a significant history of physical training, a 20 or 25 W/min protocol may be appropriate. The same protocol should be used for CPET1 and CPET2. Typically, the following cycle ergometer protocol is used for testing the ME/CFS patient:

- **START**: 3 min seated rest on cycle—monitor ECG, VO_2, and record BP and O_2 saturation at min 2.
- **EXERCISE PROTOCOL**: first minute exercise stage—begin at 0 watts (no prior warm-up) and increase 10–15 watts per min, or as appropriate.
- **DURING EXERCISE**: Measure BP/O_2 saturation/RPE every 2 min (e.g., @ 15W, 45W, 75W, etc.).
- **PEAK EXERCISE**: Obtain RPE, HR, BP at peak or immediate post exercise
- **POST EXERCISE**: Recovery measures of BP, HR/ECG, O_2sat @ minutes 1, 3, 5, etc. until recovery when HR is within 20 bpm above pretest HR, close to pretest BP, normal ECG, asymptomatic.
- **CONFIRM** reason for test termination with patient.

Test termination should comply with testing guidelines (45) and is indicated by attainment of maximal effort, or test termination due to patient safety. When testing for evidence of disability, insurers and independent medical examiners will closely scrutinize patient effort. Therefore, criteria for maximal effort should be reported which could include; plateau in oxygen consumption with increases in workload, RPE $\geq$ 18 (6–20 scale), respiratory exchange ratio (RER) $\geq$ 1.1, or peak blood lactate $\geq$ 8 mM. These criteria support evidence of maximum effort during CPET. The RER criterion is generally considered a more valid indicator of patient effort compared to the other indicators (55). Generally, satisfying two of three criteria is acceptable to determine that maximum effort was given by the patient (56). However, it would be inappropriate and unethical to prime the patient regarding effort criteria, therefore, consistency of procedures and patient motivation during both CPETs should be maintained for a valid comparison between CPETs.

Patient Risk

As with any maximal effort CPET, risk is conferred to the patient in completing such a test. Risk reduction is mitigated through standard procedures that include obtaining a relevant health history and completed cardiovascular disease risk questionnaire, a physician referral for testing, and clarifying with the patient any signs or symptoms suggestive of cardiovascular, pulmonary or metabolic diseases. Standardized guidelines for exercise testing are available and should guide decision making regarding risk classification of a patient and the need for medical oversight when conducting a CPET (7, 45, 57). When testing ME/CFS patients, it is not uncommon to find they may be well-screened for cardiovascular, pulmonary or metabolic disease risk in the course of trying to obtain a diagnosis of their illness symptoms. Due largely to the lack of knowledge and understanding of ME/CFS by medical professionals, average time from onset of ME/CFS symptoms to diagnosis is greater than 1 year, but 29 percent of patients surveyed reported that receiving a diagnosis took longer than 5 years (58, 59). Throughout efforts to obtain a diagnosis, patients commonly, but not always, visit and are screened by internists, cardiologists, rheumatologists, and others. Yet, there is insufficient evidence among this patient population to fully understand the relative risk to ME/CFS patients who complete the 2-day CPET procedure. As well, there is no evidence to suggest that the risk of untoward cardiovascular events varies from the general population. Due to the fact that many patients are well-screened prior to CPET testing, it could be suggested that risk for such an event may even be less than that of the general population. For ME/CFS patients, the greater concern of performing an exercise test is that associated with the potential for exacerbation or worsening of their typical PEM symptom profile. Because the disease is cyclic in nature, with patients often experiencing periods of remission and reactivation, and due to insufficient data on CPET testing in sufficiently large numbers of patients, it is unknown if performance of an exercise test, either submaximal or maximal, could worsen the overall illness status. Exacerbation of PEM symptoms via exercise is an inherent risk but also central to the efficacy of the 2-day CPET methodology, which should be acknowledged in the informed consent document. Most patients are well aware of their PEM symptom complex and the temporal expression of symptoms. However, particularly in patients who recently became ill, the exacerbation of symptoms due to exercise testing may coincide with the natural cyclic progression of the illness, and result in more severe and longer exacerbation of symptoms than is typical. Hence, it is difficult to predict the extent to which symptoms may flare and for how long. Patients should be fully aware of this risk prior to consenting to an exercise test. Strategies to minimize pretest energy expenditure during travel to a test site, preparation for an exercise test, and mitigating posttest symptom exacerbation are listed in **Table 2.**

Calibration and Quality Control

Calibration of the metabolic cart is essential prior to and following each CPET to assure accuracy and validity of data. Of equal importance, is biological validation for long-term stability of metabolic cart accuracy.

Quality Assurance - Biological validation for quality assurance is also essential for valid data. Reproducibility of gas exchange measurements requires consistent testing methodology. Biological quality control can identify error not detected by automated calibration of the metabolic measurement system (60). Even when automated system calibration appears accurate, results may be erroneous (61). Biological validation can be achieved by testing laboratory staff on a monthly basis at matched submaximal work rates, and for VO_2/work rate slope (62).

In general, routine maintenance based on the manufacturer's recommendation is essential for internal validity of data from the metabolic measurement system and electronic cycle ergometer.

TABLE 2 | Strategies to provide ME/CFS patients for testing.

TRAVEL
1. Avoid waiting in long security lines. Call the airline for a wheelchair in order to conserve energy and bypass the line. Be sure to check in at skycap and they will have a wheelchair waiting.
2. Preboard the flight for extra time to store belongings.
3. Sign up for TSA pre check. The security lines are shorter and there is no need to remove shoes and computers from carry-on luggage.
4. Travel with noise canceling headphones, earplugs or both.
5. Bring an eye mask and travel pillow to make the trip more restful.
6. Cover your face with a mask to avoid unwanted germs.
7. Bring healthy snacks.
8. Wear compression socks or compression calf sleeves to promote circulation and reduce fatigue.
9. Travel to your destination a day early and take a day or more to rest if needed.
HOTEL
1. Ask for a quiet room away from the ice machine.
2. Bring earplugs.
3. Use a white noise app.
4. If possible use a shower bench or sit down while showering.
5. Use a robe to dry off after showering.
6. Stay hydrated. Buy a bottle of water. If the hotel has a fitness center they usually have filtered water for free refills and often have fresh fruit.
GENERAL RECOVERY
1. Take a warm bath with Epsom salts.
2. Stretch sore muscles slowly but frequently.
3. Pace activities by planning rest breaks during the day.
4. Use diaphragmatic breathing to promote relaxation and recovery.
5. Rest until recovered.

The validity of comparison of CPET1 and CPET2 data relies on valid and reliable measurement devices.

Software Considerations - Data sampling, averaging, graphical and summary reports are determined by software supplied with metabolic measurement systems. Sampling differences can greatly affect test results. Breath by breath measurements averaged over 15–20 s intervals will reduce the effect of random noise and improve data consistency. It is essential to display data in a tabular time down format with rest, start of exercise, and peak exercise clearly delineated. Peak values should be selected from data in time down format following visual inspection of data for overt outliers due to coughing, gagging, sneezing or talking. Only data from start of exercise to peak exercise should be used to determine VAT.

CONCLUSIONS

Understanding and treating ME/CFS patients is hampered from a lack of diagnostic markers, heterogeneity in patient presentation, waxing and waning of symptoms within an individual patient, poor understanding of disease pathology, and the need to exclude other conditions. Cardiopulmonary exercise testing can provide helpful insights into this disease by better characterizing the unique post-exertional pathology of the illness.

Studies using one CPET-only are useful to elucidate immune activity and/or gene expression in ME/CFS because strenuous activity is known to induce considerable physiological changes similar to those associated with trauma (29, 63). As a quantifiable stressor, CPET has the capacity to reveal abnormalities across multiple systems that may not be apparent at rest by assessing the integrated response to exercise through comprehensive evaluation of the pulmonary, cardiovascular, haematopoietic, neuropsychological and musculo-skeletal systems (15). The inclusion of CPET could also be a primary consideration when designing clinical trials with functional endpoints (61). Determination of the respiratory exchange ratio, a measure exclusive to analysis of expired gases, provides the most accurate and reliable gauge of subject effort. This avoids problems associated with use of age-predicted maximal heart rate, which varies significantly in the general population and can be affected by both medication and pathology. Issues of response bias in self-report indictors of effort are also avoided. In the case of ME/CFS, the respiratory exchange ratio enables direct comparison between patient and control with confidence that both subjects were exposed to equivalent levels of physiological stress. Single CPET studies are also be useful for objective measurement of illness severity, pathophysiology, and for monitoring illness progression.

By comparison, the 2-day CPET methodology is useful for describing ME/CFS pathology as it provides objective and measureable changes due to impaired recovery across the two exercise tests. When the first test is conducted with a well-rested subject in a non-exacerbated state, this methodology allows for the characterization and quantification of post-exertional effects on functional capacity. Effects may be identified to correspond specifically to exercise at VAT or peak effort. Information gleaned from a 2-day CPET also offers objective evidence of impairment attributable to the effects of PEM, helps with patient management, informs therapeutic interventions, and tracks illness progression. Standardizing the 2-day CPET methodology to assess ME/CFS and other fatiguing illnesses across testing sites and study groups will allow for valid and relevant between-study comparisons. The goal is to better understand how impaired recovery impacts energy production and function, and hopefully determine the underlying pathophysiology of PEM as a disease component of ME/CFS.

AUTHOR CONTRIBUTIONS

SS designed the article and contributed to writing the manuscript and editing drafts. CS contributed to writing the background section and editing. JS, BK, and JV contributed to writing the manuscript and editing drafts.

ACKNOWLEDGMENTS

The authors would like to thank Ludovic Giloteaux, PhD, Molecular Biology and Genetics, Cornell University, for his technical assistance with preparation of the manuscript; and Simmaron Research for supporting CPET Summit meetings and the CPET Summit attendees to reach consensus on the techniques of this manuscript.

REFERENCES

1. Institute of Medicine. The National Academies Collection: Reports funded by National Institutes of Health. In: Committee on the Diagnostic Criteria for Myalgic Encephalomyelitis/Chronic Fatigue S, Board on the Health of Select P, editor. *Beyond Myalgic Encephalomyelitis/Chronic Fatigue Syndrome: Redefining an Illness*. Washington, DC: National Academies Press (2015), 82–4.
2. Carruthers BM, van de Sande MI, De Meirleir KL, Klimas NG, Broderick G, Mitchell T, et al. Myalgic encephalomyelitis: international consensus criteria. *J Intern Med.* (2011) 270:327–38. doi: 10.1111/j.1365-2796.2011.02428.x
3. Keller BA, Pryor JL, Giloteaux L. Inability of myalgic encephalomyelitis/chronic fatigue syndrome patients to reproduce VO 2 peak indicates functional impairment. *J Transl Med.* (2014) 12:104. doi: 10.1186/1479-5876-12-104
4. Snell CR, Stevens SR, Davenport TE, Van Ness JM. Discriminative validity of metabolic and workload measurements for identifying people with chronic fatigue syndrome. *Phys Ther.* (2013) 93:1484–92. doi: 10.2522/ptj.201 10368
5. VanNess JM, Snell CR, Stevens SR. Diminished cardiopulmonary capacity during post-exertional malaise. *J Chronic Fatigue Syndr.* (2007) 14:77–85. doi: 10.1300/J092v14n02_07
6. Vermeulen RC, Kurk RM, Visser FC, Sluiter W, Scholte HR. Patients with chronic fatigue syndrome performed worse than controls in a controlled repeated exercise study despite a normal oxidative phosphorylation capacity. *J Transl Med.* (2010) 8:93. doi: 10.1186/1479-58 76-8-93
7. American Thoracic Society. ATS/ACCP statement on cardiopulmonary exercise testing. *Am J Respir Crit Care Med.* (2003) 167:211–77. doi: 10.1164/rccm.167.2.211
8. Joyner MJ, Coyle EF. Endurance exercise performance: the physiology of champions. *J Physiol.* (2008) 586:35–44. doi: 10.1113/jphysiol.2007.143834
9. Mitchell JH, Sproule BJ, Chapman CB. The physiological meaning of the maximal oxygen intake test. *J Clin Invest.* (1958) 37:538–47. doi: 10.1172/JCI103636

10. Robinson S, Edwards HT, Dill DB. New records in human power. *Science* (1937) 85:409–10. doi: 10.1126/science.85.2208.409
11. Taylor HL, Buskirk E, Henschel, A. Maximal oxygen intake as an objective measure of cardio-respiratory performance. *J Appl Physiol.* (1955) 8:73–80. doi: 10.1152/jappl.1955.8.1.73
12. Blair SN, Kohl HW, Paffenbarger RS, Clark DG, Cooper KH, Gibbons LW. Physical fitness and all-cause mortality. *JAMA* (1989) 262:2395–401. doi: 10.1001/jama.1989.03430170057028
13. Bruce R, Kusumi F, Hosmer D. Maximal oxygen intake and nomographic assessment of functional aerobic impairment in cardiovascular disease. *Am Heart J.* (1973) 85:546–62. doi: 10.1016/0002-8703(73)90502-4
14. Gibbons LW, Blair SN, Cooper KH, Smith M. Association between coronary heart disease risk factors and physical fitness in healthy adult women. *Circulation* (1983) 67:977–83. doi: 10.1161/01.CIR.67.5.977
15. Forman DE, Myers J, Lavie CJ, Guazzi M, Celli B, Arena R. Cardiopulmonary exercise testing: relevant but underused. *Postgrad Med.* (2010) 122:68–86. doi: 10.3810/pgm.2010.11.2225
16. Meeusen R, Piacentini MF, Busschaert B, Buyse L, De Schutter G, Stray-Gundersen J. Hormonal responses in athletes: the use of a two bout exercise protocol to detect subtle differences in (over) training status. *Eur J Appl Physiol.* (2004) 91:140–6. doi: 10.1007/s00421-003-0940-1
17. Katch VL, Sady SS, Freedson P. Biological variability in maximum aerobic power. *Med Sci Sports Exerc.* (1982) 14:21–5. doi: 10.1249/00005768-198201000-00004
18. Weltman A, Snead D, Stein P, Seip R, Schurrer R, Rutt R, et al. Reliability and validity of a continuous incremental treadmill protocol for the determination of lactate threshold, fixed blood lactate concentrations, and VO2max. *Int J Sports Med.* (1990) 11:26–32. doi: 10.1055/s-2007-1024757
19. Welsman J, Bywater K, Farr C, Welford D, Armstrong N. Reliability of peak VO_2 and maximal cardiac output assessed using thoracic bioimpedance in children. *Eur J Appl Physiol.* (2005) 94:228–34. doi: 10.1007/s00421-004-1300-5
20. Cohen-Solal A, Zannad F, Kayanakis JG, Gueret P, Aupetit JF, Kolsky H. Multicentre study of the determination of peak oxygen uptake and ventilatory threshold during bicycle exercise in chronic heart failure. Comparison of graphical methods, interobserver variability and influence of the exercise protocol. The VO2 French Study Group. *Eur Heart J.* (1991) 12:1055–63. doi: 10.1093/oxfordjournals.eurheartj.a059837
21. Janicki JS, Gupta S, Ferris ST, McElroy PA. Long-term reproducibility of respiratory gas exchange measurements during exercise in patients with stable cardiac failure. *Chest* (1990) 97:12–7. doi: 10.1378/chest.97.1.12
22. Lehmann G, Kölling K. Reproducibility of cardiopulmonary exercise parameters in patients with valvular heart disease. *Chest* (1996) 110:685–92. doi: 10.1378/chest.110.3.685
23. Hansen JE, Sun X, Yasunobu Y, Garafano RP, Gates G, Barst RJ, et al. Reproducibility of cardiopulmonary exercise measurements in patients with pulmonary arterial hypertension. *Chest* (2004) 126:816–24. doi: 10.1378/chest.126.3.816
24. Koufaki P, Naish PF, Mercer TH. Reproducibility of exercise tolerance in patients with end-stage renal disease. *Arch Phys Med Rehabil.* (2001) 82:1421–4. doi: 10.1053/apmr.2001.26076
25. McKone EF, Barry SC, FitzGerald MX, Gallagher CG. Reproducibility of maximal exercise ergometer testing in patients with cystic fibrosis. *Chest* (1999) 116:363–8. doi: 10.1378/chest.116.2.363
26. Cox NJ, Hendriks JC, Binkhorst RA, Folgering HT, van Herwaarden CL. Reproducibility of incremental maximal cycle ergometer tests in patients with mild to moderate obstructive lung diseases. *Lung* (1989) 167:129–33. doi: 10.1007/BF02714939
27. Dobrovolny CL, Ivey FM, Rogers MA, Sorkin JD, Macko RF. Reliability of treadmill exercise testing in older patients with chronic hemiparetic stroke. *Arch Phys Med Rehabil.* (2003) 84:1308–12. doi: 10.1016/S0003-9993(03)00150-3
28. Aunola S. Rusko H. Reproducibility of aerobic and anaerobic thresholds in 20-50 year old men. *Eur J Appl Physiol Occup Physiol.* (1984) 53:260–66. doi: 10.1007/BF00776600
29. Cook DB, Nagelkirk PR, Poluri A, Mores J, Natelson BH. The influence of aerobic fitness and fibromyalgia on cardiorespiratory and perceptual responses to exercise in patients with chronic fatigue syndrome. *Arthritis Rheum.* (2006) 54:3351–62. doi: 10.1002/art.22124
30. Cook DB, Stegner AJ, Nagelkirk PR, Meyer JD, Togo F, Natelson BH. Responses to exercise differ for chronic fatigue syndrome patients with fibromyalgia. *Med Sci Sports Exerc.* (2012) 44:1186–93. doi: 10.1249/MSS.0b013e3182417b9a
31. De Becker P, Roeykens J, Reynders M, McGregor N, De Meirleir K. Exercise capacity in chronic fatigue syndrome. *Arch Internal Med.* (2006) 160:3270–77. doi: 10.1001/archinte.160.21.3270
32. Farquhar WB, Hunt BE, Taylor JA, Darling SE, Freeman, R. Blood volume and its relation to peak O(2) consumption and physical activity in patients with chronic fatigue. *Am J Physiol.* Heart *Circ Physiol.* (2002) 282:66. doi: 10.1152/ajpheart.2002.282.1.H66
33. Inbar O, Dlin R, Rotstein A, Whipp BJ. Physiological responses to incremental exercise in patients with chronic fatigue syndrome. *Med Sci Sports Exerc.* (2001) 33, 1463–70. doi: 10.1097/00005768-200109000-00007
34. Sargent C, Scroop GC, Nemeth PM, Burnet RB, Buckley JD. Maximal oxygen uptake and lactate metabolism are normal in chronic fatigue syndrome. (2002) *Med Sci Sports Exerc.* 34:51–56. doi: 10.1097/00005768-200201000-00009
35. Snell CR, Vanness JM, Strayer DR, Stevens SR. Exercise capacity and immune function in male and female patients with chronic fatigue syndrome (CFS)patients. *In vivo* (2005) 19:387–390. doi: 10.1249/00005768-200405001-01466
36. Katz BZ, Boas S, Shiraishi Y, Mears CJ, Taylor R. Exercise tolerance testing in a prospective cohort of adolescents with chronic fatigue syndrome and recovered controls following infectious mononucleosis. *J Pediatr.* (2010) 157:468–72. doi: 10.1016/j.jpeds.2010.03.025
37. Takken T, van der Net J, Helders PJM. The reliability of an aerobic and an anaerobic exercise tolerance test in patients with juvenile onset dermatomyositis. *J Rheumatol.* (2005) 32:734–39.
38. Vanness JM, Snell CR, Strayer DR, Dempsey L, Stevens SR. Subclassifying chronic fatigue syndrome through exercise testing. *Med Sci Sports Exerc.* (2003) 35:908–13. doi: 10.1249/01.MSS.0000069510.58763.E8
39. Davis JA, Vodak P, Wilmore JH, Vodak J, Kurtz P. Anaerobic threshold and maximal aerobic power for three modes of exercise. *J Appl Physiol.* (1976) 41:544–50. doi: 10.1152/jappl.1976.41.4.544
40. Chase PJ, Kenjale A, Cahalin LP, Arena R, Davis PG, Myers J, et al. Effects of respiratory exchange ratio on the prognostic value of peak oxygen consumption and ventilatory efficiency in patients with systolic heart failure. *JACC Heart Fail.* (2013) 1:427–32. doi: 10.1016/j.jchf.2013.05.008
41. Sun X, Hansen JE, Garatachea N, Storer TW, Wasserman K. Ventilatory efficiency during exercise in healthy subjects. *Am J Respir Crit Care Med.* (2002). 166:1443–8. doi: 10.1164/rccm.2202033
42. Guazzi M, Adams V, Conraads V, Halle M, Mezzani A, Vanhees L. et al. Clinical recommendations for cardiopulmonary exercise testing data assessment in specific patient populations. *Eur Heart J.* (2012) 33:2917–27. doi: 10.1093/eurheartj/ehs221
43. Hansen JE, Sue DY, Wasserman K. Predicted values for clinical exercise testing. *Am Rev Respir Dis.* (1984) 129:S49–55. doi: 10.1164/arrd.1984.129.2P2.S49
44. Brubaker PH. Kitzman DW. Chronotropic incompetence: causes, consequences, and management. *Circulation* (2011) 123:1010–20. doi: 10.1161/CIRCULATIONAHA.110.940577
45. Riebe D, Ehrman JK, Liguori G, Magal M. *ACSM's Guidelines for Exercise Testing and Prescription.* 10th ed. Philadelphia, PA: Lippincott Williams & Wilkins (2018).
46. Callahan JM. Pulse oximetry in emergency medicine. *Emerg Med Clin.* (2008) 26:869–79. doi: 10.1016/j.emc.2008.08.006
47. Haskell WL. Cardiovascular complications during exercise training of cardiac patients. *Circulation* (1978) 57:920–4. doi: 10.1161/01.CIR.57.5.920
48. Borg GA. Psychophysical bases of perceived exertion. *Med Sci Sports Exerc.* (1982) 14:377–81. doi: 10.1249/00005768-198205000-00012
49. Myers J, Arena R, Franklin B, Pina I, Kraus WE, McInnis K, et al. Recommendations for clinical exercise laboratories: a scientific statement from the american heart association. *Circulation* (2009) 119:3144–61. doi: 10.1161/CIRCULATIONAHA.109.192520
50. Beaver WL, Wasserman K, Whipp BJ. A new method for detecting anaerobic threshold by gas exchange. *J Appl Physiol.* (1986) 60:2020–7. doi: 10.1152/jappl.1986.60.6.2020

51. Bell D.S. *The doctor's guide to chronic fatigue syndrome: understanding, treating, and living with Cfids*. Boston, MA: Da Capo Lifelong Books (1993).
52. Smets EM, Garssen B, Bonke B, De Haes JC. The Multidimensional Fatigue Inventory (MFI) psychometric qualities of an instrument to assess fatigue. *J Psychosom Res.* (1995) 39:315–25. doi: 10.1016/0022-3999(94)00125-O
53. Fisk JD, Ritvo PG, Ross L, Haase DA, Marrie TJ, Schlech, WF. Measuring the functional impact of fatigue: initial validation of the fatigue impact scale. *Clin. Infect. Dis.* (1994) 18(Suppl. 1):S79–83. doi: 10.1093/clinids/18.Supplement_1.S79
54. Porszasz J, Stringer W, Casaburi R. Equipment, measurements and quality control in clinical exercise testing. *Eur Respir Monogr.* (2007) 40:108. doi: 10.1183/1025448x.00040005
55. Howley ET, Bassett DR, Welch, HG. Criteria for maximal oxygen uptake: review and commentary. *Med Sci Sports Exerc.* (1995) 27:1292–1301. doi: 10.1249/00005768-199509000-00009
56. Powers SK, Howley ET. *Exercise Physiology: Theory and Application to Fitness and Performance*. 10th ed. New York, NY: McGraw-Hill (2015)
57. Gibbons RJ, Balady GJ, Bricker JT, Chaitman BR, Fletcher GF, Froelicher VF, et al. ACC/AHA 2002 guideline update for exercise testing: summary article: a report of the American College of Cardiology/American Heart Association Task Force on Practice Guidelines (Committee to Update the 1997 Exercise Testing Guidelines). *Circulation* (2002) 106:1883–92. doi: 10.1161/01.CIR.0000034670.06526.15
58. CFIDS Association of America. *ME/CFS Road to Diagnosis Survey*. Charlotte, NC: CFIDS Association of America (2014).
59. ProHealth. *Data from: A Profile of ME/CFS Patients - How Many Years and How Many Doctors?* ProHealth.com. (2008) Available online at: http://www.prohealth.com/library/showarticle.cfm?libid=13672
60. Revill SM. Morgan MD. Biological quality control for exercise testing. *Thorax* (2000) 55:63–6. doi: 10.1136/thorax.55.1.63
61. Balady GJ, Arena R, Sietsema K, Myers J, Coke L, Fletcher GF, et al. Clinician's Guide to cardiopulmonary exercise testing in adults: a scientific statement from the American Heart Association. *Circulation* (2010) 122:191–225. doi: 10.1161/CIR.0b013e3181e52e69
62. Porszasz J, Blonshine S, Cao R, Paden HA, Casaburi R, Rossiter HB. Biological quality control for cardiopulmonary exercise testing in multicenter clinical trials. *BMC Pulm Med.* (2016) 16:13. doi: 10.1186/s12890-016-0174-8
63. White AT, Light AR, Hughen RW, Bateman L, Martins TB, Hill HR, et al. Severity of symptom flare after moderate exercise is linked to cytokine activity in chronic fatigue syndrome. *Psychophysiology* (2010) 47:615–24. doi: 10.1111/j.1469-8986.2010.00978.x

21

Estimating Prevalence, Demographics and Costs of ME/CFS Using Large Scale Medical Claims Data and Machine Learning

Ashley R. Valdez[1], *Elizabeth E. Hancock*[1], *Seyi Adebayo*[1], *David J. Kiernicki*[1], *Daniel Proskauer*[2], *John R. Attewell*[3], *Lucinda Bateman*[4], *Alfred DeMaria Jr.*[5], *Charles W. Lapp*[6], *Peter C. Rowe*[7] and *Charmian Proskauer*[8]*

[1] Optum Enterprise Analytics, UnitedHealth Group, Minneapolis, MN, United States, [2] Optum Technology, UnitedHealth Group, Minneapolis, MN, United States, [3] Innovation, Research, and Development, UnitedHealth Group, Minneapolis, MN, United States, [4] Bateman Horne Center, Salt Lake City, UT, United States, [5] Bureau of Infectious Disease and Laboratory Sciences, Massachusetts Department of Public Health, Boston, MA, United States, [6] Hunter-Hopkins Center, Charlotte, NC, United States, [7] Children's Center Chronic Fatigue Clinic, Johns Hopkins University School of Medicine, Baltimore, MD, United States, [8] Massachusetts ME/CFS & FM Association, Quincy, MA, United States

***Correspondence:**
Charmian Proskauer
charmian.proskauer@verizon.net

Techniques of data mining and machine learning were applied to a large database of medical and facility claims from commercially insured patients to determine the prevalence, gender demographics, and costs for individuals with provider-assigned diagnosis codes for myalgic encephalomyelitis (ME) or chronic fatigue syndrome (CFS). The frequency of diagnosis was 519–1,038/100,000 with the relative risk of females being diagnosed with ME or CFS compared to males 1.238 and 1.178, respectively. While the percentage of women diagnosed with ME/CFS is higher than the percentage of men, ME/CFS is not a "women's disease." Thirty-five to forty percent of diagnosed patients are men. Extrapolating from this frequency of diagnosis and based on the estimated 2017 population of the United States, a rough estimate for the number of patients who may be diagnosed with ME or CFS in the U.S. is 1.7 million to 3.38 million. Patients diagnosed with CFS appear to represent a more heterogeneous group than those diagnosed with ME. A machine learning model based on characteristics of individuals diagnosed with ME was developed and applied, resulting in a predicted prevalence of 857/100,000 ($p > 0.01$), or roughly 2.8 million in the U.S. Average annual costs for individuals with a diagnosis of ME or CFS were compared with those for lupus (all categories) and multiple sclerosis (MS), and found to be 50% higher for ME and CFS than for lupus or MS, and three to four times higher than for the general insured population. A separate aspect of the study attempted to determine if a diagnosis of ME or CFS could be predicted based on symptom codes in the insurance claims records. Due to the absence of specific codes for some core symptoms, we were unable to validate that the information in insurance claims records is sufficient to identify diagnosed patients or suggest that a diagnosis of ME or CFS should be considered based solely on looking for presence of those symptoms. These results show that a prevalence rate of 857/100,000 for ME/CFS is not unreasonable; therefore, it is not a rare disease, but in fact a relatively common one.

Keywords: ME/CFS, myalgic encephalomyelitis, chronic fatigue syndrome, prevalence, costs, machine learning, data mining

INTRODUCTION

Myalgic Encephalomyelitis (ME) and Chronic Fatigue Syndrome (CFS) are serious, debilitating conditions that impose a burden of illness on millions of people in the United States and around the world (1).

Multiple case definitions have been used to define ME and CFS. Those for ME require the presence of post-exertional malaise and tend to identify a more severely ill subset of the broader ME and CFS population (2). Although there are separate diagnostic codes for ME and CFS, the descriptions in the International Classification of Diseases (ICD)[1] listings are the same. The two terms ME and CFS have been conflated, and as of 2016, U.S. federal health agencies have used the combined term ME/CFS to refer to this disease.

ME/CFS is an acquired, chronic, multi-systemic disease characterized by significant relapse after physical, cognitive, or emotional exertion of any sort. The disease includes immune, neurological and cognitive impairment, sleep abnormalities, and autonomic dysfunction, resulting in significant functional impairment accompanied by a pathological level of fatigue. The cause of the disease remains unknown, although in many cases symptoms may have been triggered by an infection or other prodromal event [U.S. Department of Health and Human Services, (3)].

The underlying etiology is not known. There is no readily available laboratory test to diagnose ME/CFS, no FDA-approved drug for ME/CFS, and no cure. Many ME/CFS patients experience significant disability. At least one-quarter of ME/CFS patients are house- or bedbound at some point in their lives (4, 5). The direct and indirect economic costs of ME/CFS to society have been estimated at $17 to $24 billion annually (6), including $9.1 billion attributed to lost household and labor force productivity (7).

Assigning a diagnosis of ME/CFS in the clinical setting often takes years. Many physicians are uninformed or misinformed about the disease (1). It has been estimated that 84–91% of patients affected by ME/CFS are not diagnosed with the disease (8).

Thus, improving diagnosis and optimizing management can have significant economic and public health consequences (2). Without good data on the prevalence of ME/CFS, it is difficult to allocate resources for research of all kinds (etiology, pathophysiology, treatment, etc.), as well as for medical education, that would be commensurate with the burden of the disease.

This study uses data from a large sample of the general population insured by a major commercial health insurance carrier to look at characteristics of clinician-diagnosed ME and CFS patients. We applied techniques of data mining and machine learning to a large medical claims database to investigate the prevalence, characteristics, and costs for individuals with ME/CFS.

METHODS

This study examined de-identified physician and hospital data from a large claims processing database from Optum, a large healthcare information and services company, which allowed us to describe features of physician-diagnosed ME/CFS patients and to compare this group to the general insured population. The overall sequence of the study is shown in **Figure 1**.

Data Sources

The Optum database contains membership, provider, claims, and ancillary data on over 101 million former and current members. The database contains no identifying information on individuals (names, addresses, etc.), but each individual's claims data are linked. The database contains a primary diagnosis and up to four additional diagnostic codes for each claim.

The primary dataset used in this study includes medical and facility insurance claims for nearly 50 million (49,963,500) individuals age 0 through 89 who had at least one medical or one facility claim. Only medical (e.g., from doctor's offices and including any tests or procedures that were conducted or ordered there) and facility (e.g., hospital) claims were part of the data sets used in this study. Prescription drug claims were not included.

The database captured all medical and facility claims, and did not require that the individual have continuous insurance coverage over a specific period of time. The data used in this study are primarily from individuals enrolled during the years 2011–2016, 2016 being the last year for which complete enrollment data were available. All claims for these individuals were considered including claims from the year 2017 if available.

Approximately 80% of individuals in this dataset were insured by commercial health insurance; close to 20% had coverage from Medicare, the U.S. government program for individuals age 65 and over and for certain individuals with disabilities. The dataset did not include any claims associated with Medicaid, the U.S. government program for low-income individuals. For some of the topics in this study, sub-sets of the dataset were used.

We used diagnosis codes which were assigned and entered into the patient's record. From the code alone we could not determine what case definition or clinical diagnostic criteria were used to make the diagnosis.

During the years 2011–2016 two different sets of ICD codes[2] were in use, ICD-9-CM and ICD-10-CM. Both versions included codes that were used for CFS (Chronic Fatigue Syndrome) and

[1]ICD codes for ME and CFS
Available online at: https://www.icd10data.com/ICD10CM/Codes/G00-G99/G89-G99/G93-/G93.3
Available online at: https://www.icd10data.com/ICD10CM/Codes/R00-R99/R50-R69/R53-/R53.82
Available online at: http://www.icd9data.com/2014/Volume1/320-389/320-327/323/323.9.htm
Available online at: http://www.icd9data.com/2014/Volume1/780-799/780-789/780/780.71.htm

[2]ICD codes related to fatigue
Available online at: http://www.icd9data.com/2014/Volume1/780-799/780-789/780/780.79.htm
Available online at: https://www.icd10data.com/ICD10CM/Codes/R00-R99/R50-R69/R53-/R53.81
Available online at: https://www.icd10data.com/ICD10CM/Codes/R00-R99/R50-R69/R53-/R53.83

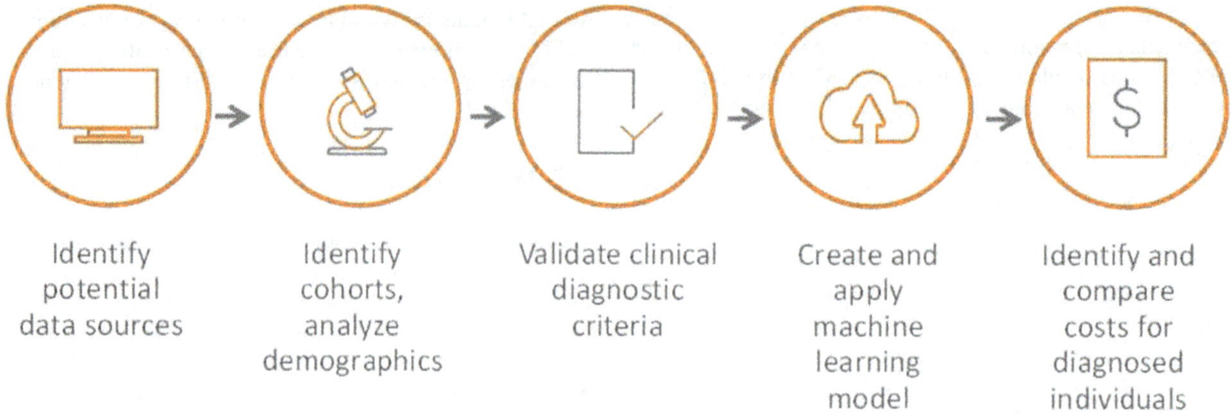

FIGURE 1 | Graphic showing sequence of steps in this study.

TABLE 1 | ICD codes used for diagnosis of ME and CFS.

Diagnosis	ICD-9-CM (retired Oct 1, 2015)	ICD-10-CM
ME (Myalgic Encephalomyelitis)	323.9	G93.3
CFS (Chronic Fatigue Syndrome)	780.71	R53.82

ME (Myalgic Encephalomyelitis) (**Table 1**). ME and CFS were analyzed separately in some analyses. The lack of specificity and interrelationships of these codes (see **Appendix 1** in Supplementary Material, Interrelationships of ICD codes used for Chronic Fatigue Syndrome (CFS) and Myalgic Encephalomyelitis (ME) in the U.S. as of October, 2018) introduce a degree of uncertainty; however, these are the diagnostic codes used for ME and CFS, and provide the best available baseline for this type of study at this point in time.

Frequency of ME/CFS Diagnosis and Demographics of Diagnosed Population

Main dataset: The general population (all individuals in the database) and the diagnosed population (all those with codes for ME or CFS) were examined for distribution by current (as of 2017) age and gender. Queries were run against the entire data set and two subsets. Separate queries were run to eliminate duplications if an individual had codes for both ME and CFS.

The initial analysis was conducted using the entire dataset of 49,963,500 individuals who had at least one medical or one facility claim. Claims associated with these individuals were examined for presence of one of the four diagnosis codes as the primary diagnosis. Length of insurance enrollment was not considered for this group.

Subset 1: The first subset analysis examined individuals who were continuously enrolled in the same insurance plan for the entire 2011–2016 period, providing longer length of enrollment, and more complete medical history.

Subset 2: The second subset consisted of individuals who were continuously enrolled in the same insurance plan for between 2 and 4 years at any time between 2011 and 2016. This group more accurately represents the central tendencies of the data and eliminates outliers. For this query we used codes from all 5 diagnosis code fields in the analysis, not just the primary diagnosis. All claims for these individuals were included. In addition to the base query, we also separately analyzed demographic data for individuals in this subset who were diagnosed with ME only, without including those diagnosed with CFS alone.

For all datasets, the reference population is all the individuals in that dataset.

Validation of Clinical Diagnostic Criteria

An important component of this study was an examination of symptom codes in medical records to determine if the diagnosis of ME/CFS could be confirmed by the presence of a unique cluster of symptoms, such as those in the diagnostic criteria proposed in the 2015 report from the National Academy of Medicine (1), which requires 4 or 5 core symptoms that were determined to be strongly supported by evidence as accurately identifying ME/CFS (**Appendix 2** in Supplementary Material).

In order to maximize the probability of being able to identify symptoms, we limited analysis to the population continuously enrolled for the entire 2011–2016 period (subset 1), since longer enrollment provides a more complete history.

Estimating Prevalence Using Machine Learning

We applied the techniques of machine learning to predict the prevalence of ME using another method of analyzing our claims data. (For more information about machine learning, see **Appendix 3** in Supplementary Material). From the cohort of individuals who were continuously enrolled for 2 to 4 years, individuals under the age of 15 years were removed in order to minimize features that would be created from predominantly pediatric care. To create the machine learning modeling cohort,

TABLE 2 | ICD codes used for the diagnosis of multiple sclerosis and lupus.

Diagnosis	ICD-9-CM (retired Oct 1, 2015)	ICD-10-CM
MS (Multiple Sclerosis)	340	G35
Lupus (includes all subcategories)	710	M32, L93

we included all members of the diagnosed population as well as a random sample of 25% from the remaining general population.

The modeling cohort was randomly split into a training, validation, and testing set per data science protocol. The training set was rebalanced for modeling with a 50–50 random split, so that the diagnosed and general population were evenly split and the model could train on positive and negative classes evenly. The training set was used to train the model. The validation set was used to tune the model. The testing set was used to do a final test on the finished model.

The model was built using XGBoost, an open source implementation of the boosted tree method of supervised learning. The final model contained 507 features which included medical claim codes, age, and gender information. The validation set was used for prevalence estimates. Prevalence was estimated from individuals that the model predicted to have ME at a 99% probability and dividing by the total number in the dataset.

Costs

To analyze the financial impact of the disease, we used data from the main data set for the years 2012 through 2016. This time period was chosen because it includes the largest number of individuals and the most years of claims data. We focused on individuals with the ME diagnosis code because we speculated that assignment of the less well-known ME diagnosis code might better represent the characteristics and diagnostic criteria of ME/CFS, and therefore this would be a more specific group. We only considered individuals from the overall cohort who were 13 years of age or older, since the incidence of ME in young children is much smaller.

Costs used were the standard allowed payment (contracted rate) for all provider services which may have ultimately been paid by either the insurer or related patient responsibility associated with the claim such as patient co-payment or deductible, if any.

We looked at the yearly costs related to claims for individuals diagnosed with ME vs. all other individuals in the reference population. The average annual cost per individual was calculated on medical claims >$0 for each year from 2012 to 2016. Costs were not adjusted for inflation. Costs included both those paid by the insurer at the standard allowed payment for all provider services and the related patient responsibility associated with the claim such as patient co-payment or deductible, if any. Only medical and facility claims were considered, and we did not analyze the content of claims that contributed to the costs.

To put the cost in context, we also looked in the same way at annual costs related to claims for two similar diseases which are often compared to ME/CFS, multiple sclerosis and lupus erythematosus. ICD codes used in these queries are shown in **Table 2**.

TABLE 3 | Prevalence of ME diagnosis for varying lengths of continuous enrollment (any years).

Continuous years enrolled	Diagnosed	General Pop.	Prevalence per 100,000
0–1	2,668	3,648,421	73
1–2	11,070	13,422,797	82
2–3	7,883	7,339,562	107
3–4	6,337	4,438,630	143
4–5	6,375	3,660,868	174
5–6	2,971	1,670,694	178
6–7	4,925	2,629,342	187
Total	42,229	36,810,314	115

RESULTS

Prevalence of ME Diagnosis vs. Average Length of Enrollment

In creating Subset 2, we compared the average length of continuous enrollment for individuals diagnosed with ME-only vs. the general insured population. The average length of enrollment of all individuals in the database is just over 2 years (980 days). Individuals with a diagnosis code for ME but not for CFS, on average, have been enrolled for just over 3 years (1,204 days). We therefore chose the length of continuous enrollment from 2 to 4 years to most accurately represent the central tendencies of the data and eliminate outliers for both the general and the ME-diagnosed population. Subset two includes individuals with a diagnosis of ME in any of the diagnosis fields in the claims (primary diagnosis plus up to four additional secondary diagnoses).

Table 3 shows the number of individuals continuously enrolled for periods of from 1 to 7 years who had a diagnosis code of ME (but not CFS). Note that as the length of continuous enrollment increases, the proportion with an ME diagnosis also increases, as would be expected as the opportunity for diagnosis is extended.

Frequency of ME/CFS Diagnosis

Tables 4, 5 show diagnostic codes for ME and CFS and prevalence of these diagnoses for the three population sets. Data columns for ME and CFS include all individuals who had that as the primary diagnosis code in any of their claims. Prevalence for each of the three groups was calculated by dividing the number of diagnosed individuals by the total in the reference population. Some individuals might have had both codes within their set of claims; separate queries were run to eliminate this duplication. **Table 4** shows the prevalence for ME and CFS separately. **Table 5** shows the prevalence for ME+CFS with and without duplication. Without duplication, prevalence of ME/CFS was 519/100,000 in the main dataset (non-continuous enrollment), 669/100,000 in Subset 1 (continuous enrollment for the entire period), and

TABLE 4 | Summary of prevalence of ME and CFS in three studied cohorts.

Population	ME				CFS			
	G93.3	323.9	Total w/Dups	per 100K	R53.82	780.71	Total w/dups	per 100K
Main dataset	16,305	9,263	25,568	51	140,947	99,929	240,876	482
Subset 1	1,044	1,030	2,074	81	6,635	10,234	16,869	661
Subset 2	10,196	3,945	14,141	121	87,282	57,614	144,896	1,236

TABLE 5 | Summary of prevalence of ME + CFS in the three studied cohorts, and with duplicates eliminated.

Population	ME+CFS		Union ME+CFS		Reference
	Total	per 100K	Total no dups	per 100K	Total
Main dataset	266,444	533	259,275	519	49,963,500
Subset 1	18,943	742	17,074	669	2,553,722
Subset 2	159,037	1,357	121,632	1,038	11,720,401

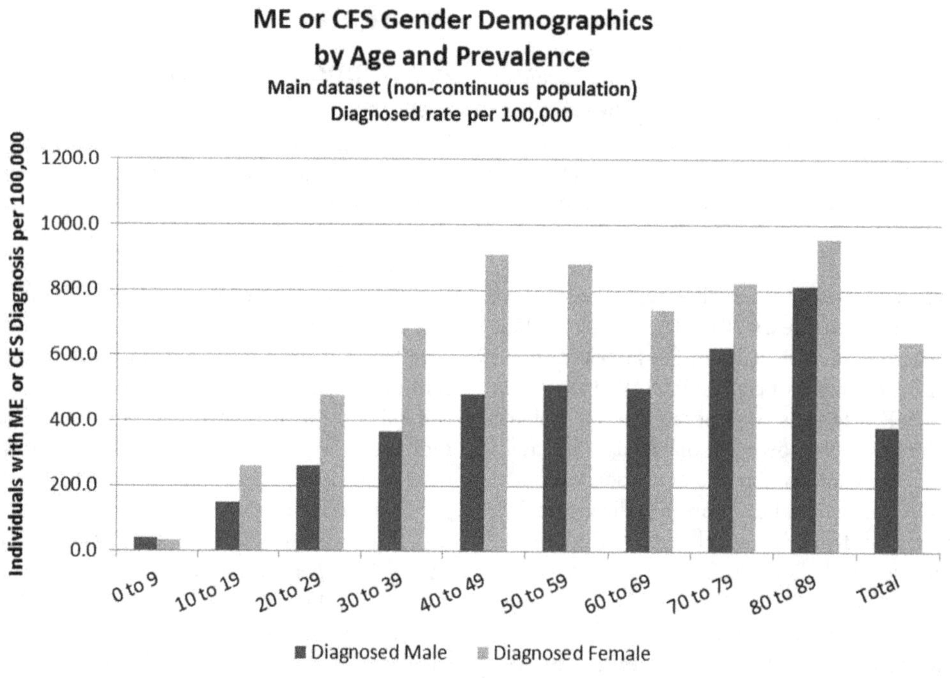

FIGURE 2 | ME or CFS gender demographics by age and prevalence (main dataset, non-continuous enrollment).

1,038/100,000 in Subset 2 (continuous enrollment for any 2–4 year period). For Subset 2 only, up to four secondary diagnosis fields were included from the claims in addition to the primary diagnosis.

Extrapolating from this frequency of diagnosis and based on the estimated 2017 population of the United States of 325,719,178 (9), a rough estimate for the number of patients who are diagnosed with ME or CFS in the U.S. is 1.7 million to 3.4 million.

Demographics of Diagnosed Population

Detailed analysis of gender distribution by age for ME or CFS diagnosed individuals (no duplicates) within the three studied population sets are shown in **Figures 2–4** and **Tables 6, 7**. Totals for the gender distribution are slightly smaller because gender information was not available for every individual. Results are normalized for each decile.

Demographics of Diagnosed Population for the Main Dataset (Non-continuous Enrollment)

Figure 2 and **Table 6** show the gender distribution by age for individuals diagnosed with ME or CFS for the population of individuals who were enrolled at any time during the period

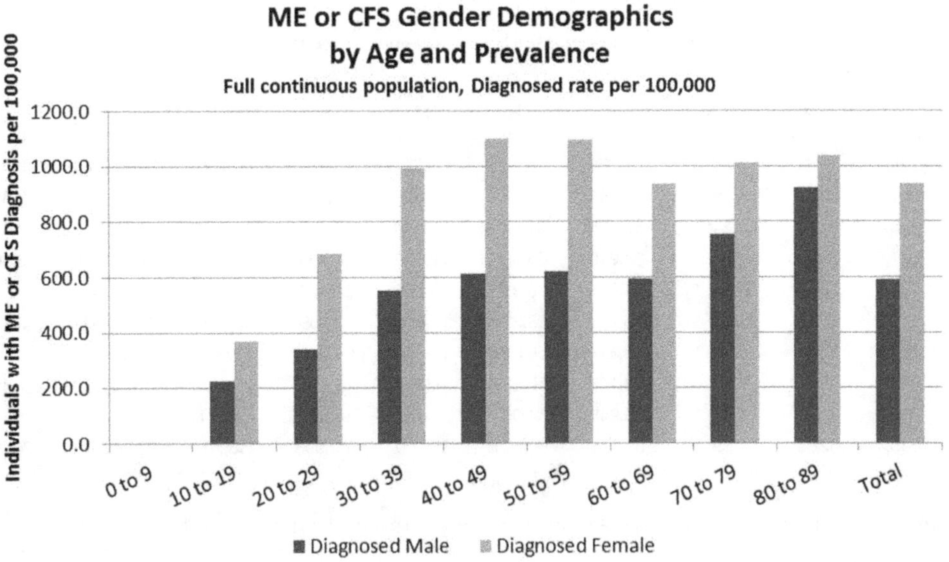

FIGURE 3 | ME or CFS gender demographics by age and prevalence (Subset 1, continuous enrollment from 2011 to 2016).

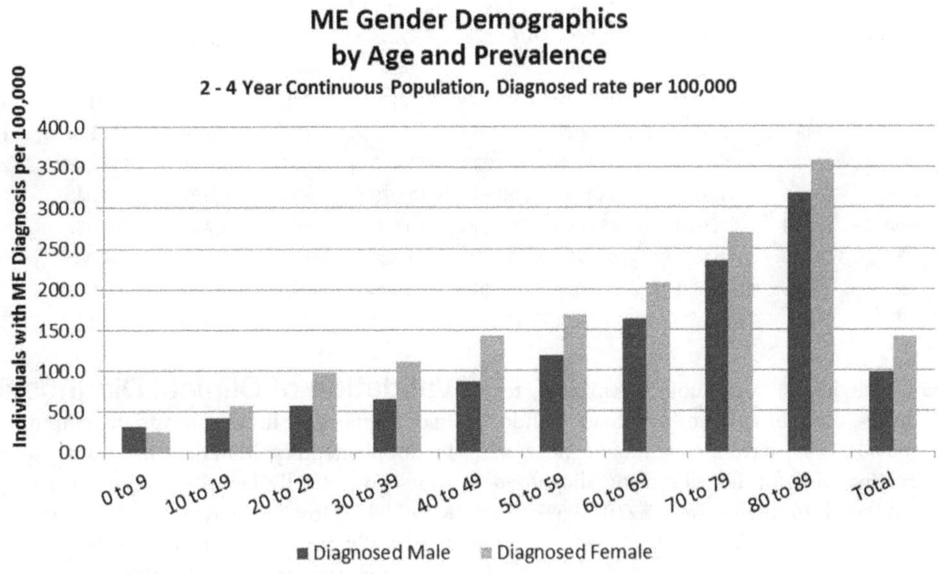

FIGURE 4 | ME gender demographics by age and prevalence (Subset 2, continuous enrollment from 2 to 4 years).

2011–2016, and the gender distribution by age and prevalence for these same individuals.

Of the 49,570,369 individuals enrolled during the period 2011–2016 for whom we have gender information, 258,702 (or 519/100,000) had a code for diagnosis of either CFS or ME. The relative risk for females being diagnosed with ME or CFS compared to males was 1.238 (95% CI: 1.235–1.242).

In the youngest age group, 0–9, boys outnumber girls; relative risk for females being diagnosed with ME or CFS compared to males in this age group was 0.922 (95% CI: 0.874–0.970).

Demographics of Diagnosed Population, Subset 1, Continuous Enrollment From 2011 to 2016

Figure 3 and **Table 7** show the gender distribution by age for individuals diagnosed with ME or CFS for the population of individuals who were continuously enrolled in their insurance for the entire period 2011–2016 (Subset 1) and the gender distribution by age and prevalence for these same individuals. In this group there were no diagnosed individuals younger than 10.

TABLE 6 | ME or CFS gender demographics by age and prevalence vs. reference population in the main dataset (Main dataset: non-continuous enrollment).

	Diagnosed-ME/CFS (count/100,000)			F: M ratio	Diagnosed-ME/CFS (% normalized)		Diagnosed-ME/CFS (count)			Data set population		
Age range	**M**	**F**	**Total**	**F: M**	**M**	**F**	**M**	**F**	**Total**	**M**	**F**	**Total**
0 to 9	40.0	34.3	37.2	0.86: 1	53.83%	46.17%	978	796	1,774	2,446,920	2,321,941	4,768,861
10 to 19	148.8	261.8	204.8	1.76: 1	36.24%	63.76%	4,023	6,934	10,957	2,702,876	2,648,306	5,351,182
20 to 29	259.5	478.1	379.3	1.84: 1	35.18%	64.82%	7,725	17,245	24,970	2,976,670	3,606,744	6,583,414
30 to 39	365.8	681.9	539.0	1.86: 1	34.91%	65.09%	11,679	26,390	38,069	3,192,640	3,869,894	7,062,534
40 to 49	482.1	909.1	708.4	1.89: 1	34.65%	65.35%	15,264	32,472	47,736	3,166,430	3,571,767	6,738,197
50 to 59	510.4	879.5	705.2	1.72: 1	36.72%	63.28%	16,865	32,459	49,324	3,304,031	3,690,758	6,994,789
60 to 69	499.6	739.6	628.1	1.48: 1	40.31%	59.69%	14,433	24,610	39,043	2,889,185	3,327,290	6,216,475
70 to 79	623.7	822.8	731.3	1.32: 1	43.12%	56.88%	9,976	15,479	25,455	1,599,520	1,881,168	3,480,688
80 to 89	814.2	958.0	900.3	1.18: 1	45.94%	54.06%	7,766	13,608	21,374	953,817	1,420,412	2,374,229
Total	381.8	645.4	521.9	1.69: 1	37.17%	62.83%	88,709	169,993	258,702	23,232,089	26,338,280	49,570,369

TABLE 7 | ME or CFS gender demographics by age and prevalence vs. reference population (Subset 1: continuous enrollment 2011–2016).

	Diagnosed-ME/CFS (count/100,000)			F: M ratio	Diagnosed-ME/CFS (% normalized)		Diagnosed-ME/CFS (count)			Data set population		
Age range	**M**	**F**	**Total**	**F: M**	**M**	**F**	**M**	**F**	**Total**	**M**	**F**	**Total**
0–9	0.0	0.0	0.0		0.00%	0.00%	0	0	0	4	5	9
10 to 19	179.7	288.7	233.1	1.61: 1	38.36%	61.64%	242	374	616	134,694	129,563	264,257
20–29	297.3	584.0	443.8	1.96: 1	33.74%	66.26%	405	831	1,236	136,205	142,303	278,508
30–39	481.6	881.7	695.9	1.83: 1	35.33%	64.67%	270	570	840	56,062	64,646	120,708
40–49	515.3	956.9	749.2	1.86: 1	35.00%	65.00%	780	1,631	2,411	151,354	170,449	321,803
50–59	530.7	947.4	749.4	1.79: 1	35.91%	64.09%	1,155	2,277	3,432	217,625	240,347	457,972
60–69	527.7	819.9	682.5	1.55: 1	39.16%	60.84%	1,073	1,877	2,950	203,345	228,921	432,266
70–79	640.2	848.8	752.9	1.33: 1	43.00%	57.00%	695	1,082	1,777	108,557	127,478	236,035
80–89	791.5	909.7	862.8	1.15: 1	46.52%	53.48%	1,385	2,420	3,805	174,985	266,008	440,993
Total	507.7	807.6	668.6	1.59: 1	38.60%	61.40%	6,005	11,062	17,067	1,182,831	1,369,720	2,552,551

Of the 2,552,551 individuals continuously enrolled for the entire period 2011–2016 for whom we have gender information, 17,067 (669/100,000) have a code for diagnosis of either CFS or ME; relative risk for females being diagnosed with ME or CFS compared to males was 1.210 (95% CI: 1.196–1.223).

Demographics of Diagnosed Population, Subset 2, Continuous Enrollment 2 to 4 Years

Figure 4 and **Table 8** show the gender distribution by age for individuals enrolled for a period of from 2 to 4 years and having a diagnosis code of ME in any diagnosis field in the claim, and the gender distribution by age and prevalence for these same individuals. The overall prevalence of a diagnosis of ME only (no CFS diagnosis) in the cohort continuously enrolled for 2 to 4 years is 121/100,000. The relative risk for females being diagnosed with ME compared to males was 1.178 (95% CI: 1.162–1.194). In the youngest age group, 0–9, boys outnumber girls once again.

Validation of Clinical Diagnostic Criteria

In developing the list of appropriate symptom codes (**Appendix 4** in Supplementary Material) it became apparent that existing codes do not fully identify symptoms that specifically describe ME/CFS. Most importantly, there is no symptom code specifically for post-exertional malaise, a core symptom, and codes for various types of fatigue do not match well with the description of another of the core symptoms, i.e., a substantial level of impairment in the ability to engage in pre-illness activities accompanied by fatigue.

Use of symptom codes relating to fatigue, sleep abnormalities, cognitive impairment and orthostatic intolerance, and without requiring codes possibly representing post-exertional malaise from consideration, resulted in a very small number of individuals who were diagnosed with ME or CFS. The vast majority of individuals who had a diagnosis code of ME or CFS did not appear in this symptomatic cohort (**Figure 5**).

Machine Learning

We were unable to create a model for ME and CFS together that could be trained and tuned to a sensitivity accuracy of

TABLE 8 | ME gender demographics by age and prevalence vs. reference population (Subset 2, continuous enrollment 2 to 4 years).

	Diagnosed-ME (count/100,000)			F: M ratio	Diagnosed-ME (% normalized)		Diagnosed-ME (count)			Data set population		
Age range	M	F	Total	F: M	M	F	M	F	Total	M	F	Total
0–9	32.7	25.9	29.4	0.79: 1	55.81%	44.19%	207	157	364	633,270	606,551	1,239,821
10–19	42.0	58.1	50.0	1.38: 1	41.97%	58.03%	307	412	719	730,324	708,729	1,439,053
20–29	57.4	97.8	77.5	1.70: 1	37.00%	63.00%	462	778	1,240	804,286	795,311	1,599,597
30–39	65.8	111.1	88.6	1.69: 1	37.20%	62.80%	545	932	1,477	827,930	838,616	1,666,546
40–49	86.9	142.5	114.7	1.64: 1	37.89%	62.11%	668	1,099	1,767	768,545	771,386	1,539,931
50–59	118.5	168.9	144.1	1.43: 1	41.22%	58.78%	903	1,335	2,238	762,241	790,364	1,552,605
60–69	164.0	207.6	187.0	1.27: 1	44.13%	55.87%	1,090	1,540	2,630	664,725	741,738	1,406,463
70–79	234.3	268.7	253.1	1.15: 1	46.58%	53.42%	824	1,135	1,959	351,709	422,440	774,149
80–89	317.9	358.1	342.5	1.13: 1	47.02%	52.98%	621	1,099	1,720	195,363	306,871	502,234
Total	98.1	141.9	120.4	1.45: 1	40.87%	59.13%	5,627	8,487	14,114	5,738,393	5,982,006	11,720,399

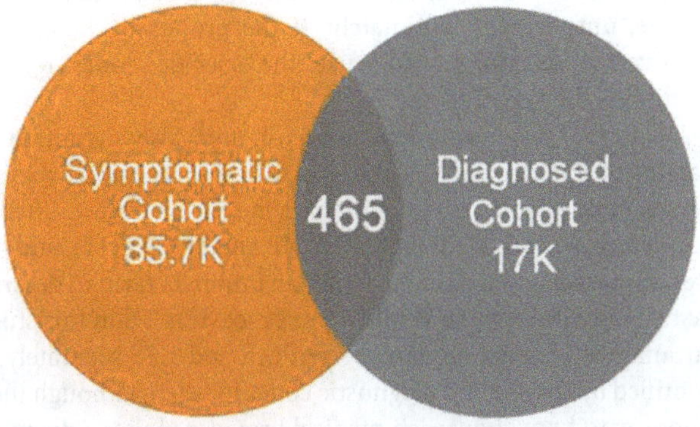

FIGURE 5 | Overlap of individuals with some symptoms of ME/CFS vs. those diagnosed.

much better than 50%. This indicated that there was insufficient correlation between the input data (features) and outcome (diagnosis of ME or CFS) for the algorithm to make a useful prediction.

After failing to have the model resolve when including common symptom data along (CFS diagnosis), we refocused on diagnosis of ME (diagnosis presumed to include assessment of impaired function and the presence of PEM as core symptoms). The ME model was able to be trained and tuned successfully to achieve sensitivity of 0.738 (95% CI: 0.721–0.754) and specificity of 0.823 (95% CI: 0.823–0.823) with the threshold set at 0.6. The threshold signifies that the model will identify an individual as having ME if they have a risk score greater than or equal to 60%.

Based on the machine learning predictive model, the projected prevalence of ME in our continuously insured population was 857/100,000, calculated from the number of individuals predicted by the model to have an ME diagnosis when the model was evaluated using 99% probability (3,989) and dividing by the total number of individuals in the dataset (465,193). This methodology was used to capture individuals who are undiagnosed, but are most likely to be living with an ME-like illness. The gender distribution, normalized to size of population by gender, was 1.38:1 (58% female and 42% male).

The top predictive features (those with the highest weights) in the model, which included both ICD and CPT codes submitted to insurance, are listed in **Table 9**.

Costs

Table 10 shows the average annual medical costs paid by insurance and the patient by year for individuals diagnosed with ME, as well as those diagnosed with lupus or multiple sclerosis, vs. those in the reference population. Costs used were the standard allowed payment (contracted rate) for all provider services which may have ultimately been paid by either the insurer or related patient responsibility associated with the claim such as patient co-payment or deductible, if any.

The average annual medical cost per individual diagnosed with ME in our dataset was $30,860, while the average annual medical cost per individual in the general population in the database was $7,760. For comparison, the average annual cost in our dataset for lupus patients was $20,160 and for multiple sclerosis patients, $21,660.

The costs varied by year, but on average, ME patients had medical costs that were three to four times greater than those in the general population, and ~50% higher than either lupus or multiple sclerosis patients.

DISCUSSION

Prevalence of ME/CFS has been difficult to estimate due to a number of factors including lack of specific diagnostic tests, multiple case definitions, different methodologies, and confusion about coding. This study offers a new approach to this problem, using a large dataset of insurance claims to examine various characteristics of the group of patients for whom health care providers have given a diagnosis code for CFS or ME. We used a variety of data analysis techniques similar to those used in commercial research, which provide a range of estimates, and compare our results to other methods which have been used to estimate prevalence.

TABLE 9 | Top predictive features for ME machine learning model.

Score	Feature	Description
0.105990	age	
0.017413	gender	
0.016377	icd_R53	Malaise and fatigue
0.014899	cpt_00175	Qualitative_or_Semiquantitative_Immunoassays
0.014763	icd_N39	Other disorders of urinary system
0.014508	icd_E55	Vitamin D deficiency
0.014083	cpt_00123	Diagnostic_Radiology_(Diagnostic_Imaging)_Procedures_of_the_Head_and_Neck
0.013081	cpt_00124	Diagnostic_Radiology_(Diagnostic_Imaging)_Procedures_of_the_Chest
0.012911	icd_R07	Pain in throat and chest
0.012452	cpt_00128	Diagnostic_Radiology_(Diagnostic_Imaging)_Procedures_of_the_Abdomen
0.011824	icd_R51	Headache
0.011824	cpt_00217	Cardiography_Procedures
0.011178	cpt_00168	Urinalysis_Procedures
0.010957	icd_R06	Abnormalities of breathing
0.010499	icd_R00	Abnormalities of heart beat
0.010465	icd_R94	Abnormal results of function studies
0.010431	cpt_00289	Subsequent_Hospital_Care_Services
0.010074	icd_R50	Fever of other and unknown origin
0.009819	icd_D64	Other anemias
0.009751	icd_E03	Other hypothyroidism
0.009429	cpt_00367	Temporary_National_Codes_(Non-Medicare)
0.009378	cpt_00220	Echocardiography_Procedures
0.008987	icd_K59	Other functional intestinal disorders
0.008885	cpt_00350	Ambulance_and_Other_Transport_Services_and_Support
0.008596	cpt_00174	Hematology_and_Coagulation_Procedures
0.008392	icd_Z51	Encounter for other aftercare and medical care
0.008307	icd_M62	Other disorders of muscle
0.00739	icd_R79	Other abnormal findings of blood chemistry
0.007339	cpt_00160	Diagnostic_Nuclear_Medicine_Procedures
0.007203	icd_R26	Abnormalities of gait and mobility

Coding and Diagnosis Considerations

The diagnostic codes for CFS (in ICD-10-CM) and for ME (in both ICD-10-CM and ICD-9-CM) are not exclusive to these diseases and can include other conditions, which introduces an unknown degree of uncertainty into any prevalence estimates based on these diagnostic codes (see **Appendix 1** in Supplementary Material, Interrelationships of ICD codes used for Chronic Fatigue Syndrome (CFS) and Myalgic Encephalomyelitis (ME) in the U.S. as of October, 2018).

A proposal to change the coding for ME, CFS, and related conditions was made at the September 12, 2018 meeting of the National Center for Health Statistics which addresses this ambiguity (10). If this proposal is approved, ME, CFS, Systemic Exercise Intolerance Disease (SEID, the new term recommended by the Institute of Medicine report in 2015), and postviral fatigue syndrome will have separate and distinct codes beginning in October 2019.

TABLE 10 | Average yearly medical costs for diagnosed vs. reference population.

Year	General population	ME	Lupus	MS
2016	$ 8,500	$ 30,600	$ 22,600	$ 23,220
2015	$ 7,800	$ 32,400	$ 21,100	$ 22,090
2014	$ 7,500	$ 31,300	$ 20,100	$ 21,050
2013	$ 7,700	$ 34,300	$ 20,100	$ 22,780
2012	$ 7,300	$ 25,700	$ 16,900	$ 19,160
Average	$ 7,760	$ 30,860	$ 20,160	$ 21,660

For better tracking of this disease, two options could be considered. In the short term, and if the new proposal is not approved, providers who diagnose ME/CFS could use the ICD-10-CM code of G93.3 for ME/CFS and *not* use R53.82 (Chronic Fatigue, unspecified). Ultimately, if the proposed changes are approved, researchers could use the specific codes for the conditions they are tracking.

Diagnosis may vary depending on the case definition or diagnostic criteria used by the provider. Furthermore, there is considerable ongoing investigation on the effect of using different case definitions on the diagnosis of ME and or CFS (11), and this affects whether it is legitimate to use an umbrella term to describe the two conditions (12). While we refer to ME/CFS in this study, our analysis is based on diagnosis of ME and CFS separately, as identified by the specific diagnostic codes for each, although there is no way to know how each medical provider makes a diagnosis and assigned a code.

Prevalence of ME/CFS Based on Frequency of Diagnosis in an Insurance Claims Database

This is the first study to determine the frequency of ME/CFS diagnosis using insurance claims data for a large number of individuals. Prevalence estimates for chronic fatigue syndrome in the U.S. have been as low as 235/100,000 (373/100,000 in women and 83/100,000 in men) (13) and as high as 2540/100,000 (14). Our prevalence estimates ranged from 519/100,000 to 1,038/100,000 (0.52% to 1.03%), which fall between those expected from large-scale health surveys and smaller scale community-based studies.

Our highest prevalence estimate for ME/CFS, 1,038/100,000 or 1.04%, was found in the group most representative of the insured population—those continuously enrolled for 2 to 4 years—and with the broadest reach: it includes all individuals with ME or CFS as either a primary or a secondary diagnosis, and all claims for these individuals. This estimate can be compared with health surveys conducted in Canada and in some states in the U.S. Recent CDC prevalence estimates of ME/CFS from the Behavioral Risk Factor Surveillance System (BRFSS) (lifetime 1.6%; current 1.2%) (15) were similar to

Canadian Community Health Survey 2003 (1.3%) 2010 (1.4%), and 2014 (1.4%) data (16–18). These survey studies do not verify that the specific diagnosis code has been entered in the patient's medical record. They only indicate that the patient is reporting having been given this diagnosis by the health care provider.

Our lowest prevalence estimate for ME/CFS, 519/100,000 or 0.52%, was calculated using all claims from individuals who have ME or CFS as the primary diagnosis and with no restriction on the length of enrollment. This group could therefore have an unknown number of individuals with only one miscellaneous claim, thereby diluting the sample. Nevertheless, the prevalence of ME/CFS in this group is higher than predicted by community-based studies which verified the diagnosis with a medical examination and verifying symptoms using an accepted ME or CFS case definition (e.g., Jason et al., (19), 0.42%; 7, 0.24%; 10, 0.2%).

Our intermediate prevalence estimate has no direct comparisons with previously published results. The prevalence of ME/CFS in the group continuously enrolled for the full 7 years and with ME or CFS as the primary diagnosis, the most restrictive group, is 669/100,000 or 0.67%. Note that this is somewhat higher than the 519/100,000 calculated from the non-continuously enrolled population. The group of individuals continuously enrolled in the same health insurance for a long period of time may include a higher proportion of sicker people than the other groups, but we did not assess this.

Using the diagnosis of ME only, prevalence in the group continuously enrolled for 2 to 4 years is 121/100,000, or 0.12%. This lower prevalence of ME compared with ME/CFS would be expected, as the case definitions for ME are much less well-known by medical providers than CFS. Nevertheless, our sample included more than 14,000 individuals with this diagnosis, which is quite large compared with most studies which examine the characteristics of this group.

Using claims data alone, it is not possible to determine what criteria health care providers are using to make a diagnosis of either ME or CFS. Likewise, a provider might tell a patient they have ME/CFS without the specific diagnostic code being entered into the patient's record.

The prevalence of ME/CFS could be **overestimated** if providers or medical coders are using the CFS diagnosis code to identify a "CFS-like" illness or condition, without reference to any case definition, or simply "chronic fatigue."

The prevalence of ME/CFS could be **underestimated** if providers or medical coders (a) use a different diagnosis that is less specific (e.g., 780.79, Other Malaise and Fatigue, R53.81 Other Malaise or R53.83 Other Fatigue); (b) do not put ME or CFS diagnosis into the record due to not wanting to expose their patients to a perceived stigma of the disease (1), due to not wanting to provide a discouraging diagnosis when there is no cure, or due to knowing that some appropriate treatments might not be covered under that diagnosis; and (c) if providers are unaware of the diagnosis of ME/CFS, since diagnosis and management of ME/CFS is not taught in most medical schools (20, 21).

It has been reported (8) that 84–91% of patients with ME/CFS are undiagnosed. However, this study is now 14 years old, and so may not reflect the increased awareness of ME/CFS in recent years, which could result in a higher rate of diagnosis. The earlier case definitions used in previous studies require the diagnosis to be one of exclusion, resulting in less likelihood of diagnosis than with more recent clinical diagnostic criteria published by the Institute of Medicine (1).

Age, Gender, and Prevalence in the Diagnosed Population

This study also shows a lower ratio of females to males diagnosed with ME/CFS than is generally reported. While many studies show a much higher percentage of females (as high as 80% female –7; 9) at least one health survey (17) shows a lower percentage of 65% female. For ME/CFS, our studies show an average of between 60 and 65% female across age groups, except in the youngest group, 0–9 years, where boys outnumber girls. For ME only, the percentage of females is lower, 60%, and again for the youngest group, boys outnumber girls.

While our numbers are based on diagnostic codes in the medical record and reflect actual clinical practice, there is no information about what criteria the providers used to assign these codes, or if they evaluate men differently than women. Nevertheless, the higher than expected number of males with this diagnosis is interesting, and the possible reasons for this need more study.

Prevalence in Children and Adolescents

There is little published data on prevalence of ME/CFS in children and adolescents. One community-based study reports a prevalence for adolescents (aged 13 to 17) of 181 per 100,000 or 0.181% (22). Our main dataset shows a prevalence of 37.2/100,000 in children 0–9 years, and 204.5/100,000 in ages 10–19 (**Table 6**).

Validation of Clinical Diagnostic Criteria

One goal of the study was to determine whether the presence of specific symptom codes within administrative medical claims data could identify individuals for whom a diagnosis of ME/CFS should be considered. Lack of specific codes for two of five core symptoms required for a diagnosis of ME/CFS using the IOM criteria made it impossible to identify individuals for whom this diagnosis should be considered from administrative claims data, or to validate that individuals diagnosed with ME/CFS had documented evidence of the required core symptoms in their claims data.

Prevalence Based on Machine Learning

Based on the 2017 population of the U.S. noted earlier, the predicted prevalence rate based on our model of 857/100,000 translates to up to 2.8 million people with ME/CFS in the U.S. This number is somewhat larger than other published estimates of 836,000 to 2.5 million Americans (19) and is significant because it is predicted based on characteristics drawn from those diagnosed with ME only, not including those with a diagnosis of CFS only.

The machine learning technique is a useful way to compensate for the lack of specific symptom codes which might otherwise be used to predict or identify undiagnosed patients. It uses a weighted analysis of a large number of "features" (over 500) derived from a known group (in this case, individuals already diagnosed with ME) to identify individuals with a similar combination of factors. The model can be "tuned" to a desired balance of specificity and sensitivity. Our model performed reasonably well at a threshold of 0.6 (sensitivity 0.82336 and specificity 0.73787). If specific symptom codes for ME were available the model could be improved. To predict the prevalence of ME from our dataset we used a probability threshold of 0.99. Using the 99% probability cut-off is a conservative approach, but provides a reasonable estimate.

The inability to train the machine learning model when CFS diagnoses were included indicates that the population of individuals diagnosed with CFS is too heterogeneous for this method. In contrast, individuals diagnosed with ME were a more homogenous population for which this approach was more effective.

The CFS diagnosis code, in the signs and symptoms section of the ICD, is perhaps being used incorrectly to indicate the symptom of chronic fatigue, which is characteristic of many different underlying conditions, or a "CFS-like" illness which may lack some of the defining features of Chronic Fatigue Syndrome. However, patients coded with ME, which has clinical information identical to Chronic Fatigue Syndrome in ICD-10-CM and is placed in a disease chapter, were significantly, and usefully, more homogeneous. This supports our supposition that clinicians using the ME code are more familiar with the disease than clinicians using the CFS code, and thus may be specifically diagnosing ME/CFS, not using the diagnosis code to cover unspecified chronic fatigue or a "CFS-like" illness.

These results show that the predicted prevalence rate of 857/100,000 based on the machine learning model is not unreasonable for ME/CFS, including the symptom of post-exertional malaise. This estimate suggests that ME/CFS is not a rare disease, but in fact a relatively common one, and offers a new benchmark for future studies.

Costs

Direct medical costs are important to insurers, who need to deliver good medical care in a cost-effective way, and to patients, who must pay both insurance premiums and out-of-pocket for co-payments, deductibles and treatments that are uninsured.

Direct medical costs for caring for ME/CFS patients are significantly higher than for the general population. Specific components contributing to increased costs (hospitalization, specialist visits, diagnostic tests, presence of other chronic conditions, etc.) were not examined.

Many patients cite a long and costly journey to receiving an accurate diagnosis of ME/CFS (23). Further, once diagnosed, most patients struggle to find primary care providers who are knowledgeable about the condition and well versed in the best practices for managing the symptoms. These twin challenges in diagnosis and treatment are certainly contributors to added cost in the healthcare system.

Direct medical costs are only one component of the total disease costs; others include disability claims, health insurance premiums, and expenses not submitted to insurance such as alternative treatments, nutritional supplements, costs to the economy due to productivity loss, costs to the family for caretaking, and possibly early death. Previous studies have estimated the total annual cost to the economy from ME/CFS to be $17–24 billion (2008 dollars) (6).

Patients with ME/CFS have a high level of disability. Despite high direct medical costs, these patients often have significant unmet health care needs (17) or forgo routine medical care (15). Health surveys have indicated that ME/CFS patients also tend to have more than one chronic condition (15). All these factors could combine and result in poorer quality of life for the patient and even higher medical costs in the future, as well as increasing the burden of illness.

The data from this study illustrate the high costs of the illness, and point to the potential for cost control if patients are diagnosed and provided with the most effective care. Good medical management also holds the promise of improving the experience of patients living with ME/CFS.

Putting the Results in Context

Prevalence

The estimated prevalence of ME/CFS in our study ranges from 519 to 1,038/100,000, and falls between the rates estimated from community health studies and self-reported health surveys. Our study uses larger samples than previous studies, and two different methodologies. Our studies show a range of gender distribution, with the lowest ratio of female to male occurring in the youngest age group, 0–9 years, where boys outnumber girls, and in groups diagnosed with ME only.

Table 11 illustrates the spectrum of prevalence studies which use a variety of techniques. Comparing these studies shows the range of prevalence and gender distribution. Bolded entries are from this study.

Generally accepted gender ratios for ME/CFS in the community are as high as 3:1 or 4:1 female to male F (75–80% female). Our data indicate that the actual rate of diagnosis is much less skewed based on gender, though still more commonly diagnosed in women, with a range of 60–65% female.

Disease Burden

The World Health Organization has pioneered the use of the Disability Adjusted Life Year (DALY) as a single measure of disease burden in a population (25) and importantly, it includes a measure of the degree of disability from the disease. Using the DALY measure, ME/CFS has been estimated to have a higher total disease burden than multiple sclerosis, autism, or HIV/AIDS (26).

Lupus and multiple sclerosis (MS) are two diseases which are better known than ME/CFS and often compared to it. Although they have different etiologies they have some similar characteristics and symptoms. Both significantly affect quality of life, may take some time to diagnose, affect more women than men, present with some of the same symptoms, and like ME/CFS are often diagnosed late and/or inaccurately initially.

TABLE 11 | Comparison of prevalence rates.

Source	Population size	Prevalence per 100,000	% Female	Method
Diagnosed with ME (subset 2, continuous enrollment 2–4 years)	11.7M	121	60.1%	Insurance Claim Data
Nacul et al. (24), (ME/CFS, U.K.)	143,000	200	51.0%	Community Health Study
Reyes et al. (13) (ME/CFS, Wichita, KS)	90,316	240	81.8%	Community Health Study
Jason et al. (19) (ME/CFS, U.S.)	18,675	420	71.9%	Community Health Study
Diagnosed with ME or CFS (main dataset, non-continuous enrollment)	50M	519	65.7%	Insurance Claim Data
Diagnosed with ME or CFS (subset 1, continuous enrollment 2011–2016)	2.5M	669	64.7%	Insurance Claim Data
Projected prevalence of ME using machine learning	2.7M	857	57.9%	Machine Learning Predictive Model
Diagnosed with ME or CFS (subset 2, continuous enrollment 2 to 4 years)	11.7M	1038	65.0%	Insurance Claim Data
National ME/FM Action Network (17) and ME Association of Ontario (16) (Canadian Community Health Surveys)	65,000	1,400	63.4%	Survey
Lin et al. (15) (BRFSS survey, ME/CFS, several states)	54,695	1,600	80.0%	Survey

TABLE 12 | Comparison of several factors relating to ME/CFS, lupus and multiple sclerosis.

Disease	# Patients based on est. 2017 U.S. population	Prevalence	Burden of illness (DALY–disability adjusted life years)	Average annual medical cost	NIH research spending 2017 (NIH categorical spending, 2017)
ME/CFS	1,726,000–3,746,000	519–1,038/100,000 0.52–1.04%	714000 (26)	$30,860	$15MM
Lupus	785,000	241/100,000 0.241% (27)	No data available	$20,160	$109MM
Multiple Sclerosis	486,000	149/100,000 0.15% (28)	300200 (26) –284171 (NIH, disease burden 2015)	$21,000	$111MM
Reference population				$7,760	

Table 12 compares the estimated prevalence and number of patients in the United States, the burden of illness, and average annual medical cost, and NIH research spending for ME/CFS, lupus, and multiple sclerosis (29, 30). As shown in **Table 12**, ME/CFS affects more than double the number of persons in the U.S. than lupus and four times as many as MS. The prevalence of lupus is less than half that of ME/CFS, and the prevalence of multiple sclerosis, in a comparable study of commercially-insured patients, is less than one-third of the prevalence of ME/CFS as found in our study.

The burden of illness for ME/CFS is more than double that of MS (26), and medical costs for ME/CFS in this study are double those for either Lupus or MS and four times higher than for the general insured (reference) population.

An additional point of comparison is the amount spent on research for these diseases by the National Institutes of Health. Looking at these comparisons for prevalence, burden of illness and annual medical cost, and the amount of NIH funding for these three similar diseases, ME/CFS, lupus, and multiple sclerosis, it is evident that research on ME/CFS is grossly underfunded ($15 vs. $109–111 MM), a point also made by Dimmock et al. (26).

Limitations of This Type of Study

This study, based on claims data including Medicare and commercial insurance, does not assess the prevalence in Medicaid recipients or the uninsured, two groups in which the prevalence of ME/CFS might be higher, as indicated by community-based studies (19). Furthermore, the financial impact of disability from ME/CFS may lead to Medicaid eligibility, thus removing some ME/CFS patients from the commercially insured population.

Since we were not able to validate ME/CFS diagnosis using codes for some (but not all) of the core symptoms, our machine learning model results must be considered preliminary.

ICD codes used for ME/CFS as of 2018 are inexact and may be applied to individuals with other conditions (see **Appendix 1** in Supplementary Material). This introduces an unknown degree of uncertainty to the estimates of prevalence of ME/CFS in this study. In doing this study, we necessarily made a number of assumptions which are stated in the Methods section and are also discussed above. The results might have been different if different assumptions were used. Since this data is from U.S. insurance claims and reflects the practices of U.S. health care providers, these results may not be valid for other countries.

Implications for the Future and Next Steps

The authors recommend use of the ME diagnosis code (G93.3) rather than CFS (R53.82), which defaults to "Chronic fatigue, unspecified," for better tracking where symptoms warrant.

The authors also recommend the creation of new symptom codes for post-exertional malaise and substantial impairment in activity levels accompanied by profound fatigue, two of the core symptoms of ME/CFS.

In Summary

This study is the first to use a large medical claims database to study the characteristics of a large group of individuals who have been diagnosed with ME or CFS and to explore the potential of mining this type of data. This study used a base data set of 50 million individuals tracked over 6 years. The next largest study referenced had a sample size of 90,316, all located in a single municipality.

While the percentage of women diagnosed with ME/CFS is higher than the percentage of men, ME/CFS is not a "women's disease." Thirty-five to forty percent of diagnosed patients are men.

It is not possible at this time to use symptom codes in medical claims data to identify individuals for whom a diagnosis of ME/CFS might be considered. Introducing new symptom codes for two of the required symptoms identified in the study published by the Institute of Medicine (1) should be considered.

Patients diagnosed with CFS may represent a more heterogeneous group than those diagnosed with ME; this study makes no conclusions about accuracy of diagnosis or quality of care given to ME/CFS patients by providers.

Annual direct medical costs for ME/CFS patients are three to four times higher than average of the reference population and fifty percent higher than for multiple sclerosis or lupus, diseases with similar characteristics.

This study is a "snapshot" and could be repeated in future years for comparison. It would also be interesting to look in more detail at the diagnosis of conditions which are co-morbid with ME/CFS, such as migraine headaches or orthostatic intolerance.

These results show that a prevalence rate 857/100,000 for ME/CFS is not unreasonable; therefore, it is not a rare disease, but in fact a relatively common one.

Based on our results and analysis, ME/CFS should get more attention in research and provider communities, and warrants more education to providers (primary care, specialties, and allied health sciences) to improve the quality of health care and quality of life for affected individuals.

AUTHOR CONTRIBUTIONS

Research for this study was carried out by AV, EH, SA, and DK, with direction and support from DP and JA. LB, AD, CL, and PR provided clinical guidance. AD advised on statistics. The manuscript was written primarily by AV, DP, and CP, with editorial suggestions from LB, AD, CL, PR, and JA.

ACKNOWLEDGMENTS

We are grateful to Optum Enterprise Analytics, Optum Technology, and UnitedHealth Group for making staff time available for this project, and to Mary Dimmock, Arthur Mirin, and Leah Williams for helpful comments. We are grateful for donations to the Massachusetts ME/CFS & FM Association which funded the publication of this manuscript.

REFERENCES

1. Institute of Medicine. *Beyond Myalgic Encephalomyelitis/Chronic Fatigue Syndrome: Redefining an Illness*. Washington, DC: The National Academies Press. (2015). Available online at: http://www.nationalacademies.org/hmd/Reports/2015/ME-CFS.aspx (Accessed September 15, 2018).
2. Smith MEB, Nelson HD, Haney E, Pappas M, Daeges M, Wasson N, et al. *Diagnosis and Treatment of Myalgic Encephalomyelitis/Chronic Fatigue Syndrome*. Agency for Healthcare Research and Quality, Evidence Reports/Technology Assessments (2014).
3. Chronic Fatigue Syndrome Advisory Committee. *CFSAC Recommendations: Recommendations and Rationale from Working Group on IOM and P2P Reports-PDF* (2015). Available online at: https://www.hhs.gov/ash/advisory-committees/cfsac/recommendations/2015-08-18/index.html and https://www.hhs.gov/sites/default/files/advcomcfs/recommendations/2015-08-18-19-recommendations.pdf (Accessed September 15, 2018).
4. Marshall R, Paul L, Wood L. The search for pain relief in people with chronic fatigue syndrome: a descriptive study. *Physiother Theor Pract.* (2011) 27: 373–83. doi: 10.3109/09593985.2010.502554
5. National Institutes of Health. *State of the Knowledge Workshop. Myalgic Encephalomyelitis/Chronic Fatigue Syndrome (ME/CFS) Research*. Workshop report. Bethesda, MD: Office of Research on Women's Health, NIH, US Department of Health and Human Services (2011). Available online at: https://www.meassociation.org.uk/wp-content/uploads/2011/08/SoK-Workshop-Report-508-compliant-8-5-11.pdf (Accessed September 15, 2018).
6. Jason LA, Benton MC, Valentine L, Johnson A, Torres-Harding S. The economic impact of ME/CFS: Individual and societal costs. *Dyn Med.* (2008) 7:6. doi: 10.1186/1476-5918-7-6
7. Reynolds KJ, Vernon SD, Bouchery E, Reeves WC. The economic impact of chronic fatigue syndrome. *Cost Effect Resour Alloc.* (2004) 2:4. doi: 10.1186/1478-7547-2-4
8. Solomon L, Reeves WC. Factors influencing the diagnosis of chronic fatigue syndrome. *Arch Intern Med.* (2004) 164:2241–5. doi: 10.1001/archinte.164.20.2241
9. United States Census Bureau (2018). *Population estimates.* Available online at: https://www.census.gov/quickfacts/fact/table/US/PST045217
10. National Center for Health Statistics. *ICD-10 Coordination and Maintenance Committee Meeting, Diagnosis Agenda Part 2* (2018). Available online at: https://www.cdc.gov/nchs/data/icd/Topic_packet_Sept_2018_part2.pdf (Accessed September 30, 2018).
11. Jason LA, Brown A, Clyne E, Bartgis L, Evans M, Brown M. Contrasting case definitions for chronic fatigue syndrome, myalgic encephalomyelitis/chronic fatigue syndrome and myalgic encephalomyelitis. *Eval Health Prof.* (2012) 35:280–304. doi: 10.1177/0163278711424281
12. Jason LA, Sunnquist M, Brown A, Evans M, Newton JL. Are myalgic encephalomyelitis and chronic fatigue syndrome different illnesses? A preliminary analysis. *J Health Psychol.* (2016) 1:3–15. doi: 10.1177/1359105313520335
13. Reyes M, Nisenbaum R, Hoaglin DC, Unger ER, Emmons C, Randall B, et al. Prevalence and incidence of chronic fatigue syndrome in Wichita, Kansas. *Arch Intern Med.* (2003) 163:1530–6. doi: 10.1001/archinte.163.13.1530
14. Reeves WC, Jones JF, Maloney E, Heim C, Hoaglin DC, Boneva RS, et al. Prevalence of chronic fatigue syndrome in metropolitan, urban, and rural Georgia. *Popul Health Metr.*(2007) 5:5. doi: 10.1186/1478-7954-5-5
15. Lin JMS, Hayes K, Brimmer D. 9630: BRFSS State-Added Questions: Leveraging an Existing Surveillance System to Monitor Prevalence and

Health Indictors for Myalgic Encephalomyelitis/Chronic Fatigue Syndrome (ME/CFS). In: *2018 CSTE Annual Conference, Council of State and Territorial Epidemiologists* Palm Beach, FL. (2018). Available online at: https://cste.confex.com/cste/2018/meetingapp.cgi/Paper/9630 (Accessed August 15, 2018).

16. ME Association of Ontario. *THE QUANTITATIVE DATA: Environmental Sensitivities/Multiple Chemical Sensitivity (ES/MCS), Fibromyalgia (FM), Myalgic Encephalomyelitis/Chronic Fatigue Syndrome (ME/CFS).* Appendix to The Ontario Centre Of Excellence in Environmental Health Business Case (2013). Available online at: http://meao.ca/files/Quantitative_Data_Report.pdf
17. National ME/FM Action Network. *Myalgic Encephalomyelitis/Chronic Fatigue Syndrome and Fibromyalgia Findings from the 2014 Canadian Community Health Survey* (2014). Available online at: https://www.mefmaction.com/docs/CCHS_Stats_2014.pdf (Accessed August 4, 2018).
18. Rusu C, Gee ME, Lagacé C, Parlor M. Chronic fatigue syndrome and fibromyalgia in Canada: prevalence and associations with six health status indicators. *Health Promot Chronic Dis Prev Can.* (2015) 35:3–11.
19. Jason LA, Richman JA, Rademaker AW, Jordan KM, Plioplys AV, Taylor R, et al. A community-based study of chronic fatigue syndrome. *Arch Intern Med.* (1999) 159:2129–37.
20. Peterson TM, Peterson TW, Emerson S, Regalbuto E, Evans MA, Jason LA. Coverage of CFS within U.S. medical schools.*Univers J Public Health* (2013) 1: 177–9. doi: 10.13189/ujph.2013.010404
21. Jason LA, Paavola E, Porter N, Morello ML. Frequency and content analysis of chronic fatigue syndrome in medical text books. *Austral J Primary Health* (2010) 16:174–8. doi: 10.1071/py09023
22. Jordan KM, Huang CF, Jason LA, Richman J, Mears CJ, McCready W, et al. Prevalence of pediatric chronic fatigue syndrome in a community-based sample. *J Chron Fatigue Syndr.* (2006) 13:75–8. doi: 10.1300/J092v13n02_04
23. ProHealth. *A Profile of ME/CFS Patients: How Many Years and How Many Doctors?* (2008). Available online at: https://www.prohealth.com/library/a-profile-of-me-cfs-patients-how-many-years-and-how-many-doctors-25211 (Accessed September 15, 2018).
24. Nacul LC, Lacerda EM, Pheby D, Campion P, Molokhia M, Fayyaz S, et al. Prevalence of myalgic encephalomyelitis/chronic fatigue syndrome (ME/CFS) in three regions of England: a repeated cross-sectional study in primary care. *BMC Med.* (2011) 9:91. doi: 10.1186/1741-7015-9-91
25. Murray CJ, Lopez AD, and Jamison DT. The global burden of disease in 1990: summary results, sensitivity analysis and future directions. *Bull World Health Organ.* (1994) 72:495–509.
26. Dimmock ME, Mirin AA, Jason LA. Estimating the disease burden of ME/CFS in the United States and its relation to research funding. *J Med Ther.* (2016) 1: 1–7. doi: 10.15761/JMT.1000102
27. Rees F, Doherty M, Grainge MJ, Lanyon P, Zhang W. The worldwide incidence and prevalence of systemic lupus erythematosus: a systematic review of epidemiological studies. *Rheumatology* (2017) 56:1945–61. doi: 10.1093/rheumatology/kex260
28. Dilokthornsakul P, Valuck RJ, Nair KV, Corboy JR, Allen RR, Campbell JD. Multiple sclerosis prevalence in the United States commercially insured population. *Neurology* (2016) 86:1014–21. doi: 10.1212/WNL.0000000000002469
29. National Institutes of Health. *Report on NIH Funding vs. Global Burden of Disease* (2015). Available online at: https://report.nih.gov/info_disease_burden.aspx (Accessed August 25, 2018).
30. National Institutes of Health. *Estimates of Funding for Various Research, Condition, and Disease Categories (RCDC)* (2018). Available online at: https://report.nih.gov/categorical_spending.aspx

Permissions

All chapters in this book were first published by Frontiers; hereby published with permission under the Creative Commons Attribution License or equivalent. Every chapter published in this book has been scrutinized by our experts. Their significance has been extensively debated. The topics covered herein carry significant findings which will fuel the growth of the discipline. They may even be implemented as practical applications or may be referred to as a beginning point for another development.

The contributors of this book come from diverse backgrounds, making this book a truly international effort. This book will bring forth new frontiers with its revolutionizing research information and detailed analysis of the nascent developments around the world.

We would like to thank all the contributing authors for lending their expertise to make the book truly unique. They have played a crucial role in the development of this book. Without their invaluable contributions this book wouldn't have been possible. They have made vital efforts to compile up to date information on the varied aspects of this subject to make this book a valuable addition to the collection of many professionals and students.

This book was conceptualized with the vision of imparting up-to-date information and advanced data in this field. To ensure the same, a matchless editorial board was set up. Every individual on the board went through rigorous rounds of assessment to prove their worth. After which they invested a large part of their time researching and compiling the most relevant data for our readers.

The editorial board has been involved in producing this book since its inception. They have spent rigorous hours researching and exploring the diverse topics which have resulted in the successful publishing of this book. They have passed on their knowledge of decades through this book. To expedite this challenging task, the publisher supported the team at every step. A small team of assistant editors was also appointed to further simplify the editing procedure and attain best results for the readers.

Apart from the editorial board, the designing team has also invested a significant amount of their time in understanding the subject and creating the most relevant covers. They scrutinized every image to scout for the most suitable representation of the subject and create an appropriate cover for the book.

The publishing team has been an ardent support to the editorial, designing and production team. Their endless efforts to recruit the best for this project, has resulted in the accomplishment of this book. They are a veteran in the field of academics and their pool of knowledge is as vast as their experience in printing. Their expertise and guidance has proved useful at every step. Their uncompromising quality standards have made this book an exceptional effort. Their encouragement from time to time has been an inspiration for everyone.

The publisher and the editorial board hope that this book will prove to be a valuable piece of knowledge for researchers, students, practitioners and scholars across the globe.

List of Contributors

Katherine S. Rowe
Department of General Medicine, Royal Children's Hospital, Melbourne, VIC, Australia

Todd E. Davenport
Department of Physical Therapy, Thomas J. Long School of Pharmacy and Health Sciences, University of the Pacific Stockton, CA, United States Workwell Foundation, Ripon, CA, United States

Mary Lehnen
Department of Physical Therapy, Thomas J. Long School of Pharmacy and Health Sciences, University of the Pacific Stockton, CA, United States

Staci R. Stevens, Jared Stevens, Chris Snell and Christopher R. Snell
Workwell Foundation, Ripon, CA, United States

J. Mark VanNess
Workwell Foundation, Ripon, CA, United States
Department of Health, Exercise, and Sport Sciences, College of the Pacific, University of the Pacific Stockton, CA, United States

Luis Carlos Nacul, Kathleen Mudie, Caroline C. Kingdon and Eliana Mattos Lacerda
Department of Clinical Research, Faculty of Infectious and Tropical Diseases, International Centre for Evidence in Disability, London School of Hygiene and Tropical Medicine, London, United Kingdom

Taane G. Clark
Department of Infectious Disease Epidemiology, Faculty of Infectious and Tropical Diseases, Faculty of Epidemiology and Population Health, London School of Hygiene and Tropical Medicine, London, United Kingdom

Amy Proal and Trevor Marshall
Autoimmunity Research Foundation, Thousand Oaks, CA, United States

Maria Roma, Colleen L. Marden, Marissa A. K. Flaherty, Samantha E. Jasion and Erica M. Cranston
Division of General Pediatrics and Adolescent Medicine, Department of Pediatrics, Johns Hopkins University School of Medicine, Baltimore, MD, United States

Kenneth J. Friedman
Retired, Plantation, FL, United States

Jonathan R. Kerr
Department of Microbiology, West Suffolk Hospital Foundation Trust, Bury St Edmunds, United Kingdom

Roumiana S. Boneva and Elizabeth R. Unger
Division of High-Consequence Pathogens and Pathology, National Center for Emerging and Zoonotic Infectious Diseases, Centers for Disease Control and Prevention, Atlanta, GA, United States

Friedrich Wieser and Robert N. Taylor
Department of Gynecology and Obstetrics, Emory University School of Medicine, Atlanta, GA, United States

Urs M. Nater and Beate Ditzen
Department of Psychiatry and Behavioral Sciences, Emory University School of Medicine, Atlanta, GA, United States

Faith R. Newton
Department of Education, Delaware State University, Dover, DE, United States

C. (Linda) M. C. van Campen and Frans C. Visser
Stichting CardioZorg, Hoofddorp, Netherlands

Peter C. Rowe
Children's Center Chronic Fatigue Clinic, Johns Hopkins University School of Medicine, Baltimore, MD, United States
Division of General Pediatrics and Adolescent Medicine, Department of Pediatrics, Johns Hopkins University School of Medicine, Baltimore, MD, United States

Keith James Geraghty and Charles Adeniji
Division of Population Health, Health Services Research and Primary Care, Centre for Primary Care, University of Manchester, Manchester, United Kingdom

Lily Chu, Ian J. Valencia, Donn W. Garvert and Jose G. Montoya
Stanford ME/CFS Initiative, Division of Infectious Diseases and Geographic Medicine, Stanford University School of Medicine, Stanford, CA, United States

Jaeyong Bae
Chronic Viral Diseases Branch, Division of High-Consequence Pathogens and Pathology, National Center for Emerging and Zoonotic Infectious Diseases, Centers for Disease Control and Prevention, Atlanta, GA, United States
Department of Health Policy and Management, Rollins School of Public Health, Emory University, Atlanta, GA, United States

Jin-Mann S. Lin
Chronic Viral Diseases Branch, Division of High-Consequence Pathogens and Pathology, National Center for Emerging and Zoonotic Infectious Diseases, Centers for Disease Control and Prevention, Atlanta, GA, United States

Melanie Perez, Kelly Hilton and Kristina Gemayel
Dr. Kiran C. Patel College of Osteopathic Medicine, Nova Southeastern University, Fort Lauderdale, FL, United States

Rajeev Jaundoo
Department of Psychology and Neuroscience, Nova Southeastern University, Fort Lauderdale, FL, United States
Institute for Neuro Immune Medicine, Nova Southeastern University, Fort Lauderdale, FL, United States

Ana Del Alamo and Lubov Nathanson
Dr. Kiran C. Patel College of Osteopathic Medicine, Nova Southeastern University, Fort Lauderdale, FL, United States
Institute for Neuro Immune Medicine, Nova Southeastern University, Fort Lauderdale, FL, United States

Nancy G. Klimas
Dr. Kiran C. Patel College of Osteopathic Medicine, Nova Southeastern University, Fort Lauderdale, FL, United States
Institute for Neuro Immune Medicine, Nova Southeastern University, Fort Lauderdale, FL, United States
Veterans Affairs Medical Center, Miami, FL, United States

Travis J. A. Craddock
Dr. Kiran C. Patel College of Osteopathic Medicine, Nova Southeastern University, Fort Lauderdale, FL, United States
Department of Psychology and Neuroscience, Nova Southeastern University, Fort Lauderdale, FL, United States
Institute for Neuro Immune Medicine, Nova Southeastern University, Fort Lauderdale, FL, United States
Department of Computer Science, Nova Southeastern University, Fort Lauderdale, FL, United States

Sarah Jenette Knight
Murdoch Children's Research Institute, Melbourne, VIC, Australia
The Royal Children's Hospital, Melbourne, VIC, Australia
Department of Pediatrics, The University of Melbourne, Melbourne, VIC, Australia

Jennifer Politis and Christine Garnham
Murdoch Children's Research Institute, Melbourne, VIC, Australia
Melbourne Graduate School of Education, The University of Melbourne, Melbourne, VIC, Australia

Adam Scheinberg
Murdoch Children's Research Institute, Melbourne, VIC, Australia
The Royal Children's Hospital, Melbourne, VIC, Australia
Department of Pediatrics, The University of Melbourne, Melbourne, VIC, Australia
Department of Pediatrics, Monash University, Melbourne, VIC, Australia

Michelle Anne Tollit
Murdoch Children's Research Institute, Melbourne, VIC, Australia
The Royal Children's Hospital, Melbourne, VIC, Australia
Melbourne Graduate School of Education, The University of Melbourne, Melbourne, VIC, Australia
The Royal Children's Hospital Education Institute, Parkville VIC Australia, Melbourne, VIC, Australia

Eliana M. Lacerda, Jack D. Butterworth, Shennae O'Boyle and Luis Nacul
Department of Clinical Research, Faculty of Infectious and Tropical Diseases, London School of Hygiene and Tropical Medicine, London, United Kingdom

Barbara B. Comerford
Law Offices of Barbara Comerford, Paramus, NJ, United States

Richard Podell
Robert Wood Johnson Medical School, Rutgers, The State University of New Jersey, New Brunswick, NJ, United States

Leonard A. Jason and Madison Sunnquist
Center for Community Research, DePaul University, Chicago, IL, United States

Betsy Keller
Department of Exercise and Sport Sciences, Ithaca College, Ithaca, NY, United States

Ashley R. Valdez, Elizabeth E. Hancock, Seyi Adebayo and David J. Kiernicki
Optum Enterprise Analytics, UnitedHealth Group, Minneapolis, MN, United States

Daniel Proskauer
Optum Technology, UnitedHealth Group, Minneapolis, MN, United States

John R. Attewell
Innovation, Research and Development, United Health Group, Minneapolis, MN, United States

Lucinda Bateman
Bateman Horne Center, Salt Lake City, UT, United States

Alfred DeMaria Jr.
Bureau of Infectious Disease and Laboratory Sciences, Massachusetts Department of Public Health, Boston, MA, United States

Charles W. Lapp
Hunter-Hopkins Center, Charlotte, NC, United States

Charmian Proskauer
Massachusetts ME/CFS & FM Association, Quincy, MA, United States

Index

www.ingramcontent.com/pod-product-compliance
Lightning Source LLC
LaVergne TN
LVHW060603210926
848485LV00005B/1362